WHY ANIMALS AREN'T FOOD

~ And How Low-Carb and Paleo Diets Sicken and Kill Us ~

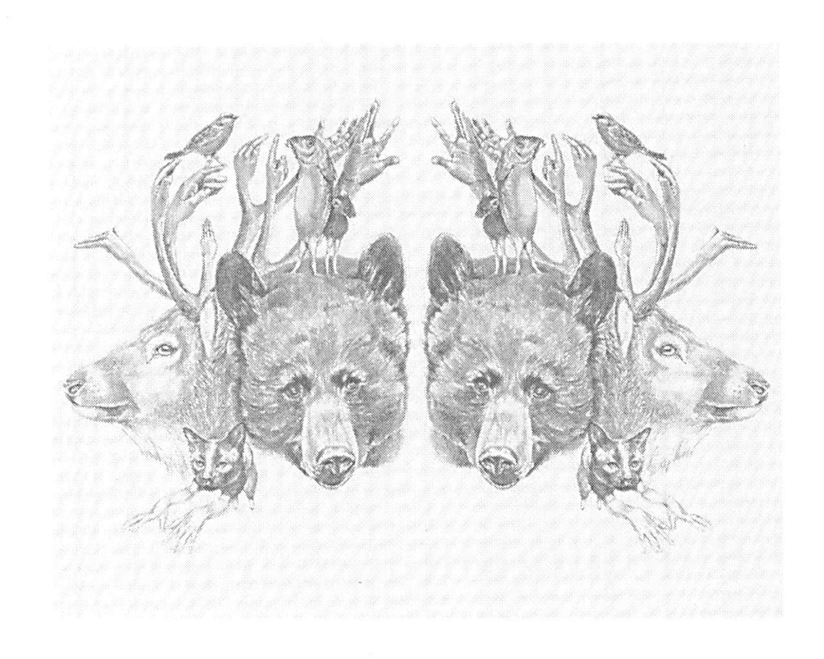

Rohan Millson

Tabularasa Press
Cape Town 2016

DISCLAIMER

The information contained in this book is for educational purposes only and is not intended to be, and should not be used by you as medical advice. **Please DO NOT delay in seeking medical advice from a licensed health care professional for any health problems you may experience. Please DO NOT base any health care decision on the information contained in this book**, no matter how strongly the author believes the evidence shows that lifestyle medicine and preventive whole-food, plants-only nutrition are the best remedy for most chronic ailments.

What people are saying about *Why Animals Aren't Food*

"With passion, wit, and facts, Rohan Millson shows why choosing to eat animals isn't bad only for them, and exposes the irony that when we rob them of their lives, we raise the risk of doing the same to ourselves."

- **Jonathan Balcombe**, PhD, author of *Pleasurable Kingdom* and *What a Fish Knows*

"Rohan is passionate about health that is honest and true and this book is an honest approach to the truth about human nutrition - we all need to read this - it can change our lives and make the world a better place."

- **Mary-Ann Shearer**, founder of The Natural Way

"I think it's going to be an important resource not just for the vegan movement but for the general public to understand the deeper picture of health on every level."

- **Will Tuttle**, PhD, author of *The World Peace Diet*

"One day every enslaved animal will obtain their freedom and the animal rights movement will succeed because no lie can live forever. As an in-the-trenches activist for nearly 20 years, I tried EVERYTHING in my power - from direct action and civil disobedience to education and advertising - to make people understand that animals have been victimized to such a degree that they aren't even considered to be victims. They aren't even considered at all. Humans have actually turned animals into inanimate objects; sandwiches and shoes. But animals are not food, clothing, entertainment or research specimens under any circumstance!

Rohan Millson, with his extraordinary book *Why Animals Aren't Food*, is doing everything in his power, as well, to expose the lies and help us understand why animals should play no part in the human diet."

- **Gary Yourofsky**, founder of ADAPTT, Animals Deserve Absolute Protection Today and Tomorrow

COPYRIGHT ACKNOWLEDGMENTS

ISBN-13: 978-1518699276
ISBN-10: 1518699278

Cover art: Details from "Kohler's Pig," with kind permission of the artist, copyright Michael Sowa 2016

Cover design: Mark van Wyk (http://earthalive.org)

Frontispiece: "Hybrid I," with kind permission of the artist, copyright Oriana Fenwick 2016

Many thanks to all the cartoonists and other artists who've given their permission to reprint their work in this book.

Special thanks for their generous support to

Dan Piraro of Bizarro.com for his brilliant cartoons
Michael Sowa for the evocative front cover image
Oriana Fenwick for the quirky frontispiece
Mary-Ann and Mark Shearer
Mark and Tarryn van Wyk
Will and Madeleine Tuttle
The Ghost of Brooklyn
Andre Phillipe Côté
Dr. Michael Greger
Evolve! Campaigns
Dr. Neal Barnard
VeganStreet.com
Nicola Vernon
Michael Haupt
John Darkow
Steve Sack
PCRM

Every effort has been made to trace other copyright holders, and the author & publishers will happily correct any omissions or errors in future editions.

No animals were harmed during the 5 years it took to make this book. 49 were adopted.

DEDICATION

I dedicate this book to Michael Greger, Will Tuttle and Nicola Vernon, crazy diamonds of the first water, who personify the beautiful difference between love of animals and love of food.

Foreword by Will Tuttle, PhD, author of *The World Peace Diet*

In looking at our contemporary situation regarding food and health, what is most obvious is that debates rage ceaselessly about nearly everything. Why is it that, besides all sides agreeing that vegetables are necessary and nutritious, we find so much disagreement regarding healthy eating? The primary reason for this dissension is that we all live in a herding culture organized at its core around eating animal-sourced foods, and yet virtually all genuine research and experience reveals that animal flesh, dairy products, and eggs are exceedingly detrimental to our health. As a result, there are two powerful forces working to convince the public that we are carnivorous by nature and adapted to thrive on animal foods. These two forces conflict with and battle against the essential truth that we are adapted to thrive on organic, whole, plant-based foods.

One of these two forces is the enormously powerful corporate financial structure built on animal agriculture: the huge food manufacturing, chemical, agricultural, medical, pharmaceutical, petroleum, grocery, and restaurant/fast food conglomerates that are enriched by the animal-based food system that we have today. The other force, ironically, is the public itself. We are all required from infancy to participate in relentless mealtime rituals eating the flesh and secretions of abused animals, and because we are all eating these foods, and being creatures of habit and social pressure, we tend to resist information that questions the food status quo into which we have been born. As I discuss in *The World Peace Diet*, it is becoming increasingly obvious that our very survival depends upon our ability to question the official food stories that have been, and continue to be, injected into us, and that are devastating not just our physical health, but our environmental, cultural, psychological, and spiritual health as well.

Fortunately, with every passing day, we are learning more about the beneficial effects of eating vegetables, fruits, legumes, and whole grains, and the damaging effects of confining and killing animals for food. Despite the enormous resistance to these basic truths, we see that what Gandhi termed Satyagraha, or "Truth Force" is ultimately irresistible. Our true nature is repulsed by gratuitous and unnecessary violence, and animal foods are not only manifestations of this type of violence toward innocent pigs, cows, chickens, fishes, and other fellow passengers on this beautiful Earth, they also cause unremitting violence to wildlife, ecosystems, hungry people, workers, and our own bodies as well. At a deeper level, this violence that we inflict and eat desensitizes our children and represses the inner wisdom and compassion that shine in our hearts and that yearn to protect and celebrate life.

This remarkable book not only summarizes the nutritional discoveries that can liberate us from the abuse that animal foods inflict on our physical health, it explains and catalogues them with an astonishing degree of depth and breadth. Anyone of us who takes the time to read and understand the empowering information contained in this book will learn how we can live more healthy and productive lives, and contribute to a more harmonious world. There is no greater gift any of us can give to our world and to ourselves than making this effort to understand the power of our food choices. Virtually all the essential information about this subject can be found in this painstakingly-researched volume, from both the inherent and bio-accumulated toxins in animal foods to the conditions that result from eating them, as well as the benefits of whole, plant-based foods, all of which we can to put into practice in our daily lives.

By understanding the many ways that animal-sourced foods harm us, and by freeing ourselves from the established narrative that forces us to abuse others and ourselves, we create the foundations of a more conscious, healthy, and sustainable world. We owe a debt of gratitude to the author and to the countless courageous researchers whose work is summarized here, who have devoted themselves to being agents of Satyagraha, the truth-force that can heal us all. May we deeply comprehend the splendid good news embodied in the pages of this book—that we can feed all of humanity on a fraction of the land we are now using—and that we can not only eliminate food shortages and malnutrition, but also the driving forces behind disease, conflict, habitat loss, and environmental devastation as well. Thank you for caring enough to help be, as Gandhi also said, the change we would like to see in our world.

~

Contents

Introduction

Forget about the Paleocene. Right here, right now in the Holocene, **more people die from eating animals than from all other causes of death combined**.

Eating processed junk also sickens and kills us.

Animals aren't food.

Only one of the three things we eat is food.

We eat:

- Processed-to-death animals
- Processed plants, and
- Whole plants.

Only whole plants qualify as food for human beings.

Every year about 2½ million Americans die. Mal-nutrition is what kills 4 out of 5 of us. Mortality stats show we die mostly from long, slow degenerative illnesses such as heart, lung, kidney or liver disease; or from cancer, stroke, hypertension, diabetes, septicemia, Alzheimer's or Parkinson's. In reality, our #1 killer goes unrecognized: it's what Dr. John McDougall calls "food poisoning" – eating animals and junk.

Obesity and most degenerative diseases aren't diseases at all. They're *symptoms of an underlying eating disorder*. If we want to carry on thinking of them as diseases, then they're zoönoses, or animal-borne diseases. As Dr. Michael Greger points out in *How Not to Die*, if we start early enough, eating whole plants has the power to prevent, arrest and even reverse our most dreaded chronic conditions, the ones we give ourselves several times a day over many years, using knife and spoon and table fork, Gandhiji's "most violent weapon on Earth." Mostly, we die from self-inflicted eating injuries.

Why Animals Aren't Food describes more than two hundred pieces of scientific evidence which prove that eating animals is our #1 killer, because of what animals themselves are made out of, and because of what they contain, both in terms of lethal chemicals and living germs and parasites.

The online *Merriam-Webster Dictionary* defines 'etiology' – '**ae**tiology' in the English-speaking world – as:

1: cause, origin; specifically: the **cause of a disease** or abnormal condition.

2: a branch of knowledge concerned with causes; specifically: a **branch of medical science concerned with the causes and origins of diseases**.

To show how eating animals and junk harms us, I've defined

EATIOLOGY

as 1: causes or origins of ill-health or death brought about by eating **"foods"** or **non-foods** (animals and junk).
2: a branch of knowledge concerned with causes; specifically: **a branch of lifestyle medicine or nutrition science concerned with the causes and origins of "diseases"**.

Whenever something we think of as a disease is really just a symptom of eating animals or junk, I'll refer to a **"disease"** or **non-disease**, or a **symptom** or **condition**. Eating animals and junk is the underlying cause. Obesity, type 2 diabetes, hypertension, stroke and auto-immune conditions such as type 1 diabetes and rheumatoid arthritis are the outcomes of mal-nutrition. If the things we eat come from animals or are processed into junk, then I'll call them **"foods"**.

As a rule I avoid "scare quotes," unless I want to make use of the ironic overtone fine wordsmiths sometimes conjure up… as in Lou Reed's "You're so "vicious"/ You hit me with a flower." (In other words, not very vicious at all, cher.) To emphasize that our current definitions of the words 'food' and 'disease' are half-baked, I crossed them out in early drafts of this book. So, food and disease became ~~food~~ and ~~disease~~. Alas for me, one dear friend commented: "I can't tell you how much this crossing out gets on my tits," and another turncoat pal agreed with her.

There are 1351 iterations of the word 'food' in the body of *Why Animals Aren't Food* - make that 1352 - and 1044 of the word 'disease.' Plus 1 = 1045. My ego said no, I'm not going to change what I've written, I like it this way, but what's the point of asking people to read our work critically if we won't heed them? Imagine my chagrin at having to search for all those 'foods' and 'diseases' to check if they needed replacing or not. It took me two days. I was vexed but I'm glad I followed their advice.

For auld lang syne I did leave a sprinkling of crossed-out words, mainly in chapter headings, hoping that they'd spring out at you, dear reader, and remind you… Oh yes, Parkinson's isn't a disease; it's a symptom of an eating disorder.

So I apologize ahead of time if you feel the same way as I do about the overuse of sarcastic quotes, those seemingly indispensible tools of paleo bloggers. If heart "disease" and Alzheimer's "disease" jar initially, it's because we haven't yet internalized the greatest truth about modern nutrition and lifestyle medicine: most so-called chronic diseases such as diabetes and multiple sclerosis and coronary artery "disease" aren't diseases at all. They're merely preventable, usually reversible symptoms of eating animals and processed junk.

To substantiate my claims about *Why Animals Aren't Food*, after a short explanation of terminology, I've created a modular book with the following parts:

In Part 1 (ANIMALS, THEMSELVES), I describe

- the COMPONENTS of animals – the substances they're made out of
- the MECHANISMS whereby eating animals and junk sicken and kill us
- and the EATIOLOGY of degenerative "diseases".

I'll show that eating animals and junk causes about 90% of the "Diseases" of Western civilization. Put differently, eating nothing but whole plants makes most chronic ailments and deaths unnecessary and postponable. Most of us are dying years before we should... from a lack of knowledge.

In Part 2 (PATHOGENS), I describe some of the unavoidable illness-causing life forms that inhabit the animal package we eat.

These include:

- Viruses
- Bacteria and their toxins
- Fungi, including yeasts
- Parasites, such as protozoa, flukes and worms, and
- Prions

I'll show that eating animals causes at least 90% of the illnesses, hospitalizations and deaths due to pathogens, because of the concentrated load of sickness-causing germs and parasites in animals.

I'll also show that eating animals creates most of the antibiotic-resistant species of bacteria which are already killing tens of thousands of people worldwide, and which will probably kill millions more of us in the future.

Besides being the strongest driver of climate change, animal agriculture is the biggest user of antimicrobial drugs and thus the leading cause of a possible "post-antibiotic" public health crisis.

In Part 3 (~~FOOD~~BORNE CONTAMINANTS), I describe the chemical pollution that saturates the animals we eat, including:

- Industrial pollutants, inserted as a side-effect of unbridled industry, and
- Drug, feed and "food" additives, inserted on purpose by unbridled industry.

I'll show how the physiological processes of bio-accumulation and bio-magnification account for the fact that eating animals contaminates our bodies with more than 90% of the environmental toxins that damage us and kill us (and deform our babies).

In Part 4 (ANIMAL DEFICIENCIES), I describe many of the vital nutrients (and processes) in which animals and junk are lacking, including fiber, minerals, vitamins and other phytochemicals, or plant nutrients.

I show that in many ways hyper-processed plants and animals are similar in their Eatiology, or diet-related disease-causing effects. Processed junk and animals behave alike in their ill-effects, while whole plants can prevent or mend what eating junk and animals causes.

~90% of the damage we inflict on ourselves when we eat comes from eating animals and junk: from animals' basic 'ingredients,' from the germs and parasites in them, and from the pollutants they amplify in their fat. Animal deficiencies add to the massacre when we behave as if we're omnivores, as do the additives in junk.

Part 5 (SUMMARY) begins with References to landmark studies in nutrition. A conventionally well-educated reader of an early draft of this book thought I was making stuff up. For example, he didn't believe that the majority of the world's people are lactose intolerant or that acne rarely exists outside of industrialized societies. So I went back and added 70-odd pages of references and commentary to show the evidence behind the greatest dangers of Meating. That's the last of the reductionist science.

Thereafter, I get *Whole*, describing what happens inside us after we've eaten an animal meal, showing how animal substances cause problems at every step of the way through our digestive tracts and elsewhere in our bodies.

It's not just the animal cholesterol that harms us (the cholesterol which low-carb, high-animal pseudoscientists are obliged to try to exonerate): It's the animal cholesterol + the animal proteins + the animal fats + the animal hormones + the animal heme iron + the animal nitrosamines + the animal *E. coli* + the animal methyl-mercury and... and... and...(x100)... plus the high fructose corn syrup and the hydrogenated vegetable oils and the refined sugar and the salt and the additives in junk, all collaborating to inflict disease, disability, birth defects and death upon us – not features we should expect or accept from real food.

Having proved with hundreds of facts why animals aren't food, I devote the latter pages of Part 5 to drawing conclusions about our behavior as animal eaters and the Consequences of our Meating for life on Earth.

In On Silver Bullets & Coffin Nails, I describe ten of the best reasons why we can be sure that animals aren't food. In The Pointlessness of Meating, I name a few dozen of humanity's destructive behaviors that stem from our false belief that animals are food. Meating and Earth's Climate is self-explanatory. In The Good News, I dispel the doom and gloom. Being at peace with our beautiful, essential natures as solar- and plant-powered beings is liberating and empowering.

In Bibliography, I list some of the wonderful thinkers whose books have formed my understanding of nutrition and much else besides. In Acknowledgments, I name and thank my major influences, and in Glossary ~ Terminal Terminology I describe some words and phrases I've found useful when thinking about nutrition.

"What's next?" describes my future goals, and "Staying in touch" gives my contact details. *Why Animals Aren't Food* ends with an Extended Table of Contents and a short Index - maps of the vast territory we'll be covering.

OK... So what's nutrition all about, really? If compassion is a "sympathetic concern for the misfortune of others, accompanied by a strong desire to relieve their suffering," then nutrition is about compassion... compassion for ourselves and other animals *in the present*, and also for our children and for our innocent *future* selves, who will reap the cumulative health effects we sow today with our meal-time empathy, or lack of it. With wisdom, love and compassion, our younger selves can prevent the suffering of our older selves.

In *The Pathway of Life: Teaching Love and Wisdom* (published posthumously in 1919), compassionate eater Leo Tolstoy writes: "We marvel that there should have been men… who slay human beings in order to eat their flesh. The time will come when our grandchildren will marvel that their grandfathers had been in the habit of killing millions of animals every day in order to eat them, although they could satisfy their hunger both wholesomely and pleasantly with the fruits of the earth and without killing."

"As long as there are slaughterhouses, there will be battlefields."
- Count Leo Tolstoy
(1828 - 1910)

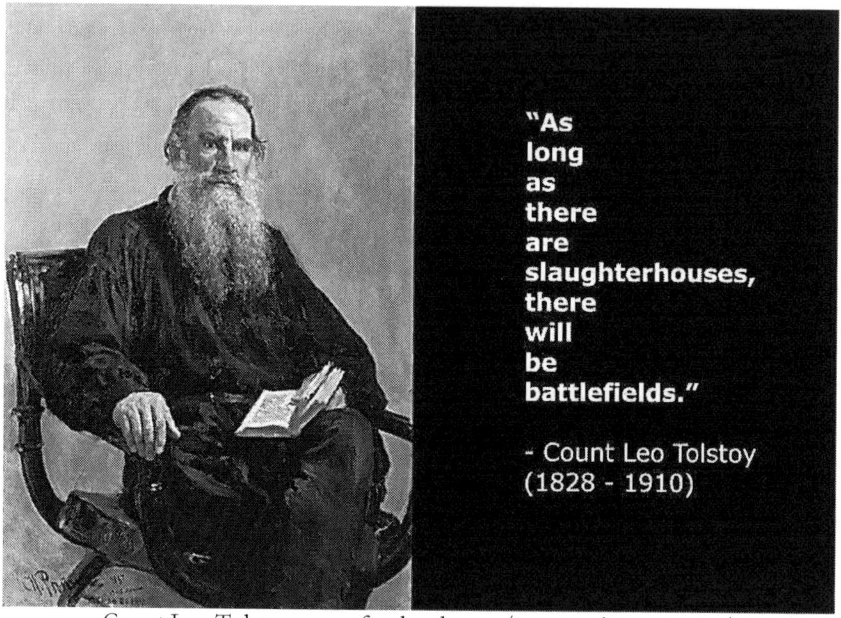

Count Leo Tolstoy. www.facebook.com/compassionateeaters/

"Give," as Luke says, "and it will be given to us. A good measure, pressed down, shaken together and running over." This book shows that when we eat with compassion, we have compassion visited upon us in return, in the form of good health, serenity and longevity. We eat ourselves whole by following the Golden Rule and doing unto others…

Conversely, even if we lose weight by eating mounds of animals, they sicken and kill us before our time. Because this is so, merchants of popular fiction, counseling us to eat animals - people like Robert Atkins, Loren Cordain, William Davis, S. Boyd Eaton, Sally Fallon, Richard Feinman, Tim Noakes, David Perlmutter, Joel Salatin, Gary Taubes, Nina Teicholz, Jeff Volek and Eric Westman - are merchants of death. They incite us to suicide.

And now for a few words…

Terminology

Here are some definitions of words I'll be using during the next few hundred pages.

Vegan and **Veganism**

Donald Watson, co-founder of The Vegan Society in the UK, was one of a group of six founder members who coined the term 'vegan' back in November 1944. World War II was raging. Americans and other Allies had recently stormed the beaches of Normandy, with thousands dying, while a million Russians would soon die on their way to Berlin.

Animals were scarce and many English people tended small Victory Gardens, growing much of their own food. Millions of Brits, somewhat grudgingly perhaps, were eating almost no animals at all. And they were healthier than before, as were the Scandinavians who'd had their livestock confiscated by their German conquerors, leading one commentator to suggest that the Germans were great "public health benefactors."

According to The Vegan Society's webpage: "When the society became a registered charity in 1979, the Memorandum and Articles of Association updated [the] definition of "veganism" to be:

"...a philosophy and way of living which seeks to exclude—as far as is possible and practicable—all forms of exploitation of, and cruelty to, animals for food, clothing or any other purpose; and by extension, promotes the development and use of animal-free alternatives for the benefit of humans, animals and the environment. In dietary terms it denotes the practice of dispensing with all products derived wholly or partly from animals."

Because veganism is an ethical system as much as a nutritional guideline, many of my heroes in the nutrition sciences have balked at using the word 'vegan' to describe a way of eating. Prof. T. Colin Campbell, for example, probably the greatest of all nutrition scientists – alongside Ancel Keys and Dean Ornish, in my estimation – doesn't like the word. So he gets in something of a tangle, talking about a Whole Food Plant-Based Diet or WFPB diet. A bit of a mouthful, no?

I don't share his qualms. Yes, I've met people who said that they "ate vegan" for a while and it didn't work for them, meaning they were never vegans to begin with. They just ate like vegans temporarily, without sharing the vegan ethos of compassion.

Another problem some people have with using vegan as a nutrition word is that candy, soda pop, tobacco, alcohol and junk in general can all be vegan, so it's possible for 'junk food vegans' to eat a vegan diet and be desperately unhealthy. That's a legitimate concern.

While I don't have a problem using veganism as a nutrition term, following the Vegan Society's words above: "in dietary terms… dispensing with… animals," I'll defer to Prof. Campbell on his reason for not using vegan, but ixnay on the 'plant-based diet' rigmarole. (That concept should amscray.) It gives the impression that the human diet is *based* on plants, with some animals thrown in for good measure. I think it's misleading. Only plants are food, as I intend to prove, so I prefer a 'plants-only' to a 'plant-based' diet.

[Editor's note: fans of The Three Stooges will know that ixnay and amscray are pig Latin for 'nix' and 'scram,' meaning 'no' and 'buzz off.']

I'll use 'vegan' now and then, but I'll use the following words more.

Just as vegan contains the first three and last two letters of 'vegetarian' - "the beginning and end of vegetarian," according to Watson – for the duration of this book I'll be talking about

Planters – whole plant eaters, and

Meaters – animal eaters;

Planting – eating whole plants, and

Meating – eating animals.

To denote the eaters of the other class of things we chuck down our necks, in a mistaken belief they're food, I'll be using the words

Junkers – 'junk food' eaters, and

Junking – eating hyper-processed muck.

Oxymorons abound within nutrition writing. 'Junk food' is one: if it's junk, it's not food. It's junk "food".

This book presents the best science showing that only whole plants qualify as food.

Processed animals and processed plants are more alike than they're different. In fact, in their shabby health outcomes, processed plants behave more like processed animals than like whole plants. For instance, Meating and Junking both cause us to be hopelessly fiber-deficient, constipated and insulin resistant. Much more on these topics later…

Having three categories of eaters – Planters, Meaters and Junkers – avoids the confusion created by vegans who may be eating junk; also the conundrum of people eating like vegans, but not buying into the vegan spirit. My three categories demarcate clearly the three things we eat.

Planters eat nothing but whole plants; no animals, no (other) junk either. I sometimes refer to Whole Planters or Pure Planters, to reinforce the importance of excellence in the diet and my contempt for "moderation."

Junkers eat highly processed non-foods of either animal or plant derivation. They may sometimes eat whole foods, probably by accident.

Meaters eat animals. Whether we eat whole plants or processed plants along with our 'meat and 2 veg' is moot. Paleo advocates are sensible, only to the extent that they recommend eating whole plants and avoiding dairy products.

There can be an overlap between Meaters and Junkers, and vegans can be Junkers. Planters are entirely separate – whole-plant eaters only.

Because animals and junk aren't food (because they make us ill), I distinguish between foods (whole plants) with beneficial effects, and non-foods, with harmful effects:

- **"Food"** or **non-food** or **unfood**; sometimes **~~food~~** – Animals or junk. When the word 'food' is used by others and appears in a quote or the title of a paper, I'll just use the word without comment, even if the authors are referring to animals or junk.
- **"Foodborne" illnesses** – By their very definition of wholesomeness, foods don't cause illness or disease. Eating may make us sick, but food doesn't.
- **"Food" poisoning** – Being poisoned by non-food or unfoods. As almost all cases of stomach upset are caused by eating animals, it's not sensible to talk about food poisoning, unless we mean our food was poisoned, not us by food. If it's food, it doesn't poison us, unless it's been cross-contaminated with animal shit and animal shit microbes.
    - **"Diseases"** or **non-diseases** or **undiseases** – Most chronic diseases aren't diseases at all; they're symptoms of Meating and Junking. Examples include obesity, type II diabetes, atherosclerosis, hypertension, heart disease, myriad cancers, auto-immune conditions and many other ailments we'll meet later. Unless it's a

recognized medical term such as Alzheimer's disease, I usually replace the word 'disease' with 'condition' or 'symptom.' Sometimes I'll just say Crohn's or Parkinson's or Lou Gehrig's, without qualifying what they're possessive of.

- **Mal-nutrition** – the condition of being ill-nourished by the animals and junk we eat; as opposed to 'malnutrition,' which we commonly misunderstand as being deprived of calories. More than two-thirds of Americans are mal-nourished, over-powered and overweight.
- **Eating disorders** – Eating non-foods is an eating disorder. We eat for fuel, for nourishment and for entertainment; animals provide excess fuel, minimal nourishment and misguided entertainment. Meating and Junking are excessive and deficient at the same time; deficient in nutrients and fiber and phytochemicals, excessive in fat, salt, sugar, proteins and calories, and much else besides.
- **Elective "diseases"** – the maladies we elect to give ourselves by electing to eat unfoods (animals and junk) instead of plants: conditions like hypertension and heart "disease", which are symptoms of Meating, not diseases. Meating and Junking are the disease vectors.

As far as possible I avoid using words like meat, chicken, fish, pork, bacon, beef, veal, mutton and lamb. Instead of hiding behind euphemisms, I'll talk about eating animals or animal flesh or animal muscles, chickens, fishes (or aquatic animals), pigs, cows, baby cows, sheep and baby sheep. Eggs is eggs. When I mention a particular kind of milk, I'll specify whether it's an animal's milk or a cow's milk or soymilk or almond milk.

That's it for now. Some of my other, more fanciful coinages appear in the Terminal Terminology glossary at book's end.

May we all phyte the good phyte and, by so doing, "live long and prosper."

While most Trekkies know that Mr. Spock, son of Sarek, was a vegan, not many people know that Dr. Benjamin Spock, the great pediatrician, in the seventh edition of his child-care manual, *Dr. Spock's Baby and Childcare* (1998) counseled us to feed our children nothing but whole plants.

Dr Benjamin Spock (1903 - 1998)
"Children who grow up getting nutrition from plant foods rather than meats have a tremendous health advantage. They are less likely to develop weight problems, diabetes, high blood pressure and some forms of cancer."

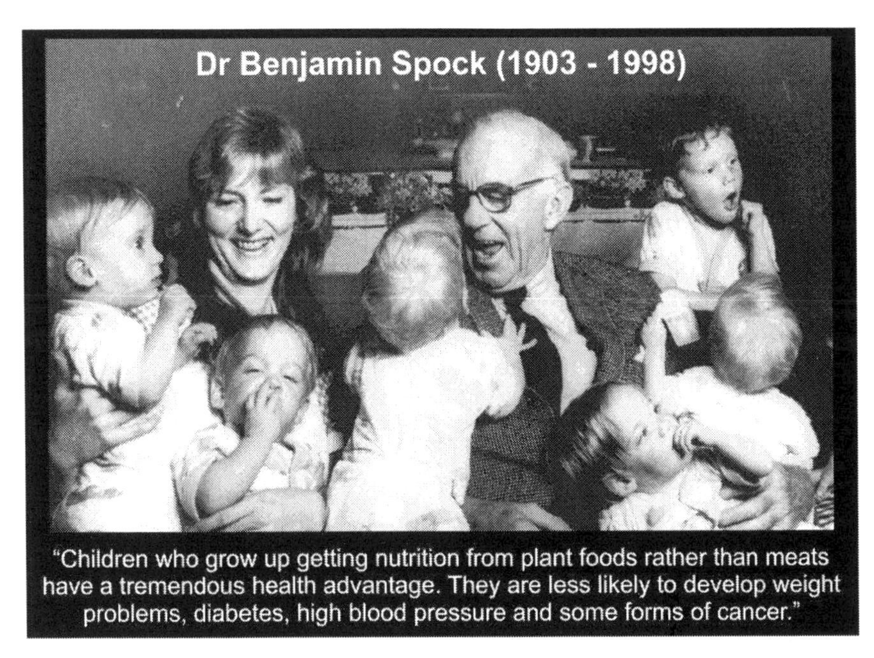

Dr. Ben Spock. https://www.facebook.com/compassionateeaters/

As Jane Brody reported (with quirky syntax) in *The New York Times* on June 20, 1998, three months after his death at age 94, the "Final Advice From Dr. Spock… [was to]… Eat Only All Your Vegetables."

Let's find out why…

Part 1 (Animals, Themselves)

Part 1A (Components): What Animals Are Made Out Of (With a side order of Junk)

Oscar Wilde on fox hunting: "The unspeakable in pursuit of the uneatable."

Here's an alphabetical listing and description of the stuff that's naturally in the non-human animals we eat (after this referred to simply as animals). I've also included some of the more noxious components of Junk.

(Part 2 deals with unavoidable animal pathogens such as bacteria, viruses, flukes and worms, and Part 3 with the environmental pollutants found massively concentrated in animals.)

Acrylamide

Acrylamide is a carcinogen and neurotoxin formed by cooking starchy carbs until they're crisp: french (or freedom) fries and potato chips mainly; baked goods like biscuits to a lesser extent. It's found in plastics and cigarette smoke too. They're a good reason why we should avoid eating junk.

AGEs

AGEs – Advanced Glycation End-products – are also known as glycotoxins or gerontotoxins, meaning 'toxins that age us.' (As in gerontology, the study of aging.)

In the words of Dr. Michael Greger (the first of many quotes from this great nutrition educator):

> "AGEs crosslink proteins together causing tissue stiffness, oxidative stress and inflammation [as measured by elevated levels of inflammatory markers such as C-reactive protein and tumor necrosis factor (TNF)]. In the brain they may contribute to dementia, in the eye, cataracts and macular degeneration. In the arteries and heart, hypertension, atherosclerosis, heart failure and stroke, then anemia, kidney disease, osteoporosis and muscle loss."

[See: http://nutritionfacts.org/video/glycotoxins/]

If we think of our bodies as big old diesel engines that can chug along for decades, then AGEs represent the quality and cleanliness of the fuel we put into ourselves. Poor-quality diesel may be full of impurities like sulfur that can clag up our injectors or cause us to need a good decoking.

All fuels – foods – cause a certain amount of pollution in our body-engines; some just way more than others.

Here's a chart showing the top 40 sources of AGEs in our diet, taken from a June 2010 paper in the *Journal of the American Dietetic Association*, now rebranded as the *Journal of the Academy of Nutrition and Dietetics*:

#	AGE kU/serving	Food item	AGE kU/100g	Serving size (g)	AGE kU/serving	Source
1	16,668	Chicken, skin, back or thigh, roasted then	18,520	90	16,668	Animal
2	11,905	Bacon, fried 5 mins no added oil	**91,577**	**13**	11,905	Animal
3	10,143	Beef, frankfurter, broiled	11,270	90	10,143	Animal
4	10,034	Chicken, skin, thigh, roasted	11,149	90	10,034	Animal
5	9,897	Chicken, skin, leg, roasted	10,997	90	9,897	Animal
6	9,052	Beef, steak, pan fried	10,058	90	9,052	Animal
7	8,965	Chicken, breast, breaded, oven fried w/ skin	9,961	90	8,965	Animal
8	8,750	Chicken, breast, breaded, deep fried	9,722	90	8,750	Animal
9	8,570	Beef, steak, strips, stir fried w oil	9,522	90	8,570	Animal
10	8,331	Chicken, selects (McDonald's)	9,257	90	8,331	Animal
11	8,044	Turkey, burger, panfried, microwaved	8,938	90	8,044	Animal
12	7,922	Chicken, roasted then BBQ	8,802	90	7,922	Animal
13	7,897	Whiting, breaded, oven fried	8,774	90	7,897	Animal
14	7,764	Chicken, nuggets, fast food (McDonald's)	8,627	90	7,764	Animal
15	7,469	Chicken, dark meat, broiled	8,299	90	7,469	Animal
16	7,426	Turkey, burger, pan fried w/ canola oil	8,251	90	7,426	Animal
17	7,420	Chicken, breast, w/ skin, 450F	8,244	90	7,420	Animal
18	7,171	Turkey, burger, pan fried w/ cooking spray	7,968	90	7,171	Animal
19	6,950	Chicken, crispy (McDonald's)	7,722	90	6,950	Animal
20	6,736	Beef, frankfurter, boiled	7,484	90	6,736	Animal
21	6,731	Beef, steak, broiled	7,479	90	6,731	Animal
22	6,687	Chicken, breast, breaded, pan fried	7,430	90	6,687	Animal
23	6,674	Beef, steak, grilled	7,416	90	6,674	Animal
24	6,651	Chicken, fried, in olive oil	7,390	90	6,651	Animal
25	6,276	Beef, steak, strips, stir fried w/out oil	6,973	90	6,276	Animal
26	6,166	Beef, steak, strips	6,851	90	6,166	Animal
27	5,975	Chicken, breast, roasted w/ skin	6,639	90	5,975	Animal
28	5,716	Turkey, ground, grilled, crust	6,351	90	5,716	Animal
29	5,706	Chicken, curry, cube skinless breast, panfry	6,340	90	5,706	Animal
30	5,510	Chicken, kebab, skinless breast, panfried	6,122	90	5,510	Animal
31	5,464	Beef, roast	6,071	90	5,464	Animal
32	5,418	Chicken, roasted	6,020	90	5,418	Animal
33	5,412	Turkey, breast, smoked, seared	6,013	90	5,412	Animal
34	5,379	Turkey, ground, grilled, interior	5,977	90	5,379	Animal
35	5,349	Sausage, pork links, microwaved	5,943	90	5,349	Animal
36	5,289	Tofu, sautéed, outside	5,877	90	5,289	Plant
37	5,245	Chicken, breast, skinless, broiled	5,828	90	5,245	Animal
38	5,157	Chisken, breast, skinless, breaded, reheated	5,730	90	5,157	Animal
39	5,071	Chicken, curry, cube skinless breast, steam	5,634	90	5,071	Animal
40	4,635	Tuna, broiled, with vinegar dressing	5,150	90	4,635	Animal

This is Table 1: The advanced glycation end product (AGE) content of 549 foods, based on carboxymethyl-lysine content, from the following paper:

Jaime Uribarri, MD, Sandra Woodruff, RD, Susan Goodman, RD, Weijing Cai, MD, Xue Chen, MD, Renata Pyzik, MA, MS, Angie Yong, MPH, Gary E. Striker, MD, and Helen Vlassara, MD – Advanced Glycation End Products in Foods and a Practical Guide to Their Reduction in the Diet. *J Am Diet Assoc.* 2010 June; 110(6): 911–16.e12.

After the top forty above, I've extracted the 50 or so worst AGE-producing things from the 549 studied in the Uribarri paper; the worst of the animal, junk and plant categories, and then added a representative sample of the least injurious real foods for comparison, ordered by their AGE content per serving (column 2). (Column one is ranking, with the worst first; Column 4 is AGE units per 100g; and column 5 is serving size.)

What's the take-home message here? Don't eat tofu? Of course it's not.

As we see, these toxins that produce rapid aging are heavily concentrated in animals, with chickens apparently being the worst source of gerontotoxins in most people's diets. But…

Although they're listed second behind chickens, based on this AGE metric, pigs must be the single most aging animal we eat. Who eats just 13g of bacon? A serving of 30g of bacon – just over an ounce; still a small portion by American standards – clocks in at 27,473 units, half again as bad as 100g of roasted chicken.

AGEs depend very much on which cooking method we use. So, for example, roasted and broiled chickens are far more damaging than boiled or raw chickens – good luck with that. Tofu is better boiled in soups than sautéed with oil in stir fries.

On the following page are the next 40 items on the list of aging toxins.

It looks like nuts are the plants that are most packed with gerontotoxins. Does that mean we should avoid nuts? If we first stopped eating the forty or so items with worse AGEing effects than nuts, should we consider cutting nuts out of our diet completely? No. We'd be crazy not to eat nuts. (It's not called nutrition for nothing.) As we'll see later, gerontotoxin intake is just one of the mechanisms by which our diet is responsible for the rate at which we age (or at which we promote cancer growth). And nuts are packed full of other nutrients that offset the effects of AGEs. The same can't be said for the animals we eat.

41	4,251	Tofu, sautéed (mean)	4,723	90	4,251	Plant
42	3,959	Shrimp frozen dinner, microwaved	4,399	90	3,959	Animal
43	3,901	Salmon, broiled with olive oil	4,334	90	3,901	Animal
44	3,696	Tofu, broiled	4,107	90	3,696	Plant
45	3,363	Pine nuts, raw	11,210	30	3,363	Plant
46	3,265	Cream cheese, Philadelphia soft	10,833	30	3,265	Animal
47	3,212	Tofu, sautéed, inside	3,569	90	3,212	Plant
48	2,942	Cashews, roasted	9,807	30	2,942	Plant
49	2,535	Cheese, parmesan, grated	16,900	15	2,535	Animal
50	2,500	Peanuts, cocktail (Planters, Kraft)	8,333	30	2,500	Plant
51	2,366	Walnuts	7,887	30	2,366	Plant
52	2,255	Peanut butter, smooth, Skippy (Unilever)	7,517	30	2,255	Plant
53	2,019	Cashews, raw	6,730	30	2,019	Plant
54	1,995	Almonds, roasted	6,650	30	1,995	Plant
55	1,934	Peanuts, dry roasted, unsalted	6,447	30	1,934	Plant
56	1,642	Almonds, blanched	5,473	30	1,642	Plant
57	1,606	Chestnut, roasted	5,353	30	1,606	Plant
58	1,522	Potato, white, french fries (McDonald's)	1,522	100	1,522	Junk
59	1,408	Sunflower seeds, roasted and salted	4,693	30	1,408	Plant
60	1,324	Butter, whipped	26,480	5	1,324	Animal
61	1,237	Egg, fried, one large	2,749	45	1,237	Animal
62	1,167	Butter, sweet cream	23,340	5	1,167	Animal
63	1,084	Oil, sesame	21,680	5	1,084	Junk
64	966	Cookie, biscotti, vanilla almond (Starbuck's)	3,220	30	966	Junk
65	965	Cheez Doodles, crunchy (Wise Foods Inc.)	3,217	30	965	Junk
66	953	Bar, Granola, peanut butter & choc. Chunk,	3,177	30	953	Junk
67	876	Margarine, tub	17,520	5	876	Junk
68	865	Chips, potato (Frito Lay)	2,883	30	865	Junk
69	843	Potatos, white, french fries, in corn oil, held	843	100	843	Junk
70	799	Fig, dried	2,663	30	799	Plant
71	709	Tofu, raw	788	90	709	Plant
72	694	Potato, white, french fries, homemade	694	100	694	Junk
73	653	Cracker, Pepperidge Farms Goldfish,	2,177	30	653	Junk
74	643	Bar, Nutrigrain, apple cinnamon (Kellogg's)	2,143	30	643	Junk
75	636	Beef, raw	707	90	636	Animal
76	600	Rice Krispies (Kellogg Co.)	2,000	30	600	Junk
77	595	Oil, olive	11,900	5	595	Junk
78	572	Oil, peanut	11,440	5	572	Junk
79	473	Avocado	1,577	30	473	Plant
80	470	Mayonnaise	9,400	5	470	Animal

Uribarri et al. Advanced glycation end-products

Even the worst Junk in this study, McDonald's french fries, can't compete with the AGEing effect of animals. Incidentally, raw beef contains far fewer AGEs than Rice Krispies. Does that mean we should eat raw cows? I'll let you decide that for yourself, particularly after you've read Part 2, which deals with animal parasites.

(Breaking news (26 October 2015): The World Health Organization is saying publicly what Planter scientists have known for decades: eating animals causes cancer, with bacon and delicatessen the wurst of the wurst.)

Here are some of the true foods we should fill our tanks with:

#	AGE kU/serving	Food item	AGE kU/100g	Serving size (g)	AGE kU/serving	Source	Category
82	298	Beans, red kidney, cooked	298	100	298	Plant	Carbohydrates
83	261	Vegetables, grilled (pepper, mushrooms)	261	100	261	Plant	Carbohydrates
84	256	Eggplant, grilled, marinated with balsamic	256	100	256	Plant	Carbohydrates
85	242	Pasta, cooked	242	100	242	Plant	Carbohydrates
86	226	Vegetables, grilled (broccoli, carrots, celery)	226	100	226	Plant	Carbohydrates
87	129	Portabella mushroom, raw, marinated with	129	100	129	Plant	Carbohydrates
88	114	Pistachios, salted	380	30	114	Plant	Fats
89	72	Potato, sweet, roasted	72	100	72	Plant	Carbohydrates
90	43	Celery	43	100	43	Plant	Carbohydrates
91	36	Raisin, from Post Raisin Bran (Kellogg Co.)	120	30	36	Plant	Carbohydrates
92	36	Onion	36	100	36	Plant	Carbohydrates
93	31	Cucumber	31	100	31	Plant	Carbohydrates
94	23	Tomato	23	100	23	Plant	Carbohydrates
95	20	Cantaloupe	20	100	20	Plant	Carbohydrates
96	18	Green beans, canned	18	100	18	Plant	Carbohydrates
97	17	Potato, white, boiled	17	100	17	Plant	Carbohydrates
98	13	Apple, Macintosh	13	100	13	Plant	Carbohydrates
99	11	Tomato sauce (Del Monte Foods)	11	100	11	Plant	Carbohydrates
100	10	Carrots, canned	10	100	10	Plant	Carbohydrates
101	9	Banana	9	100	9	Plant	Carbohydrates
102	4	Oatmeal, instant, dry (Quaker Oats)	13	30	4	Plant	Carbohydrates

Uribarri et al. Advanced glycation end-products

All of us age; all of us will die; all our engines gradually deteriorate because of the oxidative effects of the food/fuel we have to put in them to power us and to stay alive. Those who'd like to eat foods that cause the least damage should consider eating low on the AGE scale. If we eat 30g of bacon we get the damaging effects of 27,473 AGEing units. If we eat 30g of oatmeal we get 4. It's our choice.

Now, please notice that all the items on this list of low-AGEing foods (except fatty pistachios) belong to the food category known as Carbohydrates, those most demonized of macronutrients. How can this be? Well, all carbs – and especially whole carbs, not junk like table sugar or white bread – are nothing more than strung-together chains of glucose molecules, and glucose is the primary fuel of the human body, regardless of what paleo enthusiasts say about ketosis (a human survival mechanism in a low-starch environment). Is it any wonder that the cleanest fuels burn the cleanest, producing nothing but CO_2 (carbo-) and H_2O (hydrate)? As Dr John McDougall says in *The Starch Solution*, we humans are "starchivores."

And where are the carbohydrates in animals? Other than the milk sugars, lactose and galactose, whose destructive powers we'll see later; and the tiny amount of glycogen which animals, humans included, store in our muscles for quick bursts of energy, there is zero carbohydrate in the animals we eat. This is a severe deficiency. Low-carb = low life.

As Michael Stipe sings: "I'm burnin' clean… I'm gasoline."

Animals don't burn clean. To eat animals is to power ourselves with the dirtiest fuel available. 'Low-carb' is nothing to brag about.

Alpha-gal

According to Wikipedia: "Alpha-gal allergies are a reaction to Galactose-alpha-1,3-galactose, whereby the body is overloaded with immunoglobulin E antibodies on contact with the carbohydrate. Alpha-gal is found in all mammals apart from Old World monkeys and the apes (including humans)."

In plainer English, Alpha-gal is a molecule which primates, including us humans, don't make, but pigs and cows and the other animals we eat do. So when we eat animals, alpha-gal acts as an antigen – a foreign invader – and our bodies form antibodies to combat it, and inflammation results. Alpha-gal is implicated in allergic and autoimmune reactions, such as Crohn's "disease". It's also implicated in atherosclerosis and breast cancer.

If this immune response- and allergy-provoking molecule is inherent in the animals we eat, can they be considered food?

For more immune response provokers, see: Animal proteins; Cholesterol; Neu5Gc

Amides and Amines

These are nitrogen-containing organic substances which are far more common in animals than in plants and, when combined with nitrites [more later], form potent carcinogens known as nitrosamides and nitrosamines.

Conversely, the nitrates in plants, which are converted into nitrites (in the presence of vitamin C and other plant antioxidants) before being turned into NO, nitric oxide, the signaling molecule that tells our arteries to dilate, DO NOT form carcinogenic nitrosamides and –amines.

Amines are ammonia derivatives. [For more on ammonia, see Part 3 (~~Food~~borne Contaminants)]

According to Michael Greger:

> "One hot dog has as many nitrosamines and nitrosamides as 5 cigarettes. And these carcinogens are… found in fresh meat as well: beef, chicken and pork."

[See: http://nutritionfacts.org/video/can-diet-protect-against-kidney-cancer/]

Ammonia

We eat ammonia and we produce it when we eat animals. The ammonia we eat may come in the form of the "pink slime" that's injected into industrial hamburgers – you know who I'm talking about. (It's a case of: damned if we do, damned if we don't. Besides bulking up the ghastly product, the ammonia's needed to kill fecal bacteria, omnipresent in garbage like burgers.)

And ammonia's a dangerous metabolite, produced by our gut flora when deranged by animal proteins. The protein putrefies in our intestines, producing alkaline ammonia. Our colons work best in a slightly acidic state.

In the words of Michael Greger:

> "Over a lifetime on a standard Western diet, the bacteria in our colon may release the amount of ammonia found in a thousand gallons of Windex. At concentrations found day-to-day inside the colon on usual Western diets, ammonia destroys cells, alters DNA synthesis, increases cellular proliferation, may increase virus infections, favor the growth of cancerous cells, and evidently increase virus infections for a second time. It's the products of protein and fat digestion that are to blame, such that you can double ammonia concentrations in the colon by eating a lot of meat.
>
> But, put people on a plant-based diet and within just one week, the enzyme activity that creates the ammonia in the colon drops like a rock."

[See: http://nutritionfacts.org/video/putrefying-protein-and-toxifying-enzymes/]

I can't overstate how important our gut bacteria are to our health and longevity. We should do everything we can to keep them singing merrily. Fortunately, we know how to do that. We need to feed them the food they like best. Luckily, that's no hardship. It's the food we thrive on too: whole plants.

Amyloid

I've used Wikipedia's info about amyloid because it's pretty darn good:

"Amyloids are **insoluble fibrous protein aggregates** sharing specific structural traits. They are insoluble and arise from at least 18 inappropriately folded versions of proteins and polypeptides present naturally in the body.

These **mis-folded** structures alter their proper configuration such that they erroneously interact with one another or other cell components forming **insoluble fibrils**. They have been **associated with the pathology of more than 20 serious human diseases** in that abnormal accumulation of amyloid fibrils in organs may lead to **amyloidosis**, and may play a role in various **neurodegenerative disorders**."

As we'll see later, amyloid fibrils and plaques are a product of Meating, and they're more an outcome of Meating than a cause of, say, atherosclerosis or rheumatoid arthritis. The Eatiologies we already have for the latter two conditions are sufficient and predictive.

That amyloid is present in atherosclerosis and RA (but doesn't cause them) makes me certain that Meating is the major cause of Parkinson's and Alzheimer's, in which amyloid plaques feature prominently. Maybe I'm placing too much emphasis on this, but I think it's important to know that Meating causes amyloidosis as well as the other conditions it's associated with, rather than a mysterious condition of unknown origin causing the full catastrophe. Planting provides confirmation: atherosclerosis and RA (and accompanying amyloids) diminish on a pure Planter diet.

Amyloid is found particularly in foie gras, the stupendously cruel product made from the ground-up livers of force-fed, stressed-out ducks; also in the joints of stupendously stressed-out hyper-confined battery chickens, which often enter the "food" supply via pulverized chickens made into soups and fast "food" nuggets, by a process which turns chickens into benign-sounding "mechanically separated meat."

"Animal calories"

Calories and kilojoules are units we use to measure how much energy is inherent in the things we eat. Fats provide about 9 calories per gram, alcohol 7, and proteins and carbohydrates 4 each.

Traditionally, nutrition science has thought that energy must be conserved, and energy-in must equal energy-out. The thinking was that it didn't matter what source the calories come from, whether from plants or animals or junk. A calorie is a calorie.

This is wrong. Studies show that the more animal calories we eat, the more weight we gain.

This is down to two main reasons. First, **thermogenesis**. Thermogenesis means 'heat creation.' Planters burn hotter than Meaters. It's as if plant eating turns our bodily thermostats up slightly, so that isocaloric (same energy) diets produce less weight gain in plant eaters. This is borne out by the epidemiology, or population studies, especially studies of the Loma Linda 7th Day Adventist population, which show that only vegans as a group have BMIs [body mass indexes] below 25.

The second reason animal calories are more weight-producing is that plants lead to the creation of more "brown fat" than animals.

Brown fat or brown adipose tissue

Planters store fewer of our excess calories as white, or abdominal fat, the dangerous kind associated with metabolic syndrome, and more as brown fat, the kind that's responsible for temperature regulation in newly born children and which, in adults, is burned to create heat when we eat whole plants. Brown fat, which is concentrated around our necks and over our shoulders, is what turns up the thermostat on Planters' metabolism, the thermogenesis effect we've just seen, which leads to Planters laying down less fat than Meaters on an isocaloric diet.

There is absolutely zero evidence of a so-called "metabolic advantage" to eating animals, despite what various paleo writers claim. Ketogenic diets have the metabolic advantage of being energetically inefficient, in comparison to normal glucose metabolism.

Thermogenic effect 1; meatabolic advantage 0.

Animal carbohydrates

See under: Lactose

Animal fats

Well, that didn't take long. We're in cholesterol country.

There are three things we humans eat that contribute to high blood cholesterol levels. Of the three, the cholesterol we eat is the least causative of high serum (blood) cholesterol. The other two are trans fats and saturated fats – eating them stimulates our livers to produce cholesterol; damages the tight junctions between cells lining our gastrointestinal tracts, leading to a leaky gut, a non-trivial condition; and helps cause the intramuscular insulin resistance, fatty liver "disease" and pancreatic damage associated with diabetes. (Even if somehow the cholesterol theory were miraculously overturned, saturated fats are killers.)

In nature, trans fats and saturated fats occur almost entirely in animals; the unnatural (because processed) exception being vegetable oils, particularly the tropical oils, like coconut and palm.

For this, and other reasons, we'll discuss vegetable oils, which are processed plants and 100% fat, in Part 3 (~~Food~~borne Contaminants).

Trans fats also now appear in the "food" chain because Big "Food" has put them there. I'll explain, but first some facts about fats or triglycerides…

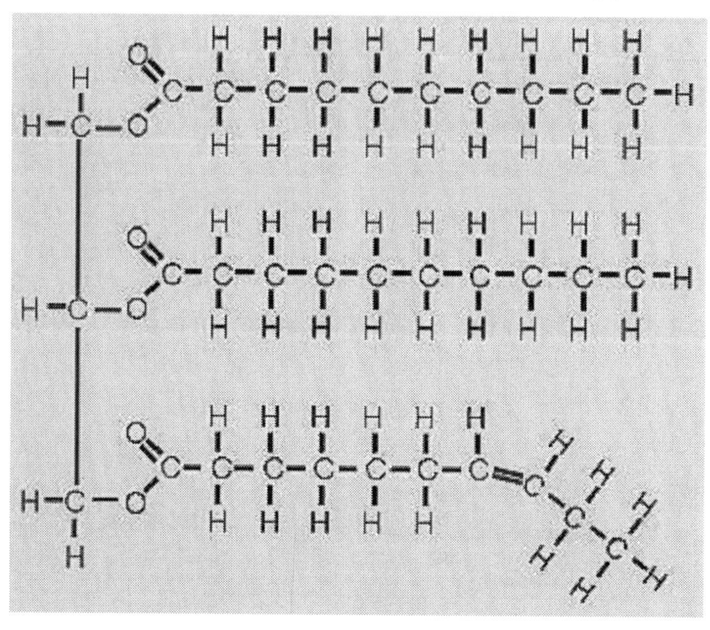

A triglyceride with 3 fatty acids, one of which is unsaturated.

https://media.lanecc.edu/users/powellt/Courses/225Lectures/05A/thumbnails/TriglycerideDetailed.jpg

Fats are different to proteins and carbohydrates in structure. Proteins and carbs are chains of similar units linked together; amino acids in proteins and sugar molecules like glucose in carbs.

Fats are made up of a bookend called GLYCEROL which can have one, two or three fatty acids attached to it (see above). Think of a capital E, with the upright being the glycerol backbone and the three horizontal lines being the fatty acids. The fatty acid chains are made up of carbon atoms, between 12 and 28 of them, each of which has four binding spots, which it uses to bind to fellow carbon atoms in a row or to hydrogen atoms off to the side.

If the carbon atoms all link to each other and have two hydrogen atoms on their other binding spots, the fat formed is called a saturated fat. Saturated, because the carbon atoms' binding spots are all saturated with as many hydrogen atoms as they can hold. These fatty chains are straight and flat, and, like plate-shaped clay molecules in soil, they can pack together very tightly. As a result, they're dense; likely to be solid at room temperature; and have a high melting point.

If the carbon atom binds to only one hydrogen atom, it can use its other binding spots to form a double bond with the next-door carbon. When this happens, the once-straight fatty acid chain gets a kink in it at the double-bond site. As a result, these fat molecules can't pack together as tightly as the saturated fats. They're known as unsaturated fats. The prefix poly-means 'many', so polyunsaturated fats are unsaturated fats that have more than one double bond and, consequently, a more higgledy piggledy shape, leading to a less dense oil that's liquid at room temperature. Polyunsaturated fats are plant fats. They oxidize and go rancid quickly.

Big "Food," as mentioned above, discovered that they could make vegetable fats behave more like animal fats through a process called 'hydrogenation.' Using chemicals they break the double bonds in unsaturated fats and add hydrogen atoms to all the carbons in the chains. The commercial benefits of hydrogenated or partially hydrogenated veggie oils include a higher melting point and longer shelf life. The disadvantage for consumers is shorter life life.

Eating saturated fats and trans fats – fats from animals and processed vegetable oils – olive oil is about 13% saturated fat – causes our livers to produce more cholesterol.

Other than to say that this isn't a good thing, we'll leave it at that until we come to cholesterol in due course.

Besides raising our cholesterol levels, animal fats (and industrial fats in junk "food") have one other brutal effect: they damage the linings of our intestines by weakening the 'tight junctions' between the single layer of enterocyte cells that is all that stands between us and the outer world.

(Our gastro-intestinal tract, if smoothed and stretched out, covers about 300-400 m^2; our lungs and other airways, $100m^2$; our skin, about $2m^2$; which means that our interface with foods and the other things we eat are by far the most relevant environmental interactions we experience. What we eat really matters.)

With the tight junctions damaged, a **'leaky gut'** ensues, which is far more serious than it sounds. If this were to happen to our skin, we'd be covered all over with oozing lesions. A leaky gut leads to unwanted molecules, such as bacteria and large protein fragments known as peptides, making their way through the gut lining. The result may be inflammatory bowel "disease", or increased allergies or auto-immune conditions, as our bodies' immune systems attack these foreign interlopers, creating inflammation, or they may instead attack parts of our own bodies that they resemble.

This 'friendly fire' or molecular mimicry is what happens, most graphically, in Type I Diabetes: facilitated by animal fats, a 17-amino acid chain from the casein in cow's milk lands up in our bloodstreams, and then our immune systems may destroy the corresponding 17-amino acid chains in the beta- or insulin producing cells of our pancreases.

We all need fat in our diets; animal and junk fats aren't the right way to go.

Here's a parting reference on animal fats, showing **how animal fats and tropical oils raise serum cholesterol**:

From: Maria Luz Fernandez and Kristy L. West. Mechanisms by which Dietary Fatty Acids Modulate Plasma Lipids. *J. Nutr.* 135: 2075–2078, 2005. [With added emphases, and my comments in square brackets.]

"**SFAs** [saturated fatty acids – animals and tropical oils] and trans fatty acids [animals and junk] have a detrimental effect on plasma lipids, whereas PUFAs of the (n-6) family [plants] and monounsaturated fatty acids [other plants] decrease plasma LDL-C concentrations [LDL or 'bad' cholesterol]. Among the SFAs, stearic acid (18:0) appears to have a neutral effect on LDL-C, while **lauric** (12:0), **myristic** (14:0), and **palmitic** (16:0) **acids** are considered to be **hypercholesterolemic** [raise cholesterol].

SFAs increase plasma LDL-C by increasing the formation of LDL in the plasma compartment and by decreasing LDL turnover."

This is a technical answer to the million dollar question: why do dietary saturated (and trans) fats spike our serum (blood) cholesterol levels? And the following shows how plant fats work to lower cholesterol (and risk of heart "disease"):

"In conclusion, fatty acids substantially affect plasma LDL-C concentrations and therefore the risk for CHD [coronary heart disease]. Although SFAs have a negative effect on LDL-C levels, unsaturated fat decreases plasma cholesterol. Possible mechanisms by which (n-6) PUFAs decrease plasma cholesterol include upregulation of the LDL receptor and increased CYP7 activity, whereas (n-3) PUFAs decrease plasma TGs [triglycerides; fats] by decreasing lipogenesis [fat creation] and VLDL secretion, increasing LPL activity, and increasing reverse cholesterol transport. By reducing plasma cholesterol and TG levels, both (n-6) and (n-3) PUFAs reduce cardiovascular risk."

Translation: animal fats raise blood cholesterol levels and the risk of coronary heart disease. And plant fats lower cholesterol and triglyceride (TG) levels and lower the risk of CHD.

What more do we need to know?

Animal proteins

One of the most risible questions of all time is: "So where do you get your protein?" As if the animal proteins the questioner eats are a good thing. They're not.

The first reason is the molecular mimicry mentioned above. Eating animals is what causes auto-immune disorders. (It's not correct to call them 'auto-immune diseases' because eating animals is the underlying cause. So, eating animals – 'Meating' – is the real disease.)

They're animals; we're animals. Our meat is very similar to their meat; our muscles are meat. When we eat their muscles (and other parts) our animal immune systems often can't tell us from them, and our immune systems end up attacking our own bodies.

The one underlying cause initiates many different symptomologies, depending on where the auto-immune response occurs. In our nerves, it's called multiple sclerosis. In our joints, it's called rheumatoid arthritis.

In Part 1B (Mechanisms), I'll cover the single important plant exception to the Meater auto-immune response rule: the complex made up of celiac disease (which is a real disease) and wheat and/or gluten sensitivities.

The second reason why animal proteins are bad for us is that they have far greater amounts of the sulfur-containing amino acids than plants do. These are two proteinogenic amino acids – meaning we make proteins out of them – cysteine and methionine, and two others, taurine and homocysteine.

All of these will feature in their own write-up, where their drawbacks are shown. For now, it's enough to say that the sulfur-containing amino acids –

found mainly in animals – lead to the production in our large intestines of hydrogen sulfide (H_2S), the gas that makes rotten eggs smell the way they do, and ammonia. This may lead to the formation of sulfuric acid; not a good idea. Systemic acidosis is the unhealthy condition of our internal milieu becoming too acidified for optimal function.

As we'll see later, sulfur metabolites harm our beneficial gut flora, encourage harmful bacteria to flourish and hinder the formation of anti-carcinogenic butyrates and other short-chain fatty acids.

Methionine intake is strongly linked both to more rapid aging and more rapid cell division, hence, more cancer. Many cancers have what's called "absolute methionine dependence," meaning that they can't grow without methionine. More later…

Thirdly, and probably most importantly, animal protein intake stimulates our liver's release of IGF1 (insulin-like growth factor 1), an absolute health calamity in adult human beings who're not in the need of growth stimulation. The consequences, both for the speed-up of aging via accelerated cell division and for the promotion of cancer cell division, make animal protein a carcinogen and gerontotoxin of note. This isn't news to nutrition scientists. (For more, see under: Cancer.)

Lastly, and not least, animal proteins put an inordinate stress on our kidneys. Plant proteins don't do this. Our kidneys are our blood filters. Their main job is to remove excess nitrogen which we pee out. All other metabolites and excesses go out in our poop. When we eat animals, we eat more, and different, proteins, which are made out of amino acids, whose definition is that they contain an amine group, which is NH_2^-. In other words, hydrogen and nitrogen.

When we eat animals, we load our kidneys with a deadly package besides large amounts of nitrogen: we shovel in the cholesterol, saturated fats and trans fats too, all of which damage our kidneys and cause them to mal-function.

Then, if we're Junkers, we're also killing our kidneys with industrial sugars like HFCS and white sugar. They increase our uric acid levels; not good for kidneys.

(In nutrition, it doesn't hurt to think 'White is Shite'… white bread, white flour, white sugar… all pure rubbish, not food for angelic humans. Colored or sweet potatoes are more nutritious than white potatoes.)

Meating and Junking both raise our blood pressure… not good anywhere, especially not for kidneys.

Animal proteins cause acidosis and inflammation in our kidneys, which stresses them out and helps cause chronic kidney "disease", characterized by hyper-filtration and protein leakage.

For hyper-filtration, think: swimming pool filter, whose intake is blocked by leaves, causing the motor to work harder and start whining. As for protein leakage, peeing out proteins is a sure sign of incipient kidney failure, and Meating and Junking are what cause it.

Chronic kidney "disease" is on the rise, with about 12% of Americans affected – ~40 million people, of whom ~30 million are oblivious that we're in danger of being on permanent dialysis or in need of a kidney transplant.

Twice as many now as a quarter-century ago.

Why?

Because of our eating habits: we're eating way more of two thing now than then – animals **and** junk.

Really, dear people, it's not just the animals. And you other dear people over there, it's not just the processed plants, or carbs, or sugar. It's both. It's the Meating and the Junking. It's the "meat + sweet" connection.

It's time we stopped talking about 'low-carb' and 'low-fat.' It's the animals and it's the junk that are killing us.

National Vital Statistics Reports Volume 60, number 4, January 11, 2012. Death, by Sherry L. Murphy, B.S.; Jiaquan Xu, M.D.; and Kenneth D. Kochanek, M.A.; Division of Vital Statistics, CDC (Centers for Disease Control).

There we are: kidney "disease" is our #8 killer, carting off 42,000 Americans each year, mostly because of our eating disorders – Meating and Junking. And, if we carry on Meating and Junking, kidney "disease" may soon be #7, with a bullet (as pop charts used to say of rapidly rising hits.)

32 National Vital Statistics Reports, Vol. 60, No. 4, January 11, 2012

Table 7. Deaths and death rates for the 10 leading causes of death in specified age groups: United States, preliminary 2010—Con.

[Data based on a continuous file of records received from the states. Rates are per 100,000 population in specified group. Rates are based on populations enumerated in the 2010 U.S. census as of April 1. For explanation of asterisks (*) preceding cause-of-death codes, see "Technical Notes." Figures are based on weighted data rounded to the nearest individual, so categories may not add to totals or subtotals]

Rank[1]	Cause of death (based on *International Classification of Diseases, Tenth Revision*, Second Edition, 2004) and age	Number	Rate
	65 years and over		
...	All causes	1,796,620	4,461.7
1	Diseases of heart (I00–I09,I11,I13,I20–I51)	476,519	1,183.4
2	Malignant neoplasms (C00–C97)	396,173	983.8
3	Chronic lower respiratory diseases (J40–J47)	117,856	292.7
4	Cerebrovascular diseases (I60–I69)	109,764	272.6
5	Alzheimer's disease (G30)	82,438	204.7
6	Diabetes mellitus (E10–E14)	49,123	122.0
7	Influenza and pneumonia (J09–J18)	42,824	106.3
8	Nephritis, nephrotic syndrome and nephrosis (N00–N07,N17–N19,N25–N27)	41,995	104.3
9	Accidents (unintentional injuries) (V01–X59,Y85–Y86)	41,160	102.2
...	Motor vehicle accidents (V02–V04,V09.0,V09.2,V12–V14,V19.0–V19.2,V19.4–V19.6,V20–V79,V80.3–V80.5, V81.0–V81.1,V82.0–V82.1,V83–V86,V87.0–V87.8,V88.0–V88.8,V89.0,V89.2)	6,376	15.8
...	All other accidents (V01,V05–V06,V09.1,V09.3–V09.9,V10–V12,V15–V18,V19.3,V19.8–V19.9,V80.0–V80.2, V80.6–V80.9,V81.2–V81.9,V82.2–V82.9,V87.9,V88.9,V89.1,V89.3,V89.9,V90–V99,W00–X59,Y85–Y86)	34,784	86.4
10	Septicemia (A40–A41)	26,322	65.4
...	All other causes (residual)	412,446	1,024.3

So, where do I get my protein? I get it 1st hand – not 2nd hand from dead animals – from the plants that make them. Yes, plants make proteins (and fats and carbs and vitamins). I get it from a low-sulfur source that doesn't derange my healthy (starch-eating) gut flora, and I get it from a source that doesn't cause my immune system to attack parts of my body, and I get it from a source that doesn't age me prematurely, or incite cancer cells to grow, or kill my kidneys.

The only safe proteins come from outside the animal kingdom. No one needs to die to supply me with their sickening proteins. With just a few components so far, I see no reason to eat animals, and every reason not to.

[See: http://nutritionfacts.org/video/which-type-of-protein-is-better-for-our-kidneys/]

In *Proteinaholic: How Our Obsession With Meat Is Killing Us and What We Can Do About It*, Garth Davis, MD, and Howard Jacobson, PhD, say: "If you are getting adequate calories in your diet, there is no such thing as protein deficiency." Well said. More isn't better; more is far, far worse.

Animals and junk aren't food, dear hearts.

Arachidonic acid

Arachidonic acid is a pro-inflammatory omega 6 fatty acid that we may eat but have no dietary requirement for. Unlike carnivores, we make the little we need, just like with the cholesterol we make. Arachidonic acid is found in animals. When it gets into our brains, it causes inflammation to the nervous tissue, not something conducive to positive mood. (Yes, vegans are happier, even though we have much to be angry about.)

Did you know that anti-inflammatory drugs like ibuprofen and aspirin have arachidonic acid as their target? So, we have a choice: avoid ingesting the arachidonic acid from animals and thereby avoid having to take drugs (which may have serious side effects, yes, even aspirin with its stomach ulcers) or… chow down and take our medicine.

If we're feeling anxious, depressed or stressed and we'd like to avoid arachidonic acid, chickens – again – and eggs are the worst culprits, but fishes have a lot too.

According to Michael Greger:

> "The pro-inflammatory metabolites of arachidonic acid from animal products are involved in more than just neuro-inflammation. They also

appear to play a role in cancer, asthma, rheumatoid arthritis, and other autoimmune disorders."

[See: http://nutritionfacts.org/video/inflammatory-remarks-about-arachidonic-acid/]

Also, inflammatory bowel "disease".

As we'll see later, aspirin (or salicylic acid) is widespread in the plant kingdom, so not only does Planting avoid the inflammation caused by the arachidonic acid in animals; it provides safe anti-inflammatory therapy from food. Other animal merchants of inflammation – characterized by heat, swelling, stiffness and pain – include heme iron, endotoxins and Neu5Gc, the "inflammatory meat molecule," each covered separately.

The fact that arachidonic acid isn't an essential nutrient for humans is yet another piece of evidence against us being adapted to eating animals.

Benzopyrene

See under: Polycyclic aromatic hydrocarbons (PAHs)

Biogenic amines

As soon as the animals we eat are killed, their bodies begin to decompose, or rot. Micro-organisms like bacteria go to work, and so-called biogenic amines arise to continue the breakdown process.

The best-known of these are **spermine** (which also gives sperm its characteristic smell), **cadaverine** and **putrescine**, which give all flesh that post-mortem smell of 'new corpse.' Cadaverine from the same root as cadaver; putrescine from the same root as putrefy.

These substances are carcinogenic and are found exclusively in animals… except for spermine, of which there's a lot in green peas, go figure. Should the presence of spermine in peas make one avoid them? I don't think so… their little green cadavers don't putrefy in quite the same way as a dead lamb, and – "Food is a package deal" – peas come packaged with plenty of offsetting positive phytonutrients. Give peas a chance.

Bones

Yes, you read me right: bones. Plants have fibrous scaffolding to counter gravity; we animals have skeletons made of bones. And every year thousands of people get bones lodged in our gullets – particularly fish bones. Sometimes they can be dislodged with a bolus of bread dough or something like that; sometimes they need to be surgically removed; occasionally, we die.

Cadaverine

One of the rotting corpse biogenic amines (see above) found in the cadavers of dead animals. It's a carcinogen.

Calcium

Cow's milk and soy milk have the same amount of calcium, and they're equally well absorbed, so a logical choice between the two must take into account what else is in them (if we're not to take into account such metaphysical issues as pain and terror.) While cow's milk is packed full of hormones that are cancer-stimulating, soy milk phytoestrogens are cancer-protective.

But one doesn't need to drink soy milk to fulfill one's calcium needs. Plants such as broccoli have calcium that is twice as absorbable as that in animal milk. As Dr Michael Klaper points out regularly: "It isn't what we eat (that's important); it's how much we absorb."

Simply checking out nutrition fact sheets to see how much of a particular nutrient is in a food isn't enough: we need to know how much of that nutrient we eat gets incorporated. (Sesame seeds are the top whole-food source of dietary calcium, according to the USDA's National Nutrient Database for Standard Reference Release 27.)

[http://ndb.nal.usda.gov/ndb/nutrients/report/nutrientsfrm?max=25&offset=0&totCount=0&nutrient1=301&nutrient2=&nutrient3=&subset=0&fg=&sort=c&measureby=m]

Calcium absorption from plant sources is a good deal higher than from animal. PLUS plant-derived calcium comes without the unwelcome baggage of IGF-raising and acid-stimulating animal proteins (among many other negatives). "Food is a package deal."

Carnitine

So, what's carnitine when it's not in some weight lifter's supplement?

Quite often people seem to forget that we're animals. As such, we do what animals of our sort do: our bodies make the same vital substances that appear in other animals. Carnitine is one of these, the carne in this case being our meat. **Arachidonic acid**, **Carnosine**, **Cholesterol**, **Choline**, **Creatine**, **Creatinine** and **Taurine** are others.

None of these substances appears in plants. Does that mean we have to eat animals or take supplements to get them? No, because we're animals and we make all the arachidonic acid, carnitine, carnosine, cholesterol, choline, creatine and taurine that we need.

Later on, in Part 1B (Mechanisms), we'll meet TMA and TMAO, trimethylamine and its oxide, and we'll find out how our gut flora interacts with some of these substances to make cholesterol's atherosclerotic effects even worse than it already is, via TMAO formation.

The take-home message from this is that eating the 6 Cs, the A and the T above, the C-C-C-C-C-C-A-T present in c-c-cats and other animals, can lead to dire health consequences and consequently show that animals aren't food.

Carnosine

See under: Carnitine, TMA(O)

Casein

Casein is the protein that makes up about 87% of cow's milk protein. Prof. T. Colin Campbell calls it "the most relevant carcinogen" known to humanity. Because low- and no-fat milks have higher concentrations of casein, they are more strongly connected to prostate and breast cancer than full cream milk. (And, no, that isn't a recommendation to drink 100%). Casein is also implicated in the Eatiology of type 1 diabetes.

A dangerous metabolite of casein, potentially lethal to infants, is:

Casomorphin

As the name indicates, casomorphins are opiate substances found in dairy products. They're formed from beta-casein, a milk protein. They bind to the same receptor sites in the brain as morphine. In a calf, this induces calmness and helps foster mother-child bonding. Swallowed by humans, casomorphins may be mildly addictive and probably explain why a vegetarian finds "*my* cheese" the hardest and last thing to give up before eating healthily.

Casomorphins are implicated in crib death or SIDS: they can shut down the respiratory centers of our babies' brains. They're not food.

Ceramide

Ceramide is a metabolite/breakdown product of animal fats that accumulates within muscle cells and contributes to muscular insulin resistance and diabetes.

For more, see under: Diabetes; Diacyl-glycerol; Insulin resistance; Lipotoxicity; Obesity

Cholesterol

Cholesterol – what is it?

Cholesterol isn't a nutrient. There's no daily recommended intake for cholesterol. We animals make all the cholesterol we need. Except in extremely rare familial, genetic conditions, there's no such thing as cholesterol deficiency. We don't need to eat any cholesterol. In fact, the safe upper limit of cholesterol consumption is zero – eat any cholesterol-containing "food" at all and there's a dose-response negative health outcome, both in heart disease and cancer risk.

Cholesterol is a waxy substance made mostly by our livers and, to a lesser extent, all our cells. Our bodies use cholesterol to make steroid hormones, like testosterone, estrogens and progesterone. When the sun shines on our skin, it's a cholesterol metabolite that gets turned into the hormone Vitamin D. Yes, cholesterol is vital to our existence. But – and I can't emphasize this strongly enough – it's not a nutrient; we're animals and we make all we need. This ain't Texas: bigger isn't better.

The simple truth about cholesterol is this: in the absence of high serum (blood) cholesterol, we don't develop heart disease and we don't die from heart attacks. Cholesterol build-up is a necessary precondition for dying of a heart attack. On autopsy, cholesterol crystals are shown to be the sharp, jagged little knives that slice open atheromas (atherosclerotic plaques) and lead to the sudden blockage in arteries that can cause heart attacks or strokes.

There is simply no way to get around this: "It's the cholesterol, ya big schtoop!"

Really. It's the cholesterol… BUT it's not just the cholesterol.

When it comes to what's in animals that's deadly, I could spot you cholesterol and still win by naming, oh, fifty, a hundred, other things that are wrong with animals to such an extent that animals aren't food, and we aren't animal-eaters.

As says Dr William Clifford Roberts, longtime editor of the *Journal of the American Heart Association* (W. C. Roberts. Twenty questions on atherosclerosis. *BUMC Proceedings* 2000;13:139–143.): "if the serum total cholesterol is 90 to 140 mg/dL, there is no evidence that cigarette smoking, systemic hypertension, diabetes mellitus, inactivity, or obesity produces atherosclerotic plaques. Hypercholesterolemia is the only *direct* atherosclerotic risk factor; the others are indirect. If, however, the total cholesterol level is >150 mg/dL and the LDL cholesterol is >100 mg/dL, the other risk factors clearly accelerate atherosclerosis."

According to Dr. Roberts, we can have all the other 8 of the 9 causes that account for 90% of heart disease and if we don't have dangerously high cholesterol levels, then it's impossible to get cardiovascular "disease", our #1 killer in the developed world. There it is, in two little words: IM POSSIBLE.

It doesn't matter if we have diabetes, or too much belly fat, or if we're stressed, or hypertensive, or don't exercise enough, or have triglycerides that are too high [blood fats]... No cholesterol, no cardiovascular disease. Atheromas – the pustular lesions in our arteries that may tear open, causing a killer clot – require the cholesterol building materials to exist.

Cholesterol is only found in animals. Trans fats are only found in nature in animals, but they and saturated fats, also appear in junk. So, no animals and no junk in the diet – no heart attacks, no strokes.

That's the real truth about cholesterol.

But sadly, here's another way we get the wool pulled over our eyes. Our largest health organizations – which are made up, like the majority of the population, of Meaters – have set dietary cholesterol intake levels way too high. (Meaning: above zero.) The crazy outcome of this is that most of the half million-odd Americans who die from heart attacks each year have so-called 'normal' cholesterol, which, depending on the organization, can be above 200! This is public health lunacy.

Our best science shows us to be inured to heart attack at less than 150. Why not set that as the safe upper limit? Because, according to their specious reasoning, the safe level might be so low that it discourages people from trying to reduce at all. Honestly, that's their lame excuse for perpetuating this public health embarrassment. (The real reason is that the only way to have optimal cholesterol levels is to stop eating animals and junk; and that's far too unpopular for a health organization to recommend.)

In a country where the norm is to die from high cholesterol, it's time to get away from normal and to embrace *ideal* cholesterol levels: a life-affirming policy of zero tolerance.

Lipoproteins

Because cholesterol is a fatty/waxy substance that's transported in our watery blood, it gets packaged into lipoproteins on moving day – carrier molecules that are fat on the inside, protein on the out. HDLs are high density lipoproteins, which have a higher protein content. VHDLs are very high density, and LDLs are more fatty low density lipoproteins. Despite what Low-Carb Bullshit Artists might tell us, under the right circumstances all lipoprotein particles can be atherogenic, i.e. cause heart and artery "disease". Some are just more dangerous than others. HDLs are generally thought to be protective, because these are the cholesterol removal vans, taking excess cholesterol to our livers for conversion into (carcinogenic) bile salts, ready for excretion into our guts, to be mixed up with fiber and shunted out.

The bullshit artists look at different lipoproteins and see that some of them – with names like 'large fluffy cholesterol' – cause less artery damage than others, say, 40% versus 60%. Then instead of saying they're both bad for us, they say that one is protective! On what planet?

As Dr. Greger so wittily puts it: "That's like saying getting stabbed with a knife is protective… compared to being shot."

[See: http://nutritionfacts.org/video/does-cholesterol-size-matter/]

The cholesterol we make is crucial; we'd be dead without it. Of the cholesterol we eat – and the animal and junk fats that promote its excess production within us – we can say (as "happy hen" promoter and nutrition ignoramus Joel Salatin says in a different context): "Folks, this ain't normal."

(Animal brains are the densest source of dietary cholesterol, followed by eggs. If we're going to eat animals and try to keep our daily cholesterol intake below the witless old US recommended maximum of 300 mg per day, and if we eat one large egg a day (~275 mg), then we'd better not eat many other animals. In truth, *there's no safe intake of animal fats and cholesterol.* The only healthy intake is none. Nil by mouth is best.)

Atherosclerosis only happens to herbivores

True functional carnivores and omnivores can't get atherosclerosis. Can't and don't, ever. We humans can and do, all the time, when we mimic carnivores and eat animals. Therefore, we're obligate herbivores… we must eat whole plants.

We have to understand that atherosclerosis – a condition in which our arteries becoming stiffened, enflamed and blocked throughout our bodies – is a natural consequence of unnaturally feeding animals to plant-eating animals such as ourselves and rabbits.

Atherosclerosis never, ever occurs in non-herbivores. If, as is claimed by Meaters, animals were suitable food for humans, not a single case of atherosclerosis would ever have been diagnosed. Not one, ever.

In the words of Dr. Roberts (W. C. Roberts. The cause of atherosclerosis. *Nutr Clin Pract,* 23(5):464-467, 2008.): "Because humans get atherosclerosis, and atherosclerosis is a disease only of herbivores, humans also must be herbivores. Most humans, of course, eat flesh, but that act does not make us carnivores."

To risk belaboring the point, because we get atherosclerosis from eating animals and junk, we're not adapted to eating animals and junk. Therefore, we must be adapted to the only remaining thing we eat, which is whole plants. This is confirmed by the fact that eating a diet of nothing but whole plants reverses heart "disease" (Ornish et al, 1990).

Burying the lead on cholesterol

Now, how's this for burying the lead, the arch-crime of journalism?

Atherosclerosis is an immune response. Cholesterol is the antigen that provokes it.

Atherosclerosis results from our body's attempt to rid itself of an alien invader. "Shriek, cholesterol!" our immune system shouts, and sends out macrophages and white blood corpuscles to deal with the perceived threat. That's what lights the touch paper, leading to inflammation, the packing of cholesterol esters into foam cells, the appearance of fatty streaks in our arteries and the gradual crippling of the endothelial layer throughout our vasculature, compromising the function of EVERY organ and tissue, setting us up for chronic symptoms of Meating.

Cholesterol causes a deadly immune response.

Understanding this, is it possible to conceive of the cholesterol-containing or cholesterol-stimulating objects we stuff into our faces as foods? If an immune reaction has occurred at every single meal eaten by every single human being who's ever existed – and it has – even though humans have eaten other animals for millennia, then, armed with this knowledge, at the beginning of this 21st Century, shouldn't we be scientists enough to admit that animals aren't food?

Animals are evolutionarily novel.

Always have been; always will be. They're not food.

Animals and junk are all about "wreck-creational" eating – we eat them for our entertainment but they have the last laugh: they kill us.

No, you're right, refined table sugar can damage our arteries and we shouldn't eat it, but it's not the single indispensable cause of the heart and artery disease pandemic swamping humanity. It's the animals.

Remember: We don't 'get' heart disease; we give ourselves heart "disease", by Junking and Meating.

Finally, cholesterol helps cause cancer and dementia. Cancer cells can feed on cholesterol, and, as we'll see later, its unexcreted metabolites, the bile acids, in excess, help cause breast cancer. Cholesterol damages the blood-brain barrier, the delicate structure which defends our brains, and, once in our brains, begins the vascular damage which sets the table for the amyloid cascade and metal inclusion typical of Alzheimer's.

There is no safe intake level of cholesterol and animal fats. Any is too much. Moderation sucks.

Choline

Desperate to justify their Meating, Meaters tend to look at animals and find 'ingredients' in them at high concentrations and then jump to the concussion that these substances are nutrients and must be good for us, and therefore we should eat animals. Egg, dairy and meat boards are particularly good at this strategy.

One example is the calcium in animal milks - never mind the toxic stew of animal proteins, animal fats, cholesterol, hormones, growth factors, bacteria and viruses such as bovine tuberculosis, aids and leukemia, and persistent organic pollutants that come along with the animal calcium, and never mind that plant calcium is better absorbed and toxin-free.

Another example is the long-chain fatty acids in fishes - never mind the saturated fats, animal proteins, methyl-mercury, et blooming cetera that pervade fishes, and never mind that we human animals convert plant-created short chain fatty acids to long chains in exactly the same way that fishes do.

Desperate to find something - anything - that is vital for us to consume from an animal source, some Low-Carb Bullshit Artists turn triumphantly to the USDA's Nutrient Database (which, to help make my point, has "The USDA Ground Beef Calculator" on their home page) and say: "Choline and cholesterol are in the USDA's list of nutrients; therefore they must be nutrients, and therefore Planters must be deficient in chili-con-carnitine and -carnosine and -choline." Hell, Planters may even be deficient in cholesterol, as the spectacularly witless Chris Kresser and nutritionally illiterate Chris Masterjohn implied in a mutual back-slapping bro-interview.

No, even though the Meater promo group known as the USDA lists them in their Nutrient Database, choline and cholesterol et al aren't nutrients (any more than the also-listed ethyl alcohol is a nutrient) - they're metabolites. The long-chain fatty acids in fishes are also metabolites, made out of shorter-chained fats they've eaten.

In fact, if we think about it clearly, animal proteins are also metabolites, not nutrients. Though they're in animals, let's not forget that we're also animals and we make them too. Like cows and other herbivores, we metabolize them from the plants we eat, and they're not healthy to eat pre-made; auto-immune conditions, metabolic acidosis and cancer initiation through IGF-1 stimulation being three glaringly obvious reasons why.

If animal proteins and fats were nutrients, and if animal proteins were indeed first class proteins because they're most like our proteins and therefore the easiest for us to assimilate, then we should all be cannibals, because the closest forms of these non-nutrients are human proteins and fats, with no or little conversion required.

By their own flawed logic, for Meaters to insist on eating non-human animal flesh instead of human flesh is to practice sub-standard nutrition.

Following this cannibal locomotive of thought brings us to the train wreck of kuru, the neurodegeneration that occurs in those who eat other people's brains.

Does the expression "reductio ad absurdum" spring to mind? It should. If we're going to eat animals, then eating humans is the ultimate best form of Meating. Is eating humans healthy? No. Therefore, eating non-humans is unhealthy too… a fact I think I've already shown, but which I'll prove over and over in the pages to come.

With respect to choline and the other so-called nutrients found only in animals, we human animals make all we need. More is decidedly, definitely, definitively not better.

For more, see under: Carnitine, TMA(O)

Copper

There are two problems with the copper found in animals. First, there's way more in animals than in plants and, second, what there is, is much better absorbed. (Or should I say worse?) Like the iron in heme (animal) iron, copper is an oxidant. Copper toxicity is associated with eating animals; also with increased risk of Alzheimer's.

Creatine

Another harmful ingredient found in animals; not a nutrient.

See under: Carnitine, TMA(O)

Creatinine

Yet another harmful metabolite found in animals; not a nutrient.

See under: Carnitine, TMA(O)

Cysteine

Cysteine is one of the four sulfur-containing amino acids found mainly in animals; much less in plants. Excess sulfur isn't beneficial.

For more, see under: Animal proteins.

Diabetogens

Diabetogens are substances which help cause diabetes via their estrogenic effects.

When we eat diets high in fat and low in fiber – that is, animals and junk – our fat cells and gut flora produce estrogens (or 'female' hormones) out of fat. This reinforces the connection between diabetes and obesity, the obese having raised estrogen levels (and, by the way, overweight men – i.e. most American males – having reduced levels of testosterone).

("Where do you get your protein now, my friend?")

Eating whole plants, rich in fiber, removes diabetes-producing estrogens.

For more, see under: Hormones; "Diabesity" and Diabetes

See also: Obesogens, in Part 3 (~~Food~~borne contaminants)

Diacyl-glycerol

Diacyl-glycerol is another metabolite/ breakdown product of animal fats that accumulates within muscle cells and contributes to muscular insulin resistance and diabetes.

For more, see under: Lipotoxicity; Obesity; Insulin resistance; Diabetes; Ceramide

Empty calories

The expression 'empty calories' is usually applied to junk. Highly processed non-foods provide oodles of calories but precious few nutrients. But stop right there: animals are the same. Both animals and junk are energy-dense but nutrient-poor.

Only whole plants are "full calories." Only whole plants are nutrient-hyper-dense while being calorically neutral: not too dense, not too feeble; right there in the sweet spot.

Endocrine disruptors (EDs)

Endocrine disruptors are human-made persistent organic pollutants that have dangerous estrogenic qualities. Although they're treated more fully in Part 3 (~~Food~~borne contaminants), I mention them here because a lot of people worry about them and I thought some perspective is in order.

The only people who should worry about EDs are Planters. Meaters should ignore them altogether; they're almost irrelevant to Meaters.

How can I say that? Well, endocrine disruptors concentrate in animal fat, and endocrine disruptors have about 0.0001 times the effect of natural estrogens like estradiol. So if we're drinking milk and thereby swamping ourselves with estrogens under Niagara Falls every time we do so, why on earth would we worry about being spritzed with the water pistol of endocrine disruptors?

To most people, endocrine disruptors are toxic pollutants that enter us from the external environment. To me, animal estrogens are toxic pollutants we deliberately take from the environment and put into ourselves, and they're far more destructive than other pollutants. The toxic environment includes the animals we eat, when we put the environment inside us, in the most intimate contact possible, a single enteric cell layer away from our delicate innards. (As an aside: if we're consuming non-foods, can what we're doing even be called 'eating'?)

The waterfall or the water pistol? Animal-made estrogens or animal-borne endocrine disruptors? It's our choice.

(I choose neither, especially considering what damage EDs can do to the insulin-producing beta cells of our pancreas, about which much more later.)

Endotoxins

When we eat macroscopic animals like cows and pigs, we also eat gazillions of invisible, microscopic bacteria and other micro-organisms. Some of these littlies are toxic in and of themselves; some of them produce toxic substances. They can cause toxemia or poisoning regardless of whether the bacteria are alive or have been killed by cooking.

Endo- means within (as opposed to exo-, from without.) We're eating endotoxins when we eat animals: they come from dead meat bacteria. Although these aren't animal components, strictly speaking, there's no way of ridding the animals of the bacteria, which poison us, alive or dead.

Reaching a peak about 4-6 hours after a meal of animals, our blood becomes riddled with bacterial endotoxins, our immune systems spring into action to ward off the onslaught of toxins, and our entire vascular trees become inflamed and stiffened.

(We know that the inflammation isn't being caused by our own gut bacteria because they're in our small intestine, and the "food" hasn't reached there yet.)

Repeated three times a day, each bout lasting 7 hours or so, Meating causes endotoxemia and leads to us living in a perpetual state of inflammation.

And inflammation, as we know, is a concomitant of most chronic conditions, either as a cause or an outcome.

(Which leads to this logical question: if inflammation causes a so-called disease, and eating animals causes the inflammation, which is the disease and which are the symptoms – the named disease, the inflammation or the animal eating which underlies them both?)

All the animals we eat harbor endotoxins. Some fermented plants do too, including chocolate, the making of which requires fermentation of cacao beans. As we'll see often, whole plants behave differently to animals even though they contain the same harmful elements. In this case, fermented whole plants don't cause systemic inflammation even though they carry endotoxins, because they're packed full of offsetting anti-inflammatory (and antioxidant) phytochemicals.

(Which is why Big "Food" tinkers constantly with their animal products, adding plant extracts in a vain attempt to make animals safe to eat.)

[For a comprehensive discussion of this topic, see Dr Greger's videos at nutritionfacts.org: "The Leaky Gut Theory of Why Animal Products Cause Inflammation" and "Dead Meat Bacteria Endotoxemia."]

'Essential' Nutrients: A Quick Rant

It's time for some straight-talking about the word "Essential" that causes so much confusion in Nutrition-land. Essential really means its exact opposite: inessential.

Substances that are essential are all the things that we humans don't make: two essential fatty acids, 13 vitamins (as they appear in the current canon) and 50-odd minerals, even though they're not called essential. Because we don't make them, it's essential that we eat them. That's usually the way it's put.

A better way to put it is this: Because we eat them, we needn't make essential nutrients. They're so pervasive in our diets that *H. sapiens* didn't bother to waste precious evolutionary energy on developing metabolic pathways for their creation.

Vitamin C is an essential nutrient because plants are full of it, so why should we make it? Carnivores make it because they don't eat plants, and they need the antioxidants to counter the oxidation caused by carnivory.

Vitamin B_{12} is an essential nutrient because the cyanobacteria that blanket the earth make it, so why should we? It's only because of the hyper-sterility of modern food that we don't get B_{12} with our plants.

We make long-chain fatty acids like EPA and DHA out of shorter chains, so why should we eat the longer versions, which come pre-made in animals like fishes who got them from algae? (If we're worried, supplementing with algae-based long chain omega-3 fatty acids is far safer than eating the fishy package, which is both inherently unhealthy and externally contaminated.)

Essential means 'essential to eat.' It also means 'absolutely inessential to make because it's everywhere.' Calling things 'essential' calls too much attention to them. On the original plant diet we're best adapted to eating, it was impossible not to get enough of these inessential trifles.

Now, Planting + B_{12} saves us from deficiency and provides peak health.

Sadly, deficiency isn't what ails us. We Meaterialists are suffering from the surplus of Affluenza; a deficiency of deficiency. The question shouldn't be: "Where do you get your _______?" It should be: "Where do you get your _______, without getting too much of it, and without getting too much other shit at the same time?"

The only reasonable answer is: "As far as possible, from whole, fresh, organic, ripe, seasonal, local plants; raw or cooked." Home-grown may be best; the safest and most nutritious.

And, if we're not getting enough dirt in our diet, we should take our B_{12}.

Estradiol

17-beta-estradiol is the most common female sex hormone in vertebrates. Not just primates. Not just mammals. Vertebrates. That's a lot of animals that use this estrogen to maintain homeostasis and to control physiological functions.

While xenoestrogens such as **phthalates** and other environmental toxins disrupt our endocrine function, the animal estradiol we eat is >10,000 times more aggressive. It's in animal eggs, animal muscles, but, particularly destructive, animal milks (and the concoctions made from it).

Animal Estrogens

Before I discuss estrogen specifically, I'm going to go on a long diversion, during which we take a look at our endocrine (or hormone) system.

The Endocrine System ~ Hormones

Although I'm going to tackle the topic of hormones in some depth, here's all we need to know about them to make sound eating choices: They're incredibly powerful chemicals and, because of their potency, we only need miniscule quantities of them. And, all mammals use the same hormones!

We make all the hormones we need… from cholesterol, as it turns out. And we make all of what we need of that too. Any excess hormones, and any excess cholesterol, damages our health. We have zero need for exogenous hormones… and animals are laced with them. We don't need to eat theirs. To put it more strongly: we shouldn't.

Hormones are subtle. To eat hormone-laden or hormone-production–provoking nonfoods is to play merry hell with our endocrine signaling. Eating endocrine disruptors is like inviting a pack of lager louts to sing 'Auld Lang Syne' while our diva sings 'Un bel di.'

And, when I say subtle, we're talking about parts per *trillion* for endocrine disruptors to cause estrogenic effects.

Earlier, in the cancer section, we met estrogen, and, later, in the obesity section, we'll come back to estrogen and we'll connect the dots, showing how obesity and cancer are linked: fat cells produce their own estrogen! (And their own IGF-1, the human growth hormone.) So many of us are overweight now, being overweight has become a greater risk factor than smoking for premature death! It's the hormones, ya big schtoop!

The *italicized* material in the following crucial introductory section on hormones is available online at this excellent website of the National Cancer Institute at the National Institutes of Health (www.cancer.gov.): http://training.seer.cancer.gov/anatomy/endocrine/. (Emphases added.)

Introduction to the Endocrine System

The ***endocrine system****, along with the nervous system, functions in the* ***regulation of body activities.*** *The nervous system acts through electrical impulses and neurotransmitters to cause muscle contraction and glandular secretion. The effect is of short duration, measured in seconds, and localized. The endocrine system acts through* ***chemical messengers*** *called hormones that influence growth, development, and metabolic activities. The action of the endocrine system is measured in* ***minutes, hours, or weeks*** *and is more* ***generalized*** *than the action of the nervous system.*

There are two major categories of glands in the body – exocrine and endocrine.

Exocrine Glands

Exocrine glands have ducts that carry their secretory product to a surface. These glands include the sweat, sebaceous, and mammary glands and, the glands that secrete digestive enzymes.

Endocrine Glands

The endocrine glands do not have ducts to carry their product to a surface. They are called ductless glands. The word endocrine is derived from the Greek terms "endo-," meaning within, and "krine," meaning to separate or secrete. ***The secretory products of endocrine glands are called hormones and are secreted directly into***

the blood and then carried throughout the body where they influence only those cells that have receptor sites for that hormone.

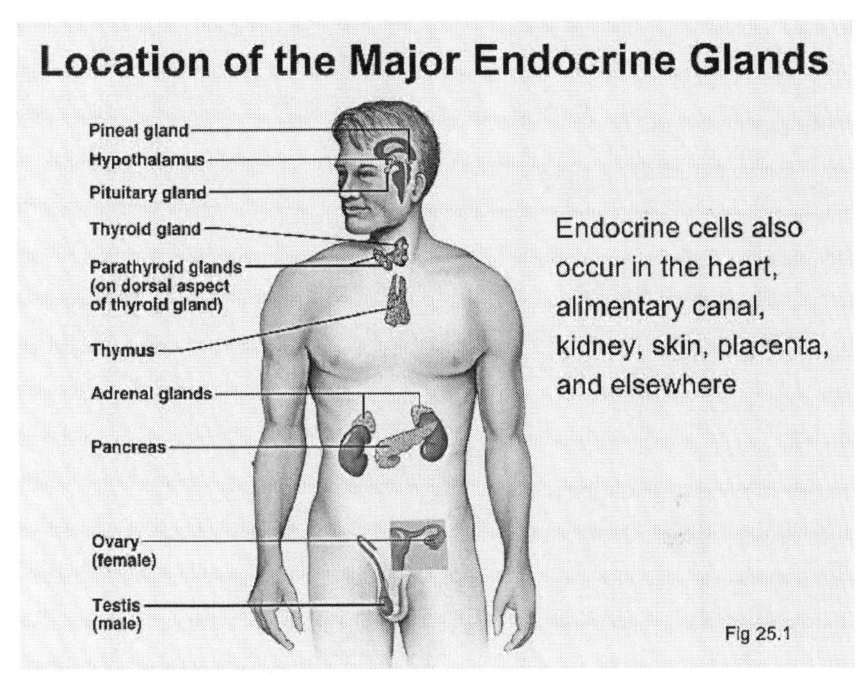

Location of the major endocrine glands. Source: www.slideshare.net

Characteristics of Hormones

Chemical Nature of Hormones
Chemically, hormones may be classified as either proteins or steroids. All of the hormones in the human body, except the sex hormones and those from the adrenal cortex, are proteins or protein derivatives.

Mechanism of Hormone
Action Hormones *are carried by the blood throughout the entire body, yet they affect only certain cells. The specific cells that respond to a given hormone have* ***receptor sites*** *for that hormone. This is sort of a lock-and-key mechanism. If the key fits the lock, then the door will open. If a hormone fits the receptor site, then there will be an effect. If a hormone and a receptor site do not match, then there is no reaction. All the cells that have receptor sites for a given hormone make up the target tissue for that hormone. In some cases, the target tissue is localized in a single gland or organ. In other cases, the target tissue is diffuse and scattered throughout the body so that many areas are affected.*

Hormones bring about their characteristic effects on target cells by modifying cellular activity.

Protein hormones react with receptors on the surface of the cell, and the sequence of events that results in hormone action is relatively rapid. Steroid hormones typically react with receptor sites inside a cell. Because this method of action actually involves synthesis of proteins, it is relatively slow.

Endocrine Glands & Their Hormones

Control of Hormone Action

Hormones are ***very potent substances****, which means that* ***very small amounts*** *of a hormone may have* ***profound effects on metabolic processes****. Because of their potency, hormone secretion must be* ***regulated within very narrow limits*** *in order to maintain homeostasis in the body.*

[I can't emphasize how important it is to understand this last paragraph. Hormones are so potent, only tiny amounts are needed for optimal control and, thus, optimal health. Regulation of hormones requires "very narrow limits."

If we understand this, we're well on our way to understanding that animals aren't food: every mouthful of animal carries a load of endocrine-disrupting hormones (i.e. natural hormones, identical to human hormones) and also xeno-estrogens (human-made chemicals that mimic human hormones). If we eat animals, the beautiful and delicate harmonies of our self-composed hormones are hard to hear above the competing blare and white noise of imported hormones.

To disturb the very fine balance of our endocrine system is to set ourselves up for ruinous outcomes such as cancer. When we understand just how powerful hormones are, and how subtle our hormonal controls are, it should make sense to us how excess steroid sex hormones often cause cancer in our sex organs: vagina, uterus, ovaries, breasts, prostate and penis. Catabolic steroids are those that break down proteins and muscle tissue. In excess, steroid hormones can be catastrophically "catabolic" to our health.]

The endocrine system is made up of the endocrine glands that secrete hormones. Although there are ***eight major endocrine glands*** *scattered throughout the body, they are still considered to be* ***one system*** *because they have similar functions, similar mechanisms of influence, and many important interrelationships.*

Some glands also have non-endocrine regions that have functions other than hormone secretion. For example, the pancreas has a major exocrine portion that secretes digestive enzymes and an endocrine portion that secretes hormones. The ovaries and testes secrete hormones and also produce the ova and sperm. Some organs, such as the stomach, intestines, and heart, produce hormones, but their primary function is not hormone secretion.

Following is a flow chart showing hormone construction from cholesterol. In this case, the 'male' sex hormones, or androgens, are highlighted in the right-hand column.

Testosterone, the best known of the 'male' hormones, and Estradiol, "the most common vertebrate estrogen" are inter-convertible. ('Male' in quotes because women also utilize these hormones, in smaller amounts.)

The cortico-steroids (those made in the cortex of the adrenal glands) are on the bottom left of the diagram.

"You see! Cholesterol is vital to life," cried the Meater. "Our sex and other hormones are made out of it. That's why eating animals is necessary."

The first three sentences are correct. The fourth is fallacious; 180° wrong; so wrong, it sounds right, to those of us who "like to hear the good news about our bad habits," as Dr. John McDougall often says.

It's precisely *because* our hormones are made out of cholesterol that we should limit cholesterol intake to an absolute minimum: zero. We make all we need. More isn't better. Remember, guys: try and think like a woman here… it's subtle. Hormones are needed in miniscule amounts.

Any time we eat animals it disrupts our delicate endocrine balance and sets us up for chronic "disease".

For more, see under: Cancer; Estrogen; Obesity; Xenoestrogens

Estrogens (continued)

Okay, welcome back. If we got anything out of that little excursion into the world of hormones, I hope it's this: we're finely tuned, subtle beings with a requirement of only minute amounts of estrogen. Hormones are powerful. More isn't better. More is far worse. Excess estrogen causes cancer.

Estrogen (from the Greek, meaning "producer of passion") is a catch phrase for many different 'female hormones,' so called because men make tiny amounts in comparison to women. Estradiol, estrone, estriol… they're all estrogens.

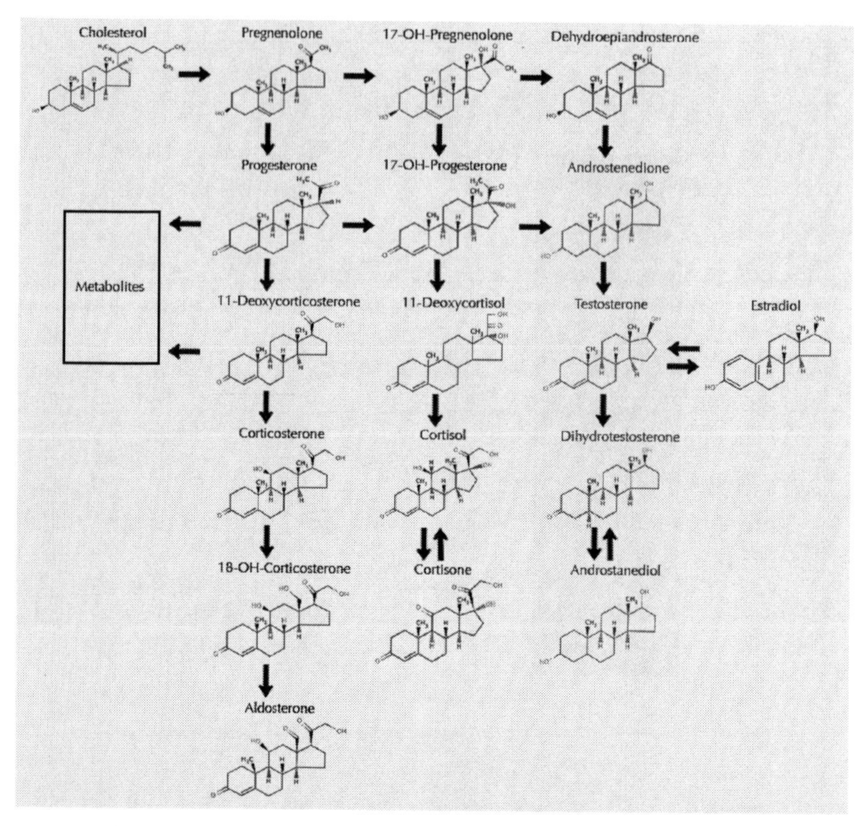

A series of chemical changes turns **cholesterol** into **androgen hormones.**
Tulane/Xavier Center for Bioenvironmental Research.

Now, everything's connected. Planting → high fiber intake → large & frequent bowel movements → more estrogen excretion (+ more cholesterol conversion into bile acids + more bile acid excretion) → less breast cancer.

Sure, cholesterol's a crucial substance. But more isn't better. The same applies to estrogen. We need no more than we make of either of these two molecules, both of which are carcinogenic in excess.

Not eating enough fiber-rich plants leads to longer transit time for our bowel contents. The resultant longer exposure to estrogens leads to more reabsorption, higher blood levels of circulating estrogens and higher concentrations in breast and other tissues. We don't know how to eat… so we don't know how to poop… so we retain the substances that should be excreted. Planting helps us poop properly, so we excrete more than twice as many estrogens than when we're Meating.

Eating animals causes cancer. I can't put it any plainer than that.

Breast cancer is an anal retentive condition. Breast cancer is a symptom of constipation. Breast cancer is a choice we make. Other than a very few genetically ordained situations, most breast cancer is a form of mal-nutrition; a form of self-mutilation. Breast cancer isn't a disease. Breast cancer is a symptom of Meating, the culturally induced form of suicide that sends millions of us thudding into our body boxes every year.

Of course, vegans sicken, age and die. Of course, some unlucky vegans get breast cancer. BUT… whole-food vegans get far less breast cancer than normal or average women. And, if any of us do get it on a plant diet, our chances of surviving it are far greater on a plant diet. The best treatment is exactly the same as the best prevention: sound Planter nutrition. In the case of breast cancer (and prostate cancer), it's the diet that minimizes carcinogenic estrogen levels (as well as carcinogenic IGF-1 levels, carcinogenic cholesterol levels, and carcinogenic bile acid re-uptake). It's the diet that maximizes fiber, water and phytonutrient intake.

And the Planter anti-cancer diet is the same diet that reverses atherosclerosis (and everything which cascades from that condition), hypertension, diabetes and dementia. It's all connected. Planting is our one-stop health food shop and doctor's office for optimum health.

Fecal contamination

See: Feces; also the entire ~~Food~~borne Pathogen section (Part 2)

Feces/Manure/Shit

There's no getting away from it: there's shit in the animals we eat. Which also means that there's fecal bacteria in the dead animals, many of which cause "food" poisoning and many of which are fast becoming resistant to our most powerful antibiotics. Animal agriculture is by far the greatest cause of death via superbug infection, dwarfing the over-prescribing of antibiotics by physicians.

Plants may also be cross-contaminated with animal shit (containing fecal bacteria) during conventional agriculture, so veganically produced plants are safer. (When "conventionally grown" cantaloupes cause an outbreak of *Listeria* poisoning, it's not because they've suddenly grown anuses.)

For more, see Part 2 (~~Food~~borne Pathogens)

Fish oil

Here's some of the latest, best science about supplementing with fish oil:

E. C. Rizos, E. E. Ntzani, E. Bika, M. S. Kostapanos, M. S. Elisaf. Association between omega-3 fatty acid supplementation and risk of major cardiovascular disease events: A systematic review and meta-analysis. *JAMA* 2012 308(10):1024 – 1033.

Rizos et al conclude: "Overall, **omega-3** PUFA supplementation was not associated with a lower risk of all-cause mortality, cardiac death, sudden death, myocardial infarction, or stroke…"

The fish oil myth came out of ML Burr et al's 1989 DART study, published in *The Lancet*, which looked promising, but which was almost immediately overturned by DART-2, a larger, better controlled study. Conveniently for vested corporate interests, but inconveniently for human health, sales based on outdated science have continued unabated.

The Inuit, exemplars of high omega-3 diets, are probably the unhealthiest population in the world, as we'd expect of people inhabiting such a grim, plant-poor landscape.

Paul Jaminet writes: "Considering that 75% to 90% of their food was acquired in the traditional way, a **life expectancy of 32 years** is not exactly a ringing endorsement of the healthfulness of the Eskimo/Inuit diet."

(http://perfecthealthdiet.com/2011/07/serum-cholesterol-among-the-eskimos-and-inuit/)

There's more. People with the highest blood levels of EPA and DHA (the long-chain omega acids) have higher risk of cancer, especially prostate cancer.

Fishes and fish oil aren't food.

For more, see under: Omega-3 fatty acids

Free fatty acids

Michael Greger has this to say about them:

> "Free fatty acids, meaning free fat circulating in the bloodstream not packaged into triglycerides, result in inflammation, toxic fat breakdown products, oxidative stress, which can gum up the insulin receptor pathway and lead to insulin resistance in our muscles. And insulin resistance is what causes prediabetes and type 2 diabetes.

> As the level of fat in the blood rises the body's ability to clear sugar from the blood drops. Where does this fat in our blood that's wreaking all this havoc come from? It comes from the fat that we eat and from the fat that we wear."

[See: http://nutritionfacts.org/video/the-spillover-effect-links-obesity-to-diabetes/]

Animals cause more free fatty acids in our blood because (1) a Meater diet contains far more fat than a Planter one, >30% as opposed to about 10%, and (2) animal fats [and junk fats] are of the saturated and trans fat varieties rather than the healthier polyunsaturated sort.

Galactose

In "Is Milk Good for Our Bones?" Dr Greger says: "The galactose in milk may explain why milk consumption is associated with significantly higher risk of hip fractures, cancer, and premature death."

Animal experimenters – a pox on their houses! – use D-galactose to age lab animals prematurely, via brain degeneration, inflammation and oxidation. Need I say more?

Gerontotoxins

See under: AGEs ~ Advanced Glycation End-Products

Gluten ~ Gliadin ~ Wheat protein (the Planter exceptions)

Gluten-free is big business. Even though only 0.7% of Americans have an auto-immune condition called celiac disease, brought about by proteins found in wheat, rye or barley, far more people than the affected 2.24 million eat gluten-free. Some have sensitivity to gluten or wheat; others have an allergic reaction, and still others have a (still powerful) psychosomatic response. (This is not to down-play the seriousness of these conditions, which are real and debilitating.)

While more than 99% of us are free of celiac disease – it only manifests in those who're "genetically pre-disposed" – some Low-Carb Bullshit Artists tell us that celiac disease proves that all grains are "evolutionarily novel" for all of us, and that we shouldn't eat them. Compare this to the 100%, no exceptions ever, immune response elicited by animal cholesterol (and the frequent auto-immune responses to animal proteins), begging the question: which is evolutionarily novel, the item that's a non-food for 2 ¼ million Americans, or the items that are non-foods for all 7.2 billion human Earthlings and counting?

Grains have been the caloric engines that have powered all civilizations, throughout human history. To claim otherwise is to look foolish in the face of reality. For an excellent overview, read Dr. John McDougall's *The Starch Solution.*

We shouldn't let the fine gluten hairs at the celiac tip of the tail wag the nutrition dog.

For more, see under: Celiac disease and Gluten, in Part 1B (Mechanisms)

Glycotoxins

See under: AGEs ~ Advanced Glycation End-Products

Harmane

An essential-tremor-inducing neurotoxin commonly found in the flesh of cooked animals, particularly chickens and pigs.

For more, see under: Heterocyclic amines

HDL Cholesterol

So-called 'good cholesterol,' HDL cholesterol is good because it's the cholesterol that's involved in 'Reverse Transport': cholesterol is bound to high density lipoprotein molecules and being ferried back to the liver for conversion into bile acids and excretion.

It seems like the only good blood cholesterol is the soon-to-be-dead-and-gone cholesterol.

Much is made of the benefits of a high HDL cholesterol level. I suppose some Meaters can seek solace in having high HDL – after all, it's cholesterol that's earmarked for removal – but high HDL is of little benefit to people with elevated LDL cholesterol. That is, low density lipoprotein or 'bad' cholesterol.

Regardless of HDL level, to be in the sweet spot, we need to have a total cholesterol reading of less than 150mg/dL and an LDL level below 70 or 75mg/dL, according to Dr. Walter Castelli of the Framingham Heart Study.

[In old money: Total less than 3.88 mmol/l; LDL less than 1.9 or so.]

Different units are used in the US and other parts of the world:

mg/dl = milligrams per deciliter, the unit used in medicine to measure the concentration of substances in the blood.

Mmol/l or mmol/L = millimoles per liter, the SI unit in medicine for measuring concentrations of substances in the blood.

HDL lipoproteins can be atherogenic at times. That is, they can take part in causing atherosclerosis.

As a vegan of six years' standing, I don't bother to check my cholesterol. I did once, and it was way below the figures I've listed here. So low, in fact, that my outstanding vegetarian doctor was concerned about my low HDL level (not an issue for me when my LDL barely made it onto the scale).

A whole plant diet lowers our cholesterol level into a zone in which no atheromas form; in fact, a zone in which "reverse atherosclerosis" takes place, like a film being run backwards: there go the lesions, there go the fatty streaks, there go the foam cells, and – voila! – bright pink shiny happy endothelium, supple and strong once again.

Cholesterol lowering and reversal of atherosclerosis (and weight loss, if we need it) all happen automatically when we become Planters.

For more, see under: Cholesterol

Heme iron

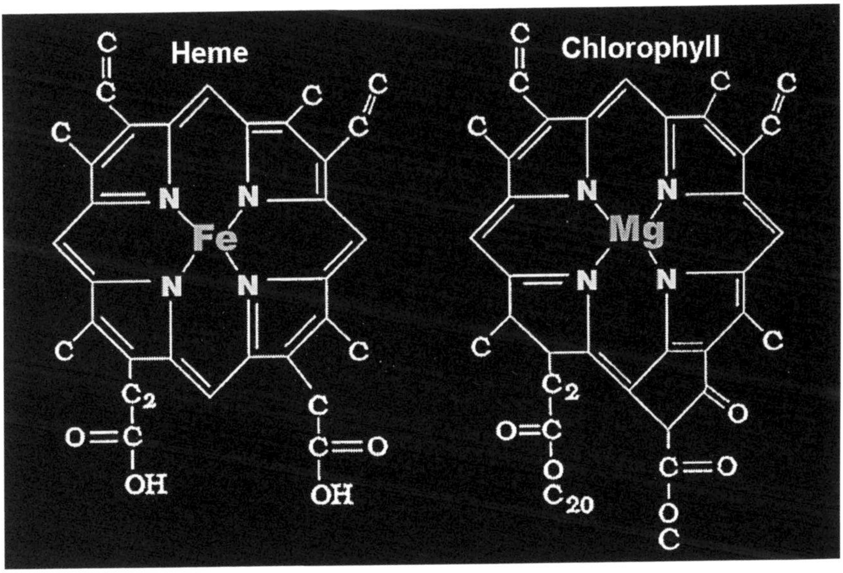

Comparison of heme and chlorophyll molecules
http://waynesword.palomar.edu/images2/Porphyrin5.jpg

Heme iron is fascinating. Heme iron is the iron we get from eating animals. It's the iron atom that's at the heart of hemoglobin, the oxygen-carrying molecule in animal blood, and it behaves very differently from the way that plant iron behaves.

Incidentally, the wonderfully nutritious and healthy green pigment in plants, chlorophyll, is made up of a near-identical molecule to the heme in hemoglobin, except that there's a magnesium ion where the iron ion is in heme. How fantastic is that! (And it can't be an accident. Heme must surely be built out of chlorophyll…? Leafy greens build blood. They're a blood tonic.)

How are they different, heme (animal) and non-heme (plant) iron? When we get our iron from plants like spinach or kale or broccoli, our enteric lining – that single layer of cells lining our guts – can regulate iron intake depending on how much we need. If we have enough, iron absorption declines; if we need more iron, absorption increases.

Heme iron blows right through our gut wall, regardless of whether we need it or not. The human body isn't able to regulate the iron it gets from animal blood.

Let that sink in for a moment.

We cannot regulate the amount of iron we absorb when we eat animals.

I find that an absolute stunner.

Why? Because paleo diet peddlers make much of a phrase they've come up with when speaking about grains: they say they're "evolutionarily novel." Meaning, they've come on the scene too recently in our human history for us to be able to digest them properly. (This they base on the fewer than 1% of us who have a genetic inability to deal with gluten or gliadin, or wheat, barley and rye in general. For more, see under: Celiac disease.)

How then is it possible for these paleo hucksters not to notice that the animals we eat are, after millions upon hundreds of millions of years, still so evolutionarily novel that we can't tolerate eating animal blood? (Shylock springs to mind, in *The Merchant of Venice*, thwarted by Portia in his desire for his pound of flesh, when not allowed to spill a single drop of blood.)

We can't regulate heme iron; never have been able to. Plant iron is what we're adapted to eating. Heme iron is damaging all on its own. However, it can also lead to the formation of carcinogenic nitrosamines, about which more later.

Heme iron is another – usually unmentioned – facer for Meating's promoters.

We've all heard of antioxidants, those wonderful substances made almost exclusively by plants. Well, heme is one of the main reasons why we need to eat antioxidant-packed plants: it's a strong oxidant or free radical producer, and, hence, a strong promoter of 'ferrotoxic' diseases such as heart "disease", diabetes, dementia and cancer.

All on its own, heme iron should be strong enough evidence that we aren't adapted to eating animals; that we are best adapted to eating whole plants.

In a sane universe, I should just be able to say these two words – heme iron – for everyone to acknowledge our frugi-/herbivorous nature, and for the paleofantasists to bugger off back to their caves and leave us alone to heal and to thrive.

Heterocyclic amines

A.k.a. the "cooked meat carcinogens"

For more, see Part 3 (~~Food~~borne contaminants)

Homocysteine

Homocysteine is an artery-damaging sulfur-containing amino acid that's a breakdown product of methionine, another amino acid that we get mainly by eating animals. (For more on methionine, see later.)

Homocysteine is a non-proteinogenic amino acid, while methionine is proteinogenic, meaning our bodies don't make proteins out of homocysteine.

In part because it damages our arteries, homocysteine helps cause dementias like Alzheimer's. It causes inflammation in our brains.

Our bodies use three B vitamins – two from plants, one made by cyanobacteria – to detoxify homocysteine and thus help keep us safe from cognitive decline. These are B_6 (pyridoxine), folate (B_9) and B_{12} (cobalamin). On the positive side, very low homocysteine levels are the main reason why whole food vegans suffer the least brain damage.

On the negative side, low vitamin B_{12} intake by many vegans may lead to increased and unnecessary Alzheimer's risk, even if we are reducing our methionine intake.

Wikipedia says: "Intrinsic factor (IF), also known as gastric intrinsic factor (GIF), is a glycoprotein produced by the parietal cells of the stomach. It is necessary for the absorption of vitamin B_{12} (cobalamin) later on in the small intestine."

All vegans – and everyone over the age of 50 or so, because of decreased production of the Intrinsic Factor needed for B_{12} absorption – should take a B_{12} supplement or eat enough fortified foods to get sufficient B_{12}. B_{12} is the crucial limiting factor of an otherwise optimal plant diet.

(I like to think B_{12} is like the one knot in Oriental rugs that's deliberately mis-tied, because only God can make a perfect thing.)

Hydrogen sulfide

H_2S isn't in the food we eat – at least, it shouldn't be. It's a toxic gas which smells like rotten eggs – I wonder why? – and which helps cause inflammatory bowel "diseases" like ulcerative colitis and Crohn's "disease". Our gut bacteria break down the sulfur-containing amino acids – methionine, homocysteine, cysteine and taurine – which, as we know by now, are concentrated in animals, less common in plants – and form this cell toxin.

H_2S is a free radical (oxidant) which can damage the DNA of the enterocytes lining our colons.

Because, by definition, amino acids are nitrogen-containing, another gut flora-produced animal amino acid metabolite is **ammonia** (NH_3); also not something we want in our guts.

IGF-1

Insulin-like Growth Factor (IGF-1) is human growth hormone. When we're young, IGF-1 secretion is what's responsible for the growth spurt we undergo after birth; our doubling and re-doubling in size. When growth is required, IGF-1 is an absolute necessity.

When we're fully grown, however, excess growth hormone is harmful. Because it promotes rapid cell division, it's associated with premature aging and all three stages of cancer: initiation, promotion & progression.

What stimulates IGF-1 production? Animal protein.

This is understandable if animals aren't food for human adults, because then the only time we're exposed to animal proteins is through our mothers' breast milk, when it's time for us to grow. Makes sense, right?

We certainly don't need extra growth hormone from cows. The IGF-1 in cows is identical to human IGF-1, though in humans the IGF-1 we have is safely inactivated by being bound to proteins. Not so in cows. And rBGH (recombinant Bovine Growth Hormone), the foul genetically modified form of BGH fed to cows to increase milk production, boosts the amount of IGF-1 in cow's milk.

Milk isn't just a species-specific nutritional fluid; it's a species-specific hormonal signaling system. When we swallow the signaling system of another species, we send all the wrong cell-dividing, cancer-stimulating signals to our bodies.

Cows aren't food – not their flesh, not their juices.

For more, see under: Aging; Animal proteins; Cancer

Insulin-like growth factor-1
See under: IGF-1

IQ and IQ4,5b
Cooked animal carcinogens.

See under: Heterocyclic amines, in Part 3 (~~Food~~borne contaminants)

Junk
This is a catch-all category for everything that's not exclusively animals or whole plants. Junk consists mainly of highly processed plants, but may include animals. (I think of all animals as junk too …) Junk has very little or no fiber left in it. Junk has lots and lots of salt, sugar and fat, the three substances modern "food" technologists [oxymoron alert] have used to "hijack our taste buds"; also lots of preservatives, fake colors and flavors, and other chemicals. Unlike apples and grapes, which require no labels, junk usually has long lists of ingredients.

Even if junk doesn't contain any animal ingredients, junk and animals behave alike: fiber-free, they both cause an insulin spike, even though animals contain no glucose, and they're both inflammatory and constipation-causing (a far more serious condition than we may understand.)

Junking is almost as big a killer as Meating, and it's a co-star in the obesity pandemic. Junk isn't food.

Lactose

A.k.a. "milk sugar."

Lactose is the sugar found in the breast milk of animals, and the only unprocessed form of carbohydrate that's universally harmful to health; breast milk to infants excepted. Lactose is a disaccharide consisting of one glucose and one galactose molecule. Galactose, lactose's bone-damaging metabolite, we met earlier.

In a case of the tail wagging the dog – brought about by Western ethnocentrism – people who can't digest lactose are termed "lactose intolerant," as if that's a bad thing. In fact, the overwhelming majority of humanity [3/4] has the good fortune to be lactose intolerant; our flatulence- and diarrhea-inducing intolerance leading us *not* to consume a noxious fluid. Being intolerant of lactose is the healthy norm for humankind.

While lactose tolerance is a genetic adaptation that probably conferred increased survival odds to Western proto-humans in the inhospitably frozen Northern climes of the past, it's outlasted its usefulness. The science is clear: milk consumption shortens the lives of both men and women, increases the risk of bone fracture in women, and helps cause prostate and breast cancer. It's not food.

Even milk's most vaunted benefit – its calcium content – is put into proper perspective when we see that calcium absorption from milk is far lower than from broccoli or leafy green vegetables… It doesn't even do its main job very well. It's acidifying and mucus-forming.

As Prof. T. Colin Campbell is wont to say, after sixty years of nutrition studies: "There is no nutrient in animals that's not better supplied by plants." That applies particularly to animal milks other than human milk.

Isolating lactose from whey and feeding it to infants should be criminalized as a form of violence against children. In an ideal future, people will look back at us and shake their heads… What were we thinking?

Lauric acid

Lauric acid is one of the four fatty acids found in animal fats, the others being myristic, palmitic and stearic acids. All of them, except stearic acid, which appears to be neutral, are cholesterolemic – meaning they give rise to increased cholesterol production.

If Dr Greger has a mantra, it's "Food is a package deal." So, if anyone tries to tell us that we can eat all the animals we like because stearic acid doesn't raise our cholesterol, ask them for a steak *with* the stearic acid, but *without* the other three. It can't be done: they come as a package deal, kind of like the Four Musketeers: "All for one, and one for all."

For more, see under: Animal fats

LDL cholesterol
A.k.a. Bad cholesterol, as if any excess cholesterol is good.

See under: Cholesterol

Leucine
We can extend our lives by minimizing protein intake in general, thereby controlling the two major aging pathways (via the hormone IGF-1 and the enzyme TOR), and by minimizing leucine intake in particular. How do we minimize leucine intake? By minimizing animal intake. Animal flesh, animal milk and animal eggs contain far more leucine than beans and greens.

(Yes, we all age; but some quicker than others. Leucine is one of many reasons why Meaters age faster than Planters.)

Leucine is covered in more depth under: Aging.

Lipoproteins
See under: Cholesterol

Meat
Now this might seem obvious, but there's meat in animals. Animal muscles are made of meat. Meat is in this list because every year a few unlucky Meaters get a chunk of animal muscle or gristle stuck in their throats, get so embarrassed about it that they stagger to the restaurant toilet, where they die in privacy from asphyxiation. The lucky ones get the Heimlich Maneuver performed on them by a fellow patron, such as Phil Connors, the Bill Murray character in *Groundhog Day*.

People tend to choke to death on chunks of animal, not fruit.

Mechanically separated meat
Ground-up chickens after they're 'spent,' used for sub-standard nonfood items such as packaged soups and chicken nuggets. Besides their normal

content of animal-only cholesterol, animal fats, animal proteins and sundry pathogens such as viruses and fecal bacteria, this macerated conglomeration of chickens contains amyloids, mis-folded protein fibrils and tangles found in association with conditions including atherosclerosis, type II diabetes, rheumatoid arthritis, mad cow disease, Parkinson's and Alzheimer's.

See also: Amyloidosis

MeIQx

A cooked flesh carcinogen.

See under: Heterocyclic amines, in Part 3 (~~Food~~borne contaminants)

Methionine

Methionine is a real doozy. As we read earlier, under Sulfur-containing amino acids, methionine is a proteinogenic amino acid found mainly in animals, giving rise to the same toxic effects as the other sulfur-containers.

As we saw under Homocysteine, methionine's breakdown leads to the formation of this toxic metabolite. The more methionine we eat, the worse our homocysteine levels, and the more arterial and brain damage we suffer.

Gerontologists – scientists who specialize in the aging process – worked out that calorie restriction leads to people living longer lives, then that protein restriction is as effective, and then that just two amino acids – leucine and methionine – do most of the heavy lifting when it comes to protein and calorie restriction as a fountain of youth. L & M are concentrated in animals; diffuse in plants.

And, as if their aging character traits aren't repellent enough, many cancers (breast, for one) exhibit "absolute methionine dependency," meaning "no money, no play;" no methionine, no cancer.

Miscellany: skin, cartilage, tendons

Nothing goes to waste from the animals in the "food" chain. Hot dogs and hamburgers are notorious for their low muscle meat content. Studies of industrial burgers show they contain between 3% and 15% of what people think of as meat. The rest – call it 90% - is a mystery. Most of what we eat from these unrestaurants consists of the parts of no-longer-economically-viable dairy cows that aren't muscles: skin, udders, snouts, some bones, tendons, cartilage, eyes… you name it.

[Note: industrialized cows are still children when they're 'spent' and sent to slaughter: they're usually totally worn out by the age of 4 or so. Beeves have a normal lifespan of about 25 years. Which makes the dairy industry more cruel than the regular animal industries: all males are slaughtered almost immediately – the dairy and veal industries are synonymous – and all calves are wrenched away from their mothers, who're then enslaved for four years until that too get the chop.]

Now, I'm as parsimonious as the next person, but the economies provided by shoving all the left-over body parts into hot dogs and burgers and other mystery meat may have dire consequences for humans dining and dying on these miscellaneous animal scraps. They're animals; we're animals; microscopically, some of our constituent parts are indistinguishable. Why should we expect our immune systems to be able to differentiate between us and them with infallibility? Eating cow tendons may cause cross-reactivity with our human tendons. Ditto, cow cartilage and human cartilage.

It's difficult for me to think of something that causes auto-immune 'friendly fire' as food.

Myoglobin

According to the NIH's Medical Encyclopedia (at https://www.nlm.nih.gov/medlineplus/ency/article/003663.htm),

"Myoglobin is a protein in heart and skeletal muscles. When you exercise, your muscles use up any available oxygen. Myoglobin has oxygen attached to it, which provides extra oxygen for the muscles to keep at a high level of activity for a longer period of time.

When muscle is damaged, myoglobin is released into the bloodstream. The kidneys help remove myoglobin from the body into the urine. **In large amounts, myoglobin can damage the kidneys.**"

There we have it, in a nutshell. Hands up, anyone who thinks that flooding our systems with myoglobin by eating animals is a good idea. Anyone with a kidney to spare?

Myristic acid

Myristic acid is another of the animal saturated fatty acids that raise our cholesterol levels.

For more, see under: Animal fats

N-nitroso-compounds (NOCs)

See under: Nitrosamines

Neu5Gc

What is it? It's "an immunogenic [and carcinogenic] non-human dietary sialic acid" that's found in human tumors and the atherosclerotic plaques in human arteries.

Human beings don't have the ability to make Neu5Gc. It's not made by micro-organisms; it's not made by plants; the only way this baleful "inflammatory meat molecule" gets into us is via eating animals.

Immunogenic means that it provokes an immune response within us. It causes inflammation, and helps cause auto-immune conditions, ischemic heart "disease" and cancer.

Cancer cells love Neu5Gc and use it to provoke the state of inflammation in which they thrive. Neu5Gc also promotes angiogenesis, the growth of new blood vessels to feed the cancerous tumor.

Neu5Gc is an antigen – a substance that causes our bodies to recognize that it doesn't belong within us and to form antibodies to fight off the alien invasion. Which begs this question: if we don't make it and it causes our immune systems to go haywire, how can the animals that contain it be considered food? Neu5Gc is another 'bred in the bone' proof of the non-foodhood of animals all on its own, just like cholesterol and heme iron.

Neu5Gc is also another piece of evidence that it's animals that are universally "evolutionarily novel," not certain grains that cause problems for a tiny (<1%) subsection of humans.

For more, see under: Xeno-autoantibodies; also Part 1B (Mechanisms)

Nitrites

Nitrites are in the animals we eat, either naturally or in additives. The additives protect against deadly bacteria and turn dead flesh from its normal grey color to a more consumer-acceptable pink, by combining with myoglobin in animal muscles.

The nitrites we ingest when eating animals have an altogether different effect than the nitrites that are formed during metabolism of the nitrates found in plants. Animal nitrites form nitrosamines, the same carcinogens found in cigarette smoke. This is one of the many ways in which eating animals and consuming junk plants have similar outcomes, the polar opposite of eating whole plants.

Eating animals is a choice between bacterial poisoning without nitrites, or cancer, with: not a choice one would expect from something called food.

Animal and added nitrites *do not* participate in the formation of nitric oxide, NO, the gas which is emitted by the endothelial cells lining our blood vessels which allows them to expand, which is what happens when we eat the nitrates in leafy green vegetables. Many animal eaters get their NO by taking nitroglycerine tablets during angina or heart attacks, in an attempt to rid themselves retroactively of crushing chest pains through drugs, rather than preventing them via plants.

This is another case of a compound or element that's found in animals having a deleterious effect on health, while being well-regulated when eating plants.

Other examples include plant vs. heme iron (above) and plant vs. animal phosphorus (below.)

Nitrosamines and Nitrosamides

As explained above (under nitrites, amides and amines), these highly carcinogenic substances are made by Meating, not Planting.

The nitrites we eat aren't carcinogenic, but that doesn't mean they're safe to eat. Animal nitrites combine with nitrogen-rich amides and amines (also from animals) to form the carcinogenic nitrosamides and nitrosamines. (Unlike plant nitrites which are formed in the presence of antioxidants such as vitamin C, and then converted into artery-dilating nitric oxide.)

These are the toxic substances that make a hot dog, for example, the cancer-causing equivalent of smoking five cigarettes. While the smoking and animal eating addictions are embedded in our culture and are thus above the law, any new products that caused a fraction of the cancer that these two do would be outlawed. Such is the power wielded by Big Smoke and Big Animal, which are owned by the same people, by and large.

Nitrosamines are in a category of compounds called N-nitroso-compounds (NOC). In their provocative *Lancet* paper on 26 October 2015, Carcinogenicity of consumption of red and processed meat, V. Bouchard et al told the world that the WHO thinks Meating causes cancer. They say: "Meat processing, such as curing and smoking, can result in formation of carcinogenic chemicals, including N-nitroso-compounds (NOC) and polycyclic aromatic hydrocarbons (PAH)."

So, it's cook them and die, or eat them raw and die. That's all the choice we get when we eat animals.

Obesogens

See Part 3 (~~Food~~borne contaminants)

Omega-3 fatty acids

Like God, and the Greek alphabet, fatty acids are described as having an alpha and an omega end. Omega-3 means that there's a double bond, three slots from the omega end, and likewise, 6 from the end, for Omega-6s. (There are also omega-7s and -9s.)

The omegas are polyunsaturated fatty acids or PUFAs, with multiple double bonds. Because they have double bonds, they're not saturated (or hydrogenated) fats, which have a full complement of hydrogen atoms on each carbon atom. The double bond puts a bend in each molecule, so they don't stack together as easily as saturated fats and they're consequently less dense, liquid at room temperature; more healthy.

Of the two Essential Fatty Acids (EFAs) – i.e. the they're-in-the-food-so-we-don't-bother-to-make-them fats – **alpha-linolenic acid (ALA)** is an omega-3 fatty acid) and **linoleic acid (LA)** is an omega-6. These are SC-PUFAs, or short-chained poly-unsaturated fatty acids.

Animals such as humans and fishes can convert the short chains into LC-PUFAs, or long-chained fats. Examples of long-chained omega-3s are **DHA (Docosahexaenoic acid)** and **EPA (Eicosapentaenoic acid)**. As such, DHA and EPA are metabolites, not nutrients. Fishes get them by eating algae and phytoplankton, which contain ALA, then convert the ALA into EPA and DHA, or they eat other fishes.

As a rule, whole Planters don't suffer from a shortage of long-chain omega-3s. Our bodies make the longer-chain fats out of shorter ones, like **ALA (α-linolenic acid)**, admittedly less common in plants; and we can turn DHA into EPA, and EPA into DHA, as well.

That said, non-vegans have higher levels of EPA and DHA than vegans. Does this mean we should eat more animals? No. More isn't better. Here's why:

T M Brasky, A K Darke, X Song, C M Tangen, P J Goodman, I M Thompson, F L Meyskens Jr, G E Goodman, L M Minasian, H L Parns, E A Klein, A R Kristal. Plasma phospholipid fatty acids and prostate cancer risk in the SELECT trial. *J Natl Cancer Inst.* 2013 Aug 7;105(15):1132-41. http://www.ncbi.nlm.nih.gov/pmc/articles/PMC3735464/pdf/djt174.pdf

"This study **confirms previous reports** of **increased prostate cancer risk** among men with **high blood concentrations of LCω-3PUFA**. The consistency of these findings suggests that these fatty acids are involved in prostate **tumorigenesis**. Recommendations to increase LCω-3PUFA intake should consider its potential risks."

According to our most up-to-date science, *confirming previous reports*: More long-chain omega-3 fatty acids? More cancer.

Also from Brasky et al:

"Long-chain ω-3 PUFAs have been widely promoted for prevention of heart disease and cancer. Both this study and a recent meta-analysis of clinical trials showing no effects of long-chain ω-3 PUFA supplementation on all-cause mortality, cardiac death, myocardial infarction, or stroke (48) suggest that general recommendations to increase long-chain ω-3 PUFA intake should consider its potential risks."

One of the biggest selling points for Meating, specifically Fishing, just got eviscerated. EPA and DHA supplements cause cancer, and they do squat for longevity, heart "disease" and stroke. Less is more.

A multi-billion dollar industry hawking a quackpot wemedy, cwushed.

Fishes or their oil as sources of omega-3s can no longer be recommended as healthy. Omega-3s aren't cardioprotective, and fish consumption is pro-inflammatory and increases our risk of diabetes, heart "disease" and stroke.

Because "food is a package deal," eating animals like fishes to get omega-3 fatty acids makes about as much sense as, well, drinking cow's milk to get calcium, or eating animals to get protein.

In other words, none whatsoever.

Besides the baked-in ill-effects of excess omega-3s, every ludicrous toxic substance humans have ever made ends up in our rivers and our seas. (About 80,000 of them, by one account; 100,000 by another, and most of them untested; and testing for cross-reactivity is impossible.) As a result, fishes and other aquatic animals, which bio-accumulate and –magnify these toxins in their body fat, are by far the most contaminated things we eat.

In a bizarre twist, we can use people's blood dioxin, PCB, arsenic or mercury levels as biomarkers to tell how many sea animals we eat. Isn't that amazing? We can tell how many animals we eat by how polluted our bodies are. These contaminant biomarkers are more accurate than the omega-3 content of fishes.

With the essential fatty acids, the nutrients themselves are necessary; the animal source isn't. Farmed fishes are the worst source, and even distilled fish oils are contaminated, and go rancid quickly. So, what we lose on the swings of the excess omega-3s from animals, we continue to lose on the roundabouts of other sickening components and contaminants of animals.

Sheer weight of evidence has led to a reversal of consensus on the benefits of fish oil to counter cardiovascular "disease". It doesn't. But medical practice seems always to operate on scientific research that's a generation out of date. This is particularly true of the continuing medical malpractice of recommending fish products to heart-diseased patients.

For more, see under: contaminants such as dioxins, mercury, other heavy metals, PBDEs, PCBs and polychlorinated naphthalenes, and parasites such as ciguatera (a sexually transmissible form of fish poisoning) and fish tapeworms.

(If I were French I'd call fish poisoning 'poissoning.')

Flax seeds, besides containing cancer-fighting lignans, are an excellent source of the shorter-chain ALA omega-3 fats, from which we can make DHA. Walnuts, hemp and kale are other good sources.

It shouldn't be necessary but if we're concerned about a deficiency of long-chain omega-3s, perhaps in older age as our ability to manufacture them from short-chain acids declines, we can supplement our plant-only diet with a clean and healthy microalgae- or yeast-based source.

Omega-6 fatty acids

As a group, the omega-6 acids are pro-inflammatory, meaning that they cause inflammation. They're found particularly in animals and in vegetable oils. **Linoleic acid** is the best-known.

Much is made of the ratio of fats, omega-3s: omega-6s. Because we skip vegetable oils (Junk), Planters' 3:6 ratio best approaches an ideal-ish 1:1.

In his "Chicken, Eggs, and Inflammation" video, Michael Greger says:

> "Chicken and eggs are the top sources of **arachidonic acid** in the diet, an omega 6 fatty acid involved in our body's inflammatory response."

'Nuff said, I think.

See also: Arachidonic acid; Homocysteine

Palmitic acid

Palmitic acid is one of the animal saturated fatty acids that raise our cholesterol levels. It's also found in tropical oils such as palm and coconut, which should be used in moderation by the healthy and not at all by anyone who eats animals (and is thus at risk of heart "disease").

For more, see under: Animal fats

PhIP

Per Wikipedia: "PhIP (2-Amino-1-methyl-6-phenylimidazo[4,5-b]pyridine) is one of the most abundant heterocyclic amines (HCAs) in cooked meat. PhIP is formed at high temperatures from the reaction between **creatine** or **creatinine** (found in muscle meats), amino acids, and sugar."

PhIP is a "cooked animal carcinogen." We get it from eating cooked animals.

For more, see under: Creatine; Creatinine; Heterocyclic amines; Cancer progression, in the discussion of cancer in Part 1B (Mechanisms)

Phosphorus

As we've seen with heme iron, there are components of animals and plants that are identical but are so arranged or bound that they have entirely different health outcomes when we eat them. Phosphorus is another of these anomalies.

We can't regulate the amount of phosphorus we get from animals as well as we do that from plants. It seems our bodies are programmed for plant phosphates, which are much less absorbable (1/3 to 1/2) than animal phosphates (3/4). More isn't better: less phos = more life.

Animal protein → declining kidney function → phosphorus build-up → calcium build-up → metastatic calcification (+ shorter lifespan.)

Once again, when we pull back from a reductionist view of nutrition… when we start by looking at a single nutrient and then place it in its larger context… we see that Meating – the underlying cause of calcification – is the etymon (the source or fountainhead) from which spring all manner of health nightmares. The derivation or etymology of chronic illness is Meating and Junking.

Loving words as I do, I'm tempted to talk about Eatymology, the derivation of nutrition terms, but I've already put Eatiology out there…

Getting back in character…

Junk (particularly soda) and animals (especially chickens) are terrible sources of phosphate additives and preservatives. (If these items were to carry all the health warnings they should… modern kids would double the amount of time they spent reading.)

See also: Metastatic calcification in Part 1B (Mechanisms)

Pink slime

For shameful additives to an already shameful product, the injection of ammonia into industrial hamburgers takes the beefcake.

For more, see under: Pink slime, in Part 3 (~~Food~~borne contaminants)

Polycyclic aromatic hydrocarbons (PAHs)

This is another class of carcinogenic substances, besides heterocyclic amines, created by cooking animals over high heat. They're found particularly in grilled, fried and barbecued birds like chickens and turkeys.

Especially dangerous are the vapors containing these chemicals, such as from frying bacon, which can cause cancer and disturb fetal development. So, pregnant women should beware.

Benzopyrene is one such mutagenic PAH that forms in barbecued animal flesh.

Prolactin

Prolactin isn't something we eat. Meating raises the level of this hormone in us; Planting lowers it. Women who suffer from dysmenorrhea (painful periods), bloating, mastalgia (breast pain) and PMS (pre-menstrual syndrome) can find relief by switching to a diet of… food.

Purge

Purge is the liquid that oozes out of aging meat, particularly packaged chicken chunks, which may contain dangerously high amounts of phosphates, injected into carcasses as a preservative and purge suppressor. Unfortunately the preservative also preserves the *Campylobacter* and other bacteria that thrive on the blood, fat and water mix that makes up purge, 'chicken juice' or 'exudate.'

It's often this "fecal soup" that's responsible for cross-contaminating kitchen surfaces, even putting at risk of infection children who ride in tainted shopping carts. Not cool.

Purines

Purines are metabolites of DNA, so they're in both animals and plants, but they're another example of how eating the same 'ingredient' from whole plants and animals (or processed junk) provides startlingly different results.

When purines break down, they form uric acid which, in excess, can crystalize out to form kidney stones or, when the jagged crystals form in our joints, painful gout. (A low uric acid level is linked to Parkinson's.)

When we eat high-purine plants such as legumes, asparagus or cauliflower, we excrete more uric acid and we have Goldilocks uric acid levels - not too high, not too low. Why? Because plant purines may be less bio-available; plants contain antioxidant, anti-inflammatory nutrients such as vitamin C; in an alkaline state, we urinate more uric acid; and plant fiber binds uric acid and increases its 'clearance rate' in our feces. Planting is protective against gout (and dementia). Gout is an elective "disease" Planters elect not to get.

When we eat an animal package of purines, we receive few antioxidants, almost no phytonutrients, and zero fiber; our urine becomes more acidic; and our uric acid levels go up. Rather like how T. Colin Campbell switched cancer on and off in rats using casein, researchers in dietary intervention trials can switch gout on and off by giving people animals to eat or taking them away. (Alcohol and Junker fructose (HFCS) have the same effect.)

Besides gout, having a high uric acid level is linked to cardiovascular and kidney "disease", hypertension, obesity, pre-diabetes and diabetes. Whole plants are protective against these Meater symptoms. Health is optional; a matter of choice. We select illness by selecting Meating and Junking.

Pus

Besides the tendons and ears, snouts and udders, and the tumors and other diseased animal bits in things like burgers and hot dogs, there is pus in "liquid meat" or milk. Not much – only about a drop per glassful – but – call me old-fashioned – I'd rather not consume any pus at all, thanks all the same. It's known euphemistically within the industry as "high somatic cell count," and it's these white blood cells that have given their lives fighting infection that give milk its distinctive color. Taste too, for all I know. Hmm.

Putrescine

Carcinogenic breakdown product that forms in putrefying animal flesh.

For more, see under: biogenic amines

Saturated fats

See under: animal fats

Sodium/salt

Animals are naturally high in sodium. Junk is unnaturally high in sodium, with massive amounts added to hook our taste buds (along with masses of added fats and sugar.) Whole plants, on the other hand, have normal, low sodium levels.

A pet gripe: Beans, among the healthiest human foods, are often made extremely unhealthy when they're canned. Why "food" companies add any salt at all to their canned beans is quite beyond me.

Excess sodium in the diet leads to millions of excess deaths worldwide by damaging our arteries and by inducing hypertension, or chronic long-term high blood pressure. High sodium intake contributes to about 100,000 deaths in the USA annually.

According to Michael Greger,

> "Sodium intake increases kidney disease risk, but is that just because it increases blood pressure? No, it appears the salt is associated with increased cancer risk even independently of hypertension."

[See: http://nutritionfacts.org/video/can-diet-protect-against-kidney-cancer/]

Thanks to the economics of chicken farming, chickens are particularly high in sodium: many farmers bulk up the chicken bodies they sell by pumping them full of salt water. Cheese is also preternaturally high in salt.

Again, according to Dr. Greger:

> "Despite evidence linking salt intake to high blood pressure, heart disease and strokes, dietary salt intake in the U.S. is on the rise. Right now we get about seven to ten grams a day, mostly from processed foods. If we were to decrease that just by three grams, which is about a thousand mg of sodium, half of a teaspoon of table salt, every year we

> could save tens of thousands of people from having a heart attack, prevent tens of thousands of strokes, and tens of thousands of deaths."

[See: http://nutritionfacts.org/video/improving-on-the-mediterranean-diet/]

There is consensus within the scientific community about the dangers of sodium. If a scientist is a 'salt denialist,' the chances are good that they have industry ties. Extremely good. Or they have a contrarian book to peddle.

High sodium comes from eating animals and other junk.

Spermidine
Carcinogenic breakdown product in rotting flesh.

For more, see under: biogenic amines

Spermine
Carcinogenic breakdown product in rotting flesh.

For more, see under: biogenic amines

Stearic acid
Stearic acid is the exceptional saturated animal fat that has no effect when it comes to raising cholesterol levels, unlike lauric, myristic and palmitic acids. Stearic acid doesn't raise blood cholesterol; neither does it lower it.

It's impossible to eat stearic acid without also eating some of the other cholesterologenic animal fats. And we have no dietary requirement for stearic acid; we're a kind of animal that makes all we need.

For more, see under: Animal fats

Steroids
See under: Hormones

Sulfur
Because of all the sulfur in animal proteins, eating animals causes a systemic acidosis. The old theory was that our bodies buffered this excess acidity by releasing calcium from our bones, which was then excreted in our urine. Inconveniently, the most recent, best science we have, using radio-actively marked dietary calcium, show this to be untrue. I say 'inconveniently' because this theory explained why animal eaters have inferior bone health; why the populations worldwide who eat the most dairy products have the highest levels of hip fractures and other manifestations of osteoporosis.

Now it turns out that our bodies buffer the high systemic acidity by releasing calcium from our muscle cells. And the mechanism that links osteoporosis to eating animals is as yet undetermined. Meanwhile, leaching calcium out of our muscle cells isn't a desirable state of affairs. '**Muscle wasting**' isn't an inevitable consequence of aging; it's a consequence of eating animals.

See also: Hydrogen sulfide, Ammonia, for the Eatiology of inflammatory bowel "diseases" linked to high animal protein/sulfur intake.

Sulfur-containing amino acids

For the ill-effects of these amino acids, highly concentrated in animals, see individual entries under: methionine, homocysteine, cysteine and taurine.

See also: Ammonia, hydrogen sulfide, sulfur.

TMA and TMAO

Trimethylamine-n-oxide (TMAO) boosts cholesterol uptake into the inflammatory foam cells that are the precursors of the fatty plaques in our arteries. It's made in our livers from TMA, itself produced by our gut bacteria from the carnitine and choline in the animals we eat.

This topic is covered in more detail in Part 1B (Mechanisms) – Deranged gut flora

Taurine

Think toro. A sulfur-containing amino acid found mainly in animals. We don't need to eat any. More sulfur, we need like another hole in the head.

Trans fats

In nature, trans fats appear only in animals. Trans fats are highly cholesterologenic – they stimulate our livers to produce excess cholesterol. Unhorrified by the horrendous health heffects of trans fats, Big "Food" has designed and created vegetable Franken-oils with the same death-dealing abilities as these animal fats. We shouldn't put hydrogenated vegetable oils into ourselves.

See under: Animal fats

Triglycerides

Blood lipids or fats, they're esters of glycerol + 3 fatty acids, such as oleic, palmitic, linolenic, all of whom we've already met.

Triglycerides look like a capital letter E, with an upright spine of glycerol and 1, 2 or 3 fatty acids forming lonnnnnngggggg horizontal bars. (I think of tri-puses instead of octopuses. Tri-pi?) When triglycerides break down, they liberate free fatty acids (see above).

Having high triglycerides is one of the four horsemen of the apocalyptic "deadly quartet" of metabolic syndrome/syndrome X. The others are abdominal obesity, high fasting sugars, and high blood pressure.

Meatabolic Syndrome, as I call it, is a product of Meating and Junking: no animals, no junk, no meatabolic syndrome.

Not only are animal and junk fats more destructive – being trans or saturated/hydrogenated – they come in far greater quantities in the Meater diet, by a ratio of at least 3:1. Therefore, lower triglyceride levels in Planters. Check.

High triglycerides → insulin resistance → higher fasting sugars in Meaters. Check.

Animal and junk fats cause more deposition of abdominal fat; less brown fat deposition. Check. Planters simply don't eat and/or wear as much fat as Meaters and Junkers.

Meater fats and Meater cholesterol → Meater atherosclerosis → Meater higher blood pressure. Check.

Uric acid

Our bodies tightly regulate uric acid production. It's a potent antioxidant, and it promotes salt and fat retention. Understandably, for these reasons, more isn't better. In our ancestral past, maybe, but not today.

Uric acid is a breakdown product of the purines in the animals we eat, and the fructose in junk. Excess uric acid causes gout, the painful arthritic condition caused by uric acid crystallizing in our joints.

If animals contain high levels of purines… and purines degrade into uric acid… and uric acid causes mayhem in our joints (and kidneys)… and *Homo sapiens* lost the ability to decontaminate uric acid several million years ago, why would we call animals food? Why would we call HFCS food?

One of the first hurdles a potential food item should clear is that it shouldn't harm us. First, do no harm. *Primum non nocere.* Bioethically, animals fail this measly entry-level requirement, over and over and over again.

VLDL

Very low density lipoprotein, one of the fat/protein molecules that transport fatty cholesterol in the watery environment of the bloodstream. All lipoproteins can be atherogenic, depending on the situation, regardless of size; some are just more so than others. (HDL is generally atheropreventive, but can be atherogenic in some circumstances.)

For more, see under: Cholesterol

Whey

No whey, no how, no-when.

The liquid portion of milk, as opposed to the solid curds. Dreadful stuff… not food.

Xeno-autoantibodies

Xeno- = foreign; auto- = self; antibodies are immune system 'soldiers' to fight off antigens (foreign invaders). So xeno-autoantibodies are antibodies we produce to combat a foreign antigen, which instead fights ourselves.

In a video essay called "How Tumors Use Meat to Grow: Xeno-Autoantibodies," Dr Michael Greger says: "Cancer may use a molecule found in animal products to trick our immune system into feeding it with inflammation."

The molecule in question is **Neu5Gc**. [See separate entry]

This Wikipedia-quote is pretty good, and I've highlighted the salient parts:

"**N-Glycolylneuraminic acid** (Neu5Gc) is a sialic acid molecule **found in most mammals. Humans cannot synthesize Neu5Gc** because the human gene CMAH is irreversibly mutated, though it is found in apes. It is absent in human tissues because of inactivation of gene encoding CMP-N-acetylneuraminic acid hydroxylase. The gene CMAH encodes for CMP-N-acetylneuraminic acid hydroxylase, which is the enzyme responsible for CMP-Neu5Gc from CMP-N-acetylneuraminic (CMP-Neu5Ac) acid. This loss of the CMAH was estimated to have **occurred two to three millions of years ago**, which occurred just **before the emergence of the genus *Homo*."**

We don't need it. We don't make it; haven't for millions of years. It's in the mammals we eat that do make it. It causes us harm. Cancer tumors may be made of mutated human cells that don't cause an immune response, so the tumors suck up Neu5Gc, a xeno-auto-antigen which does provoke an immune response and the attendant inflammation on which cancer cells thrive.

Tricky little devils. We all have cancerous cells within us, all the time. Why feed them with Neu5Gc from animals?

For more, see under: Neu5Gc

Xenoestrogens

Xeno- means 'foreign,' so, by definition, xenoestrogens act as hormones, but they're contaminants, not 'bred in the bone.' I mention them here because we can't avoid them unless we eat organic plants only. That's how toxic we've made our environment. "Food is a package deal."

Xenoestrogenic chemicals can be demasculinizing or feminizing in their effects. They aren't to be confused with phytoestrogens; plant estrogens that reduce the carcinogenic effects of real and xeno-estrogens by binding to the same estrogen receptors, without producing noxious effects. The phytoestrogens in soy and flax seeds are particularly preventive of breast and prostate cancer.

For more, see Part 3 (~~Food~~borne contaminants)

Zugzwang

Pronounced 'tsoog-tswung,' zugzwang is in here because I enjoy the word and I wanted to finish my A to Z on a Z. I'll do my best to connect it to Meating.

It's a chess term, describing a situation in which we're forced to move, and every move we make, makes our situation worse.

This aptly describes the cascade of ill-effects that flows from Meating: first we silt up our arteries, so we take a drug to counter that, then we take another drug to bring down our blood sugars, but those may raise our blood pressure (even more), and then we may have to take another drug to counteract the side-effect of that drug, and so on… which is Big Pharma's wet dream – millions of us Meaters taking multiple, symptom-palliating medications for the rest of our lives.

As Meaters, we're "compelled to move" and every step and counter-step we take makes our predicament worse. As Planters we simply eat food and step off the Big Pharma pill-popping merry-go-round.

Okay, that's it for the COMPONENTS of animals – what's naturally bred in the bone and the flesh we eat. Now let's take a look at the MECHANISMS involved in the animal Eatiology of "disease"…

~

Part 1B (Mechanisms): How Meating Sickens, Maims & Kills Us

If anyone tells us, with an air of great condescension, "Correlation isn't causation," the chances are good that we're listening to a Low-Carb Bullshit Artist, intent on justifying their High-Animal diet. It's as if they think they're the only ones privy to the unstartling truth, usually among the first words out of the lecturer's mouth in Statistics 101, that correlations between variables doesn't mean that one causes another. For example, we know that countries that have lots of telephone poles and cars and TV sets and computers have lots of cancer, but there's little evidence of a direct link between TVs and cancer. The linkages are subtle and secondary, via sedentary lifestyles and TV dinners.

We get it. We know we can't just rely on population studies. We know we have to account for the possibility of 'reverse causation' and the presence of confounding variables. We know that we have to furnish 'plausible biological mechanisms' for the etiology of diseases. I'm going to go one better. I'm going to see your plausible mechanisms, and raise you dozens of proven Meater and Junker Eatiologies.

Meating in Action

This is an incomplete list of *physiological mechanisms* whereby eating animals sickens us, maims us, kills us and deforms our children:

Inflammation

When we cut or bruise our skin, the area becomes hot, swollen, red and sore – enflamed. This is an indication that our immune system has been mobilized to come in and start repair works. A similar thing happens on our insides. While plants are strongly anti-inflammatory, animals are inflammation-causing. Chronic conditions such as cancer and atherosclerosis thrive on inflammation and so, they have ways of promoting the very inflammation they thrive on.

Eating animals enflames us from the inside out.

Planting is anti-inflammatory; mushrooms* and nuts, in particular, but plants in general, especially those containing aspirin or, rather, salicylic acid. (Fungi, but treated as plants*)

For more, see under: Arachidonic acid; Endotoxins; Neu5Gc

Oxidation or Oxidative stress

When iron rusts it forms iron oxide. In our bodies, oxidation is like rusting.

Oxidation, per se, isn't a bad thing: it's part of our normal digestive and metabolic processes. Excessive oxidation is a problem though; particularly of non-foods such as cholesterol and animal fats (a process that begins the moment the animal goes bellowing to its death). When the Low-Carb Bullshit Artists tell us that it's *oxidized* cholesterol that's the problem, not cholesterol, they're telling us a partial truth. Oxidized cholesterol is worse than cholesterol cholesterol, but if there's no cholesterol cholesterol floating around, as there isn't in a Planter diet, then what is there to oxidize? Planters have minimal amounts of oxidized cholesterol. Meaters? Maximum.

Instead of being full of health-promoting antioxidants like whole plants are, animals are packed full of oxidants or pro-oxidants, sometimes also called free radicals or reactive oxygen species (ROSs).

It shouldn't be a surprise that heme iron, the central ion of the oxygen-carrying molecule in the blood, hemoglobin, is strongly oxidizing.

Eaten animals rust us from the inside out. Unlike plants, which are packed with antioxidants. Plants *are* antioxidants.

For more, see under: Heme iron

Now let's take a look at the circulatory SNAFUs that Meating creates:

Ischemia

Ischemia is the unhealthy condition of reduced blood supply and resulting reduced oxygen and nutrient supply to the tissue beds and organs that are downstream from arteries that have been narrowed, stiffened and enflamed by eating animals and other junk. This often leads to…

Hypoperfusion

Hypoperfusion means reduced supply or irrigation. Cells are being starved of nutrients and oxygen, reducing their efficiency and health.

Hypoxia and Anoxia

Hypoxia is a condition of low oxygen saturation in which cancer thrives. Anoxia is a condition of no oxygen, which can lead to rapid tissue death (necrosis), as in myocardial (heart muscle) or other infarctions [see below.]

Rouleau(x) formation

A rouleau or clump of disc-shaped red blood cells forms in response to Meating; a reaction to increased plasma protein concentration. (More isn't better.) This is concerning because rouleaux are a general indicator or biomarker of disease.

Rouleaux can damage our peripheral blood supply by making it impossible for blood to pass through miniscule capillaries. Clumped-together red blood cells resemble densely-packed clay platelets in waterlogged soil. They're particularly seen in diabetes sufferers, and rouleaux are a proximate cause of damage to our eyes in the condition known as diabetic retinopathy.

As we'll see shortly, type 2 diabetes is usually a symptom of Meating and Junking.

Remember: "First class protein is worst class protein."

See also: Diabetes; Diabetic retinopathy; Sludging of the blood

Sludging of the blood ~ Lactescence

There are several terms used to describe how fats cause our blood to become more viscous, more difficult to pump, and more likely to cause 'postprandial' (after meal) angina.

These include:

- **Lactescence** – the milkiness that eating fat causes in our blood;
- **Lipemia** (also known as hyperlipemia, hyperlipidemia or lipidemia) – an excess of fat in the blood;
- **Sludging** of the blood – which is self-explanatory; and
- **Rouleaux formation** – the clumping together of red blood cells. As we saw above, excess fats coat our oxygen-delivering erythrocytes, making them sticky, clumping them together and reducing their oxygen-carrying ability.

Perhaps more important than excess fat's effect on our blood is the simultaneous effect it has on the endothelium, the amazing inner lining of our blood vessels. It's some 700 square yards (or meters) in area and 3 pounds (1.4 kg) in weight. Unlisted as such in most medical texts, the endothelium is our largest endocrine (hormone-releasing) organ. Our blood vessels aren't supine; they're muscular, flexible tubes that constrict and relax, controlling the blood supply throughout 100,000 km of pipes. Excess fat in our blood, whether of animal or plant origin, inflames and stiffens our endothelia, severing hampering the vasodilation and vasoconstriction they control.

Vegans shouldn't feel smug here: it doesn't matter whether the fat in the meal is of animal or vegetable origin. Excess of both make our blood fatty. Planters who remember that vegetable oils are to plant fats as white bread is to whole grains – in other words, highly processed, low-fiber empty calories – will keep their vegetable oil intake to a minimum. Even relatively healthy vegetable oils such as olive oil contain 13% saturated fat. All oils are essentially 100% fat – being carb- and protein-free, 100% of their calories come from fat. (Remember Dr Caldwell Esselstyn's stern admonition to his recovering heart patients: "No oil!")

Pure Planters get about 10% of calories from fats, and they're the fats one naturally gets from lettuce and avos and nuts and kale. Meaters of all descriptions, from dairy-slurping and egg-chomping vegetarians on up, take in three or more times as many fat calories. This difference makes Planters by far the least prone to the problems caused by blood sludging. Not only are Meaters' bodies fatter than Planters'; Meater blood is fatter than Planters' too.

When we eat fat, it enters our guts, is absorbed into lacteals (lymphatic vessels of the small intestine), enters our bloodstreams and wends its way to the liver for processing.

Peaking about five hours after a high-fat meal, our arteries become stuff and uncompliant, unable to dilate. This affects all the tissue beds and organs of our bodies, every single one of which requires oxygenation, most crucially our heart muscles. Diminished blood flow to the heart can cause frightening and painful angina, which rises to a crescendo as blood fats reach their peak, 4,5, 6 hours after we eat them.

If any of us who're practicing Meaters suffer from postprandial angina, we've got cardiovascular disease. (Well, we knew that anyway, but lactescence is the proximate cause.)

The inflammation that results from endothelial dysfunction is made worse by the swarm of endotoxins (dead or living bacteria and their products) that Meating introduces into our blood. Not to be encouraged.

For more, see under: Angina; Fatty liver "disease"; Rouleau(x) formation

[See: http://nutritionfacts.org/video/fatty-meals-may-impair-artery-function/]

Sclerosis

Sclerosis is a general term for the unhealthy condition of any bodily tissue becoming abnormally hard. The best known of the scleroses is…

Arteriosclerosis

Literally, 'artery hardening.' A major symptom of Meating.

Platelet hyperreactivity

Platelets are components of our blood which are responsible for clotting in case of injury. In their inactive state, they circulate harmlessly throughout our bloodstream. In the pathological Meater state, however, platelets are what trigger the clots that block off arteries in heart attacks and hemorrhagic strokes, after an atheroma bursts. Plus, in Meaters, activated platelets release an array of inflammatory chemicals which are implicated in inflammatory conditions such as atherosclerosis, diabetes, rheumatoid arthritis and cancer.

How do we prevent our platelets from aggregating, without reducing our emergency blood-clotting mechanisms? Planting. Fruits are great; berries are spectacular. Salicylic acid (aspirin) from whole plants also discourages platelet activity, and it's much better for us than aspirin aspirin. The Union of Concerned Scientists has estimated that if Americans just met the pathetically low dietary guidelines for fruit and veggies that 100,000 deaths could be avoided each year. Cholesterol and animal fats are platelet-activating fiends. Not eating fruit is one of our biggest killers.

Hypercholesterolemia

Hypercholesterolemia is the condition of having high levels of cholesterol circulating in our blood. It's the one inescapable consequence of Meating that Meater broscientists devote 99% of their attention to, in an attempt to make Meating appear acceptable. Entire books are written on the topic. All we have to remember is this: no one who's maintained their total cholesterol below 150 for a while has ever had a heart attack. We become what Caldwell Esselstyn calls "heart attack-proof" below Tc = 150 and LDL < 70. Easy peasy on a Planter diet; almost impossible otherwise. Which is why there's a pandemic of heart disease among Meaters and Junkers.

(I'm qualifying what I'm saying by saying 'maintained': for all I know some poor sod may have dropped their cholesterol from 300 to 150 in a couple of months on a Planter diet and dropped down dead as they went by 150. It's unlikely.)

As we'll see by the end of this book, cholesterol is only one of dozens of animal components or contaminants that rule out animals as food.

Hyperlipidemia

Lipids are fats. Hyperlipidemia = high fat levels in the blood. The term also includes cholesterol, which is a fatty/waxy substance. Because cholesterol is fatty and our blood is watery, and ne'er the twain shall mix, cholesterol is carried through the blood by lipoproteins, half-fat, half-protein molecules, which are blood-soluble.

According to the American Heart Association, "Managing hyperlipidemia means controlling cholesterol and triglycerides." Planting does that exceedingly well; Meating does a shite job of it.

Hyperlipidemia is also sometimes called hyperlipemia or lipemia.

Atherosclerosis

Atherosclerosis comes from the Greek word 'athero' meaning porridge or gruel + 'sclerosis', hardening.

Atheromas are the pustular, porridge-like lesions or sores that form in endothelial, muscle and connective tissue cells forming our blood vessels – mainly our arteries because the arterial system is a muscular, thick-walled high pressure system, while the venous return flow is a lower pressure system requiring thinner walls.

Atheromas are built out of excess cholesterol and cholesterol esters; and calcium, connective tissue and fatty acids. They start out as foam cells, which gradually get packed fuller and fuller with cholesterol, particularly low density lipoprotein (LDL) cholesterol.

According to the Mayo Clinic website: "Arteriosclerosis occurs when the blood vessels that carry oxygen and nutrients from your heart to the rest of your body (arteries) become thick and stiff — sometimes restricting blood flow to your organs and tissues. Healthy arteries are flexible and elastic, but over time, the walls in your arteries can harden, a condition commonly called hardening of the arteries.

Atherosclerosis is a specific type of arteriosclerosis, but the terms are sometimes used interchangeably. Atherosclerosis refers to the buildup of fats, cholesterol and other substances in and on your artery walls (plaques), which can restrict blood flow.

These plaques can burst, triggering a blood clot. **Although atherosclerosis is often considered a heart problem, it can affect arteries anywhere in your body**. Atherosclerosis usually is preventable and is treatable."

Cholesterol crystals, with their jagged edges, are what slice through the caps of atheromas, leading to the rapid cascade of events of clotting, infarction and death. On autopsy, every heart attack victim is found to have these cholesterol crystals in their atheromas. Super-saturated cholesterol crystals appear to be a necessary precondition for heart attack.

Health tip: don't allow cholesterol levels to get so high that there's so much cholesterol in foam cells that it reaches saturation level and precipitates out and kills us. Better still, keep one's cholesterol levels as low as possible by eating only whole plants.

While the Mayo Clinic is certainly right about atherosclerosis being preventable and treatable, they don't say how best to achieve these goals. In their description above, they say that this is a process that happens "over time," which is true, but it's not time that does it; it's eating animals and junk, leading to high cholesterol levels in our blood and high concentrations of cholesterol being incorporated into our arterial walls.

Depending on the site of a rupture, atherosclerosis is responsible for multiple, seemingly unrelated outcomes. They're all connected by the damage that atherosclerosis does to the blood supply of the region in question.

When it comes to understanding nutrition, it's important to grok how one faulty behavior can cause so many different outcomes. Meating has hundreds of seemingly unrelated fallouts, from the A of acne to the Z of zoönosis.

In the words of Jason Kovacic and Valentin Fuster:

> **"Atherosclerosis is an omnipresent pathology that involves virtually the entire human organism."**

[Kovacic Jason C. MD, PhD and Valentin Fuster MD, PhD. Atherosclerotic Risk Factors, Vascular Cognitive Impairment, and Alzheimer Disease. *Mount Sinai Journal of Medicine* Volume 79, Issue 6, pages 664–673, November/December 2012.]

This shouldn't be heard to grok. If we dam a river, we affect EVERYTHING that lies downstream from the dam. (As the High Dam at Aswan has done, cutting off the sediments that used to create the soils of the Nile delta, requiring vast inputs of artificial fertilizers, and so on.)

As Kovacic and Fuster show, hardening of the arteries leads to 'cognitive impairment' – reduced ability to think – and later, complicated by other factors, to Alzheimer's "disease".

Which begs the question: Which comes first, the 'cognitive impairment' of Meating that leads one to eat animals in the first place, or the 'cognitive impairment' that comes as a result of eating animals? Put like that, it's pretty obvious that Meating is the causative agent, and that Meating comes about via our societal cognitive impairment about what constitutes food.

Cognitive impairment → Meating → atherosclerosis → cognitive impairment.

Coming fool circle, our ignorance about how and what to eat leads to our own declining ability to think at all.

Citing the above paper, Michael Greger says:

> "One of the most poignant examples of the systemic nature of clogged arteries "is **the link between coronary artery disease (CAD), degenerative brain disease (DBD), and Alzheimer's (dementia)."** [emphasis added]
>
> Just as a heart attack or a brain attack (stroke) can be significantly prevented, one can think of Alzheimer's as a mind attack. Mind attacks, like heart attacks and strokes, need to be prevented by controlling vascular risk factors like high blood pressure and cholesterol… controlling **chronic blood hypoperfusion – the lack of adequate blood flow to the brain** in the years before the onset of Alzheimer's."

[See: http://nutritionfacts.org/video/preventing-alzheimers-with-lifestyle-changes/]

Atherosclerosis affects every cell, every tissue and every organ in our bodies. Unfoods cause atheromas; foods reverse them. That's why we need to eat nothing but whole pure plants, ever.

We shouldn't eat any unfoods, not even in moderation. There's nothing moderate about the destruction unfoods cause, even moderate amounts of them. Remember: "Moderation kills." Why should we love ourselves and our kids only moderately? Why not with complete love, devotion, surrender? In nutrition, moderate is a synonym for mediocre. It's a synonym for Meater or Junker.

Foam cells

Foam cells are what cholesterol gets packed into within the walls of our blood vessels. They're called foam cells because they look like the foamy head on beer; that's because of their fatty contents. They're precursors to the formation of atheromas, the pustular lesions characteristic of atherosclerosis. They're what make up the initial fatty streaks we see in the arteries of Meater kids.

Foam cells disappear over time when we eat a whole plant diet

Fatty streaks

'Fatty streaks' describes well the first visible signs of atherosclerosis or artery "disease". Meater children start to develop these symptoms of Meating as early as ten years old. Planter children don't. Actually, some children of Meater mothers are born with early signs of artery "disease"!

Ok, so most adults don't know how or what to eat, themselves, so we can't really call parents feeding animals to children a crime or a sin… because we do so out of loving ignorance when we practice Meating. The road to hell is paved with loving ignorance.

In its original usage, the word 'sin' meant 'missing the mark.' It came from an ancient Aramaic word for missing an archery target. It meant 'to err.' That's what we do today when we feed our kids fatty streaks of pig flesh that become fatty streaks inside us, there until the day we die, mostly likely from heart failure. We err.

Inflammation, ulceration, and calcification

These are three of the outcomes of atherosclerosis. Inflammation, as cholesterol produces an immune response in us which mobilizes macrophages – "big eaters" – to come to the rescue of our arteries, under attack by alien animals. Ulceration, as sores form on the interior walls of our arteries. Calcification, as our arteries and heart muscles become stiff and rigid, wrapped in a carapace of calcium, like coral, compromised in their ability to dilate or beat.

Metabolic acidosis

In general, our bodies work best in a slightly alkaline state. In general, only. Different body compartments have different pH requirements. While our urinary tracts work best in an alkaline milieu, our colons and vaginas need to be slightly acidic for best health.

Simplifying greatly, Meating is acid-forming while Planting is alkaline.

Eating animals produces an unhealthy amount of acid in us. Not surprising, really, when one considers the hyper-consumption of protein we Meaters indulge in, flooding our bodies with amino acids; even worse, flooding our bodies with sulfur-containing amino acids. Sulfur, as in hydrogen sulfide. Sulfur, as in sulfuric acid.

Inconveniently, it turns out that we don't buffer our systemic acid load with calcium from our bones, so we'll need to find another explanation for why Meating causes osteoporosis. For now, we'll just have to trust the epidemiology that shows that it does. (And uncommon good sense.)

Our bodies buffer Meating-provided acids by stripping calcium out of our muscles, leading to **muscle wasting** as we age. There's a double whammy here: large amounts of animal protein overtax our kidneys, worsening kidney function, making our blood more acidic with time, wasting our muscles even more.

Other consequences of acidosis include gout, gallstones and kidney stones; results of mal-nutrition, all.

Hyper-filtration and protein leakage

Continuing the kidney stress saga from acidosis, above… Animal proteins (along with animal fats and animal cholesterol) cause our kidneys to work harder – or hyper-filter – and to lose function, by releasing whole proteins into our urine, instead of breaking them down.

Metastatic calcification

Segen's Medical Dictionary describes metastatic calcification as "deposition of calcium in otherwise normal, non-osseous [non-bone] tissue—e.g., kidneys, blood vessels (vascular media), lungs, stomach, heart and eyes… due to increased levels of calcium in the serum."

Although it's calcium that builds up on our heart valves and other inappropriate sites, phosphorus is the problematic ingredient that leads to hypercalcemia (high calcium).

MC is a condition OF calcium build-up caused BY animal phosphorus build-up, as a result of declining kidney function, as a result often of chronic overexposure to animal proteins. This should remind us of type II diabetes, a condition OF excess glucose and insulin caused BY excess animal fat and junk. It should also remind us of the crucial difference between healthy plant and unhealthy animal iron.

As we've seen, our bodies can dispose of plant phosphorus much better than animal phosphorus.

Here's the Meater cascade leading to metabolic calcification: Excess, animal proteins → excess nitrogen → decline in kidney function → phosphorus build-up → calcium deposition.

Wikipedia tells us: "Metastatic calcification can occur widely throughout the body but principally affects the interstitial tissues of the vasculature, kidneys, lungs, and gastric mucosa."

The outcomes of calcification aren't pretty: calcification is what really puts the stiff in artery stiffening. Our arteries are supposed to be supple and elastic; meating causes them to become rigid and enflamed and full of lesions. If only we could see the internal damage we do ourselves by eating animals, we'd… probably still eat bacon. It seems we need to survive a massive first health scare to become imaginative. Good luck.

If we're in danger of kidney failure, doctors put us on low-phos diets. A low-phos diet *has to be* a low-protein diet. Which non-foods are beneficial? Meating is high-phos (and bad-phos too); Planting has the right amount and the right kind of protein; and the Goldilocks amount and kind of phosphorus.

Stenosis

In general, a stenosis is the abnormal narrowing of any bodily passage. Most germane to nutrition science is the narrowing of arteries via atherosclerosis, induced by eating animals. For example, Meating causes spinal stenosis, in the cervical or lumbar regions, leading to lower back pain. It causes penile stenosis, leading to erectile dysfunction. It causes clitoral stenosis, leading to decreased sexual function in women. It causes sciatic stenosis, narrowing of the arteries that feed the nerves that run down our legs, resulting in painful sciatica. And on and on.

Atherosclerosis causes stenoses EVERYWHERE in our circulation, but mainly in our high pressure arteries. If blood flows there, it'll take cholesterol there and there'll be atheromas.

Stenoses are preventable, stoppable, even reversible by not eating animals and junk.

Embolism

Per Wikipedia: "An embolism is the lodging of an embolus, which may be a blood clot, fat globule, gas bubble or foreign material in the bloodstream. This can cause a blockage in a blood vessel. Such a blockage (vascular occlusion) may affect a part of the body distanced from the actual site of the embolism."

This is a good thing to know – but it's something cardiac surgeons rarely reveal to their patients beforehand – that during the course of procedures such as bypass surgery, there's inevitably debris that enters the blood stream, some of which may lodge in cerebral arteries. Cognitive decline is a common result of heart surgery. Fact.

Pulmonary embolisms are those that form in the lungs.

Thrombosis

Unlike an embolism, a thrombus forms locally to create a thrombosis. For example, the classic mechanism of plaque rupture entails the cap of a pimple-like atheroma tearing off, spilling debris into the artery. Platelets and other clotting factors spring to our defense, and it's our own self-healing mechanisms that cause the clot that blocks off the entire artery.

Infarction

The Wikipedia-definition of an infarction is: "tissue death (**necrosis**) caused by a local lack of oxygen, due to an obstruction of the tissue's blood supply."

If an atherosclerotic plaque bursts in an artery, the tissues and organs it supplies may lose their oxygen supply. Myocardial infarction is the cut-off of oxygen to a region of the heart muscle, leading to its rapid death, often to be followed in quick order by the death of its eating-disordered owner.

The most common place this happens is the anterior interventricular branch of the left coronary artery, which has earned it among cardiologists the unhappy nickname of "the widow maker."

The next time we eat a cow, perhaps we should remember how ghouls die: a steak through the heart. If, as *Merriam-Webster* tells us, a ghoul is "a legendary evil being that robs graves and feeds on corpses," is that not us when we're Meaters?

Endothelial dysfunction

Let's talk briefly about the endothelium before we dysfunct it up with dead animals and junk.

The endothelium is a layer of flat or squamous cells that line our blood and lymph vessels, and the chambers of our hearts. Keeping in mind that we have about 100,000 km of blood vessels in our bodies, or 60,000 miles' worth, enough to go around the Equator 2½ times, it seems right that we have about 700m^2 of endothelium. (Compare this to 300 to 400 m^2 of gut, 100m^2 of lung, and 2m^2 of skin.)

With a combined weight of 3 pounds, our vasculature is our largest endocrine organ. Our blood vessels actively emit nitric oxide, constrict and relax, regulate our blood viscosity, release hormones and feed every single cell in us. A healthy, whole endothelium is crucial to health. The damage we do our endothelium has massive repercussions throughout our bodies.

According to Michael Greger:

> "We used to think the endothelium was just an inert layer lining our vascular tree, but now we know better. The endothelium is directly involved in peripheral vascular disease, stroke, heart disease, diabetes, insulin resistance, chronic kidney failure, tumor growth, metastasis, venous thrombosis (blood clots), and severe viral infectious diseases. Dysfunction of the vascular endothelium is thus a hallmark of human diseases."

[See: http://nutritionfacts.org/video/fatty-meals-may-impair-artery-function/]

Healthy blood vessels, particularly our arteries, which are more muscular than our veins, can change diameter on demand, depending on how much oxygenated blood is required by our muscles. During exercise, the endothelial cells – the single layer of cells that line our arteries, separating inside from out – emit a gas called nitric oxide (NO) which causes the artery to widen, or dilate.

When we eat high-fat meals, either of plant or animal origin, our endothelium is crippled for hours afterwards. A BART (brachial artery reflex test) after a SAD (Standard American Diet) meal shows that normal function is just beginning to return six hour later… when we choke down another SAD meal. Meaters spend almost 24 hours a day in a state of low-grade arterial inflammation. Planting – naturally low in fats and high in nitrates – engenders peak endothelial function.

The following diagram shows what happens in the arteries of animal eaters over time.

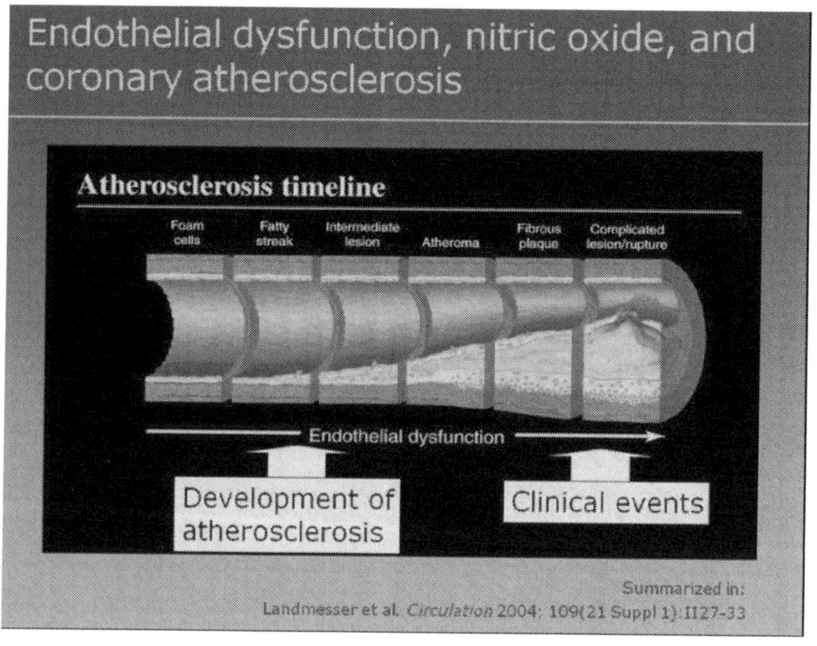

http://www.pace-cme.org/legacy/images/Endothelial-dysfunction-nitric-oxide-and-coronary-atheroscle-003251-800x600px.png

This is what Meating causes. The 'before' artery on the left is relatively healthy, flexible and supple, with the first cholesterol-filled foam cells beginning to appear. The artery on the right is diseased; narrowed, inflamed, ulcerated, stiff and hard. It's vital to understand this: this crippling happens to every single artery in us, not just in our hearts.

With time and repeated injury, the endothelial function of Meaters becomes severely compromised. NO is made from nitrates, common in plants (particularly leafy green veggies) but severely lacking in the animals we eat. But, even with all the NO in the world, the stiff, sick artery on the right would have great difficulty in expanding.

Not just by the way – crucially – the opposite process, moving from right to left, is what happens over time on a whole plant diet, if one stops Meating and Junking. The calcification of our blood vessels stops; the ulceration gets healed; the inflammation vanishes, and even the fatty streaks disappear as the cholesterol and other debris get unpacked from the foam cells.

A remarkable demonstration of this appeared in this paper from the July 4th 1985 edition of the *New England Journal of Medicine*, called Nathan Pritikin's Heart:

Hubbard JD, Inkeles S, Barnard RJ. Nathan Pritikin's heart. *N Engl J Med.* 1985 Jul 4;313(1):52.

Nathan Pritikin was the remarkable engineer who got the heart-healing ball rolling in the US in the 1970s, showing that a diet of whole plants is sufficient to reverse heart disease. When he was diagnosed in middle age with severe coronary artery disease, he refused his doctors' recommendation of surgery. Instead, he followed the advice of the African "fiber deficiency theorists" – Denis Burkitt et al, mentioned elsewhere in this book – who showed that chronic Western ailments are a function of diet. Pritikin reversed his own mal-nutritional-caused non-disease, wrote many influential books on the topics of nutrition, weight loss, fitness and health, and founded the chain of clinics that today bears his name and continues his life-saving work.

The Pritikin website says that "he was among the first worldwide to assert that diet and exercise, not drugs and surgery, should be the first line of defense against cardiovascular disease." How right he was.

https://www.pritikin.com/home-the-basics/about-pritikin/38-nathan-pritikin.html

On autopsy, the 69-year-old Pritikin was found to have the arteries of a healthy child, with only a few fatty streaks. Pritikin had eaten his heart and arteries well by becoming a Planter.

Getting technical for a moment, a later review paper summed up:

[Barry A. Franklin & Joel K. Kahn. Delayed Progression or Regression of Coronary Atherosclerosis with Intensive Risk Factor Modification: Effects of Diet, Drugs, and Exercise. *Sports Medicine* November 1996, Volume 22, Issue 5, pp. 306-320.]

"Contemporary studies now suggest that **multifactorial risk factor modification**, and especially more intensive measures to control hyperlipidaemia with diet, drugs, and exercise, may slow, halt, and even **reverse the progression of atherosclerotic coronary artery disease**. Added benefits include a **reduction in anginal symptoms**, decreases in exercise-induced **myocardial ischaemia**, fewer recurrent **cardiac events**, and a diminished need for **coronary revascularisation procedures**. Several mechanisms may contribute to these improved clinical outcomes, including partial (albeit small) **anatomic regression of coronary artery stenoses**, a reduced incidence of **plaque rupture**, and improved **coronary artery vasomotor function**. These findings suggest **a new paradigm** in the treatment of patients with coronary artery disease."

No "may" about it: Planting is the best cure for cardiovascular "disease", and Meating and Junking are what cause it. A whole plant diet is anti-atherosclerotic. A plant diet returns peak endothelial function; drugs may or may not be required, depending on the severity of the dis-ease. Sadly, this "new paradigm" is yet to make its way into the mainstream of medical practice. Inchworm, inchworm…

[By the way, that the *New England Journal of Medicine* keeps studies such as the Pritikin autopsy paper behind a pay wall 30 years after its publication is a disgrace. The same, in spades, goes for the Enos paper detailing the omnipresent atherosclerosis in young soldiers killed in the Korean War, published in the *Journal of the American Medical Association* on 18 July 1953. Why do they do that? Surely this information should be available to all?]

Endothelial dysfunction: summary

The endothelium is the single layer of cells that lines our blood vessels. During exercise or sex, when our arteries need to dilate to accommodate greater blood flow, endothelial cells release molecules of nitric oxide gas, the signaling molecule which causes the muscular layer of the blood vessel to relax and dilate, thus allowing increased blood flow.

Pro-oxidants or free radicals in what we eat can use up NO and prevent NO creation (from nitrates in plants) by taking over NO-synthase, the enzyme that makes NO. Meating creates torrents of the free radicals responsible for endothelial dysfunction. Only whole plants are packed full of nitrates and antioxidants, which promote peak arterial function.

Endotoxemia

An inflammatory response to the dead or living bacteria in the animals we eat.

See under: Endotoxins, in Part 1A (Components)

Claudication

According to medicinenet.com, "Claudication is pain and/or cramping in the lower leg due to inadequate blood flow to the muscles. The pain usually causes the person to limp. The word "claudication" comes from the Latin "claudicare" meaning to limp [like the lame ('claudus') Emperor Claudius]. Claudication typically is felt while walking, and subsides with rest."

Because the pain comes and goes, this condition is also called Intermittent Claudication. Some definitions say that claudication is caused by exercise. I have to disagree. Claudication is most apparent during exercise, true, but, baby, we were born to run. The underlying atherosclerosis (induced by eating animals) is what causes muscle pain and this is more prevalent during the stress of exercise.

Claudication can also happen in our arms.

OK, that's it for the circulatory disorders promoted by eating animals. Let's move on to our intestines:

Water deficiency ~ dehydration

There's relatively little water in animals by the time we eat them. Most of what there is has been cooked out. (Or should be if we want to kill what's lurking or burrowing in the flesh.) This causes the blood of Meaters to be sludgy in comparison to Planters, especially "postprandially," especially after high-fat meals. (Post-prandial lipemia.)

It also causes one's poop to become dryer and harder and more difficult to squeeze along by the muscles of our intestines.

More later.

Fiber deficiency
There's no fiber in animals; they have bones to hold them up. And fiber deficiency is general in the Western diet. 97% of Americans don't eat enough, even by the USDA'S pitifully low standards. Fiber deficiency leads to several harmful consequences, more serious than they sound: e.g. constipation, increased transit time and a deranged gut flora.

(More on each later.)

Fiber deficiency is also directly related to increased toxicity from carcinogenic cholesterol metabolites – the bile acids – which play such a role in breast and prostate cancer.

In a normal, fiber-filled gut, bile acids are diluted and swiftly moved out of the system. Meater diets keep these fecal mutagens in us for far longer, allowing them to be reabsorbed and to accumulate in the breast, for one, where they exert strong estrogenic cancer-causing effects.

Which goes to show: Everything's connected – not pooping properly can cause cancer.

(As a culture, we Westerners don't know shit.)

Fiber-associated nutrient deficiency
Folate et al.

Naysayers of the Fiber Theory, espoused by such brave researchers as my personal hero, Denis Burkitt, point out that experiments using fiber supplements have failed to show benefits against colorectal cancer.

This isn't an accident. The Low Carb Bullshit Artists operate in a one-nutrient-at-a-time manner. **Reductionism** is what these people thrive on to bamboozle people. [Prof. T. Colin Campbell's *Whole* should be required reading for anyone with an interest in nutrition.]

But the fiber in fiber supplements isn't equivalent to fiber as it appears in whole plants. Remember Michael Greger's great words: "Food is a package deal." Many of the benefits of high-fiber diets come from substances that are bound to the fiber.

When eating food – whole plants – if we're getting fiber, we're also getting a whole raft of phytonutrients that come along for the ride. Folate is a good example. We can't *not* get folate when we eat fiber-rich plants… unless we process the plants first and turn them into junk.

As we'll see later, Diverticulitis is a fiber deficiency condition.

Constipation

Because of Meating and Junking, the whole of Western civilization is chronically constipated. We're all uptight, even a lot of vegans… except for those amongst us who're Planters (who can be considered Orientalists). That's a strong statement, I know. But if we're not having *at least* one glorious bowel movement a day, we're constipated. We're full of shit – hard, compacted, disease-promoting shit.

And we can still be constipated if we are having a bowel movement every day. Huh? Here's how… Meaters have long transit times. It can take days, sometimes more than a week, for the contents of a high-animal-fat and –protein meal to move from oral lips to anal lips. Michael Greger suggests a 'beet test.' Eat lots of beets and see how long it takes for our poop to turn purple – if it doesn't happen in 24 hours, we're constipated.

Constipation is a fiber- (and water- and phytonutrient-) deficiency *symptom* of eating animals and junk, both notoriously fiber- and nutrient-free and dehydrating. Good luck eating an Atkins diet without taking the nutrient-free fiber supplements they peddle. (Good luck, with.)

The consequences of being constipated are legion and serious. Here are a few, some of which are merely unpleasant and painful, and some which can be deadly:

- Anal fissure and rectal inflammation
- Aneurysm
- Appendicitis
- Breast cancer
- Colorectal cancer
- Diverticulitis
- Hiatal hernia
- Hemorrhagic stroke
- Hemorrhoids
- Prostate cancer
- Varicose veins

Each of these symptoms of constipation – itself the outcome of Mal-nutrition – will be treated separately in the Eatiology section. Anyone who thinks I'm overstating the seriousness of constipation, or doubts the connection between unhealthy infrequent (or long-delayed) bowel movements and, say, breast cancer, should read the relevant sections to find out how the dots are connected.

(Looking at us Westerners prancing around like the lords of creation, playing bwana to all the ignorant darkies around the world, when we're so full of shit ourselves, and don't know it, makes me laugh to recall a passage from Salman Rushdie's *Midnight's Children*. During the Raj, the epitome of benevolent racism, the Indians discover, to their horror, that English folk wipe their asses with paper – they don't clean themselves with water. I can picture the English, not being noted for the fervor with which they embrace foreign languages (or, some used to say, personal hygiene), forever ignorant of the fact they're secretly being called "Smelly bottoms" or "Stinky bums" by a smiling, head-bobbing local populace.)

"'…for two months we must live like those Britishers? You've looked in the bathrooms? No water near the pot. I never believed, but it's true, my God, they wipe their bottoms with paper only!…'"

Truly, our ignorance of nutrition, and our self-satisfaction about what we think we do know, is vast and deadly. We don't even know what is and what isn't food. We don't even know how to shit properly.

Yes, we are what we eat. But there's more…

We are what we absorb. But, again, there's more…

We are what we don't excrete… or sheet. And that's a killer.

We can even think of cardiovascular disease as a kind of constipation; a failure to excrete cholesterol. When we eat animals, we create more cholesterol than our livers can convert into bile acids and excrete… the rest ends up lining our arteries, preparing us micron by micron for our #1 and #2 killers, heart attack and stroke.

Everything's connected.

Even obesity. Especially obesity.

Obese people are walking around with the residues of dead animals and other junk packed into their bellies and butts and thighs. To be obese is to be a walking charnel house garbage disposal unit. We eat animals and junk, then we don't shit them out. We pack them into ourselves then carry them around like satchels of fat for the rest of our truncated lives, like we're thoroughbreds being handicapped.

I forget who said it, John McDougall probably: "The fat we eat is the fat we wear." Biopsies of adipose tissue (fat) taken from our butts show the source of discrete pockets of fat: pig fat, olive oil fat, baby cow fat. We can tell what we ate at a particular meal. Here's McDonald's; here's KFC; here's Sarah Lee.

Obesity is a form of constipation. And from there it's all downhill…

Obesity connects to diabetes and hypertension and heart disease and cancer… the whole schmeer, Zorba's "full catastrophe."

Putrefaction

When we feed our gut flora the wrong foods (for them and for us), we can expect bad outcomes. Most animal proteins are completely digested in the small intestine, but a small amount makes it through to our colons, where our trillions of gut flora are living.

Here, quite literally, the stuff rots, or putrefies, giving rise to poisonous metabolites such as hydrogen sulfide and ammonia and TMAO (trimethylamine oxide), and deranging our gut flora so that they no longer produce beneficial products like butyrate and propionate.

If we eat animals, we select for animal-eating bacteria in our colons. The result? Koyaanisqatsi – Life out of balance, disease and misery. Mutually Assured Destruction.

If we eat whole plants, we select for happy, healthy plant-eating bacteria. The result? Mutually Assured Construction.

(I'm reminded of Charles Dickens. Mr. Micawber sums up what modern central planners have forgotten: "Annual income twenty pounds, annual expenditure nineteen six, result happiness. Annual income twenty pounds, annual expenditure twenty pound ought and six, result misery."

Something similar can be said of our gut flora, with happiness the result of eating food, and misery the result of eating unfoods, even in moderation. (Cut to scene of Dr Caldwell Esselstyn Jr. saying: "Moderation kills!")

[Hopeless sidetrack: Did you know that the full title of Dickens' book is *The Personal History, Adventures, Experience and Observation of David Copperfield the Younger of Blunderstone Rookery (Which He Never Meant to Publish on Any Account)*?]

No extra charge for the trivia…

For more on butyrate, acetate and propionate, see under: Deranged gut flora; Animal Deficiencies

Fermentation (a Planter mechanism)

By way of contrast to the putrefaction that animal protein undergoes in our guts to form sulfurous alkaline compounds like ammonia, fermentation is the healthy bacterial breakdown of fiber in the intestines to form slightly acidic compounds such as lactic acid.

Not to be confused with Meater- and Junker-induced fermentation used by anaerobic cancer cells to produce lactic acid from sugar.

Deranged gut flora, or microbiome

This may be the most important section in the book. To me, it's the most fascinating, and it shows how two things go hand in hand in nutrition. Our health depends on the **presence of the good Planter effects** PLUS the **absence of the bad Meater and Junker effects.**

Although, strictly speaking, much of this material belongs in the Animal Deficiencies section, I'm going to deal with the Planter benefits and the Meater deficits at the same time here, because they're inseparable. I'd love to just lay out my conclusions right now but we need some background. Bear with me as I start from basement level.

Microbiome research, or microbiomics, is an exciting and important new field of study, about which whole books will soon be written. As with other sub-sciences, such as epidemiology, epigenetics and nutrigenomics, Planting blows Meating and Junking out of the water. Meating and Junking really stuff up our intestinal flora, and our intestinal flora are far more important to our health than most of us realize.

If there are somewhere between 10^{13} and 10^{14} (ten and one hundred trillion) human body cells, there are many more bacteria living on and in us. Without them we can't exist; we work together to mutual benefit and survival. Together, we make up the super-organism that is human, but "more than human," as in Theodore Sturgeon's tale of human symbionts who complete each other. They are us, and we are them.

In "Among Trillions of Microbes in the Gut, a Few Are Special," Moises Velasquez-Manoff says:

"Each of us harbors a teeming ecosystem of microbes that outnumbers the total number of cells in the human body by a factor of 10 to one and whose collective genome is at least 150 times larger than our own." (*Scientific American* Volume 312, Issue 3 Feb 17, 2015.)

In other words, there's >150 times as much bacterial DNA in us than human DNA. Perhaps 300 times. That's mindboggling, and should keep the NIH's Human Microbiome Project busy for a while.

Different species of bacteria colonize different parts of our bodies – our mouths, our skins, our placentas (formerly thought to be sterile environments, now known to be awash with life) but mainly our moist, warm, nutrient-rich, bacteria-friendly large intestines.

In the olden days – meaning about ten, fifteen years ago – we used to think our colons just reabsorbed water and electrolytes, and that no digestion took place there. Now we know better. Our colons are amazing "anaerobic digestion chambers" and they're about a whole lot more than reabsorption.

Our gut flora (or intestinal bacteria) are truly remarkable. They're so numerous and they perform such important functions that they amount to a separate, virtual human organ, weighing several pounds.

In a paper called "Feed Your T_{regs} More Fiber" (*Science* vol. 341 Aug 2 2013 463-4), Julia Bollrath and Fiona Powrie write:

"The human intestine harbors up to 10^{11} [100 billion] bacteria per gram of intestinal content, comprising over 500 different species that have coevolved with their hosts in a mutually beneficial relationship."

Think about that for a mo'. Humans coevolved with bacteria over billions of years, through all the species that preceded us, until today we could no more separate us from them than we could stop breathing. We are them, and they are us (and we are all together, as sang John Lennon.)

Successful coevolution requires that we be mutually beneficial. The good bacteria in our colons aren't parasites – they do stuff for us that we can't do ourselves. Unlike termites, we lack the cellulase enzyme which allows them to digest cellulose. So the main thing our friendly gut bacteria do for us is to digest indigestible plant fiber.

In "Microbes in the Gut Are Essential to Our Well-Being" (*Scientific American* Volume 312, Issue 3 Feb 17, 2015), David Grogan writes:

"They are not freeloaders but rather perform many functions vital to health and survival: **they digest food, produce anti-inflammatory**

chemicals and compounds, and train the immune system to distinguish friend from foe. [Emphasis added.] Revelations about the role of the human microbiome in our lives have begun to shake the foundations of medicine and nutrition. Leading scientists… now think of humans not as self-sufficient organisms but as complex ecosystems colonized by numerous collaborating and competing microbial species. From this perspective, human health is a form of ecology in which care for the body also involves tending its teeming population of resident animalcules."

Among numerous other functions, they make vitamins and they keep competing pathogenic bacteria in check.

Let's deal with the three functions of the gut flora Grogan listed above. Our microbiome

1. **digests fiber**
2. **produces anti-inflammatory compounds**
3. **regulates the immune system**

Fiber isn't just inert stuff that passes through us undigested, as we believed not very long ago. (Really, we're in the infancy of nutrition science.) In the low-oxygen environment of our colons, bacteria ferment fiber. It's their food. They break down fiber anaerobically, gaining energy from it. In so doing, they produce waste products, or metabolites.

Here's where the symbiosis occurs. The bacterial wastes feed and power the endothelial cells lining our gut walls. (Unlike the majority of our cells which are powered by glucose, these cells are powered by bacterial poop: short-chain fatty acids (SCFAs) such as butyrate, lactate, acetate and propionate, created as by-products by bacteria as they ferment fiber.)

We power our gut bacteria with fiber, and they power us with butyrate. (Or we feed them good shit; they feed us good shit right back.)

Goldsmith and Sartor say: "Of the SCFAs, butyrate in particular is considered to be the preferred fuel of colonocytes" [colon cells.]

J R Goldsmith, R B Sartor. The role of diet on intestinal microbiota metabolism: downstream impacts on host immune function and health, and therapeutic implications. *J Gastroenterol.* 2014 May;49(5):785-98.

2. That's not all. Not only does butyrate power our endothelial cells, it's a powerful anti-inflammatory compound.

Here's how it works, according to Bollrath and Powrie:

"Microbes that metabolize dietary fiber can generate key fatty acids that enforce regulatory T cells in the gut."

It looks like this:

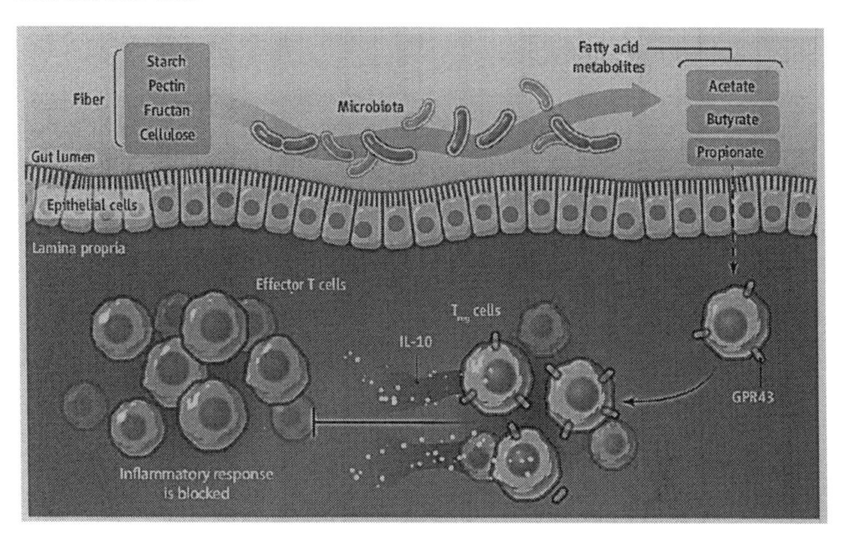

Why we *must* eat "carbs." Image: Bollrath and Powrie

The full caption reads: "**Bacterial metabolites fight intestinal inflammation.** Commensal bacteria metabolize fiber and generate short-chain fatty acids. These fatty acids are ligands for GPR43 expressed by T_{reg} cells and stimulate their expansion and immune-suppressive properties such as the production of IL-10, thereby controlling proinflammatory responses in the gut."

Put simply: our good gut bacteria make beneficial compounds out of fiber which block our immune system from causing inflammation (which covers point 3 above – regulation of immune function).

Our intestinal bacteria control our intestinal immune systems. *We're* not in charge. *They* are. I find that amazing. Essentially, a few species of non-human life forms regulate the immune functioning of our human colons.

Let's lay out the facts, so there can be no misunderstanding. If we want an efficient immune system, one which doesn't cause inflammation (and set us up for inflammatory bowel "diseases" such as ulcerative colitis and Crohn's "disease", or possibly colorectal cancer), we need to supply our colon-dwellers with lots of fiber. In other words, lots of whole plants.

Some colon-dwellers are more equal than others.

Faecalibacterium prausnitzii, and a group of related bacteria, known as 'clostridial clusters,' are the ones that live in symbiosis with our colon walls and make butyrate, acetate and propionate for us. They benefit us by maintaining a thick mucus layer which protects our gut lining, and in which they make their home. They help maintain the tight junctions between gut cells, keeping foreign interlopers out, and thus preventing inflammatory allergic or immune reactions. They make the anti-inflammatory molecules, which power our gut cells and also keep our immune systems damped down.

And, finally, we've reached the crux of the matter.

In the presence of butyrate (et al), our immune systems lie dormant. Butyrate is the signaling molecule that lets our immune system know that all is well. The absence of butyrate is what switches our immune function on, and which leads to inflammation, and inflammatory bowel "diseases".

The absence of fiber = the absence of whole plants = the absence of *Faecalibacterium prausnitzii* and the clostridial clusters = the absence of butyrate = the absence of immune function suppression = inflammation and chronic disease. These ill-effects are all synonyms for Meating.

The absence of Planting is what causes inflammatory bowel "diseases".

If we take a look at the following terrific infographic from *Scientific American* called "How Microbes Keep Us Healthy," we can see a clear difference between Planting health (on the left) and Meating/Junking sickness (on the right). It's the difference between high-fiber and low-fiber diets.

Epidemiology tells us that Meaters and Junkers suffer more colitis and colorectal cancer. As we can see, depletion of the microbiome's *F. prausnitzii* is certainly a plausible biological mechanism that explains why.

The absence of *F. prausnitzii* and/or fiber in the disease state of the disrupted biome is what Meating and Junking cause. Both animals and junk are notoriously fiber-free. What better demonstration do we need than this that animals and (other) junk aren't food?

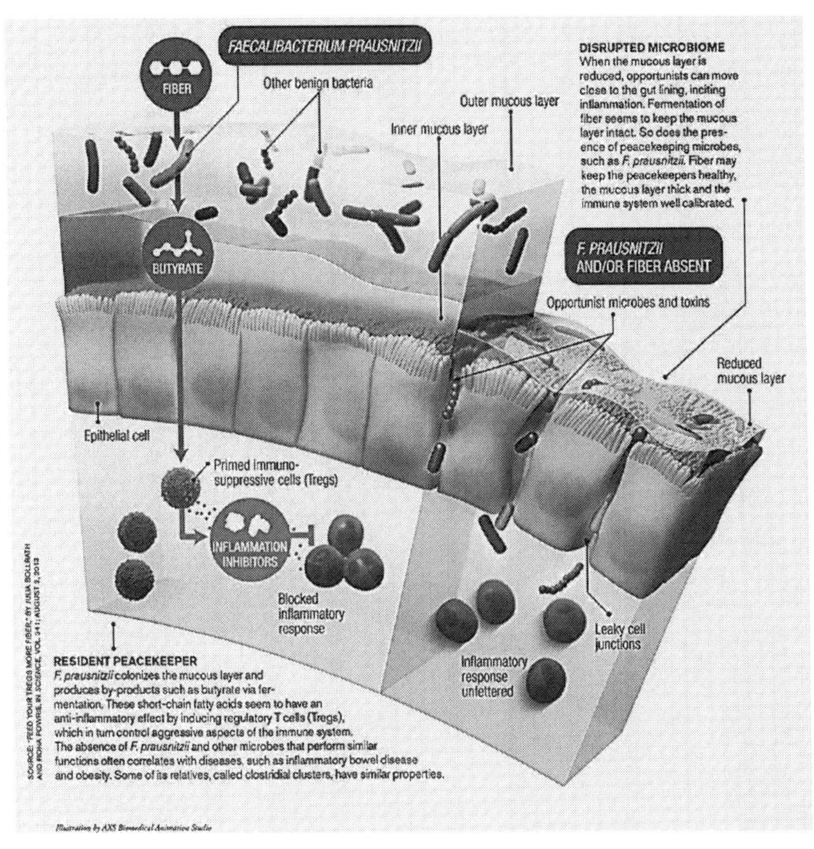

How Microbes Keep Us Healthy [Infographic]
Scientific American Volume 312, Issue 3. 17 February 2015.

As we see above under "disrupted microbiome," Meating and Junking derange our gut flora. *Scientific American* says: "When the mucous layer is reduced, opportunists can move close to the gut lining, inciting inflammation. Fermentation of fiber seems to keep the mucous layer intact. So does the presence of peacekeeping microbes, such as *F. prausnitzii*. Fiber may keep the peacekeepers healthy, the mucous layer thick and the immune system well-calibrated."

Our gut bacteria keep the "immune system well-calibrated" and "train the immune system to distinguish friend from foe." This is wild stuff, and it proves that we're Planters from way, way back, not Meaters, and definitely not Junkers.

When we eat whole plants – fiber-packed items that our bodies have come to recognize as food over eons – our microbiome produces butyrate, and our immune systems stay relaxed and go, "Ok, everything's fine, there's nothing for us to do." The presence of butyrate suppresses our immune system… not in a bad way. Butyrate is a signaling molecule that tells our immune cells to stay off or 'hypo-responsive,' saying there are no antigens to react to. So there's no inflammation.

However, in the absence of butyrate – fiber – whole plants – our immune systems throw their toys out the cot and start attacking our gut bacteria, left, right and center; in effect, trying to wipe out *F. prausnitzii*'s low- or non-butyrate-producing competitors and restore homeostasis. Inflammation and "disease" are the result.

This tells us that our bodies only recognize high-fiber plants as food. Everything else causes an inflammatory immune response in our colons. Everything else being… Junk and Animals. QED, neither is food. Our ancient enteric immune systems tell us so. Animals are antigens.

Meaters' and Junkers' failure to eat enough fiber (causing them to not make enough butyrate) leaves their immunes system in a chronic hyper-reactive state. Fiber deficiency misinforms their immune systems that they've got an overgrowth of bad bacteria in their colons, and the resulting immune attack leaves their bowels in a constant, simmering state of inflammation, setting them up for inflammatory bowel "diseases".

It's absolutely vital that we eat fiber-rich whole plants, not junk.

[See: http://nutritionfacts.org/video/prebiotics-tending-our-inner-garden/]

Sadly, there are two obstacles microbiome research faces. One, the researchers are researchers, by which I mean they're paid by Big Money to look for silver bullet, patentable, profitable drug cures, while Planting is for free and in the public domain and by far the most effective prevention. Two, the researchers are probably mostly Meaters, so even though the solution is fiber, i.e. Planting, they're looking for ways of carrying on eating 'normally' while ignoring the dangers of Meating.

Let's take **fecal transplants** as an example. I kid you not, they're taking microbes from the shit of healthy people and stuffing them up the butts of people with colitis and Crohn's "disease". For six months or so, they see that the gut flora does well, but then the effect goes away. Why? Planters will have no difficulty answering this question. The answer is that the patients aren't Planters. Why would we expect the gut flora of newly treated fecal transplantees to stay healthy when they carry on eating fiber-depleted junk and animals, which are what caused the initial microbiome disruption and the resultant illness?

This isn't stupidity. Microbiome researchers are very bright people. It's the Meater mindset at work. There are none so blind as those who can't see past their Meating.

Meating and Junking → fiber depletion → ↓ *F. prausnitzii* and clostridial clusters → ↓ butyrate → ↓ T_{reg} cells → ↓ immune system modulation → ↑ inflammation → ↑ inflammatory bowel ~~diseases~~.

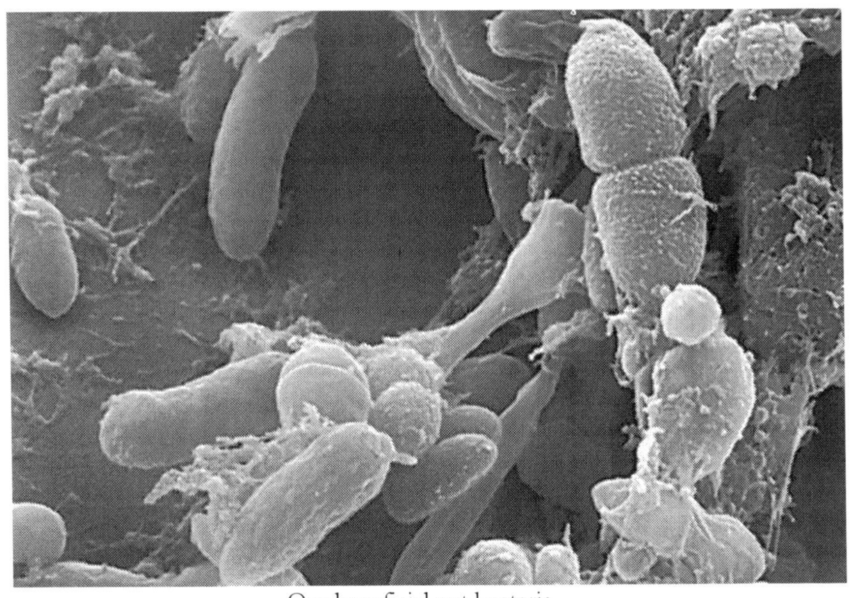

Our beneficial gut bacteria
http://www.nature.com/polopoly_fs/1.15730!/menu/main/topColumns/topLeftColumn/pdf/512247a.pdf

Apparently this Planter truth is too foreign for the Meater rocket scientists to grasp. The word 'vegan' doesn't appear once in the dozen or so microbiomics papers I've read.

Meanwhile, even scientifically illiterate Planters are practicing practical (and optimal) microbiomics at every meal, feeding our intestinal bacteria the fiber on which they thrive, making butyrate, damping down inflammation and lowering our risk of colon "disease". Forget about twin studies; forget about gene sequencing; forget about pharma-cures; forget also fecal transplants, perleez. Why not just eat the food? If we build it out of fiber, they will come… they being our beneficial gut flora.

We saw what they looked like on the previous page…

…and very pretty they are too:

So far we've seen that the absence of a fiber-fueled Planter microbiome causes inflammation and "disease". Now we'll see how the presence of some Meater substances also deranges the microbiome, causing inflammation and "disease".

When we give our gut bacteria animals to eat, a certain amount of animal protein, roughly 12g a day, may reach our colons, where it rots, forming poisonous hydrogen sulfide out of the sulfur-containing amino acids in animal proteins. H_2S smells like rotten eggs or, rather, I should say that eggs smell of H_2S. Ammonia is cytotoxic; a cell-poisoning metabolite.

Carnitine and **choline**, two similarly structured components of animals, when acted upon by our gut flora, amplify the ill effects of three other components of the animals we eat: **saturated fats**, **trans fats** and **cholesterol**. The ill effects of animals aren't confined to cholesterol.

What happens is this: our gut flora convert carnitine and choline into a substance called trimethylamine (TMA). Our livers then oxidize TMA into poisonous trimethylamine-n-oxide, TMAO. In our blood vessels, TMAO boosts cholesterol uptake into the inflammatory foam cells that are the precursors of the fatty plaques in our arteries that kill us through heart attacks and strokes.

It's important to see that:

Planters and Meaters – vegans and carnivore wanna-bes – **have fundamentally different digestive tracts**.

Having different gut flora is tantamount to having our cars run on different types of fuel, one more efficient than the other. We eat different things. The things we eat provide food for different species of bacteria in our guts. Meater *Bacteroides* bacteria produce harmful TMAO.

Planter *Prevotella* bacteria don't. Planter bacteria produce anti-inflammatory, anti-cancer agents, such as propionate, acetate and butyrate. Meater bacteria like *Bilophila wadsworthia* don't do that very well. Instead they produce hydrogen sulfide. This is part of the reason why

Meaters have more inflammatory "diseases", die more often from strokes and heart failure, and live shorter lives.

(Fancy that: a failure of heart leading to heart failure.)

As noted before, we have no dietary need for carnitine – we make it ourselves, like the good little animals we are. It's found mainly in animal red meat, but there's a little carnitine in fruits, grains and vegetables. Does our gut flora form TMAO out of Planter carnitine? No, it doesn't, because it's packaged in a gut-flora-feeding fiber package, and because Planters have different species of plant-fed bacteria living in our colons.

We do need some choline but, again, Planter gut bacteria don't produce TMAO out of the choline in plants like beans, fruit, grains and vegetables. Besides 'red meat,' choline is found in dairy, eggs, livers, poultry and sea animals (the same places cholesterol is found).

It doesn't matter that the same TMAO progenitors, carnitine and choline, are found in both animals and plants. Habitual plant eaters couldn't form TMAO even if they wanted to; habitual animal eaters couldn't stop forming TMAO, even though they should want to.

TMAO formation from carnitine supplements, or energy drinks with carnitine in them, or lecithin supplements with choline in them means they qualify as dangerous junk.

TMAO is also linked to prostate cancer initiation, metastasis and death, particularly from the choline in eggs, milk and animal flesh. Their high choline content is a good reason never to eat eggs: 2.5 eggs per week increases our risk of prostate cancer by 81%.

[See: http://nutritionfacts.org/video/carnitine-choline-cancer-and-cholesterol-the-tmao-connection/

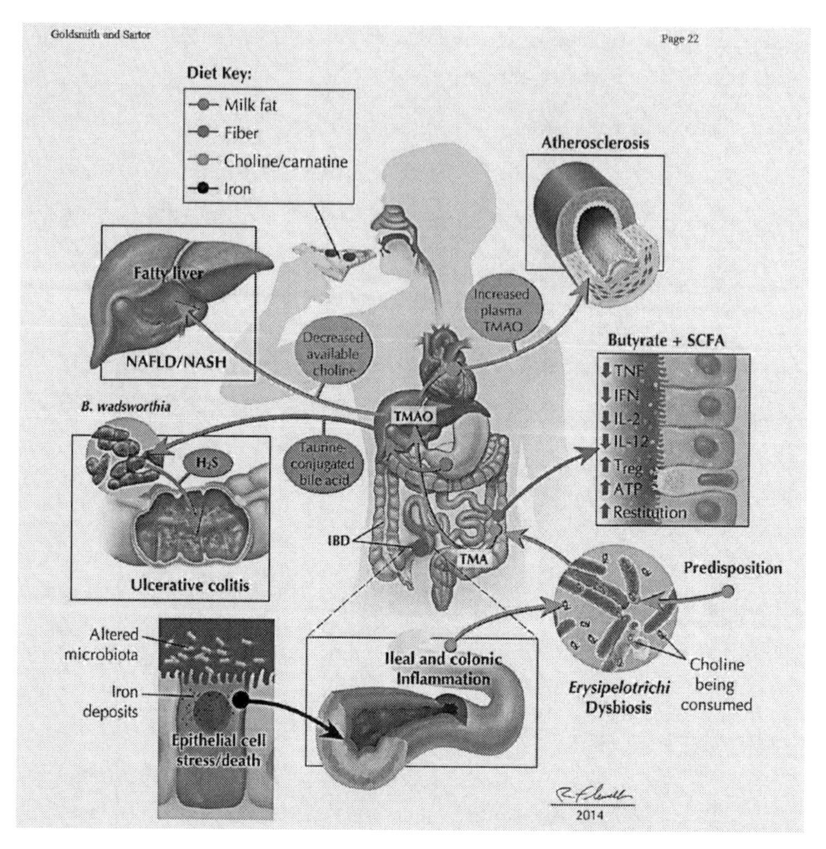

Goldsmith et al: Figure 1. The complex interplay of dietary elements, the microbiota, and the host can be beneficial or detrimental to host health.

Let's take a look now at a graphic representation of how Planting heals while Meating ills or kills, via their beneficial or detrimental effects on our microbiome.

J R Goldsmith, R B Sartor. The role of diet on intestinal microbiota metabolism: downstream impacts on host immune function and health, and therapeutic implications. *J Gastroenterol.* 2014 May;49(5):785-98.

This study shows:

"**Milk fat** (blue): increased consumption of milk fat leads to increased levels of taurine conjugated **bile acids**, which result in a **bloom** of *Bilophila wadsworthia*, a **colitogenic, H_2S**-producing bacteria. [VERY BAD]

Fiber (pink): Consumption of fiber leads to the production of **butyrate** and other short-chain fatty acids by colonic bacteria. These SCFAs promote **epithelial healing** and **decrease intestinal inflammation**, in part through induction of Tregs. [VERY GOOD]

Choline/carnitine (green): Dysbiotic states, as found naturally in a subset of patients or in patients with IBD, results in the increased bacterial metabolism of choline and/or carnitine to TMA. This decreases the bioavailability of choline, leading to NAFLD/NASH, while increased levels of TMA are metabolized by the liver to **TMAO**, an **atherosclerotic** compound. [VERY BAD]

Iron (black): Increased oral iron intake is associated with increased **intestinal epithelial cell stress** and **cell death** and altered microbiota profiles, which may exacerbate active **IBD**." [VERY BAD]

These researchers didn't make this stuff up. Animal fats and animal iron are bad for us, and there are none in whole plants. Fiber is fantastic food, and there's none in animals. And iron, carnitine and choline from plants don't harm us. Animals contain what's bad for us, and they lack what's good.

SNAFU.

I said it up front, and I'll say it again: Meating stuffs up our gut flora. The "downstream impacts" of Meating on our microbiome are severe and life-shortening.

Meating and Junking kill our gut bacteria and us, both by what's in them and by what they lack that's in whole plants.

Carbohydrate resistance

What's that, you may well ask? It's a concept touted by Low-Carb Bullshit Artist Prof. (not of nutrition) Tim Noakes to explain why he has a decreased ability to digest plants, or "can't handle carbs." It's an excuse to eat more animals and fewer grains; an alibi for Meating. A GoogleScholar quest for a peer-reviewed explanation of the idea comes up empty.

LCBAs want us to believe that carbohydrate resistance → Meating.

In truth, Meating → carbohydrate resistance.

As usual, LCBAs are 180° wrong, misrepresenting effect as cause.

Still, if we rescue it from its low-carb origins, CR can be a useful concept, because it describes what we do to ourselves when we eat animals – we diminish our ability to digest plants. When we feed animals to our gut flora, we set off an explosion in the population of harmful, animal-rotting bacteria in our colons, and we cause a simultaneous implosion in the population of beneficial, fiber-fermenting bacteria. In effect, we cause cirrhosis of the little livers in our gut, by decimating species such as *Faecalibacterium prausnitzii* which are responsible for digesting fiber, and which use fiber to produce cancer-combatting short-chain fatty acids such as propionate and butyrate, which modulate our intestinal immune function.

Meating *leads to* carbohydrate resistance; not the other way round. This LCBA Meats himself into being resistant to carbohydrate, then turns around and tells us to Meat *because* we're carb-resistant. CR in Meaters and Junkers helps explain why their fiber-deficient diets give them more inflammatory bowel "diseases" and colorectal cancer. Thank you for the term, Prof. Noakes – I think I'll prise it from your paws and put it to better use.

Thinking that 'we' can't handle carbs is to be egocentrically ignorant or ignore-ant of the fact that it's our trillions of gut bacteria which can and do handle carbs on our behalf, and, when we poison our gut bacteria with animals, we do damage to the amazing virtual organ known as the microbiome, and we make ourselves less carbohydrate-sensitive, just as we make ourselves less insulin-sensitive and more diabetic by Meating and Junking. The *combination* of "meat + sweet" is what makes us carbohydrate-resistant, insulin-resistant and diabetic, as Noakes is at the time of writing. It's not just one; it's both, making each other worse.

We can all overcome our carbohydrate resistance by repopulating our intestines with bacteria that eat plant fibers. We upregulate our genes for amylase, the starch-cracking enzyme, by eating more starch. To improve our ability to digest fiber… we need to eat more fiber! The more whole carbs we eat, the better we digest carbs. This isn't news to Planter nutritionists: 98% of Americans are fiber-deficient, because of Meating and Junking. (And, remember, fiber lowers our carcinogenic cholesterol, estrogen and bile acid levels too.)

To think we can feed animals to our microbiome without serious ill-effects is to ignore human anatomy, physiology and (co)evolutionary biology; and to snub the splendid new sciences of microbiomics, epigenetics and nutrigenomics (each of which will receive more attention later).

Leaky gut

As mentioned under Animal Fats, Meater fats damage the tight junctions between the enterocytes making up the single layer of cells that separates us from the world outside, responsible for absorbing what's needed, excluding what's harmful, and excreting what's unneeded.

Saturated fat is a big cause of leaky guts. So too, as we've just seen, is a lack of good bacteria in our colons, brought about by the fiber deficiency innate in Meating and Junking.

With holes in our gut walls, inflammation-causing proteins, malefic microbes, endotoxins and environmental toxins can enter where they don't belong. Nothing good results from this…

Toxemia

See under: Pre-eclampsia, in Part 1C (Eatiology)

Allergic responses

A leaky gut helps bring about allergic and auto-immune responses. Eating animals, especially animal fats, diminishes our enteric ("relating to or occurring in the intestines") integrity, allowing larger-than-usual peptides or bugs to pass through into our blood, setting up an immune reaction. Fiber-free diets also contribute to gut leakiness.

Immune and Auto-immune responses

Immune responses are good. They protect us against pathogens (disease-causing agents) like bacteria and viruses. Our bodies detect a foreign invader – called an antigen – and creates antibodies to deal with the specific threat. We'd die very quickly without an efficient immune system.

It doesn't matter what we think or say or write, consciously. If our bodies say animals are foreign, then they're foreign. There's no way to get around that fact. (And that should be the end of the discussion about whether or not animals are food. Our bodies say they're not.)

Our saying otherwise – that animals are food – means nothing in the face of our bodies' utter rejection of them as food; outright rejection of their mere presence or their continued existence. When animals show up in our blood, it's a fight to the death, until the manxome foe is slain, or we die trying.

The collateral damage of this savage war within us – the wantonly slaughtered and drone-struck civilian population – is:

- our joint cartilage and bone (where it's known as the Rheumatoid Arthritis war);
- the myelin sheaths of our nerve cells (multiple sclerosis);
- the beta cells of our pancreases (type I diabetes);
- the mucosa of our mouths (aphthous ulcers (canker sores));
- our nervous systems (acute inflammatory demyelinating polyneuropathy, a.k.a. Guillain-Barré syndrome – or myasthenia gravis, also a neurological autoimmune response);
- our intestinal walls (Crohn's "disease", an inflammatory bowel condition).

Immune responses create inflammation… and some cancers grow best in inflamed environments… so they co-opt our immune systems to help them grow. So cancer can be thought of as an auto-immune response.

These auto-immune battles are all part of the global conflict of Us vs. the Animals. Animals are the antigens that invade our country and we are the antibodies that get conscripted to combat them. When we eat animals regularly, they win. Eating them creates an army with limitless reinforcements, while we're all we've got. Every meal, another brigade gets thrown into battle against us, so we're losing… and our joints become stiffer and more painful and deformed; our nerves more inflamed; our insulin-producing ability impaired or destroyed.

Auto-immune conditions are the animals' revenge against us for eating them.

Auto-immune conditions prove conclusively that animals-as-food aren't just evolutionarily novel; they're novel right now, with every meal, with every bite we take.

Eating whole plants prevents, stops, and can even reverse the damage caused by auto-immune conditions. Planting undoes what Meating causes.

With the one notable exception of gluten-induced celiac disease, a genetically determined condition affecting fewer than 1% of Americans,

Planting doesn't cause auto-immune conditions. Bacteria can (e.g. rheumatic fever and heart damage from staph infection) and animals do, all the time.

The reason we have antibodies against fishes and pigs and chickens and cows circulating through us constantly, vigilantly, is simple.

Animals are *not* food. They're alien threats.

Molecular Mimicry
Molecular mimicry is sometimes also called 'friendly fire.' It's equivalent to getting fragged by one's own soldiers.

This is how auto-immune conditions start: A molecule that's not supposed to be in our bloodstream is identified by a member of our immune system and tagged for destruction. Other immune molecules, called antibodies, bind to the outsider (called an antigen) and rip it apart. The problem starts when the antigen molecule is made out of something that closely resembles or mimics a part of us. That's when an immune reaction becomes an auto-immune reaction – an immune reaction attacking and destroying our own bodies. Understandably, this happens more often when the antigen is an animal like us.

Auto-immune conditions arise almost entirely in reaction to dietary animal protein antigens.

Friendly fire
A condition in which one's immune system attacks one's own tissues, fooled into doing so by the mimicry of human proteins by the non-human animal proteins we eat.

See under: Auto-immune conditions; Molecular mimicry

Auto-immune conditions
See: Immune and Auto-immune responses, above

Celiac disease, gluten sensitivity and wheat allergy
Celiac disease is the exception to the rule of auto-immune conditions caused by Meating. As such, it's used by some Meater apologists to claim that all grains should be called non-foods.

I'll try to cover, in one page, a subject that others have written books about.

Celiac disease occurs in a small subset of people who have a genetic mutation (to chromosome #6 (the short arm, to be more precise)) which causes their immune systems to react to glutamine and a class of proteins called prolamins. These incur the wrath of both the innate and adaptive arms of our immune systems – the standing armies and the mobilized reserves, such as T-helper cells.

The prolamins include gluten proteins such as gliadins (in wheat), hordein (in barley) and secalin (in rye). As animal and junk fats do to us all, gliadin can damage the tight junctions between the enterocytes lining the small intestine of some sensitive people, allowing unusually large peptides (amino acid fragments) to penetrate the gut wall. Here, they can induce an auto-immune "friendly fire" reaction, with resulting inflammation and damage to intestinal villi – the finger-like projections of the mucosa through which absorption takes place.

It's way more complicated than this, but that's the nutshell version.

If we remember from our earlier encounter with gluten, celiac disease affects ¾ of 1% of Americans; roughly 2 ¼ million people. These unfortunates have no recourse except to avoid all grains that contain the prolamins that cause them to suffer from chronic diarrhea, cramping, fatigue, abdominal pain and diminished nutrient absorption (such as vitamins D, K and B_{12}, iron, folic acid, carbs, calcium, copper and zinc). They also have increased risk of developing lymphomas.

Those on a gluten-free diet should avoid barley, rye and wheat (including durum, kamut and spelt); triticale too; and a small minority of people may respond to oats. Grains and near-grains safe for eating include amaranth, buckwheat, corn, millet, quinoa [pronounced keen-wha], rice, sorghum, teff and wild rice. Of course, gluten-free, high-carb vegetables such as sweet potatoes cause no problems.

But…

If only it were this simple. There's another, larger group of people who have other issues with gluten or wheat than this small group of genetically unique celiac'ers with their **gluten intolerance**.

Some people who have chronic diarrhea, but who don't have celiac disease get better on a gluten-free diet. So, they're genetically unmutated, yet they have **non-celiac gluten sensitivity**. It's real – they don't "need a check-up from the neck up," as doctors used to think.

And then there's another group of people who have **wheat sensitivity**, unrelated to gluten.

And then there's a whole lot of people who think they have sensitivities… so they do, even when what they've eaten contains nothing remotely resembling a gliadin or a wheat protein. These people often have other sensitivities, particularly to dairy, so it may be difficult for them to pinpoint the exact antigen; it makes life easier for them to round up all the usual suspects and cut them all from their diets.

There's a wide spectrum of gluten and/or grain intolerance, allergy, sensitivity and psychosomatic response, and all of them affect our health for the worse. People who only think that gluten's bad for them are missing out on excellent food. The number of people experiencing actual physical reactions to grains or their proteins is probably low… about five or six million Americans, or less than 2% of the populace.

There are those (many with vested interests in a multi-billion dollar bun fight) who bandy about much higher numbers. The science doesn't back their claims. If I'm "misunderestimating" the numbers, it's not by an order of magnitude.

(Incidentally, does anyone remember what **meat glue**'s made out of? Transglutaminase. As we've just seen, glutamine can cause celiac disease as well as gluten. Put those two facts together and we get a pretty ugly scenario: Meaters chowing down on a juicy steak-through-the-heart, not knowing it's been stitched together with an enzyme that could set off their immune response to wheat. How weird is that?

This is another reason, besides a sat fat-induced leaky gut, that celiac sufferers should become Planters. I love these little details; there's no detail so fine that it doesn't slam Meating to the mat.)

For more than 95% of us, gluten is real good protein from real good food. Our beneficial gut bacteria *hate* not having gluten to eat. Grains, with or without gluten, protect us against a welter of constipation-related conditions and Alzheimer's. (*Grain Brain*? Pfft.) For non-gluten sensitives to avoid gluten is to limit our ability to eat (and be) well.

Dr. Michael Greger has a fine trio of videos dealing with this topic:

- "Is Gluten Sensitivity Real?"
- "Gluten Free Diets: Separating the Wheat from the Chat," and
- "How to Diagnose Gluten Intolerance."

Obesity ~ Diabesity ~ Diabetes

I'm going to make an exception of obesity and diabetes, and deal with their multiple mechanisms together in the Eatiology, or dietary causes, section. That's because, by the time I've finished describing the mechanisms of obesity and the different forms of diabetes, I'll have described the "diseases" themselves.

The mechanisms and diabetes-related topics I'll be covering in Part 1C (Eatiology) are:

- Obesity – excess body fat caused by Meating and Junking
- Obesogens – Meater viruses and chemicals that cause obesity
- Infectobesity – infectious obesity of animal origin
- Diabesity – the obesity-diabetes connection
- Cholesterol – a diabetogenic (diabetes-causing) Meater substance
- Saturated and trans fats – diabetogenic Meater and Junker fats
- Circulating sex hormones, such as estrogens, elevated by Meating
- Reduced sex hormone binding proteins, caused by Meating
- Oxidation and inflammation – outcomes of Meating and Junking
- Insulin resistance – an outcome of Meating and Junking
- Hyperglycemia – high blood sugar levels caused by M&J
- Hyperinsulinemia – high blood insulin levels, ditto
- Prediabetes – the unhealthy early stage of diabetes, ditto
- Type 1 diabetes – an 'irreversible' Meater condition
- Pancreatitis – how Meating and Junking damage our pancreases
- Type 2 diabetes – an easily reversible Meater/Junker condition
- Gestational diabetes – diabetes we give ourselves during pregnancy
- Type 1 ½ diabetes – a combination of types 1 and 2
- Lipotoxicity – fat poisoning, caused by M&J's saturated and trans fats
- Bio-accumulation – how animals magnify environmental pollutants
- Endocrine disruptors – chemicals biomagnified in animal flesh
- Diabetogens – gut flora-created estrogens that help cause diabetes
- The spillover effect – how being fat makes matters worse

Ketosis

Ketosis isn't a subject I find particularly interesting, except insofar as my body may go into a ketogenic, or ketone-producing state during my periodic fasts. It's certainly not a state we should remain in indefinitely. If, as this book shows, we can see hundreds of reasons why animals aren't food, why would I eat animals for the paltry supposed benefit of ketosis and weight loss? Especially when Planters are already the slenderest people in the world. And the healthiest. And the longest-lived. Still, I guess I should say something about it. (I cover the topic in more depth in *The Low-Carb Bullshit Artists Are Lying Us to Death* (Cape Town: Tabularasa Press, 2016).)

A ketone-producing diet is an alternative way to stay alive when the opportunities for glycolysis (glucose burning) are limited, e.g. for cave dwellers during icebound winters when plant sources of glucose weren't available. It's a back-up generator for our solar system, i.e. sunlight → chlorophyll → photosynthesis → glucose → carbohydrates, our primary fuel.

Glucose is so fundamental to our survival that we have a redundant system for converting fats and proteins, even nucleic acids, into glucose for burning, a process known as Gluconeogenesis – "Making new glucose."

What is ketosis, and how does it work? In *Atkins Exposed*, Michael Greger tells us:

> "In biochemistry class, doctors learn that fat "burns in the flame of carbohydrate." When one is eating enough carbohydrates, fat can be completely broken down as well. But when one's body runs out of carb fuel to burn, its only choice is to burn fat inefficiently using a pathway that produces toxic byproducts like acetone and other so-called "ketones." The acetone escapes through the lungs – giving Atkins followers what one weight-loss expert calls "rotten-apple breath" – and the other ketones have to be excreted by the kidneys. We burn fat all the time; it's only when we are carbohydrate deficient and have to burn fat ineffectively that we go into what's called a state of ketosis, defined as having so much acetone in our blood it noticeably spills out into our lungs or so many other ketones they spill out into our urine.

> To wash these toxic waste products out of our system our body uses a lot of water. The diuretic effect of low carb diets can result in people losing a gallon of water in pounds the first week. This precipitous early weight loss encourages dieters to continue the diet even though they have lost mostly water weight and the state of ketosis may be making them nauseous or worse...
>
> The Director of Yale University's Center for Eating and Weight Disorders explains the miracle formula used by diet books to become bestsellers for over a century now: "easy, rapid weight loss; the opportunity to eat your favorite foods and some scientific 'breakthrough' that usually doesn't exist." The rapid loss of initial water weight seen particularly on low carb diets has an additional sales benefit. By the time people gain back the weight, they may have already told all their friends to buy the book, and the cycle continues. This has been used to explain why low carb diets have been such "cash cows" for publishers over the last 140 years. As one weight loss expert notes, "Rapid water loss is the $33-billion diet gimmick."

That doesn't sound particularly healthy... or even safe. MG continues:

> "The immediate concern [about Atkins and other animal diets] centers on the state of ketosis. Pregnant women are the most at risk. Based on detailed data from 55,000 pregnancies, acetone and other ketones may cause brain damage in the fetus, which may result in the baby being born mentally retarded. The fact that ketones seemed to cause "significant neurological impairment" and an average loss of about 10 IQ points was well known and aroused "considerable concern" years before Atkins published his first book. Atkins nonetheless wrote. "I recommend this diet to all my pregnant patients.""

"Show me the money."

Planting is the safest diet for all humans, but especially for pregnant women and unborn babies. Why would we ever consider eating a ketogenic diet, when it's so harmful to mothers and children?

Proponents of ketogenic diets are telling us we should disconnect our beautiful solar arrays and run our stinky, inefficient diesel back-up generator full-time instead.

Herein lies the daft logic of the paleo and low-carb crowd. Because they're concerned almost entirely with weight loss, they call the built-in inefficiency of ketogenesis a "metabolic advantage."

Low-Carb Bullshit Artists cover up the inefficiency (and the dangers) of ketosis with a marketing ploy: Hey, this stuff is so bad, it'll make you lose weight.

A ketogenic diet may keep us alive in starvation situations. Long-term high-animal, high-fat, low-carb ketosis is dangerous – at the very least, it makes us insulin resistant; also raises LDL cholesterol, while not raising HDL. And ketoacidosis can be lethal.

Whole food veganism, high in carbohydrates and fiber, causes the weight to drop off obese people. Unlike carb restriction it also lowers triglycerides and cholesterol, and removes insulin resistance better than mere weight loss. The science is clear: people eating extremely high-plant diets live the longest.

The science is equally clear: **low-carb diets shorten our lives.**

Check out this study, one of many showing the same result:

Noto H, Goto A, Tsujimoto T, Noda M (2013) Low-Carbohydrate Diets and All-Cause Mortality: A Systematic Review and Meta-Analysis of Observational Studies. *PloS ONE* 8(1): e55030.

Noto et al conclude: "Our systematic review and meta-analyses of worldwide reports suggested that low-carbohydrate diets are associated with a **significantly higher risk of all-cause mortality** in the long run."

There is, according to PlantPositive, a "similarity between ketogenic diets and starvation, but starvation is not the only circumstance in which ketosis takes place. Ketosis also takes place during uncontrolled diabetes and chronic alcoholism… Also producing ketosis are anorexia nervosa, prolonged vomiting, and several gastrointestinal diseases."

"Of course," he understates, "these all are unique in their own ways, but these associations should provoke a little skepticism of these diets."

Being low in carbs isn't something to be proud of. Low-carb diets kill, because what they're low in is… food.

It seems only fair that if we want to eat in a selfish (and pointless) way that cuts short the lives of hundreds of animals during our lifetimes, that our lives should be truncated too. They are. When we eat animals, we age faster and we die younger.

There has never been, nor will there ever be, a study showing that a low-carb (high-animal) diet can boost longevity. How can joy or peace come out of cruelty and despair? It's metaphysically impossible. As the author of *The World Peace* Diet, Will Tuttle says: "You can't build a tower of love out of bricks of cruelty."

On the flip side, there has never been, nor will there ever be, a study showing that a high-whole-carb (no animal) diet doesn't have a kaleidoscope of benefits, including longer life.

Cancer

Cancer is either incredibly complex and unfathomable, or it's simple and, like I imagine enlightenment to be, so simple – like how banksters create money out of thin air – that the mind balks at understanding.

Cancer is a Gargantuan topic that will expand to fit any amount of space allotted to it. Here's my Lilliputian version.

Cancer is cancer is cancer.

Cancer of the prostate = cancer of the bone marrow = bowel cancer = testicular cancer = liver cancer. There's only one cancer. Cancer isn't a thing; it's a process, and we need to stop the process from starting or continuing.

Remember, what we eat accounts for more than 90% of environmental effects we experience. Cigarette and spliff smoking probably account for most of the rest, with exposure to radiation like nuclear fallout and medico-dental x-rays a distant third.

Genetically programmed cancers account for only 2 or 3% of cancers, 5% max, and even if we have 'bad' genes we can eat in such ways that we up- or down-regulate them in beneficial ways. (For more, see under: Epigenetics and Nutrigenomics.)

Overwhelmingly, *we don't get cancer; we give ourselves cancer* by Meating and Junking.

Here's how it works:

Researchers usually divide the cancer process into three distinct phases:

- Initiation
- Promotion
- Progression

Just as the majority of oncologists used to smoke cigarettes before we worked out that, yes, inhaling superheated industrial smoke containing thousands of lethal toxins probably wasn't good for us – although that's still never been proven by randomized, placebo-controlled, double-blind, crossover trials, and never will be – so too today, most oncologists are Meaters.

It takes a generation for clinicians to incorporate new treatments into general practice. Who has time to read all the new science? Science must await a new generation of healers to make lifestyle medicine the norm.

Until the amazing new Planter principle of primordial prevention and healing enters and overturns the ruling medical zeitgeist of symptom treatment and disease management – Jesus in the Temple, routing the sacrificial animal salesmen and the money changers springs to mind – we will still have researchers and doctors who're wasting their time (and our lives) because they're starting from the wrong place, and we can't get here from there.

In chaos theory, SDIC (sensitive dependence on initial conditions) means that small local differences can lead to incredibly different outcomes. It's sometimes called the "butterfly effect." I like to think that there may be one square meter of land up in the Rockies at the Continental Divide, at the edges of which two raindrops may fall, and one may end up in the Pacific Ocean and one may make its way to the Gulf of Mexico (if that river still reaches the Gulf); and yet another drop may snake its way into the St Lawrence and return to the North Atlantic.

So too, health is very sensitively dependent on initial nutrition conditions. Eating is that square meter up at the Continental Divide – think continence or incontinence – and the difference between eating foods and non-foods – Planting or Meating and Junking – makes the difference between arriving at a balmy Caribbean resort or a frigid northern wasteland.

Like fishes unaware of water, or humans oblivious of air, Meater scientists and physicians are unconscious of their bred-in-the-bone

Meater bias and so CANNOT see what's plain to Planters: that the habit of Meating is what's causing most of the health problems they're straining so hard, mentally constipated, to remediate.

It takes decades for change to happen, even under the best of conditions. But these aren't the best of conditions: medical training hasn't changed in a century, and the medical establishment is resisting, tooth and claw, nutrition education for its acolytes (i.e. only our most effective method of healing); Big Pharma is one of the most lucrative agents of un-change ever, along with Big Chem and Big "Food".

Behemoth forces have captured our society, with Dairy and Egg and Meat Board and soda company teaching materials in our schools, fast unfood unrestaurants in our hospitals; truly gigantic advertising campaigns for unfoods and undrinks, saturating a media owned by the same corporate owners promoting Meating; scientific journals more and more captured by corporate advertisers; our government captured by corporate lobbyists; a revolving door policy that allows corporateers to run government departments. I'm sure you could add to the list.

Still, change is coming. It's inevitable. People would like to be healthy, and like the mythical kraken, we're awakening from our slumbers. Lifestyle medicine is on the way; we just have to work out how to recompense doctors for giving advice to do things that are essentially free: eat food; pray; love; exercise; relax; breathe fresh air; drink clean water; sleep; get out in the sun (but not of the noon-day variety like a mad dog or an Englishman).

It's that simple. Most importantly: Eat only food; no animals, no junk.

As more scientists become willing to follow the nutrition evidence to its logical conclusion, we're reading more often words such as these in scientific journals, sometimes in the section where conflicts of interest are supposed to be noted:

"So powerful was the vegan/plant diet in reversing ___________ that this researcher became a vegan during the course of this trial." [Fill in the blank with our choice of condition, from A for acne to Z for zoönosis.]

Which brings this longwinded scrivener back to cancer.

The best science today shows that Meating is implicated in all three stages of cancer. It initiates cancer. It promotes cancer, and it causes cancers to progress, invade and spread.

Here's how…

Oncogenesis or Carcinogenesis

We all have cancer cells in us all the time. Every second of every day, many of our tens of trillions of cells are mutating. Most of them get wiped out by our immune system. Some may not.

All cancer growths start with one cell whose DNA has become deranged by a carcinogen. That's not saying much: something that causes cancer causes cancer to start.

Carcinogens or oncogens are environmental agents – chemicals, viruses, radiation – that enter our bodies and damage our DNA. For a long life, we should avoid giving these mutagens access to our bodies. In that case we shouldn't eat animals, because they too are environmental agents that initiate cancer.

Here are some animal ingredients (and unavoidable contaminants) that initiate, promote and progressify cancer:

- Animal fats, both saturated and trans
- Animal proteins
- Arachidonic acid
- Cholesterol and excess bile acids
- Drug residues, such as antibiotics
- Endotoxins
- Heme iron
- Heterocyclic amines, such as IQ4,5b, MeIQx and PhIP: "cooked meat carcinogens"
- Industrial pollutants, such as dieldrin, dioxins, DDE and DDT, to name just a few deadly Ds.
- Neu5Gc
- Nitrosamines and nitrosamides
- Chicken, pig and other oncogenic viruses
- Polycyclic aromatic hydrocarbons
- Steroid hormones such as estrogen

Yes, you read that right: animal protein is carcinogenic. Much-ballyhooed animal protein causes the production and release of IGF-1 (insulin-like growth factor-1), the growth hormone that's responsible for our necessary rapid growth when we're babies, which responds to the only animal protein we should ever receive in our lives, our mothers' breast milk, by telling our bodies: okay, fellers, here's the bricks, get building. Fine in babies, but in adulthood, excess IGF-1 production leads to cancer promotion and premature aging via accelerated cell division.

And that's just one of the pranks our impish little Meater poster child gets up to.

Really, once that's said and accepted, that animal protein is a major cause of cancer, that should be it for animals as food… game over… what more needs to be said? What else do I have to say to make us all nod our heads sagely and say, "Gosh, Ro. You're right. Stop right there; don't bother to finish writing your book. We're convinced. If the proteins in animals cause cancer, then animals can't be food. Thanks for letting me know, I think I'll go work out now and grab me a salad on the way home. It's vegan all the way for me from now on."

Sigh. The vegan dream.

(Wouldn't you be surprised if you turned the page and found the rest were all blank?)

Probably the most lethal animal protein is the cow milk protein, casein. Read the Campbells, T. Colin and son Thomas M, about the Cornell Oxford China Study, to see how Campbell Sr. (unveganly) used casein to switch cancer on and off in lab rats – not conclusive about humans, I know – but suggestive enough for him to change course dramatically from the accepted wisdom of animal protein being the food messiah. His casein research while trying to understand how high protein intake was causing liver cancer in Pilipino kids was instrumental in his reaching the understanding that first class, animal protein is really wurst class protein.

[See: T. Colin Campbell and Thomas Campbell II. *The China Study: The Most Comprehensive Study of Nutrition Ever Conducted and the Startling Implications for Diet, Weight Loss, and Long-term Health* (Dallas, BenBella: 2006), which Dean Ornish calls "one of the most important books about nutrition ever written – reading it may save your life."]

On page 59, under the heading 'Not all proteins are alike,' the Campbells write: "So the next logical question was whether plant protein, tested in the same way, has the same effect on cancer promotion as casein. The answer is an astonishing "NO." *In these experiments, plant protein did not promote cancer growth, even at the higher levels of intake.*"

Animal and plant proteins are different, and have different health effects; positive in the case of plants, negative in the case of animals.

Because animals' star performer, animal protein, is a carcinogen, to eat animals is to commit decades-long, freeze-frame, slow-motion seppuku using a an animal dagger, a tantō or wakizashi of animal flesh, to rip open our own belly flesh, while a deadly assistant waits behind us to behead us with a stroke of an animal katana, or sword. [stroke pun alert]

Yet, even if animal proteins weren't deadly, even if first class protein rocked the casbah, animals are still carcinogens because of animal fats, arachidonic acid, cholesterol, drug residues, endotoxins, heme iron, heterocyclic amines, industrial pollutants, Neu5Gc, nitrosamines and nitrosamides, polycyclic aromatic hydrocarbons, animal viruses and estrogenic hormones. And probably a few other gremlins that lurk undetected.

Cancer is baked into the Meater pie. The Meater pie is made out of cancer. Meating causes cancer. Meating is cancer. "Meat is the new smoking." This parrot is dead. It's shuffled off. It's joined the choir invisible. It is no more.

There's absolutely no way of separating eating animals from cancer initiation, promotion and progression. It's an absolute impossibility.

No matter how many new ways I say it, the truth remains... this is how the Meater cookie crumbles: Animals aren't food.

Each of the items in the list above, from animal fats to steroid hormones, is tackled in a section of its own. Here follows a short discussion of the mechanisms of cancer, previewing a few of the roles our zoö-villains play. (Many of the mechanisms appear also in the Eatiology section when I take on breast cancer as an example of cancers in general.)

Initiation

Cancer begins as a sneaky crime. A silent outlaw slinks in and steals or vandalizes a small piece of the genetic code of a single cell. The cell survives and reproduces by division. One cell becomes two, becomes 4, 8, 16, 32, 64, 128, 256, 512, 1024. Ten generations after the original mutation, there are roughly a thousand demented cells. After twenty doublings, there are a million cancer cells. Thirty; a billion.

With a doubling time of up to two years (in, say, prostate cancer) and as short as three weeks (in, say, aggressive blood cancers after a nuclear explosion), a billion cancer cells can form in anywhere between about two and sixty years. (The doubling time also depends on how many animals we eat!)

A million cancer cells form a clump about the size of a pinhead, and, according to Dr. John McDougall is 6 years old, on average.

Recorded Webinar The Dietary Treatment of Cancer – https://www.drmcdougall.com/health/education/webinars/webinar-09-26-15/].

This is about the absolute smallest tumor we can detect with MRI or other fancy equipment. After ten years, on average, a billion cells will make a lump about 10mm in size. A breast tumor detected by mammography may have been initiated twenty years earlier.

Early detection is not.

If a "malignant neoplasm" has been growing for decades, the chances are good that it's been promoted and may even have progressed to the stage where it's metastasized and spread to, say, our bone marrow, lungs or brain. It isn't breast cancer that kills us; it's the metastases.

This is why early detection is actually very late detection, and a waste of time and resources; it's shutting the barn door after the cow's already jumped over the moon. We need to take pity on our future selves right now and prevent a later dread diagnosis by making our bodies so inhospitable to carcinoma that no cancerous seed can find purchase in us.

We do this by Planting.

It's called Primordial Prevention. We don't wait around for symptoms to appear and then spring into frantic action with drugs and chemicals and radiation and surgical instruments, trying to stuff the billowing cancer genie back into the lamp it's already escaped from. We co-dedicate the holy temples of our Planter bodies as mountain fortresses, crenellated walls secure against the siege engines and scaling ladders of Meating. (Flowery, moi?)

Initiation is relatively simple. It's the opening salvo of the cancer war. It's the stage at which an initial **DNA mutation** occurs in a cell. Cancer-inducing **oxidation** is built into Meating; anti-oxidation into Planting.

IGF-1 (Insulin-like growth factor-1) is the human growth hormone that is switched on by eating **animal proteins**. Animal proteins also contain more sulfur-containing amino acids, which supply the acidic conditions in which cancers prefer to grow.

IGF-1 is involved in all 3 stages of the Eatiology of cancer: after being an initiator, it helps the cancer grow and spread, invade and metastasize.

What price animal protein now?

Traditionally, we've tended to think of a cancer initiator as being radiation or an environmental chemical. That's so last century. The most relevant environmental toxins we regularly introduce into our selves are animals, what's in them naturally and what they've come to contain. This is what the archetype will be in ten, twenty years from now. Planters are "early adopters" of the Eatiology of cancer. When we're Meaterialists, we eat our most common carcinogens, mutagens, oncogens… they come from the animals we consume in the mistaken belief they're food.

Casein is an excellent cancer initiator, and so are the cooked animal flesh carcinogens, like IQ4,5b, MeIQx and PhIP.

Animals ARE the environment. They're vast. They contain multitudes of carcinogens of their own making. Plus, animals biomagnify and accumulate environmental mutagens to pathological levels, particularly in their fat. And cooking them creates even more.

Plants are past masters at preventing DNA damage by the elements, especially the sun, because we callously leave most of them out in the sun all day, making them provide their own shade even. ALL plants have the ability to counter DNA damage; some are more equal than others. Allium family members (especially garlic, also onions, leeks, shallots, like that, because of their allicin content, amongst others) and Crucifers (like broccoli, Brussels sprouts and cauliflower, because of their sulforaphane content, ditto) are especially powerful anti-cancer agents. Bog-standard white button mushrooms, high in ergothioneine, are potent breast cancer opponents. Non-GM soybeans and flax seeds counter animal estrogens. Chlorophyll is an amazing **carcinogen interceptor**.

Whole plants fix what animals cause.

Cancer stem cells
For an extended discussion of cancer stem cells, please see Part 4 (Missing in Action) #51, Natural Products That Target Cancer Stem Cells. Suffice it to say for now that phoods – plants – are what eradicate cancer stem cells, while Meating and chemo make matters worse or, at best, have no effect. Chemo and radiation shrink tumors because they target daughter cells, while the parent or stem cells usually remain unharmed or become more virulent and metastasize elsewhere.

Apoptosis
Once cancer cells have been initiated, our immune systems usually step in and wipe them out. T cells initiate a process called apoptosis, which means 'programmed cell death.' They interact with the cancer cells and give them a revolver with one cartridge in it, and say, "Go ahead, do the honorable thing."

We all have immune systems that are doing this countless times every second of every day. Here's the thing: Planters' immune systems are far more apoptotic than Meaters'. Improved apoptosis is one of the reasons why Planters get far less cancer than Meaters and Junkers.

Promotion
While cancer initiation can be the work of a moment, cancer promotion takes place over years and decades. It's the incubation stage.

Estrogenic effects
During promotion, hormones are particularly good at helping cancers grow faster, by speeding up **cell division**; endogenous hormones like **estrogen** and exogenous xenoestrogens from the environmental toxins that build up in animals and their estrogenic effects make them **endocrine disruptors** when we eat them.

During this stage, cancers thrive on **inflammation** – and animal-borne arachidonic acid, endotoxins, heme iron and Neu5Gc are experts at causing that. An **immune response** produces inflammation which in turn leads to more blood supply tubules being built. New tumors need either to co-opt existing blood supplies or, in a process called **angiogenesis** – "blood vessel new making" – they… make new capillaries to ensure their surthrival.

Cancer cells, according to some sources, are our bodies' attempt to stay alive in low oxygen environments; instead of aerobic respiration, they rely on a far less efficient anaerobic mechanism. Not only do some cancers feed on cholesterol, cholesterol also provides anaerobic conditions through the atherosclerotic **ischemia** it causes. Cancer cells now begin to ferment sugar in the low-oxygen conditions brought on by atherosclerosis.

Progression

The final stage of cancer is progression, in which Junior leaves home. Cancers **invade** surrounding tissues, and **metastases** form which enter the bloodstream and can spread anywhere in the body, where they find a foothold and continue growing. Metastases are secondary malignant growths that develop "at a distance from a primary site of cancer."

As pointed out by Kathy Freston (and Michael Greger), the carcinogens we create when we cook animal flesh over high heat are "three strikes" carcinogens: they participate in all three stages, initiation, promotion and progression. They mutate cells, they help them grow, and then they make tumors more invasive, an aide to their metastasis. Meating makes tumors more mobile.

Eating chickens quadruples our risk of prostate cancer, and less than one egg a day doubles our risk.

Plants, on the other hand, are anti-angiogenic; they contain phytonutrients such as **apigenin**, **fisitin** and **luteolin** which stop angiogenesis, cutting off the blood supply to tumors. Eating phood can prevent any cancers we have from growing further and can also reverse them.

Phytonutrients called **phytates**, found particularly in whole grains and legumes, nuts and seeds, can stop polyps developing into colorectal cancer, by preventing any potential cancer cells producing the matrix metalloproteinase enzymes they need for the job of burrowing into and invading surrounding tissues.

And, lastly, Meating's cancer-causing effects aren't confined to the *presence* of baleful ingredients and recipes; it's also got a full menu of *absent* Planter anti-cancer benefits:

- Anti-inflammatory nutrients
- Antioxidant defenders against cellular stress
- DNA repair molecules
- Immune enhancers
- Estrogen- and cholesterol-binding fiber
- Angiogenesis-combatting phytates
- Phytoestrogens in soy and flax, such as lignans
- Plant proteins (low in sulfur; non-IGF-1-stimulating)
- Anti-proliferative, anti-invasive phytonutrients
- Anti-ischemic phytonutrients

Planting has been shown to prevent, halt and reverse cancer. Planting is our best defense against getting cancer; also our best chance of surviving cancer should we give it to ourselves (more likely) or get it by chance.

Eating an ordinary apple a day really does help keep the doctor away: it contains phytonutrients that improve our immune function, prevent mutations, prevent oxidation and inflammation. Of these plants' anti-cancer effects, Dr. Greger says:

> "Which steps do apples block? All of them. Anti-mutagenic, antioxidant, anti-inflammatory effects, and even immune enhancement to help clear out any budding tumors. Eat at least an apple a day."

[See: http://nutritionfacts.org/video/apples-breast-cancer/]

All whole plants are beneficial, but Amla (Chinese gooseberry), apples, flax seeds [lignans], broccoli (and other cruciferous plants) [sulforaphane], alliums [allicins (organosulfurs)], cinnamon, turmeric [curcumin], soy [isoflavones], sweet potatoes and legumes [phytates] contain particularly powerful anti-cancer nutrients: anti-mutagenic, anti-angiogenic, anti-invasive, anti-proliferative, anti-metastatic.

In the Eatiology section, I've provided a short summary of the Eatiology of how plants unfriend cancer, under the example of:

Breast cancer healed.

Melatonin suppression

Melatonin is the hormone produced by our pineal gland that's in charge of regulating our sleep patterns. Melatonin also suppresses cancer.

So, if something were to suppress the cancer-suppressor that wouldn't be good. Light pollution suppresses melatonin, leading to increased risk of breast cancer in urban women. And – this is the kind of thing that makes me love studying nutrition – blind women are benefitted by not being affected by light pollution, so they have high melatonin levels and correspondingly low risk of breast cancer. Swings and roundabouts.

What else affects our melatonin levels? Meating. All animals. The more animal muscles and milk we swallow when we're young, the greater our cancer risk later in life.

Moving on from cancer…

Amyloidosis

In Part 1A (Components), we saw that amyloids are misfolded proteins that interact with each other to form insoluble fibrils.

Here are some amyloids and the conditions in which they're implicated:

- Beta amyloid (Aβ) appears in Alzheimer's
- Apolipoprotein AI (AapoA1) in atherosclerosis
- IAPP (Amylin) (AIAPP) in type 2 diabetes
- Alpha-synuclein in Parkinson's
- Serum amyloid A (AA) in rheumatoid arthritis
- PrPSc (AprP) in transmissible spongiform encephalopathies e.g. BSE (bovine)

As I'll show later in Part 1C (Eatiology), these 6 amyloid-related conditions are animal-borne eating disorders. I'll lay out convincing evidence that atherosclerosis, type II diabetes, Creutzfeldt-Jakob disease, Parkinson's, Alzheimer's and rheumatoid arthritis are all caused by Meating, and all arrested by Planting, and, some of them, reversible by Planting (depending on how much Meater damage has been done).

Because these chronic debilitating conditions are all caused or exacerbated by Meating, the chances are very high that Meating is also responsible for the mis-folding of the proteins that characterize their accompanying amyloidosis.

It's a mistake to find amyloid fibrils or plaques appearing along with a "disease" and to think that they cause the "disease". Instead, Meating is the ur-cause of amyloidosis, atherosclerosis, ischemia, oxidation, acidosis, molecular mimicry, and on and on… all of which are the mechanisms whereby Meating trashes us.

Amyloid is in all the animals we eat, particularly the most stressed-out ones – ducks whose livers get ground up for foie gras and poultry in general.

Here follows a list of "Amyloidosis Related Diseases & Conditions" from MedicineNet.

http://www.medicinenet.com/amyloidosis/related-conditions/index.htm

"Medical conditions are often related to other diseases and conditions. Our doctors have compiled a list of ailments related to the topic of Amyloidosis. These conditions may be a **cause or symptom** of Amyloidosis or be a condition for which you may be at increased risk."

We'd understand the situation better if we saw that when Amyloidosis causes an ill-effect, Amyloidosis itself is caused by Meating, so there's a knock-on effect of one symptom domino knocking over the next.

Here's MedicineNet's list of ailments related to amyloidosis:

- Ankylosing Spondylitis
- Carpal Tunnel Syndrome & Tarsal Tunnel Syndrome
- Creutzfeldt-Jakob Disease
- Multiple Myeloma
- Peripheral Neuropathy
- Pseudogout
- Rheumatoid Arthritis (RA)
- Tuberculosis (TB)
- Diarrhea
- Congestive Heart Failure (CHF)
- Kidney Failure
- Sudden Cardiac Arrest
- Heart Failure
- Cardiomyopathy (Restrictive)

- Tongue Problems
- Alzheimer's Disease
- Orthostatic Hypotension
- Osteomyelitis
- Stem Cells
- Fatigue
- Brain Lesions (Lesions on the Brain)

Many of these conditions have a Meater Eatiology.

In later sections of this book, I demonstrate the Meater Eatiology of ankylosing spondylitis, Creutzfeldt-Jakob "disease", multiple myeloma, rheumatoid arthritis (RA), diarrhea, congestive heart failure (CHF), kidney failure, sudden cardiac arrest, heart failure, Alzheimer's "disease", fatigue and non-trauma brain lesions, although not always under these names.

Let's take a quick look at the rest:

Peripheral neuropathy, "a problem with the functioning of the nerves outside of the spinal cord," is probably caused the same way sciatica is caused: Meaters' atherosclerotic damage to the blood vessels supplying the sciatic (peripheral) nerve. Neuropathy is common among diabetics – in other words, among Meaters and Junkers.

Pseudogout, "a form of arthritis [which] results when deposits of crystals collect in and around the joints," sounds very like other Meating-induced conditions: gout, kidney stones, gallstones. It's also reminiscent of atherosclerosis, in which lethal, jagged cholesterol crystals form within and pop atheromas like weasels.

Carpal Tunnel Syndrome & **Tarsal Tunnel Syndrome**: causes listed include "obesity, pregnancy, hypothyroidism, arthritis, diabetes, trauma, repetitive work, amyloidosis, multiple myeloma, and leukemia." When we remove pregnancy, hypothyroidism, trauma and repetitive work as irrelevant, why not just say Meating? All the rest are Meater symptoms.

Tuberculosis (TB): Spread by the *Mycobacterium tuberculosis* bacterium, TB is a classic zoönosis, a disease transmitted from cattle to humans; now transmissible between humans. Most cattle herds in the USA harbor bovine TB. Need I say more?

Sarcoidosis: Who knows? Not the NIH: they call it "a disease of unknown cause that leads to inflammation." Well, we know that Meating causes inflammation, and that Planting is anti-inflammatory, so maybe there's a link there?

Restrictive cardiomyopathy, "the rarest form of cardiomyopathy, is a condition in which the walls of the lower chambers of the heart (the ventricles) are abnormally rigid and lack the flexibility to expand as the ventricles fill with blood." Hmm, abnormally rigid and lacking flexibility are the hallmarks of Meating-induced arteriosclerosis, metastatic calcification and cardiovascular dysfunction. Look: not every chronic condition is caused by Meating – there are the occasional uncommon exceptions like celiac/gluten/wheat issues which serve to prove the general Meater rule – but RC doesn't sound like one of them.

Tongue Problems: Meating causes aphthous ulcers/canker sores and oral lichen planus in the mouth; also furry white tongue and bad breath because of deranged oral bacteria. While berries stain Planter tongues and lips delightful colors.

Orthostatic Hypotension is the lightheaded feeling we get if we stand up quickly and have the blood rush out of our brainpans. I don't know its cause, and will only say that as Planters have zero to few atherosclerotic plaques, have ideal endothelial function, have zero to no cardiovascular unease or *hypertension*, I'm not sure I'd begin my search for the cause of Orthostatic Hypotension within the Planter community.

Osteomyelitis is an infection of the bone, which may or may not be Meating-related. Sometimes it occurs as a result of injury, with an open wound or fracture; sometimes as a result of an infection elsewhere in the body. Considering the source of fecal bacteria is animals, Meaters are far more prone to bacterial infections than Planters.

And **Stem Cells**. Phytonutrients such as sulforaphane, found in broccoli and other cruciferous vegetables have been shown to selectively target and destroy cancer stem cells. Chemotherapy and radiation may temporarily shrink tumors, because they target and kill only daughter cells. Phytonutrients target cancer stem cells and may return them to working order. For more on cancer stem cells, see: Natural Products on pp. 634-6, in Part 5 (Summary): *Why Animals Aren't Food.*

Almost without exception, **amyloidosis** is an outcome of Meating. We shouldn't be surprised. As we'll see, animal proteins are toxic in many different ways. Knowing that, it shouldn't come as a shock if we found that animal proteins have a penchant for misfolding themselves or a penchant for causing others to be misfolded.

Epigenetics

Low-Carb Bullshit Artists don't like the exciting new field of epigenetics. So what is it? If the LCBAs don't like it, it interests me.

Epi- means "above, on, in addition to." It's like the meta- in metaphysics. It goes beyond.

If genetics is the study of the consequences of changes or mutations in our DNA sequences, epigenetics is the study of how our genes are expressed, without any change to the DNA itself. Environmental factors can up- or down-regulate hundreds or thousands of genes, producing vastly different outcomes. Genes aren't rigid; they can be switched on and off.

Said better: *we* can switch our genes on and off. We're not helpless victims of our genetic heritage. Not only do we inherit our parents' and grandparents' DNA arrangements; we inherit their genes with switch settings positioned in the way our forebears set them. But we don't have to leave them set that way; we can change the settings (!) by eating food (yay, good!) or unfood (boo, hiss, bad!) and either boost or damage our health.

(Isn't that amazing? Wouldn't you like your nutrition counselor to tell you this fantastic news? Well, the LCBAs won't tell you, because Meating cries 'Havoc!' and lets slip the epigenetic dogs of war.)

How do we switch our genes off and on? By changing the environment around our DNA.

How do we do that? Well, we breathe, and we put stuff on our skin, but mostly… we eat.

Eating the environment is how we bring the external environment into its closest contact with our "milieu intérieur," which is how the great Claude Bernard described our innards.

(It's helpful to think of our digestive tracts as being *outside* our bodies. Nutrients have to be absorbed through the lining of our gut walls before they're truly inside us.)

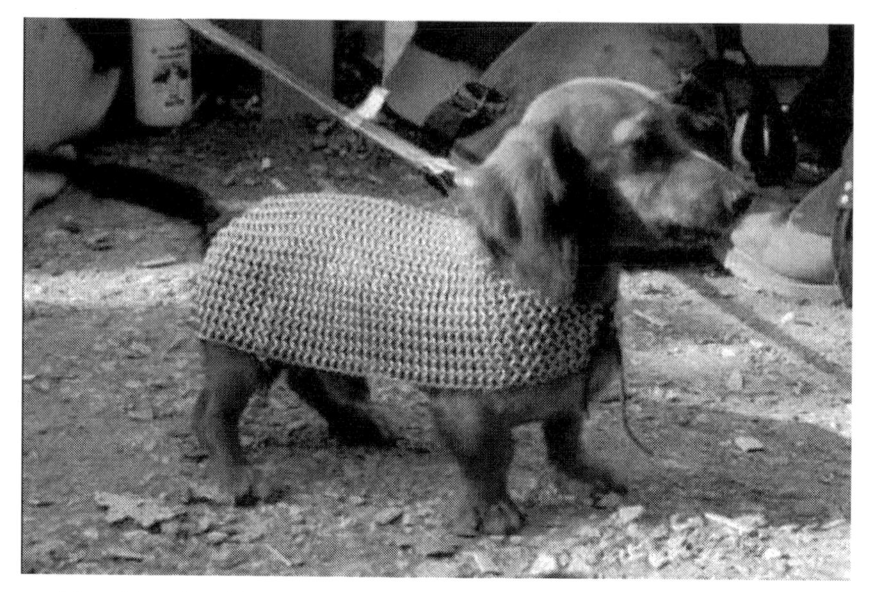

"Cry 'Havoc!' and let slip the dogs of war": http//:www.veryemotional.com

According to this paper: D M Saulnier, S Kolida, G R Gibson. Microbiology of the human intestinal tract and approaches for its dietary modulation. *Curr Pharm Des*. 2009;15(13):1403-14,

"The total surface are of the gastrointestinal system is approximately 300 to 400 m^2. Only a single epithelial layer separates the individual from enormous amounts of antigens of both dietary and microbial origin."

As mentioned before, we have <2 square meters of skin; ~100m^2 of respiratory passages; ~300 to 400 m^2 of gut, all – this part's new – backed up by ~700m^2 of blood vessels. Foods and nonfoods make up at least ¾ of our exposure to nature; more when one factors in the toxic fumes we inhale when we cook animal muscles at high temperatures.

What we eat… is the environment. (Prophetic words, in a different context, when we grok how Gaia-cidal Meating is.)

Later, under Aging, we'll hear about how Planting causes the up-regulation of a set of genes that codes for protein production, in this case an enzyme called telomerase, which leads to our chromosomes having longer telomeres (protective caps, which stop our genes from getting frayed) and us leading longer lives, and being protected against cancer-causing mutations.

Meating leads to telomere shortening, more rapid aging and shorter lifespans.

One of the most influential humans of the last millennium is Dr. Dean Ornish. He's the man who first demonstrated back in 1990 how Planting can reverse heart "disease";

Can lifestyle changes reverse coronary heart disease? The Lifestyle Heart Trial (*Lancet* 1990);

who showed in 2005 how Planting can reverse prostate cancer;

Intensive lifestyle changes may affect the progression of prostate cancer (*Journal of Urology* 2005);

and who proved in 2008 how Planting extends our lifespan through epigenetically beneficial gene expression, leading to increased enzyme activity and telomere lengthening;

Increased telomerase activity and comprehensive lifestyle changes: a pilot study (*Lancet Oncology* 2008).

Ok, but what have you done for us lately, Dr Ornish? Why should we honor you with a Nobel Prize for Medicine? All you've done is proven how to prevent or heal heart disease, stroke, cancer (and time!)... only our biggest killers. (That Ornish hasn't received a Nobel Prize, while Barrack Obama has, for Peace no less, is symptomatic of our Age.)

Planting regulates thousands of genes, using our fixed, inherited DNA words in new ways to express beautiful healthy thoughts. Meating uses the same vocab to grunt and snarl.

To me, the indisputable bedrock fact that Planting is epigenetically beneficial, while Meating is epigenetically detrimental, proves that we are best adapted to Planting. Meating is an aberration: the environment (and our genetic code!) tell us so. Animals aren't food.

Nutrigenomics

Nutrigenomics is Epigenetics, Applied. It's the nutritional manipulation of our genome. It could just as easily be called Phytogenomics, because it's all about how plants up- and down-regulate our genes beneficially. Junking and Meating aren't part of nutrigenomics: there are no processed animals or plants that are good for us in this way. None. Not ever. Some are just less bad than others.

In episode 2 of a video series called *The Truth About Cancer – A Global Quest*, available on YouTube, there's an interesting discussion of Nutrigenomics. Unfortunately, Ty Bollinger, the series director, and many of the >100 experts he interviewed seem to be Meaters, and they appear to think of Nutrigenomics as an adjunct cancer therapy, after the fact, instead of primordial prevention, before the fact. So they search out plants with powerful anti-cancer properties to reverse cancer in Meaters who're already ill, without seeing that it's the Meating that's the root cause.

Our cancer may have many different causes – genetics (only about 5% of the time), while our environment and lifestyle providing the rest – the chemicals and pathogens we expose ourselves to. Cigarette smoke, industrial sugars, alcohol, and (other) environmental toxins such as dioxins and PCBs; plus oncogenic viruses and other harmful organisms. As I'll prove later, 90% of our exposure to carcinogens comes from Meating and Junking.

Mr. Bollinger's experts get so much right, saying that cancer is a systemic problem, and that burning, cutting or chemo'ing it out locally doesn't work, because it's sure to return elsewhere, causing patients to relapse.

If only they could see that nutrigenomics *is* the answer to preventing and reversing cancer… when taken to its logical conclusion. That is, we should eat an entirely positive nutrigenomic diet – a pure Planter diet. And then, by all means, we can seek out the especially wonderful plants such as gold (turmeric), frankincense and myrrh. We don't need to resurrect special therapies, many of which the medical authorities have indeed conspired to suppress over the years – we just need to eat food.

Because it lacks a Planting foundation, *The Truth About Cancer* contains brilliance and outright stupidity, in equal measure. Only Planting allows us to tell which is which. For example, at 44.15 of episode 2, Jonathan V. Wright MD says, in response to the question: "Bio-identical hormones… do they cause cancer?" "Okay, let's see, did your own hormones cause you cancer yet? No. Bio-identical hormones are no more dangerous and no more safe than a person's own hormones…" which, as we'll see later, is not very safe at all.

Veronique Desaulniers, D.C. then says: "Breast cancer myth #1 is that women's hormones cause breast cancer… that's the biggest fallacy ever. First of all, if our hormones caused cancer, then every twenty-year-old on the planet would have cancer. So it's not our hormones."

That's just plain wrong. It can take decades for cancer to manifest. Just because 20- or 30-year-olds don't have cancer yet doesn't absolve high hormone levels. For more on the Meater Eatiology of breast cancer, and the Planter Eatiology of breast cancer prevention, skip ahead to Part 1C (Eatiology), for Breast Cancer and Breast Cancer Healed.

Dr. Desaulniers herself recovered from breast cancer, but probably not for the reasons she believes. She ate lots of whole plants and got better despite her misunderstanding the eatiology of animal hormones.

Breast cancer is largely an animal-borne eating disorder. Estrogens, whether our own or introduced, are made lethal by Meater constipation.

The Meaters who follow Mr. Bollinger's recommendations, summed up in a good publication called "22 Ways to Cancer-Proof Your Life Today," will undoubtedly benefit. The sections on household and personal care products, and the section on factory-farmed animals, are very good indeed.

However, when it comes to food Mr. Bollinger gets it spectacularly wrong.

He says: "Here's something to always remember: *If you want to live a long and healthy, cancer-free life, eat foods with a shorter shelf life*… Instead of Processed Foods Eat Whole Foods." That's outstanding. That's extraordinarily good advice… We can all benefit from this information. Bravo!

…but he doesn't know what food is. If only he thought of animals as being processed non-foods. He thinks "Whole foods are foods that exist in nature, and for the most part as nature intended. Foods such as fruits, vegetables, grains, nuts, seeds, and **animal foods including beef, fish, poultry, pork, and eggs are all whole foods**." But then he presents no evidence to support this claim about animals. We should shun them, just "as nature intended."

There is nothing natural about eating animals. Animals aren't food, and animals aren't whole: they're among the most processed things we eat.

To say, as Mr. Bollinger does, that "…if you eat animal products (i.e. meat, eggs, and milk) you must choose varieties derived from livestock and poultry raised on clean pasture rather than in commercial feedlots. This will ensure that you get the nutrients you need to steer clear of chronic diseases such as cancer," is crass. As we'll see by the end of this book, it's just plain wrong. At least he says "if."

Promoting animals as healthy because they contain omega-3 fats, while ignoring the full catastrophe of what else is in them, makes as much sense as me saying that Abrams tanks are great for peace because they're painted green, while ignoring that they're powerful weapons. We don't eat isolated nutrients, Mr. B: we eat food, which is a package deal.

Mr. Bollinger says that "chickens that forage on pasture produce eggs with rich, orange yolks that naturally contain some of the highest known levels of lutein and zeaxanthin. [Bollocks.] Both of these nutrients have been scientifically shown to protect against colon cancer." The anti-cancer part is true, but the "eggs for L+Z" story is ridiculous, as I'll show. Why eat the middle-chicken to get plant nutrients? Eating chickens and their eggs isn't a smart thing to do.

So, does Mr. Bollinger earn an A for his efforts, seeing as he's got 90% right, or does he get an F, because the 10% he gets wrong – Meating – even when garagiste and grass-fed – accounts for 90% of our cancer, and our heart "disease" and… and… and…? I'll leave it up to you to decide.

If we have a Meater mindset, we'll think this series is pretty good, and we'll benefit greatly by following its high-plant wisdom. However, it takes a Planter mindset to really cancer-proof our lives. We need to understand that eating animals is the single major initiator, promoter and spreader of cancer.

When they speak of "clean foods," in episode 6, we should realize that animals are the dirtiest non-foods we eat, by several orders of magnitude.

"The quest for the cure continues," according to this worthy Meater explorer, Ty Bollinger. The quest for the prevention is over. It's already with us: it's called Planting.

Cooking animals at high temperatures

The method we use to cook our animals can make a bad situation worse. For example, raw cows and pigs contain far fewer geronto- or glycotoxins – AGEs – than cooked ones. But then we'd run the risk of not killing potentially lethal toxic micro-organisms. Boiling produces more of these Advanced Glycation End-products, but fewer than sautéing, broiling, frying and barbecuing.

The higher temperatures we cook animals at, the quicker we die.

Recipes that contain the words Barbecuing, Grilling, Frying, Roasting or Deep frying are recipes for nutrition disaster.

For more, see under: Heterocyclic amines; Polycyclic aromatic hydrocarbons; Acrylamide

Cross-contamination

No, cross contamination isn't a sprig of parsley infesting a steak platter. Cross-contamination is what Meating can do to everyone in the world, Meaters and Planters alike. When we're Meaters, our eating addiction harms not just ourselves; it puts everyone at risk of the damage we're inflicting on ourselves.

Cross-contamination is the 2nd and 3rd hand cigarette smoke of the nutrition world.

Just as passive smokers can breathe in noxious 2nd hand cigarette fumes, and everyone can pick up the 3rd hand carcinogens that stick to indoor surfaces where people smoke, Meaters' eating habits can infect and kill innocent bystanders.

One can be a Pure Planter and still die from Meater mal-nutrition via:

- carcinogens in the smoke from animals cooked at high temperature
- toxins from animal fecal bacteria
- parasites such as worms
- animal-borne viruses
- sexually transmitted animal-borne viruses and parasites.

And, of course, cross-contamination is what we do to naturally Planter kids, when we indoctrinate them into Meating when they're not yet conscious.

Washing one's kitchen counters and one's hands, and cooking animals at über-temperatures isn't enough to prevent Meater contamination of the environment.

On a macro-level, Meating is cross-contaminating our entire natural and social environment:

- Eutrophication of lakes
- Acidification of oceans
- Species extinction
- Habitat destruction
- Climate change
- Microbial drug resistance
- Sociopathic societal violence.

Future survivors may look back at us and say: What the…? They may say: "Do you know, back in the 21st Century they used to eat animals, can you believe it?"

I just hope they don't look back at us and say, wistfully: "There used to be fellow creatures on this planet called animals, who people used to eat."

theGHOSTofBROOKLYN
Once upon a time life was so barbaric that people ate animals

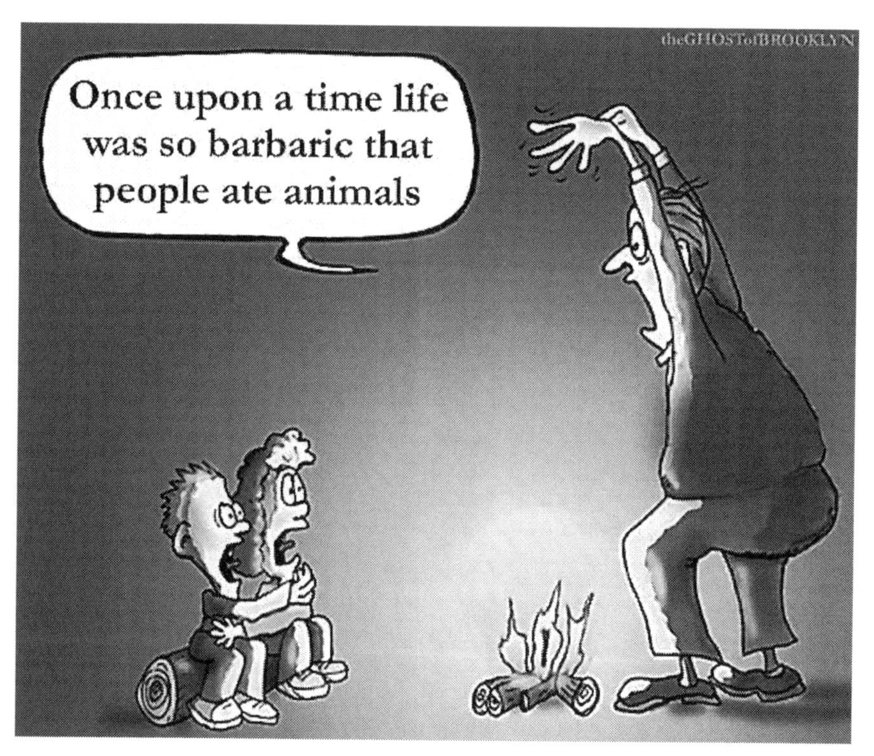

Cartoon credit: The GHOST of BROOKLYN

~

Part 1C (Eatiology): Some "Diseases" Meating Causes

So far we've looked at the COMPONENTS of animals – what they're made of – and the MECHANISMS whereby the components act to damage our health. In this section, we're going to look at the Eatiology or animal-borne causes of chronic "disease", which turn out not to be diseases, but SYMPTOMS of Meating.

The same Meater diet causes all the following conditions, via the multiple processes explained in the Mechanisms section above and expanded upon below.

If we like, we can imagine that these conditions are single players in an opposing sports team. To gain an understanding of Meating's Eatiology we're watching film clips of individual players, to see how we're going to counteract them: one player at a time. Come game (or meal) time, we'll be going up against the whole team of Meater mechanisms, working together. In reality, Meating's setting us up for all of these conditions at the same time… atherosclerosis and diabetes and dementia and… and… and… Which one arrives first is merely a matter of chance. (All the opposing team are coming at us, but only one gets credited with scoring each goal, though others will almost certainly also score later.)

Here we go:

Abdominal aortic aneurysm
MEATERS have much higher blood pressure than PLANTERS. That's because Meating stiffens and narrows our arteries, forcing our hearts to work harder to push blood around our bodies. The extra pressure, and the weakened state of the artery itself from atheromas, and the decreased flexibility of the artery due to its hardening from arteriosclerosis, often causes our mainline artery, the aorta, to stretch into a small thin balloon, which can then later suffer a blowout. It's a very quick death, I believe, from massive internal bleeding.

Sadly, Albert Einstein became a vegan too late in life to prevent or reverse this condition. It's what killed him. The smoking didn't help.

Unbeknownst to us, a million of us Americans have latent or dormant aortic aneurysms. Tick tock. Planting eases the pressure; stops the clock.

Eating animals doubles our risk of AAA; eating plants like fruits, nuts and vegetables halves our AAA risk. A million Americans have the opportunity to save our own lives by Planting.

Abdominal fat

Abdominal fat is considered the most dangerous kind of body fat; it's far more implicated in disease creation than fat carried on other parts of our bodies. This makes sense because our abdomens are where most of our organs are, and it's where digestion takes place, and our digestive tracts are our prime interface with the outside environment. Our abdomens contain our biggest link between inner and outer worlds.

Animals, in particular milk, because of the casein in it, cause increased abdominal fat storage. There are phytonutrients that decrease abdominal fat, especially in soy foods.

Accidents

Bear with me now as I make a case for Planters having fewer accidents than Meaters and Junkers. By the time you reach the end of this book, you'll have encountered hundreds of different ingredients, physiological mechanisms, pathogens and contaminants which cause Meaters to be sicker, both in body and mind, more frail and closer to death than their Planter chronological peers.

When it comes to avoiding accidents caused by others, surely Planters, being less disabled (and more conscious?) have an advantage over Meaters?

When it comes to causing accidents, don't Planters, with better agility, and superior physical and mental strength, cause fewer accidents?

I don't know… It's just a thought I'm throwing out there. Perhaps someone will do a study…

Acne

Acne doesn't exist outside of populations eating a Western diet. The billions of people who're lucky enough to be lactose intolerant (i.e., normal) don't get acne, because they don't eat or drink dairy products. They're spared the deadly assault of more than a dozen different hormones that come pre-packaged in cow's milk.

We're in no need of exogenous hormones; even in tiny concentrations they're enough to derange our subtle internal **hormone signaling system**. We don't need cows bossing our endocrine system around.

Severe acne, particularly on the back, is a very strong predictor of adult cardiovascular "disease".

Acne, back pain and erectile dysfunction are all predictors of heart attack. Why? Because they're all symptoms of the same underlying mal-nutrition.

ADHD

Attention Deficit Hyperactivity Disorder. The SAD Standard American Diet, based on animals and processed junk, packed with salt, sugar and fat, and laden with environmental pollutants, is lowering norepinephrine and dopamine levels in kids' brains. Artificial food colors in junk [oxymoron alert – if it's artificially dyed, it ain't food] are particularly damaging. The usual medical response is to pump kids full of amphetamines like Ritalin to boost the neurotransmitter levels in their brains and make them more manageable.

Exercise works better than drugs though, without negative side-effects, and acts immediately to boost norepinephrine and dopamine (besides having other positive benefits).

One study "found about a 50 to 70% increase in the odds of ADHD among children with pesticide levels in their urine common among US children." So children who eat a whole plant diet, grown veganically, shouldn't have lowered neurotransmitter concentrations to begin with; there being no disruptive chemicals like organotin or organochlorine pesticides in pure fruits and vegetables.

See also: Hyperactivity

Aggression

In "Trans Fat in Meat and Dairy," Dr. Michael Greger says: "Trans fats are bad. They may increase one's risks of heart disease, sudden death, diabetes—and perhaps even aggression. Trans fat intake has been associated with overt aggressive behavior, impatience, and irritability."

See the Golomb study on page 653 linking eating trans fats to belligerence, tetchiness and all-round Meater/Junker curmudgeonly behavior.

For more, see under: Mental health

Aging

Meaters age more rapidly than Planters. There are many mechanisms that account for this. In every case, Planting improves what Meating and Junking make worse.

1. IGF-1 levels

Animal proteins stimulate the release of Insulin-like Growth Factor #1, leading to higher concentration of this growth hormone in our blood and throughout our bodies. This stimulates faster cell division, leading to both increased cancer growth and to faster cellular aging.

Getting one's protein from animals doesn't seem like a particularly smart option… if we'd like to live a long and healthy life.

2. Oxidation

In Part 1B (Mechanisms), oxidation was compared to rusting. Oxidants age us via injury by free radicals, leading to slow-motion systems breakdown like the gradual formation of white hair and wrinkles; anti-oxidants in plants counter free radicals.

In the words of E.R. Stadtman, an NIH researcher into aging: "Aging is a disease. The human life span simply reflects the level of free radical oxidative damage that accumulates in cells. When enough damage accumulates, cells can't survive properly anymore and they just give up."

Plants 2 Animals 0.

3. Inflammation

Inflamed tissues age faster. Inflammation is a hallmark of Meating (thanks to saturated fats et al); Planting is anti-inflammatory.

4. Ischemia

Tissues that are deprived of sufficient blood flow age faster. Ischemia is a hallmark of Meating (thanks to cholesterol et al, and atherosclerosis); whole plants are anti-ischemic.

5. Calorie restriction boosts longevity

Whole-food Planters get about 10% of their energy needs from fat. The SAD (Standard American Diet), made up mostly of animals and junk, rarely comes in below 35%. Meaters eat more calories than they need; this speeds up the aging process.

Michael Greger explains how this works:

"The way caloric restriction extends lifespan appears to be mainly through the inhibition of TOR." [TOR is the so-called "aging enzyme," and TOR stands for "Target of Rapamycin."]

> "When food is abundant, TOR activity goes up, prompting the cells in our body to divide. When TOR detects that food is scarce, it shifts the body into conservation mode, slows down cell division and kicks in a

> process called **autophagy**, from the Greek auto meaning self, phagy meaning to eat, autophagy: eating one's self. Our body realizes there isn't much food around and starts rummaging through our cells looking for anything we don't need. Defective proteins, malfunctioning mitochondria, stuff that isn't working any more and cleans house. Clears out all the junk and recycles it into fuel or new building materials, renewing our cells."

See: Michael Greger's "Why Do We Age?" video, and his other fascinating material on TOR.

6. Protein restriction boosts longevity

While calorie restriction leads to greater longevity, protein restriction does the same thing, which is a good thing because starving one's self is uncomfortable and unsustainable. Whole-food Planters again get about 10% of calories from protein. Meaters rarely get less than 16%. Excess protein leads to quicker aging. So the old question, "Where do you get your protein?" should really be, "What should I eat to avoid getting too much protein?" That is, if we'd like to live longer.

Protein restriction works through the TOR pathway, in the same way as calorie restriction. Animal protein also provokes IGF-1 secretion.

7. Leucine restriction boosts longevity

It's been found that one particular amino acid accounts for most of protein's harmful aging effect. Leucine restriction works almost as well to combat aging, because leucine also accelerates aging via the TOR pathway. There's some leucine in all the things we commonly call food. There's far more leucine in animals than there is in plants – particularly in dairy and eggs, but all animals really. Practically, leucine restriction means animal restriction, unless we think that eating a hundred apples is worse for us than, say, one breast muscle from a chicken? (They have equivalent amounts of leucine.)

8. Methionine restriction also boosts longevity

Methionine restriction also slows aging. Methionine is one of the sulfur-containing amino acids found predominantly in animals. While plants abound with antioxidants, methionine is one of the many "pro-oxidants" in animals.

Increased methionine intake → increased free radical production (reactive oxygen) → increased DNA damage → more mutations → more cancer & shorter life.

(Under Breast cancer, we also see that several cancers have "absolute methionine dependency," meaning that they die when starved of methionine. I second that emotion.)

Unsurprisingly, Methionine restriction also works as an anti-cancer strategy. May low methionine be a biomarker for a healthy whole plant diet (naturally low in all four sulfur-containing amino acids)?

[See: http://nutritionfacts.org/video/methionine-restriction-as-a-life-extension-strategy/]

9. DHEA retention boosts longevity in the same way as calorie restriction

Our most plentiful steroid hormone is **dehydroepiandrosterone (DHEA)**, which boosts longevity by being an antagonist of cortisol, the so-called "stress hormone." Our DHEA levels tend to drop as we age, but calorie restriction leads to less DHEA loss. Fortunately, a Planter diet also boosts DHEA retention; one study showing a 20% improvement in less than a week. Planting is powerful.

10. The Sub-Optimal Hormone Level Theory of Aging

DHEA isn't the only hormone whose levels drop with age. Others on the decline over time include androstenedione, estrogen, melatonin, progesterone and testosterone. The theory goes that if we keep our hormone levels topped up, we'll age slower.

DHEA regulation plays a key role in maintaining optimum levels of the other steroid hormones: after conversion to an intermediary, androstenedione, estrogen and testosterone are formed.

While the steroid hormones need boosting, we need to maintain lower levels of insulin and cortisol. As we saw above, higher DHEA levels means lower cortisol levels. Planting maintains cortisol at optimum levels and, as we'll see when we cover insulin resistance and diabetes, insulin too. Meating is detrimental for both.

As for melatonin, plants make human neurotransmitters: dopamine, tryptophan, the "happiness hormone" serotonin, and melatonin. This is part of the reason why Planters experience better overall mood and improved mental health in comparison to Meaters. Now we see that Planting also provides longevity by maintaining hormones at optimal levels. Higher melatonin levels in Planters means better sleep patterns in old age, probably another reason for both improved mood and lifespan.

11. Hyperinsulinemia cuts years off our lives

Hyperinsulinemia, insulin resistance and diabetes are Meater symptoms that cause serious damage to our arteries, shortening our lives by years. If one were to list all of the physiological damage that Meating causes, they could all be included in this list of factors affecting aging. Let's just say: Meating ages us.

12. High phosphate content

The phosphorus found in animals and junk also damages our blood vessels, causing systemic damage and speeding up aging. Heme (animal) iron has the same ill-effect. Context is everything, animal or plant.

13. Telomere length and telomerase activity

Aglets are the little metal caps on shoelaces that stop them from unraveling. Our chromosomes have 'caps' too to keep our strands of genetic material from coming apart. They're called **telomeres** and, the longer they are, the longer our cells survive and the longer we live. Plant eaters have longer telomeres than Meaters. **Telomerase** is an enzyme that lengthens our telomeres. Meating down-regulates telomerase; whole plant eating increases its activity.

[D. Ornish et al. Increased telomerase activity and comprehensive lifestyle changes: a pilot study. *Lancet Oncol*, 9(11):1048-1057, 2008.]

The most aging, telomere-shortening non-foods are fishes and processed animals like lunch meats and bacon, aging DNA by 6 years and 14 years respectively.

Stress slices years off our lives by slicing nucleotides off our telomeres. Conversely, meditation and other stress relief techniques lengthen telomeres.

And, would you believe, smoking ages us? Go figure.

14. Mitochondrial efficiency

In our cells there are organelles known as mitochondria which act as our power plants. They burn glucose and oxygen to power us with ATP molecules, in a process known as oxidative phosphorylation. This high-energy system generates free radicals like **superoxide** which damage our mitochondria over time, making them less efficient and aging us.

We have an anti-aging enzyme that counters these powerful free radicals; it's known as **superoxide dismutase**. As with telomerase, Meating makes matter worse; Planting makes things better by dismantling superoxide – a 300% increase in SD action by eating whole plants.

This makes sense. As with general, systemic oxidation in 1 above… animals are full of oxidants (free radicals); plants are packed with phytonutrient antioxidants. In our mitochondria we have antioxidant enzymes to prevent oxidant damage and slow down aging.

Superoxide dismutase is also an anti-Alzheimer's and anti-cancer enzyme. Again, this makes sense, because cancer and Alzheimer's are very oxidative conditions.

When the underlying mechanism is the same, interventions on behalf of one condition benefit many others. There isn't a separate good diet for one's heart, one's brain, one's tripes… One (whole plant) diet fits all.

15. AGEs

AGEs = Advanced Glycation End-products = gerontotoxins = glycotoxins. These 'eponymous' compounds speed up aging. As shown in Part 1 (Animals, Themselves), 39 of the top 40 most aging edibles are animals. The lowest, by a country mile – and therefore the least aging – are fruits, grains and vegetables.

In "Reducing Glycotoxin Intake to Prevent Alzheimer's," Michael Greger says, too brilliantly for me to paraphrase:

> "Advanced glycation end-products in our diet may suppress sirtuin enzyme activity and play a role in age-related brain volume loss.
>
> Each of us has 6 billion miles of DNA. How does our body keep it from getting all tangled up? There are special proteins called histones, which act like spools and DNA is the thread. Enzymes called SIRtuins wrap the DNA around the histones and by doing so silence whatever genes were in that stretch of DNA, hence their name SIRtuins, which stands for silencing information regulator.
>
> Although they were discovered only about a decade ago, the study of SIRtuins has become one of the most promising areas of biomedicine,

since they appear to be involved in promoting healthy aging and longevity."

Absolutely fascinating. I wonder why info like this doesn't sneak into the Low-Carb Bullshit Artists' nutrition comic books?

[See: http://nutritionfacts.org/video/reducing-glycotoxin-intake-to-prevent-alzheimers/]

16. DNA damage

Certainly not least, damage to our DNA ages us, as seen with free radicals in #1, Oxidation above. Natural components of animals such as animal fats and animal proteins damage our DNA; the POPs (persistent organic pollutants) and heavy metals they biomagnify are added mutagens; and let's not forget the "cooked meat carcinogens" like the PAHs and HAs (polycyclic aromatic hydrocarbons and heterocyclic amines).

Planting causes orders of magnitude less DNA damage than Meating.

Like Borges' Library, this list of Meater aging mechanisms appears interminable. No doubt there are others, not covered here, but I think we're beginning to get the picture: There isn't a single aging mechanism which Meating doesn't 'win' by a landslide over Planting.

Show me a nutrition writer who says eating plants causes accelerated aging, while eating animals reverses aging, and I'll show you a crackpot with a book to sell to people "who like to hear the good news about their bad habits," as Dr John McDougall often says.

We all age and die… let's not commit slow-motion suicide by knife and fork and hasten the inevitable.

[As a whole-food vegan, I very rarely need to use a knife: spoon and fork (or fingers!) usually suffice when we eat phood. We're repaid by very rarely needing surgeons to use their knives on us, during the extra years we should live.]

Allergies

Allergens are substances that cause an allergic reaction. They can be chemicals, drugs or environmental contaminants. What's the worst allergen in America? Dairy products cause more allergic reactions than anything else. (Which is a strange thing for food to do.)

Planters also get allergies, but to a far lesser extent than Meaters. For one thing, animals bio-accumulate and –magnify all sorts of toxins in their flesh, like drug residues, heavy metals, environmental pollutants and other allergens. There are even parasitic worms in fishes that cause allergic reactions.

Plant-eating mothers give birth to children who're less susceptible to allergies, and continued planting during life confers continued protection.

Those who have nut or nightshade allergies should try becoming Planters, because various allergies can resolve as one's leaky gut mends after years of Meater abuse.

For more, see under: Atopic "diseases"

ALS

A.k.a. Lou Gehrig's disease or amyotrophic lateral sclerosis, ALS is a nasty neurodegenerative disorder that attacks the brains of middle-aged people, causing a creeping paralysis that eventually stops our breathing and kills us. There is no cure and it may affect about 1 in 400 Americans. That's a lot.

What causes it? Eating aquatic creatures like fishes and shellfishes.

How? Fishes bioaccumulate a neurotoxic amino acid called BMAA (β-methylamino-L-alanine), made by blue-green algae, which we then consume in high concentrations when eating the animals. BMAA is also found in the brains of Alzheimer's and Parkinson's sufferers.

Alzheimer's "disease"

Alzheimer's "disease", named for a physician not a patient, is set up by **arterial "disease"**, and is then complicated by the formation of **amyloid plaques** and **neurofibrillary tangles**, and then made even worse by the incorporation of **metals such as copper, iron and aluminum**.

Cholesterol is implicated both in damaging the blood-brain barrier, the delicate structure which blocks out unwanted toxins, and also causing the atherosclerotic, hypoperfused conditions in which Alzheimer's begins. Just as animal and junk fats can cause a 'leaky gut,' animal cholesterol can cause a 'leaky brain.'

This is why Planters suffer far less from this terrible condition (and from other forms of dementia) than Meaters: eating whole plants improves endothelial and blood-brain barrier function; Meating damages endothelial function, and the blood-brain barrier.

Like severe strokes, Alzheimer's may already have caused great physical damage to our brains, so the effects aren't always reversible. However, once one has Alzheimer's its progression can be slowed down by Planting. The best way to cure Alzheimer's is never to get it in the first place, and we do that by not eating animals or junk.

Our best chances of avoiding Alzheimer's is to adopt an entirely plant diet, in early in life as possible – the benefits are incremental, so the sooner, the better.

As with ALS and Parkinson's, BMAA (β-Methylamino-L-alanine), made by blue-green algae and bio-magnified in the flesh of fishes, can play a role in Alzheimer's.

The epidemiology of Alzheimer's and other forms of dementia supports the theory that Meating is causative. And, to the extent that Junking contributes to atherosclerosis and insulin resistance – the full catastrophe – epidemiology confirms their ill-effects too. It's not just the cholesterol (processed animals)… it's not just the sugar (processed plants)… it's both. Neither is food. For optimal brain health in old age, we need to start eating nothing but phyto-phood as early as possible.

Ferro- and other metal toxicities

We all need iron in our diets. The form of the iron is crucial. As we saw earlier, under Heme iron, iron from animals is dangerous to our health: we can't regulate our intake of iron from animals. Anemia is the fairly uncommon condition associated with iron deficiency; ferrotoxicity is the less well known but far more rampant state of excess iron causing the free radicals that are associated with inflammatory conditions such as diabetes, heart "disease" and cancer.

Iron, copper and aluminum build-up is common in the brains of Alzheimer's patients.

Alzheimer's – In closing…

I once had the unfortunate experience of attending a talk given at our local retirement village by a world-renowned Alzheimer's researcher. To rapturous closing applause, this eminent scientist left her audience feeling that the drug industry was on the verge of a breakthrough any day now that would make Alzheimer's a thing of the past. In response to my question, she said she thought that nutrition played a limited role in the etiology of this condition, rife in the westernized world, yet almost unknown in Planter societies.

In conversation with her afterwards, she used words which make vegans despair: "I suppose being vegan wouldn't be a bad thing, but it's **a little extreme**..."

Extreme? Her field of study is a brain-eating "disease", yet *not* eating animals is extreme?

Shazbat, as Mork used to say. How can such smart people be so dumb? Talk about a wasted professional life! This poor booby's sensitive dependence to her initial Meater condition makes any meaningful progress in her chosen career almost impossible, and... she'll never be able to hear it, unless she wakes up.

The total ignorance or ignore-ance of Planter nutrition among our predominantly Meater scientists and physicians is one of the biggest stumbling blocks we humans face in our quest for health of body and mind. The inability or refusal of physicians who do know to pass on info about the benefits of Planting to their patients is hard to stomach – claiming that patients wouldn't be able to comply with a 'draconian' diet is no excuse. It's hubris to decide for patients what they might or might not be willing to do to save their lives. Get a grip.

Amputations

Meating is the main cause of non-traumatic limb amputations... those not caused in accidents or violence such as war. Type II diabetes [much more later] is caused by eating animals and junk.

Low-Carb Bullshit Artists tell us that carbs cause an insulin release from our pancreases into our blood to deal with the glucose spike that carbs cause.

There are two things they omit. First, eating animal flesh causes as big a release of insulin as white bread. Second, not all carbs are the same and, while junk carbs do cause a rapid injection of insulin, whole-food carbs don't: they're released slowly and over a long time.

Meating and junking cause Type II Diabetes. Consequently, Meating and junking are the main reason why malnourished people are getting their gangrenous legs and arms chopped off in frightening numbers.

Pure Planting should remove T2D entirely within a month, thus preventing loss of limb and life.

For more, see under: Diabetes

Amyotrophic lateral sclerosis

See under: ALS (Lou Gehrig's disease)

Amyotrophic lateral sclerosis Parkinsonism dementia

Suggesting that they all share the same Eatiology, ALS Parkinsonism dementia is ALS, Parkinson's and Alzheimer's all manifesting together in the same brain. That the brains of all these patients can contain β-Methylamino-L-alanine (BMAA), a neurotoxic amino acid that's made by cyanobacteria and bioconcentrated in fishes' muscles, is stretching coincidence beyond breaking point.

For more, see under: ALS; Alzheimer's; Dementia; Parkinson's

Anal fissure

A torn anus that often accompanies severe constipation in children. Removing dairy products from the diet eliminates the constipation and allows for healing of painful anal fissures. Milk doesn't tear the ring out of calves. For them it's breast milk.

See also: Constipation

Angina

Angina is the frightening chest-constricting pain associated with heart "disease". Angina is a Meater condition. Planters don't get it, because we're not eating the non-food ingredients that cause it – animal fats (both trans and saturated), animal proteins and animal cholesterol – and we're not exacerbating the condition with junk containing sugar and hydrogenated vegetable oils.

For the condition known as postprandial angina:

High-fat meal → lactescence → endothelial dysfunction (impaired artery function) → decreased vasodilation → postprandial (after meal) angina.

Just one fatty meal is enough to cripple our heart's arteries, reducing their ability to flex and widen, causing an angina attack in a cardiac-compromised person… in other words, someone not a Planter.

Time for a bad joke? Newly married 80-year-olds. She says: "I gotta tell you, I've got acute angina." He says: "Your tits are great too."

For more, see under: Atherosclerosis; Lactescence

Ankylosing spondylitis

Ankylosing spondylitis is an arthritic auto-immune condition that causes chronic inflammation of the spine. Instead of treating the inflammation with TNF blocking drugs, we can eat a naturally anti-inflammatory Planter diet and prevent the formation of Tumor Necrosis Factors in the first place. Necrosis = the death of body tissue.

Primordial prevention is much better than symptom suppression.

For more, see under: Auto-immune conditions.

Antisocial Personality Disorders (ASPDs)

See under: Psychopathy and Sociopathy

Aphthous ulcers

Four times out of five, canker sores in our mouths are an auto-immune response to proteins in cow's milk like casein. If we cut dairy from our diet, there's no antigen (foreign invader) to incite antibodies to mistakenly attack and damage our oral mucosa. Simple.

Arthritis

There's two basic kinds: rheumatoid arthritis, an auto-immune condition, and osteoarthritis, an inflammatory degenerative joint condition. A Planter diet significantly improves both, once we have it. Even better, it can help prevent both from happening.

See: Osteoarthritis; Rheumatoid arthritis

Asthma

This atopic disease is also on the rise worldwide. Asthma fits the general nutrition pattern: Planting improves asthma; Meating and Junking make it worse. Particularly bad for asthma sufferers is fish consumption, fishes being the most polluted of the nonfoods.

"Intakes of high fat and sodium, and low fiber and carbohydrates are linked with asthma, while traditional and vegetarian diets are associated with lower rates."

[Michael Greger – Preventing Asthma With Fruits and Vegetables.]

Whole Planters suffer far less from asthma than Meaters.

For more, see under: Atopic diseases

Atheromas

Atheromas are the porridgy lesions that eating animals causes to form in our arteries. Eating nothing but whole plants causes these pimples to disappear over time. Dr Dean Ornish demonstrated this conclusively just over a quarter-century ago, in the 21 July 1990 edition of *The Lancet.*

Atherosclerosis

We encountered a 2012 paper by Kovacic and Fuster earlier, under MECHANISMS. This sentence is so important I'm going to repeat it, and ask you to look at it carefully:

"Atherosclerosis is an omnipresent pathology that involves virtually the entire human organism."

Once we get it, really get it, that animal- and junk-borne atherosclerosis damages our entire body, we'll understand why even "moderate" amounts of Meating and Junking (like the "moderate" terrorists the US supports in the Middle East) are dangerous to our health.

Atopic dermatitis

A.k.a. Eczema

Eczema follows the general pattern of allergic reactions: the more animals in the diet, the more eczema.

See under: Atopic "disease"

Atopic "diseases"

An online search shows atopic means "a form of allergy in which a hypersensitivity reaction such as eczema or asthma may occur in a part of the body not in contact with the allergen."

Atopic "diseases" include: asthma, eczema (atopic dermatitis), food allergies and hay fever. They're becoming ever more prevalent, doubling and re-doubling. Why? Increase in animal consumption. Mothers eating animals give birth to children more prone to childhood allergies. We don't know yet what it is in the animals; only that it's something in the animals, either themselves or contaminants.

One of my votes goes to saturated fats, which can damage the tight junctions between the enterocytes lining our gastro-intestinal tracts, allowing foreign interlopers to lope in.

Who has the most asthma? People who eat lots of sodium and fat. Meaters and Junkers.

Who has the least asthma? People who eat the most antioxidants, carbs and fiber. Planters. Fresh fruits and vegetables protect against atopic "diseases".

Autism

Are these the two worst non-foods of all? Cow's milk and fishes?

Fishes are so contaminated with mercury, no one should be eating them: the neurological damage they can cause includes autism.

Human casomorphins differ from bovine (cow) casomorphin. The human kind, in pure breast milk, produces "normal psychomotor development and muscle tone." Cow casomorphin, the kind found in infant formula, can cause "delay in psychomotor development and other diseases such as autism."

[Michael Greger: Cow's Milk Casomorphin and Autism.]

Auto-immune conditions

Each auto-immune condition is a localized physical manifestation of which the underlying cause is Meating. With the obvious exception of the gluten-associated immune response, celiac disease, auto-immune conditions are caused by "friendly fire" or "molecular mimicry" produced by the animals we eat. If the animal proteins too closely resemble the animal proteins that make up our bodies, our immune systems sometimes get confused by the similarity.

The poster child for auto-immune "diseases" is Type I Diabetes (a.k.a. insulin-dependent diabetes, because one has to supplement insulin.) There are complications including genetic susceptibility and viral infection, but the main cause of T1D is dairy consumption. There's a 17-amino acid chain in casein that mimics a similar peptide chain in the beta- or insulin-producing cells of our pancreases. Sadly, our immune systems can't tell the difference and end up wiping out our insulin-making cells.

Contentious statement #1, but one which is borne out by the facts:

The overwhelming majority of auto-immune conditions occur in response to eating animals. Meating is the underlying cause – the real disease – that causes auto-immune "diseases".

We can see that this is true: Dr Roy Swank's whole plant diet has had spectacular success against MS (multiple sclerosis.) Rheumatoid arthritis responds similarly to a diet of whole plants, as does Lupus.

Contentious statement #2:

There is only one auto-immune condition. There aren't dozens of different, separately named auto-immune "diseases". They're all immune responses to assaults by foreign proteins or pathogens appearing in our bloodstreams. Our immune systems see strangers like "Cow!" or "Pig!" that aren't supposed to be there, and so they sound the alarm and go to war. (And, as usual, it's the civilian population that bears the brunt, the "collateral damage.")

The underlying cause is the same every time. What differs is where the war takes place. In our joints it gets called 'rheumatoid arthritis.' In our nerves 'multiple sclerosis.' In our spines ankylosing spondylitis.

The names are different, but the prevention and the cure are the same every time. To avoid coming down with an auto-immune condition, or to reverse one once we have one, is relatively simple: stop Meating and Junking, and start Planting.

To treat auto-immune conditions with medications while continuing to eat animals is like taking painkillers to ease the pain of banging one's head against the wall, while continuing… to bang one's head against the wall, every mealtime.

Back pain

In the absence of mechanical damage, a symptom of Meating due to atherosclerotic narrowing or stenosis of vertebral arteries.

For more, see under: Lower back pain

Bacterial vaginosis

3 out of 10 American women get a vaginal infection each year. That's almost 50 million cases.

Why? Because of high animal intake, combined with low plant intake.

Whole plant diets, naturally rich in antioxidants like beta-carotene and vitamin C, are protective against vaginal infection.

Animals, naturally high in saturated fats, promote vaginosis. Sat fats lower the pH of the vagina, whose healthy bacteria flourish at a pH of about 4. At a more alkaline level, different 'bad' bacteria take over and cause infection.

To prevent vaginosis, we should load up on fresh fruit and veggies, and cut out animals like cows (and cow juice), chickens and pigs, and junk like cake, doughnuts and vegetable oils.

Optimal nutrition brings optimal vaginal health.

Bad breath

Bad breath or halitosis is caused by a derangement of one's sub-lingual bacteria, the micro-organisms that live under one's tongue, which take part in digestion, particularly in NO synthesis. It's caused by feeding them things they don't thrive on: animals and junk.

Birth defects

Birth defects are strongly linked to POPs (persistent organic pollutants) and heavy metals. Most of these environmental pollutants are lipophilic (fat-seeking) so they bio-accumulate in animal fat, and are then bio-magnified by the animals constantly storing more of them. To eat animals is to eat prodigious quantities of teratogenic substances. Our world has become so polluted that no one is 100% safe, but avoiding animals and junk provides the best protection.

Fishes are particularly teratogenic. To prevent birth defects, Meaters who're intending to have a child should stop Fishing at least a year beforehand. Fishes are *not* brain food.

See also under: Hypospadias; Infertility; Lower IQ; Penis size; Spina bifida

Bladder infections

Bladder or urinary tract infections come from eating chickens. True story. Other animals, too, but mainly poultry.

The bacteria that come along for the ride when we eat chickens migrate from the colon to the bladder, causing infection.

Genetic markers allowed tracking of infectious *E. coli* bacteria from farm animals to meat to mouth to colon to anus to perineum to bladder.

A vegan diet removes the possibility of infection, except through cross-contamination from kitchen surfaces and the like. No animals, no cry, mon.

For more, see under: Urinary tract infections

Blindness

There are five main causes of blindness and vision loss beside trauma: Cataracts, Diabetic Retinopathy, Glaucoma, Hypertensive Retinopathy and Age-related Macular Degeneration. Another animal-caused condition, Multiple Sclerosis, can also bring about vision loss.

Eating animals plays a central role in the Eatiology of each of these conditions, particularly through their high content of AGEs or Advanced Glycation End-products, the same gerontotoxins that accelerate aging and dementia. Ischemia, inflammation and oxidation are other Meater mechanisms involved.

At best, animals are severely lacking in the powerful sight-protective substances that are made by plants, lutein and zeaxanthin in particular.

A whole plant diet can prevent, arrest or reverse all six of these blindness-causing symptoms, bringing hope to the million-odd Americans who are blind.

See under: Cataracts, Diabetic Retinopathy, Glaucoma, Hypertensive Retinopathy, Macular Degeneration, Multiple Sclerosis.

Blood cancers

Here's a description of the three kinds of blood cancer from Leukaemia Foundation Australia:

"**Leukaemias** are cancers that affect the **blood and bone marrow**. Leukaemia starts in the bone marrow where developing blood cells, usually white cells, undergo a malignant change. The cells multiply in an uncontrolled way and crowd the marrow, affecting the body's ability to make normal blood cells. [They spell funny Down Under: they mean 'Leukemias.']

Lymphomas are a type of blood cancer that affects the **lymphatic system**. Lymphomas occur when developing lymphocytes (a type of white blood cell) undergo a malignant change and multiply in an uncontrolled way. Increasing numbers of abnormal lymphocytes, called lymphoma cells accumulate and form collections of cancer cells called tumors in lymph nodes (glands) and other parts of the body. Over time, lymphoma cells replace normal lymphocytes, weakening the immune system's ability to fight infection.

Myeloma (also known as multiple myeloma) is a cancer of **plasma cells** (a type of white blood cell) that help fight infection."

There are two lifestyle factors that are responsible for most blood cancers: smoking cigarettes and eating animals. A competing risks study showed that eating two chicken breasts carries the same risk for developing leukemia as smoking ten cigarettes. Animals and cigarettes have carcinogenic nitrosamines in common, and animal flesh also harbors mutagenic viruses and other carcinogenic substances.

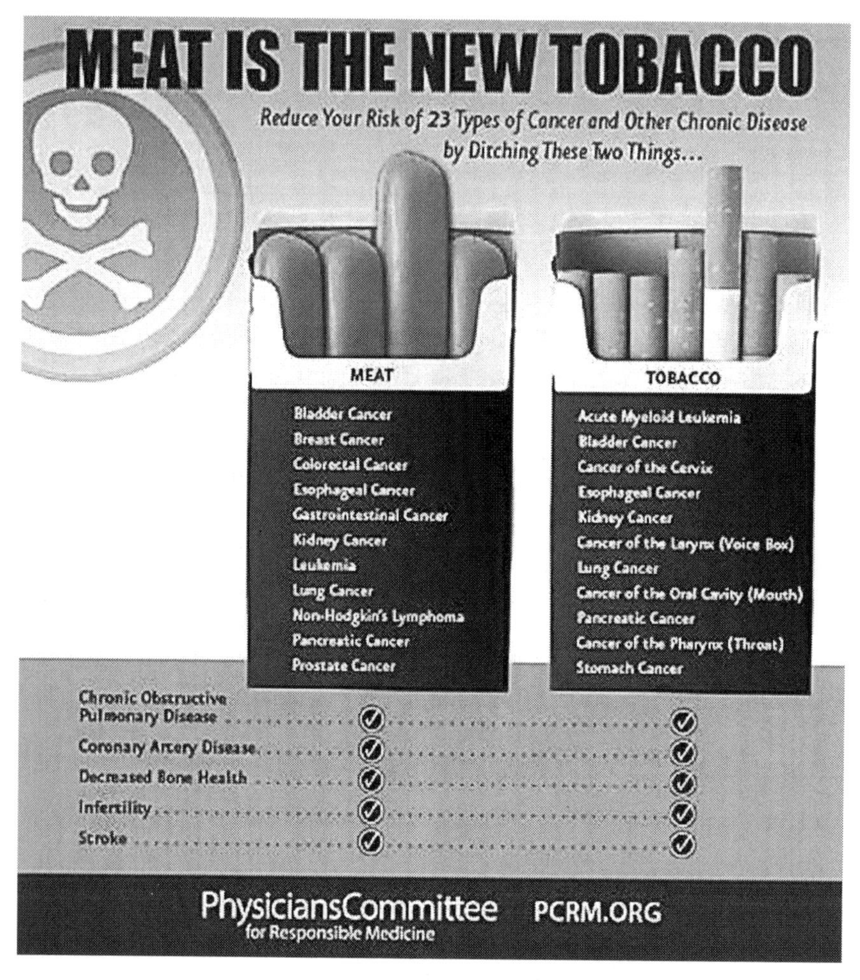

MEAT IS THE NEW TOBACCO
Reduce Your Risk of 23 Types of Cancer and Other Chronic Disease
by Ditching These Two Things...
MEAT
Bladder Cancer
Breast Cancer
Colorectal Cancer
Esophageal Cancer
Gastrointestinal Cancer
Kidney Cancer
Leukemia
Lung Cancer
Non-Hodgkin's Lymphoma
Pancreatic Cancer
Prostate Cancer
TOBACCO
Acute Myeloid Leukemia
Bladder Cancer
Cancer of the Cervix
Esophageal Cancer
Kidney Cancer
Cancer of the Larynx (Voice Box)
Lung Cancer
Cancer of the Oral Cavity (Mouth)
Pancreatic Cancer
Cancer of the Pharynx (Throat)
Stomach Cancer
Chronic Obstructive Pulmonary Disease
Coronary Artery Disease
Decreased Bone Health
Infertility
Stroke
PhysiciansCommittee
for Responsible Medicine
PCRM.ORG

Meat is the new tobacco
Source: PCRM (Physicians Committee for Responsible Medicine)

Blood cancers appear to be elective "food"- and cigarette-borne conditions, with Meaters having four times the risk of getting them as Planters.

Perhaps the "Meat is the new tobacco" graphic from Dr Neal Barnard's PCRM puts matters into perspective: Meating = Smoking.

For more, see under: Cancer; Leukemias; Lymphomas; Multiple myeloma

Blood clots

Animal eaters have high risk of heart "disease" and they're often counseled by their doctors to take a baby aspirin a day to prevent blood clots, or venous thromboses. This is pretty daft. For one thing, aspirin can be harmful to the linings of our stomachs. For another, why treat a symptom rather than the underlying cause?

Plant eaters (a) aren't at risk of heart "disease", because their diet prevents atherosclerosis and (b) wouldn't need to take aspirin anyway, because aspirin (salicylic acid) is a natural component of many plants (not just the willow bark from which it was first isolated).

Body odor

People who eat animals smell bad. Because, as the overwhelming weight of evidence will show, animals aren't food, our bodies have to contrive novel mechanisms for disposing of waste products of items they're not well-adapted to handling. The result is halitosis (bad breath) and furry tongue, when excretion takes place through the nasal passages and mouth, unpleasant body odor when waste products are ejected via the skin, and smelly feces.

(It's not that vegans' shit don't stink; it just doesn't smell so bad – it hasn't got all those excess proteins and fats and odoriferous breakdown products like hydrogen sulfide and ammonia, and it's also free of unhealthy, dead meat-eating gut bacteria.)

Bone fractures

Low-Carb Bullshit Artists cannot stand Epidemiology, the study of disease in populations. It's easy to understand why: the results of epidemiological studies are inconvenient to such people, to say the least. Sensible scientists appreciate what epidemiology can tell us: oh, like smoking cigarettes causes lung cancer, for example. There's still never been a randomized controlled trial showing the link between smoking and cancer, and nor will there ever be – it would be criminally unethical to perform such a trial. Still, we know it to be true… thanks to epidemiology. Not all smokers get cancer, but more than 90% of lung cancer patients are smokers. That's convincing evidence. And we have plausible biological mechanisms that show how.

Bone fractures – especially hip fractures – are used as a measure of bone ill-health. The more bone fractures in a population, the higher the prevalence of osteoporosis. And here's the inconvenient part for milk promoters: the countries in the world with the highest milk consumption have the highest rates of bone fractures and osteoporosis. Lactose-intolerant Asians who don't drink milk have the least.

"Correlation isn't causation!" shout the animal apologists, hell-bent on persuading us that correlation *never* implies causation (because the correlation never works in their favor). Still, what is it about the populations of New Zealand, Oz, the UK, the USA, the Netherlands and some Scandoid countries that makes their bones so brittle despite the vast quantities of dairy they consume? Why isn't the stuff working?

Bone health is more a function of load-bearing exercise than calcium intake: Use 'em or lose 'em. And, food being "a package deal," there are far healthier sources of calcium than cow's milk, the calcium from broccoli and leafy greens being twice as well absorbed, for example.

A quick aside: If a board or a council or an association or a corporation spends billions of dollars each year advertising something we eat, it's probably not food: not milk, not eggs, not flesh, not junk.

For more, see under: Osteoporosis

Bovine Spongiform Encephalopathy (BSE)
See: Mad cow "disease"

Inadequate bowel movements
Eating animals causes one's bowel movements to be infrequent and to be of much smaller volume. The increased transit time leads to longer exposure to fecal mutagens, which are best excreted quickly, and more opportunity for their reabsorption.

The smaller volume and greater density of poop produced from eaten animals leads to increased pressure being necessary to propel it along the length of the intestines. Diverticula [more later] or outpouchings in the gut wall may arise because of this high pressure or as a result of "straining at stool." Infection then becomes a possibility.

An animal diet is essentially a constipating diet. The Atkins diet, for example, requires fiber supplements to help move things along… a sure sign of its silliness.

Any way of eating that doesn't produce at least one humongous bowel movement a day is unhealthy and unnatural. An ideal diet of whole plants may even produce one bowel movement per meal. Plants take hours to digest completely; animals take days.

Once one realizes animals aren't food, it's uncomfortable looking around at people walking around full of shit that's been there for days, sometimes more than a week, animal proteins putrefying in their poor guts…

"This ain't natural, people."

As smart as we are, we don't know how to eat… and we don't even know how to poop.

BPH (Benign prostatic hyperplasia)

Enlarged prostate affects tens of millions in the West and almost no one in unwesternized parts of the world. What causes it? Eating animals, particularly chickens and eggs. Refined grains (junk) are also implicated.

What benefits BPH? Flax seeds, the onion family including garlic, and legumes, including soy.

Brain "disease"

In general, we achieve optimal brain health by maximizing the benefits of Planting, while minimizing the opposite effects produced by Meating.

Meating can use the following mechanisms to damage our brains:

- Atherosclerosis, via animal proteins, fats and cholesterol; potentiated by TMAO.
- 'Leaky brain,' caused by cholesterol damaging the blood-brain barrier
- Inflammation, via arachidonic acid and Neu5Gc.
- Oxidation, via endotoxins and heme iron.
- Amyloidosis, via animal proteins.
- Ferro- and other metal-toxicities.
- Heavy metal contamination, via animal fats.
- Contamination with persistent organic pollutants, also via animal fats.
- Molecular mimicry, via animal proteins.

(Is anyone sensing a pattern when it comes to animal proteins?)

For more, see under: Alzheimer's; Mood; Parkinson's

Breast cancer

Here's some information about the "Eatiology" of breast cancer

1. Most breast tumors are "estrogen-receptor positive." Increased estrogen exposure increases our breast cancer risk. Our bodies make estrogen from cholesterol, which cancerous cells feed on. Excess cholesterol comes from eating saturated fats, trans fats and cholesterol, found in animals and processed junk.

Our livers get rid of extra cholesterol by forming bile acids which are excreted into our tripes. If our mouth-to-anus transit time is prolonged because of inadequate fiber intake from whole plants, then our gut enterocytes may reabsorb excreted bile. These fecal mutagens may then concentrate in breast tissue at 100 times surrounding plasma levels. Bile salts exhibit estrogen-like cancer-promoting effects within the breast.

2. Cooked meat carcinogens with estrogenic effects include polycyclic aromatic hydrocarbons (PAHs) and heterocyclic amines (HAs). These arise from cooking animal muscles at high temperatures, such as broiling, frying or barbecuing. Acrylamide, a product of deep-fried carbs like chips or fries, may also be carcinogenic.

3. Earlier menarche in girls and later menopause in older women (brought about principally by the intense hormone burden of dairy products) lead to longer lifetime estrogen exposures and consequent higher risk of breast cancer. (The appalling consequences of early, immature sex include STDs, teen pregnancies and abortions in mind-numbing numbers.)

4. IGF-1 (insulin-like growth factor-1) is a growth hormone secreted by the liver when we eat animal proteins. IGF-1 tells abnormal cells to grow, multiply, and spread.

5. Neu5Gc is a so-called "inflammatory meat molecule" which breast cancer cells use to create the inflammation that promotes their own growth.

6. Breast cancer cells have "absolute methionine dependency." They die without it. This sulfur-containing amino acid (and its metabolite, homocysteine) are found mostly in animals.

7. Animal fats bio-accumulate and bio-magnify environmental toxins and heavy metals.

I could go on, but how much is enough?... Nitrosamines and sundry viruses are other animal-borne promoters of cancer in general. And heme iron and arachidonic acid, like Neu5Gc, cause immense amounts of inflammation, a condition in which breast cancer thrives.

The take-home message? To avoid breast cancer, we should avoid eating animals and processed junk.

For more, see under: Constipation

Breast cancer healed

Here's an update of a 300-odd-word piece I wrote for my local newspaper, encapsulating how Planting slaps breast cancer around.

"Eating Ourselves Healthy #19: Breast cancer, part 2

How can we chop our breast cancer risk – or boost our survival odds – not by a paltry half, but by a spectacular 90%?

Here's an incomplete list of whole, unprocessed, high-fiber, anti-inflammatory, antioxidant, phytochemical-packed foods that repel breast cancer in powerful ways:

1. Flax seeds. Lignans are plant- or phyto-estrogens. One gets 8 times more of these polyphenols from flax seeds than the next best food, sesame seeds. A tablespoon or two a day of ground flax may halve one's risk of breast cancer.

2. Sunflower and pumpkin seeds are great. They probably work via their cholesterol-lowering phytosterols.

3. Nuts, including peanuts, are outstanding, for more than their high fiber and magnesium content, as are black and other beans.

4. Speaking of beans, soy consumption is part of the reason Eastern women historically had miniscule breast cancer rates. The isoflavones in soy are phytoestrogens, which are also spectacular at preventing ovarian cancer.

5. Mushrooms. Bog-standard white buttons are best. Aromatase is the enzyme cancer cells use to create their own estrogen – mushrooms are powerful aromatase inhibitors. Strawberries and grapes work well too.

6. Seaweed. Nori and dulse are effective at lowering estrogen levels.

7. Curcumin, the multi-pathway-triggering or 'promiscuous' phytonutrient in curry-spice turmeric, may be one reason why India has such low cancer rates.

8. Teas, especially green tea without milk (or white tea with lemon) are strongly protective against breast cancer. Perhaps it's the theanine?

9. Fruits, especially berries, combat DNA damage, and strawberries also block breast cancer cell growth. Apples, particularly their peels, are anti-mutagenic.

10. Two classes of vegetable are absolute cancer nemeses: the sulforaphane-packing crucifers – broccoli, cabbage, cauliflower et al – and the allicin-wielding alliums – garlic, onions, leeks, like that. (For best results, these heat-sensitive-enzyme-activated foods should be chopped or blended half an hour before cooking.)

Each of these whole foods is powerful on its own; when combined, their synergy has the power to blast breast cancer to smithereens."

Dang! I didn't mention sweet potatoes… or… or… (You get the picture.)

For more, see: Natural Products That Target Cancer Stem Cells, p. 634.

Butcher's warts

People who handle dead animals are prone to a contagious viral skin condition known as butcher's warts. The viruses in question may be related to HPV (human papilloma virus), the virus known to cause cervical cancer. And, indeed, the sex partners of butchers are at far greater risk of cervical cancer than regular people.

Calories

There's far more energy (as measured in calories) in animals and junk than there is in whole plants. Also, animal calories are more weight gain-causing than plant calories. This is because of the absence of the thermogenic effect, which causes Planters to expend more energy in heat. There is no such thing as a "meatobolic advantage." Plant calories are to be preferred.

Cancer

Cancer is one of the scariest words in the dictionary. Carcinoma and malignant neoplasm aren't pleasant either.

Would you feel better if I told you that most cancers are caused by an eating disorder, more than double what smoking does to us (the #2 cause)? That, if we act in time, we can prevent, stop and reverse most cancers by (1) not eating any animals, (2) not consuming any junk (which includes alcohol and tobacco smoke), (3) eating whole plants and (4) changing our lifestyles to include plenty of exercise, sunshine, relaxation, peace, fresh air and clean water?

Obviously even plant nutrition can't fix the ~5-10% of cancers that are genetically ordained… *only* the ~90-95% of cancers that are caused by eating non-foods and other behavioral quirks like smoking and drinking. (And yet epigenetics shows that even genetic traits aren't destiny.)

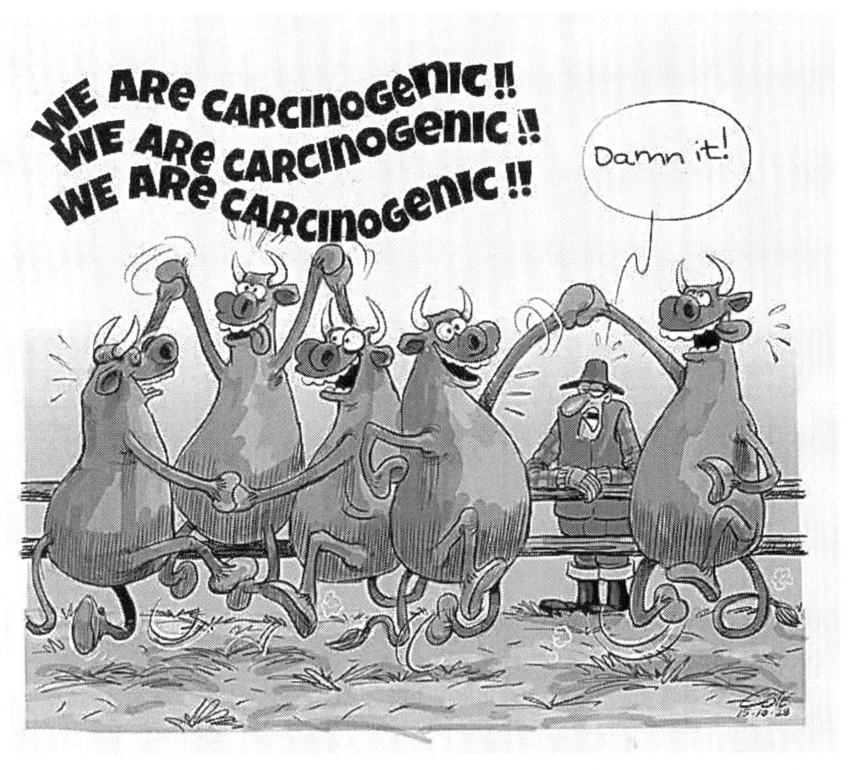

Cartoon courtesy of Andre Phillipe Côté, Quebec, following IARC's 26 October 2015 announcement of the carcinogenicity of animal flesh, particularly 'processed meat' and 'red meat.'

Yes, environmental carcinogens are often to blame: all the more reason not to put them inside our bodies by eating the animals that bio-accumulate these toxins in their flesh and secretions. By far our greatest interaction with the environment comes through what we eat, followed by the air we breathe, with what falls on our skin a miniscule third.

(Flensed and steamrollered flat, we have about ~2 m^2 of skin, ~100 m^2 of airways in our lungs and ~300-400 m^2 of gastro-intestinal tract cells.)

~~Food~~borne cancer kills millions of people worldwide every year. Most of these deaths are preventable through eating a proper human diet.

The scourge or plague or pandemic of cancer is a Western pastime; a lifestyle choice of affluent societies – it doesn't exist in populations that don't eat animals and junk.

We all have cancer cells growing in us all the time… the trick is not to promote their growth. The trick is to live so long that we die *with* harmless little cancerous growths, not *from* humungous metastasized tumors riddling our bones and lungs and other organs.

Trust me: non-genetic cancer is an elective symptom of the underlying disease, which is the eating of animals. (How can I be sure? Because Dean Ornish and others have reversed prostate cancer using a whole plant diet. Other cancers too. Also heart "disease". Also aging. It's all connected.)

Here's a crucial thing we need to know about cancers. We've been told that there's breast cancer and colorectal cancer and brain cancer and pancreatic cancer and penis cancer and… and… and… This isn't quite true.

There's only cancer. And some tissues, like breast and prostate, are more susceptible to damage than others.

Follow me here: Cancer isn't a cause of anything; it's the result of something. Okay? That means that cancer isn't the disease. Cancer is a symptom of a life out of balance. So all the differently named cancers are actually local manifestations of an underlying systemic disease or cause. We don't die from our primary cancers, where they start… we die from secondary cancers, which have metastasized from elsewhere.

As with auto-immune conditions, cancer is given a different name each time it's sighted. (As might happen if hundreds of birdwatchers were to give different names to the same bird species if they weren't to communicate with each other.)

The lifestyle modification that reverses one kind of cancer is the same one that can reverse another. (And the same one that routinely reverses atherosclerosis and type II diabetes and hypertension and… and… and…)

The anti-cancer lifestyle is Planting, with a capital P. Meating and, to a lesser extent, Junking cause cancer; Planting can prevent it, stop it in its tracks, heal it.

Most cancer is nothing more than a severe form of "food" poisoning.

So, take heart, dear human: eating human food can heal us of our inhumanely caused condition.

That's all for now, under the general heading of cancer. I'll follow tradition by writing about some individual cancers under their separate headings. Please remember, though, that while the mechanisms involved in their causation may differ, their Meater Eatiology is the same… and so is their Planter remedy.

Candida

According to the National Institutes of Health, "Candida is the scientific name for yeast. It is a fungus that lives almost everywhere, including in your body. Usually, your immune system keeps yeast under control. If you are sick or taking antibiotics, it can multiply and cause an infection.

Yeast infections affect different parts of the body in different ways:

- Thrush is a yeast infection that causes white patches in your mouth.
- Candida esophagitis is thrush that spreads to your esophagus... It can make it hard or painful to swallow.
- Women can get vaginal yeast infections, causing itchiness, pain and discharge.
- Yeast infections of the skin cause itching and rashes.
- Yeast infections in your bloodstream can be life-threatening." [Systemic infections are called candidemia or invasive candidiasis.]

[https://www.nlm.nih.gov/medlineplus/yeastinfections.html]

Who gets candida infections?

Mainly the very old, the very young, people with AIDS, people who're undergoing chemotherapy and people who're taking antibiotics. And diabetics. In other words, **people with suppressed immune systems and disturbed microbiomes** (a.k.a. intestinal bacteria or gut flora).

Well, get this: **Meating and Junking mess up our gut flora**. And **Meating and Junking compromise our immune systems**.

See: Deranged Gut Flora for a full discussion of this topic.

Animals and Junk are antibiotics! They kill our beneficial microbes; through their presence, and through their total absence of fiber.

Candida albicans (and others) are normal members of a healthy microbiome. It's perfectly natural to have these yeasts in us. Killing off the beneficial bacteria which keep yeasts in check is what causes candida infections.

When we pervert our colon microbiome by not eating a high-fiber diet, and, in so doing, stop producing butyrate and the other short-chain fatty acids that feed the peace-keeping bacteria such as *F. prausnitzii* that maintain the protective mucus barrier in our colons, maintain the tight junctions between colon wall cells (i.e. prevent leaky guts), and boost the population of T_{reg} cells in our gut walls, which in turn regulate our immune function, prevent inflammation and maintain optimal levels of beneficial bacteria within the gut cavity… then quiescent yeasts can go on a rampage, penetrating our leaky guts, entering our blood and causing systemic infections.

What to do if we've given ourselves candida?

We need to re-establish optimal immune function and restore peak intestinal health, including getting rid of leaky guts and repopulating our colons with friendly bacteria.

How do we do that? Not with special PRObiotics; with PREbiotic high-fiber whole plants. Planting has multiple benefits. Coconuts, for example, contain caprylic acid, which pokes holes in yeast cell walls.

But yeasts feed on sugar, so how can we eat all that sugar in fruit? Okay, just this once, *maybe* we need to tone down the fruit consumption initially. Only maybe, because fruits are full of beneficial fiber. And *maybe* we need to take an antifungal drug for a month to get things under control. *Maybe.*

We *definitely* need to cut out all Junking. No industrial, processed, fiber-free sugars, meaning nothing with table sugar or high-fructose corn syrup in it. Nothing that comes from a box with a list of ingredients. Nothing fast. We're doing this to stop the yeasts from multiplying.

Then, to remove the underlying problems of depleted gut flora, suppressed immune systems and leaky guts, we *definitely* need to stop all Meating. Meating produces hydrogen sulfide gas, stuffs up the colon's pH, kills our beneficial bacteria, damages intestinal tight junctions, sets off an immune response and causes inflammation. (Animals aren't food.)

What's left? What we should have been doing in the first place to prevent candida overgrowths – Planting, the original high-fiber, gut flora-friendly, immune system-maximizing whole plant diet. When we cut out the 'meat + sweet' collaboration of Meating and Junking, and eat nothing but whole plants, candidiasis subsides, and normal service resumes.

Cardiac arrest

Heart failure. Sudden Cardiac Death (SCD) is what happens to roughly half of all men and 2/3 of all women who suffer cardiac arrest for the first time. This is an elective Meater condition.

Cardiovascular "disease" ~ heart "disease" ~ stroke

Cardiovascular "disease" involves our heart (or cardium) and our vasculature, or blood vessels. Stroke, or cerebrovascular "disease" – a failure of the brain's blood supply – is included under cardiovascular "disease".

CVD is a foodborne illness. Or it would be if what causes cardiovascular "disease" were food. CVD is a nonfood-borne illness. It's the result of eating animals and other junk. It's a zoönosis. If animals were food, they wouldn't cause cardiovascular disease. QED.

Cholesterol is the single necessary building block for the creation of the atheromas and emboli that lead to heart attacks and strokes. Animals are the vehicle of blood cholesterol-raising dietary cholesterol, saturated fats and trans fats, as well as cholesterol-potentiating carnitine and choline.

Pure plant eating is anti-atherosclerotic, anti-ischemic and anti-inflammatory. Pure plant eating reverses cardiovascular "disease".

The following is about par for the course when Meaters are doing the writing. We won't hear much about prevention, because prevention entails taking up Planting and giving up Meating and Junking.

This is a piece from the American Heart Association's website, called "What Is Cardiovascular Disease?" which can be found at http://www.heart.org/HEARTORG/Caregiver/Resources/WhatisCardiovascularDisease/.

"Heart and blood vessel disease — also called heart disease — includes numerous problems, many of which are related to a process called atherosclerosis… a condition that develops when a substance called plaque builds up in the walls of the arteries. This buildup narrows the arteries, making it harder for blood to flow through. If a blood clot forms, it can stop the blood flow. This can cause a heart attack or stroke."

How do you like that? A "substance called plaque builds up in the walls of the arteries," they say, without mentioning that it can't build up if we don't supply the cholesterol from which the 'substance called plaque' is made.

"A heart attack occurs when the blood flow to a part of the heart is blocked by a blood clot. If this clot cuts off the blood flow completely, the part of the heart muscle supplied by that artery begins to die. **Most people survive their first heart attack** and return to their normal lives to enjoy many more years of productive activity."

That's very peculiar, because it doesn't agree with the AHA's own findings. "A Report From the American Heart Association - Heart Disease and Stroke Statistics 2010 Update" by D Lloyd-Jones et al (*Circulation* 2010; 121: e46-e215) says: "50% of men and 64% of women who die suddenly of CHD [coronary heart disease] have no previous symptoms of this disease" and "the estimated average number of years of life lost… is 15."

So, actually, no, the AHA's own 2010 paper tells us "**most people [don't] survive their first heart attack**…" We succumb to Sudden Cardiac Death, about half of us men, and almost two thirds of us women, death being the very first symptom we're given to let us know we have heart "disease".

"But having a heart attack does mean you have to make some changes," the AHA website continues. "The doctor will advise you of medications and lifestyle changes according to how badly the heart was damaged and what degree of heart disease caused the heart attack."

And this really tees me off: "But having a heart attack does mean you have to make some changes." Really? Why wait until we've sustained potentially irreversible heart muscle damage before making changes? Why roll the dice? Why not promote Planting, to make it impossible for us to have heart attacks or strokes because we're eating no harmful animal substances?

And this takes the cake: "The doctor will advise you of medications and lifestyle changes according to how badly the heart was damaged…" Really? The same doctor who didn't advise us to prevent our heart attack by Planting, we're now going to trust this schmuck to fix us up after their negligence or ignorance or Meater bias prevented their telling us how to prevent the life-threatening condition we've been lucky to survive?

God help us, for the American Heart Association is supposed to be an oracle when it comes to heart "disease", yet their description of cardiovascular "disease" doesn't contain word one on prevention of our biggest killer – heart attacks – and our second leading killer – strokes. We've known for a quarter century now: we can prevent our two most lethal eating disorders with a pure plant diet (Ornish et al, *Lancet* 1990).

How bad is Meating for our hearts? Pregnant mothers with high cholesterol levels can cause heart "disease" in the beloved unborn fetuses they're carrying.

"...early atherogenesis is prevalent in human fetal aortas, and... it is greatly enhanced by maternal hypercholesterolemia..."

C Napoli et al. Fatty streak formation occurs in human fetal aortas and is greatly enhanced by maternal hypercholesterolemia. *J Clin Invest.* 1997 Dec 1;100(11):2680-90.

As says the President of the American College of Cardiology, Dr. Kim Williams: "There are two kinds of cardiologists: vegans, and those who haven't read the data." The AHA should start reading their own data.

Cataracts

According to the NIH: "A cataract is a clouding of the lens in the eye that affects vision. Most cataracts are related to aging. Cataracts are very common in older people. By age 80, more than half of all Americans either have a cataract or have had cataract surgery."

They make it sound as if cataracts develop naturally with age. Maybe that's the case in the US where the overwhelming majority of us eat lots of junk and animals, but it's not true in traditional societies that eat no junk and hardly any animals. Residents of the Blue Zones, for example, stay healthy and vital, and keep their eyesight way past their 80s. Optometry isn't a booming business among the vegans in Loma Linda, California.

Cataracts form as the result of mal-nutrition. This form of blindness is an eating disorder, entailing a deficiency in plant nutrients.

According to the Egg Nutrition Center website, "Both lutein and zeaxanthin are *carotenoids* called *xanthophylls*, yellow-orange plant pigments. These carotenoids have been shown to reduce the risks of cataracts and age-related macular degeneration, the leading cause of blindness in those 65 and older. **Lutein and zeaxanthin accumulate in the eye's lens** and in the macular region of the retina. Scientists believe high levels of lutein and zeaxanthin in these areas may protect the eye from damage due to oxidation.

Lutein and zeaxanthin are commonly found in dark-green leafy vegetables, such as spinach and kale, and are well-absorbed from egg yolk. A Large egg yolk contains 166 mcg of lutein and zeaxanthin."

Thanks for the info, dear eggheads.

Now, it's recommended that we eat about 10,000 micrograms of lutein + zeaxanthin a day to maintain eye health. And the ENC has told us that L+Z are "well-absorbed from egg yolk." Let's go ahead and assume that 100% of these plant nutrients are absorbed from the eggs of the supplement-fed middle-chickens. Dividing 10,000 by 166 mcg gives 60.24. Wow, that's a sales bonanza for egg producers, if people follow that advice!

This would be the most amazing marketing ploy of all time, if people were to eat eggs to meet their daily requirement of two plant nutrients: we'd all have to eat 60 ¼ large eggs every day… or maybe 40 jumbos. Congratulations, fellahs. You're making a good case for phytonutrients…

But you're not making a good case for eggs. No one is ever going to be able to rely on eggs – with their pathetically low concentrations of phytonutrients – any nutrients! – to get what we need.

Really, are you this desperate? Is this the best reason you can come up why people should eat your toxic little cholesterol and *Salmonella* bombs? Just one egg takes us close to our daily recommended intake of cholesterol (which is pretty crazy, frankly, advising any intake at all). Can you imagine what 60 would do to us? Even Cool Hand Luke couldn't eat that many.

50g of kale – less than 2oz – provides 10,000 mcg of lutein and zeaxanthin… without the "full catastrophe" of animal fats, animal proteins and cholesterol.

Thank you muchly for drawing our attention to these vital phytonutrients, dear Meaters – you've done a public service there – but now it's back to the drawing board for you, I think.

To show you just **how abysmal eggs are at supplying the very nutrients the Egg Nutrition Center has chosen to highlight**, here's a list of the top plant sources of L+Z from the U.S. Department of Agriculture, Agricultural Research Service. 2010. USDA National Nutrient Database for Standard Reference, Release 23. Nutrient Data Laboratory Home Page:

Kale, the top performer (and they were using frozen kale, not fresh), contains 25,606 mcg of lutein + zeaxanthin per cup. Ladies and gents, that's the same amount of L+Z as is in 154.3 large eggs. In just one cup.

NDL #	Description	Weight (g)	Measure	L+Z (μg)
11791	Kale	130	1.0 cup	25606
11461	Spinach	214	1.0 cup	22630
11575	Turnip greens	164	1.0 cup	19541
11765	Chard, swiss	175	1.0 cup	19276
11164	Collards	170	1.0 cup	18527
11577	Turnip greens and turnips	163	1.0 cup	15537
11271	Mustard greens	140	1.0 cup	14560
11781	Cress, garden	135	1.0 cup	11343

Lutein+zeaxanthin content of foods. USDA National Nutrient Database

For their health's sake, I hope there's no one out there eating 154 eggs *a year*, but there probably are. If people average an egg a day, then that one cup of kale – something I easily eat in one meal – represents 5 months of egg eating. Just imagine how badly our arteries are getting gunged up, the harm that's being caused to our eyes by ischemia, inflammation and oxidation, and the deposits of drusen debris, far outweighing the benefits of the pitiful amount of *plant nutrients* we're receiving.

The marketing of eggs to preserve vision is fatuous beyond belief. Just how bad are eggs for us if this is their best sales point?

Cataracts are the leading cause of blindness worldwide. I should say the leading *proximate* cause. I wouldn't go so far as to declare definitively that Meating is the only cause of cataracts, smoking and radiation also taking their toll, but…

The more animals we eat, the greater our risk of cataracts. Vegans have the lowest risk; carnivore eat-alikes, the highest; with those wishy-washy vegetarians and flexitarians somewhere in between. Those with diabetes – another Meater malady – are at increased risk of cataract formation.

"Have you no sense of decency, sir? At long last, have you left no sense of decency?"

That's what Joseph Welch said to Senator Joseph McCarthy, effectively ending the Washington Communist Witch Hunt of the '50s. It's what someone should say to the Egg Marketing Board.

Incredible! Indeed. The incredible indigestible egg.

Cellulite

The fancy name for cellulite is gynoid lipodystrophy. It's the lumpy, bumpy, dimpled-like-a-golf-ball look that butts and thighs can get when they store excess fat.

Its etymology is [Gr. Gyne- Related to the female form + lipo- fat + G. dys-, bad, difficult, + trophē, nourishment]. It's a result of defective fat metabolism.

Wikipedia says: "Cellulite (also known as *adiposis edematosa*, *dermopanniculosis deformans*, *status protrusus cutis*, *gynoid lipodystrophy*, and orange peel syndrome) is the herniation of subcutaneous fat within fibrous connective tissue that manifests topographically as skin dimpling and nodularity, often on the pelvic region (specifically the buttocks), lower limbs, and abdomen. Cellulite occurs in most post-pubescent females. A review gives a prevalence of 85%-98% of women, indicating that it is physiologic rather than pathologic. It can result from a complex combination of factors ranging from hormones to heredity."

Hormones and heredity… Not diet then? What happened to dystrophy?

When our Wikipediaologists say 'because it happens 85 to 98% of the time; therefore it must be natural and normal, and not something wrong,' I think they're suffering from Meater over-reach.

Hell, that's like saying that because 98% (or whatever) of the (Meater) population has a total cholesterol level above 150, that must be healthy.

They're wrong on both counts.

Planters naturally have total cholesterol below 150 and LDL cholesterol below 70, without going on a restrictive diet to do it – the only restriction is to eat food. Phood.

Planters also tend not to get cellulite. Which is what one would expect from the only sub-group of the population that have optimal BMIs, coming in at about 23, compared to about 28 for Meaters; a difference of 15-odd kilos (> 35 pounds).

I don't think we have to look very far to find the 2 to 15% of the population who don't have cellulite. Planters are naturally slender. Why would slender people suffer from cellulite?

Cervical cancer

Animals are full of wart viruses, particularly pigs. Butchers handle lots of dead animals. Butchers' sex partners are in great danger of cervical cancer. To have safe sex, the kind that doesn't cause cancer of the cervix, we should choose partners who don't touch dead animals.

Another vector of this sexually transmitted cancer is Human Papilloma Virus (HPV). Not all HPV infections lead to cancer. Planting leads to improved immune protection, and thus greater viral clearing and decreased viral load than Meating does, meaning far less persistence of the virus in Planters, and consequent lower cancer incidence.

The Planter diet in general (because of the phytates in grains, legumes, nuts and seeds) and, in particular, amla (Indian gooseberries), broccoli, chamomile tea, green tea, raspberries, strawberries and sweet potatoes are all protective against cervical cancer.

Planting, a source of antioxidants and other anti-carcinogens, causes Planter women to have far fewer cervical and all other cancers than Meater women.

Fact.

The "Cheese Effect"

In their paper, **Hypertensive crisis and cheese** (*Indian J Psychiatry*. 2009 Jan-Mar; 51(1): 65–66), T. S. Sathyanarayana Rao and Vikram K. Yeragani write [with my emphases]:

"The **tyramine** connection was discovered by a British pharmacist whose wife was taking a monoamine oxidase inhibitor (MAOI). He noticed that every time they had a meal with cheese, she would get a severe headache. **Cheese, especially aged cheese, contains substantial amount of tyramine**. For this reason, persons taking MAOI antidepressants are cautioned to avoid foods that are rich in tyramine so that the hypertensive crises can be avoided… **In majority that had the reaction, cooked or raw cheese was the precipitating agent. Increases in blood pressure (BP) ranged from 160/90 to 220/115 mm Hg.** The onset of the episode was usually one to two hours after the food intake. **Headache was the main symptom associated with heart pounding and palpitations and the complications included subarachnoid hemorrhage, hemiplegia, intracranial hemorrhage, cardiac arrhythmias, cardiac failure, pulmonary edema, and death.**"

The authors conclude: "For clinicians, the differentiation of true hypertensive crises from rebound headaches caused by MAOI-induced postural hypotension is **important to treat the hypertensive crises early**." In other words, our doctors should act quickly when we present with hypertension…

Or we could stop eating animals already and avoid that tricky little complication called death.

Child neglect and child maltreatment

If, as we'll understand by book's end, animals aren't food – and especially not for infants, whose digestive tracts are still developing – what can one call the withholding of human breast milk and, later, pure plants, except child neglect, and what can one call the feeding of animals to infants, particularly the milks from other species, except maltreatment? (Sexual abuse of children can only happen among those who commodify animals.)

Choking

9 will get us 10 that if we're choking to death it's on a gobbet of animal flesh, not a banana. Here's a valuable YouTube video we should watch if we're practicing Meaters. It shows in 30 seconds how to perform the Heimlich Maneuver on ourselves, in case we ever choke on a chunk of animal while we're alone.

[Jeff] Goldblum Teaches Self-Heimlich: https://www.youtube.com/watch?v=bKnHdICifuw.

Chronic "diseases"

Acute conditions are those that have a single cause and they happen in one fell swoop. Examples are infections and injuries like breaking one's arm. Their etiology is relatively simple; there's an apparent cause-and-effect relationship between agent and outcome.

Modern medicine is absolutely brilliant at dealing with injuries and infections. For now. We'll talk again in 20 years to see if what the discoverer of penicillin, Alexander Fleming, warned has come true: that we would lose antibiotics by overusing them. Animal agriculture seems to be achieving that sorry outcome in a hurry.

Unlike acute conditions, chronic illnesses are the result of multiple exposures or assaults over a long period of time. They're lifestyle issues. My thesis throughout this book is that we can't talk about chronic diseases, because they're symptoms of underlying causes, most often Meating and Junking. Smoking, drinking and being couch potatoes, too.

Included in a list of chronic diseases would be such conditions as cardiovascular disease, diabetes, hypertension, stroke and dementia. In all of these cases, the repetitive blow is a meal of animals.

A vegan diet wipes out type II diabetes in less than a month, almost every time. Hypertension vanishes on a whole plant diet, also in a matter of weeks or months. And, as Dean Ornish and company proved back on 21 July 1990 with their Lifestyle Heart Trial, published in *The Lancet*, coronary artery disease too is a reversible, elective non-disease. It's an eating disorder. It's a form of mal-nutrition. Eating real food – whole plants – can prevent, arrest or reverse most chronic conditions; the exceptions being strokes or hearts attack or dementias that have caused too much irreversible tissue damage.

Chronic diseases are not.

Not what? They're not diseases. They're the symptoms or outward manifestations of the underlying cultural diseases known as eating animals and animal agriculture. Those who're able to cast off the shackles of Meater cultural programming may achieve true peak health.

Cirrhosis

The Mayo Clinic website defines cirrhosis as: "a late stage of scarring (fibrosis) of the liver caused by many forms of liver diseases and conditions, such as hepatitis and chronic alcohol abuse. The liver carries out several necessary functions, including detoxifying harmful substances in your body, cleaning your blood and making vital nutrients.

Cirrhosis occurs in response to damage to your liver. The liver damage done by cirrhosis can't be undone. But if liver cirrhosis is diagnosed early and the cause is treated, further damage can be limited. As cirrhosis progresses, more and more scar tissue forms, making it difficult for the liver to function (decompensated cirrhosis). Advanced cirrhosis is life-threatening."

The classic cause of cirrhosis is overuse of the classic vegan Junk: alcohol. To add Meater-induced atherosclerosis to Junk-compromised livers is to fight fire with aviation fuel. Good luck with that – Meating is why non-alcoholic fatty liver "disease" is now more common than alcoholic.

Intermittent claudication

"Claudication is pain and/or cramping in the lower leg due to inadequate blood flow to the muscles." It's a Meater condition brought on by atherosclerosis, stenoses and peripheral artery "disease".

Colon cancer

See under: Colorectal cancer

Colorectal cancer

Our 2nd leading cause of cancer death, after lung cancer. So, Junking with tobacco's #1; Meating's #2.

(Sorry, but my infantile sense of humor obviously gelled when I was about six, so when I see a phrase like "colorectal cancer, number two cause of cancer death," I snigger. But it's true: we get colorectal cancer because we're eating animals and other junk, and our inability to take a proper 'number two' is killing us with cancer in response.)

Increased transit time, with Meaters taking about 1/6th as many dumps as Planters, with very low volume of excreta to boot, and thus hugely longer exposure to the carcinogens our livers have worked so hard to detoxify and expel… no wonder we get cancer of the colon and of the rectum.

(My inner 6-year-old pipes up: "It's the processed meats that wrecked 'um." Apologies all round.) Processed meats *are* prodigious causers of cancer.

Sadly, our livers' detox work may have been in vain. Meating causes a deranged gut flora, which in turn reconverts some detoxed metabolites back into a baleful de-detoxed form. Also, animal-fed gut bacteria make toxic TMAO, and another drawback is their inefficiency at making anti-cancer substances like propionate, which fiber-rich foods make very well.

The negatives of Meating are compounded by the negatives of its deficiency. Meaning, it's all bad. Junking too.

Polyps [and diverticula] are how colorectal cancer begins – harmless little lumps. If untreated with Planting, polyps can become cancerous and may metastasize or move elsewhere in our bodies, where they may prove fatal, leading our doctor to think we died of, say, liver cancer. (There is only cancer.)

While a chunk of animal rots in our colons, or **putrefies**, releasing alkaline-forming or high-pH hydrogen sulfide and ammonia, the fiber in plants

ferments, releasing healthy, slightly acidic substances, like lactic acid, produced by *lactobacillus* bacteria.

Our feces should be slightly basic or alkaline, unlike our urine, which should be slightly acidic.

Ever the rebel without a clue, Meating gets this all wrong, and makes our urine acidic (through excess nitrogen from excess protein/amino acids) and our feces alkaline. In this milieu, with pH above 8, bile acids (the packages which allow the safe disposal of carcinogenic cholesterol) are turned into carcinogens, and polyps may form in the colon's enteric lining.

Planting causes a beneficial pH of less than 6, and this doesn't favor bile acid conversion or polyp formation.

As with all other chronic conditions, Pure Planters suffer a miniscule number of colorectal cancer deaths in comparison to Meaters. In part this is due to beneficial plant substances such as fiber and propionate (and other short-chain fatty acids); in part, the relative absence of harmful animal substances like sulfur-rich methionine and its sulfide by-products.

The positives of Planting are synergized by the positives of its deficiencies. Meaning, it's all good.

As usual, epidemiology serves to confirm the benefits of Planting: People in India (with 40% of the population vegetarian) have less than 1/10th the CRC of Americans. And rural Africans, who eat a very starchy diet, have about 1/50th the colon cancer rate.

And no heart disease… hypertension… diabetes… stroke… appendicitis… et cetera.

Put that in your pipe… but don't smoke it.

See also: Ulcerative colitis

Colic

Is there anything more attention-riveting than a baby's cries? Is there anything that can drive anxious, often sleep-deprived parents to distraction or dementia more than a child who cries incessantly? "Shaken baby syndrome" is how some children die. It's very sad and it's almost always entirely preventable:, because the behavior that needs changing isn't the infant's, it's the parents'.

When we stop feeding cows' milk to babies, their colic goes away, almost instantaneously, and they stop crying because they're no longer in pain, because the cows' milk-induced bloating and intestinal cramps are gone.

For more havoc that dairy products can inflict upon infants, see...

Constipation

Constipation is almost unknown outside the West or those areas infected with Western eating habits.

As noted earlier, constipation is a serious health issue, affecting one in five SAD-eating Americans and causing a buttload of other serious problems. Low-carb [high animal] diets are, by definition, constipating.

If you didn't believe me before about the connection between constipation and breast cancer, check this out:

Petrakis NL, King EB. Cytological abnormalities in nipple aspirates of breast fluid from women with severe constipation. *Lancet.* 1981 Nov 28;2(8257):1203-4.

"Cytological [cell] abnormalities in breast epithelium associated with severe constipation may be relevant to studies of diet and breast disease since the intestinal flora has been reported to metabolise bile salts and oestrogens secreted by the liver into the gastrointestinal tract – a process which may be enhanced by severe constipation."

This is old news – 1981 – and from our most prestigious medical journal, so why aren't our doctors prescribing a constipation-preventing vegan diet for primordial prevention of breast cancer?

Childhood constipation is almost 100% associated with dairy products. Got milk? Got havoc. Chronic idiopathic [of-unknown-origin] constipation turns out to be chronic milk-induced constipation. We know the Eatiology. If everyone were to understand the damage that feeding milk to children can cause, to do so would be seen as committing a physical attack against a child. As matters stand, it's merely battery through ignorance.

Milk also causes atopic conditions such as asthma and eczema. Anyone who doesn't believe me, if you've got a spare snotty, wheezy, itchy kid slurking around the place, try getting them to cut out the dairy products... you'll be amazed and pleased.

(Milk is a pediatrician's meal ticket, probably providing more business than all other causes combined. That's my guess.)

With our current nutrition understanding, dairy products supplied to school lunch programs… is a national disgrace. Come on, all you class action lawyers, where are you? There's a heap of moolah to be made out of this suit.

Constipation-type IBS (Irritable Bowel Syndrome)

Think New York City in August, with the sanitation engineers out on strike. When the waste disposal system grinds to a halt, everything else gets worse.

Contagious pustular dermatitis

When scientists look for large concentrations of people infected with animal-caused conditions, where better to look than in slaughterhouses and meatpacking factories? CPD – a nasty state in which pustules from on the skin, and which we can transfer to those we touch – is caused by constantly handling raw dead animals.

Ok, so those of us who wear our HAZ MAT suits in our sterile kitchens won't get this very often. Just to let you know that this virus-borne condition exists.

We won't get it from carrots, no matter how many bajillions we peel.

COPD

Chronic obstructive pulmonary disease. Respiratory diseases like emphysema are a terrible way to die, sucking and gasping for air, but again, COPD's not really a disease; it's a symptom of the destructive lifestyle choices that cause it: smoking plants and eating animals.

If we don't smoke and if we don't eat animals, we cut way back on the nitros-amines and –amides that are partly responsible for this dreadful condition. There are as many of these dreadful compounds in five nasty cigarettes as there are in one horrid hot dog.

Caveat emptor and eater.

Crib death

Crib death is also known as Sudden Infant Death Syndrome (SIDS).

Crib death is caused by foisting cow's milk on infants.

Let me put it differently: cow's milk kills many infants.

Here's what happens. The casein in milk is converted into an opiate called casomorphin. Casomorphin suppresses the brain's breathing center: in a condition known as "**milk apnea**," the child stops breathing, turns blue and, if not resuscitated in time, dies.

Muscular atony is another symptom of milk drinking these infants may display during this ordeal: they go completely limp like an old rag doll. Their muscles lose all tone.

Milk isn't food. It's that simple. It's only food if we're a calf: even adult cows don't drink milk.

If meat is murder, milk is mayhem.

Crohn's "disease"

Crohn's is a so-called inflammatory bowel disease (IBD), an auto-immune condition in which our immune system attacks our own bowels.

As with many other auto-immune conditions, it's probably animal proteins that are causing cross-reactivity, our immune cells unable to distinguish between amino-acid sequences in un-human and human proteins.

Unsurprisingly then, an intervention trial shows that Crohn's patients respond well to treatment with an all-plant diet, leading to remission in more than 90% of cases after two years. Meating increases our risk of IBD, with fishes and eggs and dairy all worsening symptoms.

Inflammatory bowel conditions are symptoms of a Meaterialist lifestyle. Once we stop the three- times daily injury with toxic animal products, we give our intestines the opportunity to heal.

Dehydration

Animal and junk diets are low in water, high in sodium, and thus dehydrating. Our brain efficiency in particular drops off dramatically when we're deprived of water.

If our kids are finding it hard to concentrate, they're not necessarily Ritalin-deficient – maybe they just need to drink water. Indeed, studies have shown that drinking a glass of water before school each day works wonders with attention deficit. (And just 15 minutes of exercise does wonders for hyperactivity.)

As Sir Toby Belch says to Sir Andrew Aguecheek in *12th Night*:

"He is a prodigious eater of meat. Methinks it doth harm to his wit."

Besides the hypoperfusion (reduced oxygen and nutrient supply) in the brain brought about by atherosclerosis and ischemia, Meating makes things worse for our brains via diminished water supply.

Delayed Menopause

The hormones in the animals we eat and drink cause us to reach menopause far later than "normal." Combined with premature puberty, brought about by the same Meating mechanism, it means that Western women are exposed to excess carcinogenic estrogens for up to a decade longer than this time last century.

Is it any wonder that breast cancer is rampant? Got milk? Got mutagens.

For more, see under: Premature puberty; hormones; estrogen

Dementia

According to the Alzheimer's Association website at alz.org, "Dementia is a general term for a decline in mental ability severe enough to interfere with daily life. Memory loss is an example. **Alzheimer's** is the most common type of dementia.

Dementia isn't a specific disease. It's an overall term that describes a wide range of symptoms associated with a decline in memory or other thinking skills severe enough to reduce a person's ability to perform everyday activities. Alzheimer's disease accounts for 60 to 80 percent of cases.

Vascular dementia, which occurs after a stroke, is the second most common dementia type. But there are many other conditions that can cause symptoms of dementia, including some that are reversible, such as **thyroid problems** and **vitamin deficiencies**.

Dementia is often incorrectly referred to as "senility" or "senile dementia," which reflects the formerly widespread but incorrect belief that serious mental decline is a normal part of aging."

The Mayo Clinic says: "Dementia isn't a specific disease. Instead, dementia describes a group of symptoms affecting memory, thinking and social abilities severely enough to interfere with daily functioning.

Dementia indicates problems with at least two brain functions, such as memory loss and impaired judgment or language, and the inability to perform some daily activities such as paying bills or becoming lost while driving.

Many causes of dementia symptoms exist. Alzheimer's disease is the most common cause of a progressive dementia. Some causes of dementia may be reversible. [Yes, even preventable. Author]

Though memory loss generally occurs in dementia, memory loss alone doesn't mean you have dementia. There is a certain extent of memory loss that is a normal part of aging."

Clear as mud, right? We have two definitive assertions that memory loss isn't and is a normal part of aging.

It's a trivial point.

A major point is that neither of these august organizations says diddly about nutrition or prevention.

There are 2 pdf files one can download from alz.org: 10 Warning Signs of Alzheimer's and a Doctor's Appointment Checklist.

In preparing for a doctor's appointment, they suggest we:

- List vitamins and herbal supplements
- List current medical conditions
- List past medical conditions

Nowhere does it say: what are you eating? Or, are you eating food? Unless they're botanicals, vitamins and supplements are junk.

According to alz.org, the 10 Warning Signs of Alzheimer's are:

1. Memory loss that disrupts daily life.
2. Challenges in planning or solving problems.
3. Difficulty completing familiar tasks at home, at work or at leisure.
4. Confusion with time or place.
5. Trouble understanding visual images and spatial relationships.
6. New problems with words in speaking or writing.
7. Misplacing things and losing the ability to retrace steps.
8. Decreased or poor judgment.
9. Withdrawal from work or social activities.
10. Changes in mood and personality.

I guess those warning signs are appropriate for people who already have Alzheimer's.

The #1 warning sign of Alzheimer's in the above list should be:

1. The mistaken belief that animals are food.

How about these questions, if we'd like to prevent Alzheimer's?

1. Are you eating animals?
2. If so, how many? And if not, how long ago did you stop?
3. Are you eating junk?
4. Are you eating at least 12 servings of fruit and veg a day?
5. Do you think that taking vitamins makes up for eating a poor diet?
6. Do you think that taking medications makes up for eating a poor diet?
7. Do you think that suppressing symptoms with medications will remove the underlying cause?
8. How many hours of exercise are you getting every day?
9. How much mental stimulation are you getting every day?
10. How many hours do you spend watching the boob tube?

The Wikipedia entry for dementia reads as follows:

"Dementia, also known as senility, is a broad category of brain diseases that cause a long term and often gradual decrease in the ability to think and remember such that a person's daily functioning is affected. Other common symptoms include emotional problems, problems with language, and a decrease in motivation. A person's consciousness isn't affected. For the diagnosis to be present it must be a change from a person's usual mental functioning and a greater decline than one would expect due to aging. These diseases also have a significant effect on a person's caregivers.

The most common type of dementia is Alzheimer's disease which makes up 50% to 70% of cases. Other common types include **vascular dementia** (25%), **Lewy body dementia** (15%), and **frontotemporal dementia**. Less common causes include **normal pressure hydrocephalus**, **Parkinson's disease**, **syphilis**, and **Creutzfeldt–Jakob disease** among others. More than one type of dementia may exist in the same person. A small proportion of cases run in families."

Their Wikipedianesses continue: "Efforts to prevent dementia include trying to decrease risk factors such as high blood pressure, smoking, diabetes and obesity."

Wow. Sounds to me like they're talking about nutrition, except they don't say so. This is a fairly standard representation of conventional thinking – control the risk factors, not the precursors of the risk factors. How about removing the risk factors altogether by getting rid of the ur-cause: Meating and Junking? If we stub out smoking – "And then you do what with it, Walt?" – and if we become Planters, with down-to-zero hypertension, obesity and diabetes, then we achieve what we already know from population studies (epidemiology): the most plant-strong peoples (such as the Okinawans and Hunzas and vegan Loma Lindans) have the least dementia. (Or at least they did, when they weren't Meating and Junking.)

It's the non-foods, ya big schtoop.

As the Wikipedia quote says: "More than one type of dementia may exist in the same person." Why? Because the underlying cause – Meating – causes more than one system to fail.

Meating = atherosclerosis = ischemia = oxidation = inflammation = molecular mimicry = … They're all the same thing, in the end. Different dementias may have the same Eatiology, even if they're caused by different mechanisms of un-foods.

And we shouldn't be surprised if "a small proportion of cases run in families": families, besides sharing genes, share breakfast, lunch and supper, and drive-through windows at fast-"food," fast-death un-restaurants.

The reason why dementias appear to be "age-related" is that it takes time for us to wreck our vasculature via Meating and Junking. Atherosclerosis proceeds micron by micron. Dementia and cardiovascular symptoms go hand in hand. They too are essentially the same thing, although they present differently; biomarkers of Meating.

As the Alzheimer's Organization says above: Vascular dementia is the second leading cause of dementia, and it's a common outcome of stroke. As we know, stroke is a common outcome of Meating, and Planting is protective against stroke. Stroke is a symptom of Meating. That makes Meating the leading cause of the second leading cause of dementia.

Meating → atherosclerosis + hypertension → ischemic and hemorrhagic stroke → vascular dementia.

This makes dementia a form of chronic in-digestion caused by mistaking animals for food.

For a discussion of the leading form of dementia, see under: Alzheimer's disease.

See also: Mad cow "disease"; Parkinson's "disease"

Depression
Yep, Meating makes it worse through a cascade of oxidation and inflammation, particularly as a result of animal-only arachidonic acid.

For more, see under: Mental health

Diabetes ~ Diabesity ~ Obesity
Next up? Diabetes. And here I'm going to make my sole exception to the alphabetical order of Meater Eatiological conditions. Because obesity and diabetes go together like low-carb diets and low life expectancy, I'm going to treat obesity and diabetes together in one long section, as befits their importance, their public interest and the level of ignorance, misinformation, disinformation and outright lies sown by low-carb mischief-makers.

Obesity, a "disease" of Meater and Junker malnutrition
In a nutshell, here's why Planters are slender, while Meaters and Junkers tend to be overweight or obese*:

- Planters eat a greater volume than Meaters and Junkers, because whole plants are packed with fiber. Animals and junk are fiber-free wastelands
- Planters eat fewer calories, while eating more nutrients
- Planter calories aren't as fattening as Meater/Junker calories
- Planters eat far less fat, which is easily converted to body fat
- Planter fats are less fattening than Meater/Junker fats
- Animal fats can contain thousands of times more environmental pollutants than plant fats; they help make us fat
- Animals may play host to viruses that cause infectious obesity, and some viruses are diabetogenic
- Planters have much better insulin sensitivity than M&Js
- Planting benefits us epigenetically - via its effects on our genes - while Meating and Junking cause detrimental gene expression.

* Some paleo and low-carb eaters are a temporary exception to the rule of overweight Meaters. We can, if we choose to shorten our lives by eating lots of animals, lose weight in the short term by starving ourselves of our carbohydrate fuel. I'll treat these unhealthy specimens in a separate section.

Till then, please keep in mind that low-carbers (and their paleo sub-ilk) die young, just like their role models, the cave dwellers of old and present-day Inuit. And keep in mind: low-carb means ultra-high animal protein, ultra-high animal fat, ultra-high animal cholesterol and ultra-low plant fiber (with an accompanying ultra-derangement of gut flora), whose ill-effects are only slightly muted, if at all, by the beneficial weight loss of ultra-Meating and by whatever whole plants are eaten.

Let's look at where we are.

In late 2015, more than 2/3 of Americans are overweight, with 38% obese – more than 210 million sick people. That's a strange norm.

Overweight is defined as having a BMI (body mass index) between 25 and 30, while obesity is over 30, and morbid obesity begins at 40. (Our BMI = our weight in kilograms divided by the square of our height in meters (kg/m^2).)

The only healthy eaters, with BMIs averaging below 25, are vegans.

Vegans are protected against a Meatiological super-storm that costs employers more than $70 billion a year.

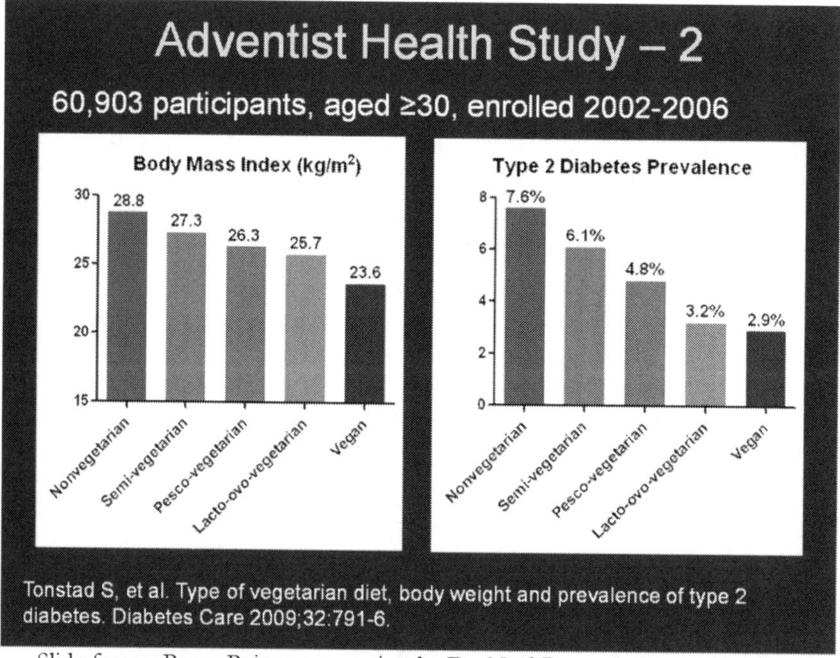

Slide from a PowerPoint presentation by Dr. Neal Barnard: "Food for Life – Healthy Eating to Tackle Weight Problems, Cholesterol, and Diabetes."

Despite what Low-Carb Bullshit Artists say, **the people who eat the most carbohydrates have the least problems with obesity and diabetes.** This includes Planters in the West, all Asian populations who're still eating their traditional rice diets and many other populations who're powered by whole grains other than rice. These are the slenderest people in the world.

In this information taken from a 2009 study of 89,000 7th Day Adventists from around Loma Linda, CA, we can see the BMIs and the risks (in %) of diabetes produced by different eating patterns:

- Meaters (Nonvegetarians) 28.8 7.6%
- Semivegetarians 27.3 6.1%
- Pescovegetarians 26.3 4.8%
- Lacto-ovo-vegetarians 25.7 3.2%`
- Vegans (Planters , but some Junkers too) 23.6 2.9%

Semivegetarians, or flexitarians, are plant-eaters who eat animals a couple of times a month. Pescovegetarians think fishes are vegetables, and lacto-ovos think animal milks and eggs qualify.

Dr. Barnard's graphic shows beautifully how obesity ramps up as we add animals to our diet. There's a 5-point Body Mass Index spread between the vegans (who may not have been pure Planters) and the Meaters (who were probably also Junkers) which equates to a huge difference in body weight. On average, vegans weigh 40 pounds (18kg) less than Meaters and Junkers. Pure Planters would weigh even less.

Come on, dear hearts. Once we know this, why would we even consider buying another diet book?

Each added animal "food" ratchets up the risk of obesity and diabetes. Compared to Meaters, vegan 7th Day Adventists have less than 40% of the diabetes risk.

(To account for the possible confounding effects of Junking in Adventist-2, which was controlled for but not specifically studied, Michael Greger refers to a study which compared animal-eating to vegan Buddhists, eating a traditional Taiwanese diet with no sodas or other added sugars, i.e. no junk. Even though the non-vegan men were only eating only ~8% of American animal intakes, and women, ~3%, the vegan men had half the diabetes and the women only a quarter. Meating, even at extremely low levels, is extremely diabetogenic.)

[See: http://nutritionfacts.org/video/plant-based-diets-for-diabetes/]

T H T Chiu, H Y Huang, Y F Chiu, W H Pan, H Y Kao, J P C Chiu, M N Lin, C L Lin. Taiwanese Vegetarians and Omnivores: Dietary Composition, Prevalence of Diabetes and IFG. *PLOS* February 2014 Volume 9 Issue 2.

Let's take a quick look at the Adventists.

They're an excellent population to study. Their moral code includes strictures on alcohol, tobacco, drugs… and (the most basic drug) animals as food. Adventists, being human, show a wide range of behavior within a relatively homogeneous community. Their homogeneity allows us to discount genetic and non-dietary environmental variations as confounding factors, while studying differences in diet.

The more animals we eat, the more we suffer from obesity and diabetes. Other Adventist studies show that the same applies to osteoporosis, hypertension, heart disease and mortality: the more animals, the worse the outcome.

The vegan Adventists are the most-studied Blue Zoners in the world. (Blue Zones are areas whose residents appear to live abnormally long lives.) And the results of the studies show that the vegan Adventists of Loma Linda are the healthiest and longest-lived people ever studied.

G E Fraser, D J Shavlik. Ten years of life: Is it a matter of choice? *Arch Intern Med.* 2001 Jul 9;161(13):1645-52.

Fraser and Shavlik say: "Adventist vegetarian men and women have expected ages at death of 83.3 and 85.7 years, respectively. These are 9.5 and 6.1 years, respectively, greater than those of the 1985 California population… [the best data available as the time]. "

Non-smoking, exercising Adventist Planters did even better, outliving the general American population by 10 to 14 years.

Slenderness and longevity are Siamese twins – they're not easily separated. When we're overweight, we don't live as long as when we're slender. *All* population studies show that we shouldn't eat animals if we want to be skinny old people one day. There never has been – and never will be – a population study that shows a benefit of Meating over Planting… unless it's about B_{12}. Moving on…

Epidemiology

Epidemiology, the study of health and disease at the population level, as in this Adventist-2 study, is a wonderful tool of scientific discovery. It shows us where to look for plausible biological mechanisms to explain the etiology, or root causes, of disease. Epidemiology is a telescope which shows us where to use our microscopes. In this case, it points us towards Eatiology; symptoms caused by Meater mal-nutrition.

After seeing that mere non-Planter vegans weigh 40 pounds less than Meaters (and have <40% of the diabetes), surely no sane person would start studying Planters for the causes of obesity and diabetes? We need to study the obesity- and diabetes-riddled Meaters and Junkers for the mechanisms of disease. 'Meat + sweet' is the prime suspect. If we put Planters under the microscope, it's to look for mechanisms that prevent obesity and diabetes.

We can study Meaters to see why they're sick or Planters to see why they're well. We're going to do both.

The Eatiology of Obesity

We know from the epidemiology that Meaters and Junkers are far fatter than Planters. Here are some of the reasons why:

1. Energy density vs. Nutrient density

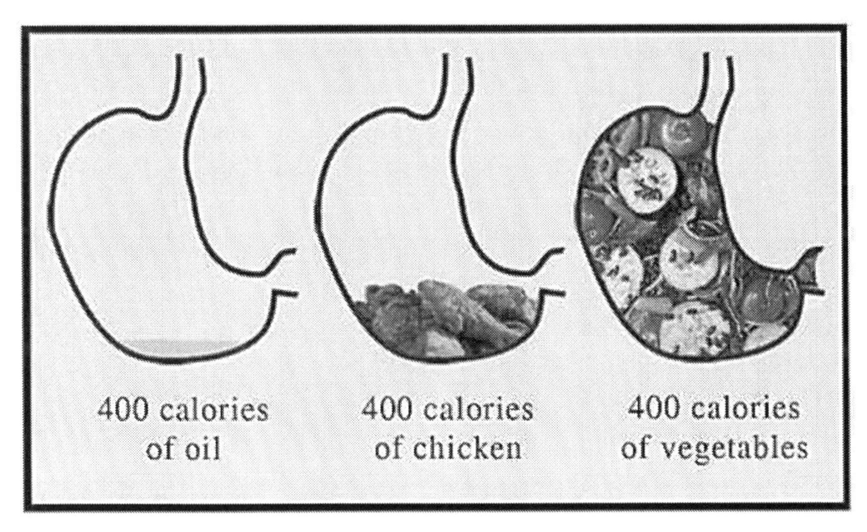

Ali Miller RD: Volumetrics

Plants are low in energy, high in nutrients. Animals and Junk are high in energy, low in nutrients. Dr. Joel Fuhrman talks about nutrient density and a Nutritarian diet. Barbara J. Rolls, PhD, has coined the word 'Volumetrics' to describe this reality.

In an unusual rear view of the stomach, above, we see how many plants it takes to be and feel full. We take in far more calories than we need when we eat junk (vegetable oil) and animals. Adding just a tablespoon of olive oil to our salads undoes much of the low-energy benefit of pure veggies.

Our stomachs have nutrient density sensors (called 'nutrient receptors') that let us know how rich a food is in nutrients, and therefore how much to eat.

2. Animals and Junk are fiber-deficient

Planters eat plenty of virtually calorie-free fiber, which fills us up without making us fat. Meaters and Junkers don't feel as full as soon, because there's not enough bulk to activate pressure sensors in our stomachs (called 'stretch receptors') which tell us when we've eaten enough volume of food.

3. Planters eat fewer fats

Perfect for their role as energy stores, fats are energy-dense, supplying 9 calories per gram, while protein and carbohydrate supply 4. Meaters and Junkers get easily 30, 35% or more of their calories from fats. Pure Planters get about 10 to 15%, unless we're avoricious avoholics or olive junkies.

Low-Carb Bullshit Artists tell us that eating fat doesn't make us fat - it's the sugar, they say. Well, okay, eating sugar-filled junk in excess, carrying on eating after we should be feeling satiated, can provide excess calories which can be stored as fat. There are two problems with this theory though. The first is that the conversion of carbohydrate to fat is an inefficient process, with much of the energy being lost as heat. Not so with laying down body fat from dietary fat - that's very efficient; almost no losses at all.

The second problem is that when scientists take biopsies of actual fat deposits from real people's thighs and butts (instead of from LCBA's theoretical bullshit), they can tell exactly where the fat comes from, and it's not from sugar: researchers can identify pig fat and cow fat and milk fat and egg fat and fish fat and… Junker alert… fat from vegetable oils. As Dr. John McDougall says, "The fat we eat is the fat we wear."

Dr. Neal Barnard's book *Turn Off the Fat Genes* contains a wonderful explanation of why this is so. "The more fat there is in your diet, the more fat passes into your blood. And the more fat in your blood, the more passes into your fat cells."

Why? Our bodies became adapted over millions of years to eating plants that contain very small amounts of fat in comparison to animals. In our blood vessels lurks a very efficient fat-grabbing enzyme called lipoprotein lipase or LPL. Let's unpack the name. Lipoproteins are fat/protein combination molecules which carry fats in our watery blood. The -ase suffix in an enzyme name means it's a splitter, so LPL is a splitter of fats carried by lipoproteins in the blood. Where does LPL hang out? In arteries that supply our fat cells and our muscle cells.

Planting suppresses LPL's action of laying down fat into our fat cells, while boosting fat uptake into our muscles for burning as fuel and creating heat. Planting turns off our fat storage genes. Meating has the opposite epigenetic effect: it boosts fat deposition in fat cells and lowers what Dr. Barnard calls the "after-meal burn" in our muscle cells. Whole carbohydrates cause TEF, the "thermic effect of food," or thermogenesis, which causes more calories to be lost as heat than calories from fats do. More on this topic later...

We can already see why eating ultra-high whole-carb diets make Asian people slender and prevents Meater and Junker fats from showing up in biopsies of body fat - there's precious little fat in whole plants. As Dr. Barnard says: "Fat in foods - not carbohydrate or protein or anything else - provides the principal raw material for building body fat."

In general, eating fat IS what makes us fat. Overeating junk doesn't help. Later on, we'll look at the unhealthy way high-fat, high-protein, low-carb diets cause weight loss.

4. Planters eat fewer saturated fats

Saturated fats are inflammatory as well as calorie-dense, and cause more weight gain. Planters eat no animal fats, and also avoid vegetable oils and other processed junk, which contain saturated fats.

5. Planters eat fewer trans or hydrogenated fats

Trans fats from animals and hydrogenated vegetable oils help cause obesity, and Planters don't eat them.

6. Planters tend to eat fewer calories

Because Planters eat fewer fats and more fiber, Planters eat slightly fewer calories than Meaters and Junkers. Yet, even when eating high-calorie plants such as dried fruits and nuts, Planters eat more but weigh less.

7. Change in animal fat content over time

In the last century, American chicken breeders have bred chickens to be obese. Chicken flesh has gone from about 2 grams of fat per serving to 23, with a change in the type of fat too. Because the birds now grow so fast and get slaughtered so young, they don't produce DHA, a long-chain fatty acid.

Michael Greger asks, "does eating obesity cause obesity in the consumer?" Certainly, it's crazy to think that chicken parts can be a low-calorie substitute for redder alternatives. Chickens and fishes are probably the two most obesogenic and diabetogenic things we eat.

As far as I'm aware, the fat content of pistachios and peaches has stayed pretty much the same during the same period, and they've never made us fat or diabetic.

[See: http://nutritionfacts.org/video/does-eating-obesity-cause-obesity/]

8. Satiety and overindulgence

Feeling satiated, or full, has several mechanisms, some healthy, some not. In a healthy state, pressure sensors in our stomachs and intestines send messages to our brains, via nerves and hormones, to say halt, enough. High-fiber whole plants do this far sooner than low- or no-fiber junk and animals. As we'll see shortly, high-fiber diets also slow down the rates our stomachs empty.

However, people on extremely high-fat animal diets also report feeling satiated, and ketogenic diets thus become calorie restriction diets – they just can't choke down any more fat. These people's bodies mimic starvation and they're essentially sick, which is why they too lose weight, except on a high-calorie, low-nutrient diet. They feel better because they lose weight, while raising their risk of all-cause mortality.

The benefits are temporary – we can't maintain calorie restriction diets indefinitely. At some point, we have to stop losing weight. The National Weight Control Registry shows that only about 1 in 10 people who've managed to lose 30 pounds and maintain the weight loss for a year is a low-carber or paleo type.

Via different mechanisms, and with different long-term health outcomes, the two far ends of the spectrum – no-animal eaters and maximum animal eaters – have the lowest tendencies to overindulge.

9. Plant calories ≠ Animal calories

Planters and Meaters who eat 'isocaloric' diets don't put on the same amount of weight. After 5 years of eating the same number of calories, Planters can weigh between 1.5 and 2.7 kg less than Meaters, or 3.3 to 6 pounds less.

According to Vergnaud AC et al. Meat consumption and prospective weight change in participants of the EPIC-PANACEA study. *Am J Clin Nutr.* 2010 Aug;92(2):398-407:

A study of almost 374,000 men and women showed that "total meat consumption was positively associated with weight gain in men and women, in normal-weight and overweight subjects, and in smokers and nonsmokers. With adjustment for estimated energy intake, an increase in meat intake of 250 g/d (e.g., one steak at ≈450 kcal) would lead to a 2-kg higher weight gain after 5 y (95% CI: 1.5, 2.7 kg). Positive associations were observed for red meat, poultry, and processed meat." [And never mind their carcinogenic effect.]

There's something about eating the same amount of energy in animal form that makes us pack on the pounds.

10. Thermogenesis

Planters generate more heat from their meals than Meaters do, which means there's less unused energy to be stored as fat. In other words, Planting has a metabolic advantage over Meating. Planters' thermostats are cranked up ever so slightly and, over time, as we saw in the EPIC-PANACEA Study, it means the difference between winning the battle of the bulge and losing.

I'll cover the 'thermic effect of food' in more detail in #32 below, when we see how carbs generate heat when they're stored as glycogen in our muscles.

11. Brown fat vs. White fat ~ Abdominal obesity

Planters store more of their fat as brown fat, the kind that is spread thinly over our shoulders and around our necks. Meaters and Junkers store their fat in their buttocks, legs and abdomens as white fat. Abdominal fat is the kind that's part of the "Deadly Quartet" of metabolic syndrome, which we'll meet again later when we discuss diabetes.

Cayenne pepper and other spices are great for laying down brown fat.

12. Flavonoids

Flavonoids are a family of >5,000 phytonutrients that boost our metabolism, preventing weight gain, via thermogenesis. There are cancer- and Alzheimer's-suppressing isoflavones in soy which also help us regulate our weight. Other good sources are beans, berries, citrus, cocoa, grapes, green tea and red onions.

13. Arginine

Arginine is a plant nutrient that turns up our thermostats, causing us to burn more calories. Arginine is involved in the creation of thermoregulatory brown fat, above. It's also what our bodies use to create NO, nitric oxide, which causes our arteries to dilate. Beans (especially soy), nuts (especially pistachios) and seeds are the best sources of arginine.

14. Citrulline

Citrulline is a precursor to arginine, so it also helps with vasodilation, and it helps us maintain an ideal body weight. As vasodilators, citrulline and arginine are antidotes to erectile dysfunction. There's lots of citrulline in watermelons, *Citrullus lanatus*. We should juice the green and white rinds – that's where most of the citrulline is. (Of course it is - antioxidant phytonutrients are plants' sunblock.)

15. Enterotypes: unhealthy gut flora in Meaters and Junkers

While there are a thousand or more species of bacteria in our enteric systems – gastroenterology is the study of our stomachs and intestines – all humans have just two families of bacteria which predominate within our digestive tracts.

Why do different people have different types of enteric bacteria?

It depends on what we eat. It depends on what we feed *them*, our microscopic partners and cohabitants in our human/non-human bodies.

An enterotype is a classification of which species has the upper hand in our colons. Meaters feed animals to their gut flora, so animal-rotting *Bacteroides* predominate. Planters feed fiber and phytonutrients to their bacteria, so plant-fermenting *Prevotella* species prevail.

This matters for several reasons, above and beyond obesity.

Because they're fiber-deficient, Meaters and Junkers lack beneficial bacteria in the colon such as *Faecalibacterium prausnitzii* which produce anti-obesity and anti-carcinogenic short-chain fatty acids such as acetate, butyrate and propionate. Meaters' suppression of *F. prausnitzii* sets off an immune response within the colon, resulting in inflammation. Our gut flora *must* have huge amounts of fiber to be healthy – especially beans and grains.

Because they feed animals to their bacteria, Meaters encourage unhealthy species such as *Bilophila wadsworthia* to flourish, and they act on animal amino acids, particularly taurine, to produce mutation-causing hydrogen sulfide (H_2S), which is one of the reasons why Meaters suffer more from inflammatory bowel "diseases", such as ulcerative colitis, and more colorectal cancer.

Not only do Meater gut bacteria produce more estrogens, strongly linked to many different cancers, including breast and prostate; they're also responsible for producing secondary bile acids like deoxycholic acid (DCA) which can damage our DNA and cause cancer, especially in the liver, which is where bile is made.

Meaters have a deranged microbiome – they have the wrong enterotype.

The good news is that the remedy is simple: if we stop Meating and start Planting, a healthy population of *Prevotella* is attainable in a matter of days.

How we disrupt our microbiome by eating animals helps explain why Dr. Caldwell Esselstyn's saying "Moderation kills" is so true.

16. Propionate

Healthy gut bacteria, especially when fed plenty of fibrous beans, produce a short-chain fatty acid called propionate, which, besides its cholesterol-lowering effect, has great weight control properties. Propionate is an anti-obesity agent which can suppress the creation of new fat cells.

17. Delayed gastric emptying

Our gut flora make propionate for us in our small intestines. It gets into our bloodstreams and makes its way to our stomachs, where it slows down the rate at which our stomachs empty. This is great for slowing down glucose absorption and insulin release into our blood, as we'll see later when we tackle diabetes.

18. The Second Meal Effect

Also known as the '**lentil effect**,' the second meal effect looks like this: Say we had beans or lentils for supper last night, and we eat white bread toast at breakfast. The propionate we generated last night blunts the glucose spike 12 hours later. Wow. The benefits of one Planter meal continue into the next meal.

19. Hypophagic effect

Hypo- means less; phagic means eating. Because of delayed stomach emptying and increased stool bulk to activate stomach wall pressure receptors, Planting naturally means that we eat less. Meating strikes out on both counts.

20. Butyrate

Butyrate is another of the short-chain fatty acids produced by our good gut bacteria from fiber, like propionate. Butyrate is a powerful anti-inflammatory compound, countering general inflammation, and germane to this list, the inflammation that's associated with obesity. Butyrate is a powerful anti-cancer agent. Its deficiency in both Meaters and Planters is one of the reasons why they suffer more colorectal cancer than Planters.

21. Polyphenols

These are phytonutrients that also contribute towards a healthy gut flora, shifting the balance of bacteria towards non-obesogenic species. They're found particularly in fruits, apple and grape vinegars, and green tea.

22. Carnitine palmitoyltransferase

When we burn fat, CPT is the main enzyme involved in transporting fat into our cells' mitochondria. Planting upregulates the genes that produce this enzyme by 60% over Meating, so Planters burn more fat.

23. Mitochondrial biogenesis

Arginine stimulates the creation of more of our cells' power plant organelles, the mitochondria. The more mitochondria we have in each cell, the more fuel we can burn, and the less weight we gain.

24. Uric acid

Hominins lost the ability to detox uric acid in a then-benevolent mutation 15 million years ago. Today, Meating and Junking – via the purines in animals and the fructose in High Fructose Corn Syrup – lead to elevated uric acid levels, which lead in turn to increased sodium and fat retention; also gout, diabetes, kidney and cardiovascular disease, among others.

25. Endogenous hormones

Every animal product humans eat has animal hormones in it – estrogens such as estradiol and androgens such as testosterone. Estrogen is estrogen; meaning that human and animal estrogen are identical. Our hormones are signaling molecules; they tell our bodies what to do. Do we need chicken hormones in us, bossing us around? Phytoestrogens, e.g. from flax and soy, counter the obesogenic and carcinogenic effects of animal estrogens.

26. Obesogenic chemicals

There are thousands of endocrine-disrupting chemicals, or xeno-estrogens, such as PCBs and dioxins which are bioaccumulated to extraordinary levels in animal fat, and they cause inflammation and make us fat when we eat them. They often cause cancer and birth defects too. Fishes are the worst of the worst when it comes to almost all environmental pollutants.

Organotin compounds in particular cause obesity by turning fat stem cells (or pre-adipocytes) into fat cells. Normal people have the same number of fat cells throughout life, and our weight is determined by how much fat is crammed into our constant number of fat cells. Meaters who're contaminated with obesogens may grow more fat cells into which to stuff fat. This is one explanation for why there are now more morbidly obese people than ever.

Girls exposed to DDE, a metabolite of DDE, in the womb are more likely to become fat later on in life. Other ill-effects of prenatal exposure to toxic waste in Meater mothers include smaller brain size, lower IQ, diminished attention, other cognitive issues, and increased risk of diabetes and cancer.

[See: http://nutritionfacts.org/video/obesity-causing-pollutants-in-food/]

27. Obesogenic viruses

Chickens, in particular, are laden with viruses such as Adenovirus-36 that can cause obesity in humans. We don't have to be infected with a virus to be obese, but it doesn't help. One in five obese people is infected, and they're up to 15kg (33 pounds) heavier than other obese people, while eating the same amount of food. Another term for this is…

28. Infectobesity

Obesity caused by viral infection from animals. It would be dreadfully unfair if Planters were to be infected with one of these animal-borne viruses, causing us not to be able to lose weight even while eating an optimal animal-free diet. Modern chickens, themselves obese, are the most fattening animals we eat, because of their own fat and because of the viruses that infest them.

29. Genetics and Epigenetics

Our genetic heritage plays an important role in obesity. Still, environment trumps genes by beneficially regulating the expression of genes that code for obesity – while Planting is epigenetically beneficial, Meating undoes the good work. We saw this earlier in point (2) Planters eat fewer fats, in which I described how LPL, or lipoprotein lipase, either lays down fat when we eat animals and junk or sends it to our muscles to burn off when we eat whole plants.

In *Turn Off the Fat Genes*, Dr. Neal Barnard describes "*five key gene effects*. First, taste genes influence which foods you prefer. Second, the leptin system... [can] increase or decrease your appetite. Third, the fat builder enzyme, known as LPL, plays a key role in whether calories are stored as fat or lost as body heat. Fourth, insulin, the chromosome 11 hormone, regulates your calorie-burning speed in several ways. Finally, your ability to exercise is influenced by genes for your muscle type."

Let's take a look at the four remaining ways that our genes set us up for obesity or slenderness, and how we can eat to change the way we express our genes to bring about improved weight management.

30. Taste preferences

According to Dr. Barnard, "About one fifth of your taste preference comes straight from Mom and Dad," so whether we have a sweet tooth or prefer savory or fatty tastes is determined 20% by genetics and 80% by our own behavior - how we eat.

The good news is that taste requires reinforcement, so if we change what we eat, say, by putting less salt on our food, it doesn't take long before salted foods taste obnoxious to us. The same goes for fat and sugar.

We have all new taste buds in three weeks, and we can program our new taste buds to like the foods we eat during those three weeks.

31. Appetite control through leptin and ghrelin

Working in opposition, leptin, our "satiety hormone," and ghrelin, our "hunger hormone," regulate our appetites. Amazingly, our fat cells themselves secrete leptin and ghrelin; leptin to tell our brains we've had enough to eat, ghrelin to say 'Please, sir, may I have some more?'

If we become obese, while our pancreases become insulin-insensitive, our fat cells become leptin-insensitive, unable to tell when we're sated.

Dr. Barnard says: "This is the critical take-home message: While an *increase* in leptin is not especially powerful at reducing your appetite or trimming you down, you definitely do not want to court a *decrease* in leptin. It could make your appetite soar."

Calorie restriction is particularly damaging to the leptin/ghrelin combo: "...your leptin system is disrupted by diets that cut way down on calories. Avoid them... people who were intentionally restraining their eating were set for a binge... Diets lead to binges... Your body thought you were starving, and it demanded a binge to save your life. This is called the *restrained eater phenomenon.*

Rather than cut calories, it is much easier over the long run to change the *type* of food you eat... Fiber reduces your appetite and helps you lose weight... even modest increases in vegetables, beans, and other fiber-rich foods led to weight loss. People whose diets were richest in fiber weighed eight pounds less, on average, than those with the least."

Fiber - whole plants - controls our appetites and our body weight via multiple mechanisms. As we know, there is zero fiber in animals and junk. With 4 calories per gram from carbohydrates and nine from fats, even long chain omega-3 fats, it takes far more calories for Meating to achieve satiety or diminish appetite.

Low-fiber diets, which is what low-carb diets usually are, are effectively calorie restriction diets. When we drop one entire macronutrient from our plates, we're forced to consume über-quantities of the other two, proteins and fats, to make up the difference.

Because eating mass quantities of animal proteins and animal fats is making us sick - how can it not? we're depriving ourselves of plant fiber, antioxidants, phytonutrients and calories - most people can't tolerate this high-animal regime in the long run, even after losing large amounts of weight, and they return to their less insane, still bad ways of eating. Long-term low-level depression of leptin sets these poor people up for bingeing, regaining some or all of the weight they'd lost and setting up the well-known 'yo-yo effect' common among calorie-restriction dieters.

As mentioned earlier, this is why there are so few low-carbers and paleofantasists in the National Weight Control Registry - going without real food is unsustainable for most people except for short periods. A year or two, yes. Decades, no. A lifetime, don't make me laugh. Planters are Planters for life, easy peasy, and Planters are the leanest people in the world, and they live the longest. It turns out that über-high-carb works better than low-carb at absolutely everything.

32. Insulin, glycogen, calorie-burning speed and resting metabolic rate (RMR)

Carrying on with the thought that über-high-carb eating, a.k.a. Planting, is better at everything than low-carb Meating, let's take a quick look at the hormone insulin. Low-Carb Bullshit Artists tell us this part of the insulin story: eating sugar makes our blood glucose levels rise, which makes our insulin levels rise to take the glucose out of our blood and into our cells.

In other words, they're saying Junking is bad for us. Then, without even mentioning Planting, they ram Meating down our throats: because sugar causes an insulin spike we should all eat lots of animals. And most people buy their fraudulent logic.

Here it is again, in slow motion. Because white bread and white sugar and sodas cause us to release too much sugar and insulin too quickly, we should cut out ALL carbohydrate-containing foods. On which planet?

As we'll see over and over and over again, Planters are the slenderest people in the world. Planters - people who eat up to 80% carbohydrates! - have the least problems with glucose and insulin. Planters are the most insulin-sensitive, the least insulin-resistant people on Earth (in the Universe, for all I know), and Planters are the least affected by diabetes. This is so because when we're Planters (1) we wear so little fat on our bodies and (2) because we eat so little fat; both of which cause problems for insulin, and again for two reasons: because (1) the fat which Meaters and Junkers eat and wear itself impedes insulin, causing resistance to its action, and (2) because when we're M&Js the fats we eat and wear contain thousands or tens of thousands of times more environmental poisons that damage the insulin-producing cells in our pancreases.

These are undebatable truths, and the Low-Carb Bullshit Artists know it. Yet they persist with their foul scribblings.

But that's not all... Here's something else the LCBAs somehow forget to mention. Insulin is a hormone with 'stacked functions.' It doesn't do just one thing. It's not just about ushering glucose into our cells to provide us with fuel. Insulin also ferries amino acids into cells to build tissues. In other words, when we eat proteins our pancreases release insulin.

Eating animals, with their heavy loads of proteins and fats, causes as much or more insulin release as eating fractionated carbohydrate-packed plants. And way, way, way more insulin than whole, carb-packed plants. Meating causes most of our insulin resistance, and Meating causes most of the damage to our pancreases leading to insulin insufficiency as well.

It turns out that the LCBAs are liars both of commission and omission.

The LCBAs chose insulin on which to fight their battle for the stomachs of the world (and for more than their share of book royalties and lecture fees). Why? Because they can sow some doubt there, blaming the kitchen sink on Plants by pretending that Junking and Planting are one and the same, and because every other health outcome like heart disease and hypertension and dementia and cancer and auto-immunity and stroke and... and... and... makes them look even more stupid than they already do ... to those trained in nutrition.

I cover low-carbers and their 'terminological inexactitudes' about glucose and insulin in microscopic detail in my book *The Low-Carb Bullshit Artists Are Lying Us to Death.*

(And a more detailed explanation of insulin and insulin resistance follows shortly when we take a look at Diabetes.)

Anyway, getting back to the topic, which is how insulin and body weight are connected...

Each of us needs to eat, let's say 2000 calories a day to power our metabolisms, even if we're doing no more than languishing on a chaise-longue and asking Beulah to peel us a grape. Our hearts go pitter-pat, our lungs do their bellows job, and our brains do their mysterious dreamy thing, all of which functions need powering.

Eating too little causes our bodies to think that food is scarce, and so our brains slow down our metabolic rates to compensate for the perceived shortage. Evolutionarily, this was of great benefit.

We all have what's called a Resting Metabolic Rate (RMR). Leptin, as we saw above, communicates with our brains and helps suppress our appetites when our fat stores are large enough. It also acts on body tissues to increase metabolism. This is a superb negative feedback loop, because we eat less and we also burn more calories, both of which help lower the fat stores which caused the creation of leptin in the first place. (When leptin levels fall too low, our appetites return and we're urged to eat more.)

Where does insulin come in? Insulin helps manage the speed with which we burn calories.

On page 21 of *Turn Off the Fat Genes* we read that "The hormone insulin, coded on chromosome 11, is part of your body's system for turning on your metabolism after meals. Depending on the type of foods you choose, you can influence insulin's ability to spark a pronounced after-meal burn that releases calories as body heat, rather than storing them as fat."

On page 71, Dr. Barnard writes, politely echoing my thoughts about Low-Carb Bullshit Artists: "Easily the most misunderstood part of our nutrient-managing machinery starts on chromosome 11, where a gene makes insulin, one of the busiest hormones in the body. Many popular diet books have demonized insulin and the carbohydrates that elicit its secretion into the bloodstream. Bread is bad. Rice is fattening. Beware of pasta. The image conjured up is that carbs elicit insulin release, and it, in turn, drives sugars into the cells where they become fat. The truth is, insulin is your best friend when it is working properly."

And when, pray, does insulin work properly? In an extremely low-fat (<10%), low-protein (<10%) environment - an extremely high-carb (>80%) environment, as long as those carbs take the form of whole plants - fruits, vegetables, legumes and whole grains (and, if we're overweight, go lightly on the high-fat plants like avos and olives). About this, there is unanimity in Nutritionland. Carb confusion only arises in the blogosphere and in our local book stores. [An aside: Shouldn't low-carb and paleo (and blood type diet) books be awarded their own category, somewhere between science fiction and fantasy? Notrition, perhaps?]

Your RMR or resting metabolic rate shows "how fast your body at rest burns calories. RMR is critical to your body weight. It accounts for 60 to 75 percent of all the calories you burn in a day, all without moving a muscle [except the involuntary muscles of our hearts and lungs et al]. Another 10 percent comes from the effort required to absorb and digest food. Physical activity adds the remainder.

If you have a fast metabolism, it means your cells are burning a lot of calories to run these various functions. The more calories they burn, the easier it is to stay slim. If your metabolism is slow, your cells have plenty of leftover calories to store as fat. Turning up your RMR, even slightly, can have a major effect on your weight. If it slows down, weight control is a challenge."

Calorie restriction, as in dieting or starvation, slows down our metabolisms so that we conserve energy, and our RMRs can stay suppressed for weeks after we end a low-calorie diet. Almost invariably this means that when we stop dieting we rebound and pack on the weight again. Our bodies have reasons that our reason can't understand - we cannot starve them into weight loss submission.

How then do we tweak our metabolic rates? Well, I have no spoiler alert to issue, because we already saw how under (9) Thermogenesis above. Here's a section from *Fat Genes* called "Insulin and the after-meal burn."

"You can rev up a slow metabolism, and this is where insulin comes in... insulin's job is to push proteins and sugars into cells of your body to build body parts and energize your movements. [I hope you caught the part about proteins...] These nutrients come from the foods you eat. They trigger your pancreas to release insulin into your bloodstream... Insulin travels to your muscles, liver, and fat tissues, where it pushes proteins and sugars into your cells." [Again with the proteins...]

In the process, your metabolism rises dramatically. The reason is that, inside the cell, these natural sugars are building glycogen, the quick energy "batteries"... [Glycogen is sugar stored in our muscles for quick response.] Building glycogen is a big job, causing your cells to actually release calories in the form of heat... This is called the *thermic effect of food*, or TEF. It's a nice way to burn calories. All you do is eat, and your body does the rest. These calories are gone forever - they never get the chance to turn into fat.

This after-meal metabolism boost depends on two things. First, some foods spark a terrific burn, while others provide none at all. Glycogen is made from natural sugars that come from carbohydrates. So spaghetti delivers a nice after-meal burn. So do most vegetables and beans. They are glycogen builders. The foods that cause the best burn are those that contain plenty of complex carbs (e.g., pasta, rice), or foods containing both carbs and protein. For example, broccoli and other vegetables are about 50 percent complex carbs and 40 percent protein, a mix for a good burn."

It takes work, or physical energy, to build something, in this case glycogen out of sugar molecules. Energy is expended in the form of heat. As mentioned above, fat is stored almost effortlessly, as is. Hence the thermic advantage of eating carbohydrates for weight loss - it's not converted into fat as efficiently as fat is.

Dr. Barnard continues: "On the other hand, butter, chicken grease, and olive oil are just fat, and they deliver a much poorer burn. In an experiment, Swiss researchers fed seven young men high-fat meals, with fat totaling 52 percent of their calories, roughly the amount found in fried chicken or french fries. They looked for any evidence that the men's bodies would respond by burning off some of this excess fat. No dice. Excess fat is mainly stored. It goes from fork to lips to your body fat. Replacing healthy complex carbs with a load of fat in this study, robs you of much of your after-meal burn. So the first key is to choose foods that supply the right raw material.

Second, the after-meal burn depends on insulin getting nutrients into your cells... and unfortunately some people poison their insulin. By eating fatty foods, or by accumulating a fair amount of body fat... ["the fat we eat or the fat we wear."]... insulin is awash in grease. The cell's tiny machinery that is supposed to convey nutrients inside becomes resistant to insulin, as if insulin's hand is slipping on a greasy doorknob. The pancreas then responds by sending more and more insulin into the blood to try to get proteins [!] and sugars into the cells... and to pack fat into fat cells... and this is when insulin becomes a problem."

What's the problem with elevated insulin levels brought on by eating animals and junk? Insulin's job "is to push nutrients into your cells. As it does so, *it temporarily shuts down your fat-burning machinery*... In the short run, this is no problem. Insulin pushes sugar **and protein** [!] into the cells and then goes away. The interruption in fat-burning is brief. But when insulin resistance develops, the body produces more and more insulin, and it shuts off fat-burning more effectively than it should... A persistent insulin rise actually increases LPL in your fat tissues, with that result that you can store fat more and more easily, and decreases LPL in your muscles, impairing your ability to burn fat.

A lack of fiber adds to the problem. Normally, fiber - plant roughage - helps keep insulin levels in check by slowing the release of sugars from the foods you eat, among other functions. When researchers track people's diets and measure insulin in their blood, those with the most fiber have the lowest insulin levels."

When Planters eat, everything we swallow has fiber in it. That's why Planters have the best glucose control... optimum body weights... the best insulin control... the least diabetes... and it's why we live years longer than Meaters and Junkers with their fiber-depleted diets.

In a sane world, that should be all we need to know for it to be game over, with low-carbers and paleonutters confined to the trashcan of history. The low-grain Planting that post-Atkins low-carbers have added to their verkakte diets has made them slightly better than they once were (i.e., awful). **The only good thing about low-carb diets is the Planting.**

I've quoted at length from Dr. Barnard here, and why not? He's probably the world's foremost expert at reversing type 2 diabetes, using (as all excellent diabetes exorcists do) an extremely high-carb whole-plant diet. He's the man who coined the term 'intramyocellular lipids, the 'inside-muscle-cell fats' that cause insulin resistance and diabetes.

Unlike Low-Carb Bullshit Artists Dr. Barnard has actually cured thousands of people PLUS he's documented his Planter techniques with rigorous peer-reviewed research. All the best, Dr. B, with your new Barnard Medical Center. May you go from healing strength to strength.

Isn't it great? Plant-based nutrition is fast becoming mainstream medicine.

[As an aside, I'm proud to be a graduate of the Food for Life training program provided by Dr. Barnard's Physicians Committee for Responsible Medicine in conjunction with The Plantrician Project.]

I'm going to let Dr. Barnard have the last word on the topics of insulin, glycogen and body weight:

"So how do we get this metabolic boost? The best foods for an after-meal burn are those that are

- high in healthy carbohydrates to build glycogen
- high in fiber to keep insulin on track
- low in fat to make insulin efficient

This means that our best choices for building glycogen, while keeping insulin efficient, are

- Beans, peas, and lentils of any variety
- Fruit - e.g., apples, bananas, oranges, pears
- Green vegetables - e.g., asparagus, broccoli, spinach
- Pasta (despite having lost fiber, it releases its sugars slowly…)
- Sweet potatoes or yams
- Whole grains: brown rice, barley, bulgur, pumpernickel bread, or oatmeal.

[In other words: Planting.]

Poor choices include

• Dairy products and eggs - they have no fiber and most are high in fat
• Foods with added fat, such as french fries and salad oils
• Olives, nuts, seeds, and avocados, as they are among the few plant foods that are naturally high in fat
• Poultry, beef, or other meats - they have no fiber or complex carbohydrates and have more fat than you need
• Sugar candies and sodas - lots of sugar, but no fiber
• White bread, and most other refined grain products, as they have lost most of their fiber...

[In other words: Meating and Junking. (We'll add avos when we're skinny.)]

Rather than avoid carbs, it is better to fix our body's natural ability to process them. It is worth remembering that carbohydrates have only four calories per gram, while fats have nine. Carbohydrates are not the enemy. They are, in fact, our natural energy source."

33. Genes and the effects of exercise

Regardless of our genetic heritage, whether our parents gifted us with Type I muscle fibers for increased endurance or more sedentary Type IIs, we all benefit from regular, moderate exercise.

Exercise has multiple benefits. Among others, physical activity

• burns calories
• builds and invigorates muscles, a process that requires energy
• improves our immune function
• improves our mood, combatting depression
• combats ADHD in children
• raises our HDL cholesterol levels without fail, unless we're low-carbers
• improves our insulin sensitivity
• boosts our resting metabolic rate for hours afterwards
• controls our appetite, and
• "counteracts the fat-storage effect of LPL [lipoprotein lipase]."

In Dr. Barnard's words: "LPL extracts fat from the bloodstream and passes it either into fat tissue for storage - which means more body fat - or into muscle cells where it is burned for energy. Exercise does exactly what you might hope. It slows down the LPL enzyme in fat tissues, making it harder to store fat, and increases LPL's activity in muscles, pushing fat into muscle cells to be burned."

For best weight control, we do best when we do just these few things:

Boost the amount of fiber we eat - plenty of whole plants
Keep fat to a minimum - no animals or junk
Get an hour or so of moderate aerobic exercise, every day if possible. The more we exercise, the more we can exercise.

Simple. Planting plus physical activity.

34. Lack of exercise ~ sedentary behavior

Inactivity is an important part of the "multi-factorial obesity model." Here's a study showing how sedentary vegans have less obesity where it counts – in our arteries – than multiple-decade Meater endurance athletes (80 km (50 miles) per week for 21 years):

S. Murakami et al. Common carotid intima-media thickness is predictive of all-cause and cardiovascular mortality in elderly community-dwelling people: Longitudinal Investigation for the Longevity and Aging in Hokkaido County (LILAC) study. *Biomed. Pharmacother.* 2005 59(Suppl 1):S49 – S53.

The equation of energy in = energy out is heavily skewed towards what we take in. There are very few of us who offset the amount of energy we take in with exercise. We have to exercise for tens of minutes to account for what may take only seconds to consume.

Still, we're built to move, and exercise has multiple benefits beyond helping us, as a junior partner to what we eat, to maintain a healthy body weight – exercise is beneficial "medicine" in preventing depression, osteoporosis, hypertension, diabetes, cardiovascular disease and cancer.

Because Meaters and Junkers tend to be overweight, they may become self-fulfilling prophets, and exercise even less. Complacency may set in for vegans, who tend to be slender without exercising. Not to exercise regularly is to live a shorter (and less eventful!) life.

35. Stress

Stress is a risk factor for obesity. From the cellular level on up, Planting mitigates stress, while Meating exacerbates it.

36. Sleep deprivation

Not sleeping enough is stressful, and it's a risk factor for obesity. Especially in later years, Planters have the best sleep patterns, probably because they have optimal melatonin levels in their brains. Meating seriously lowers our melatonin levels. Meaters suffer far more from sleep disturbances such as sleep apnea (and it's my unsupported observation and opinion that we also snore more when we Meat).

37. Dopamine deficiency and anhedonia

Obese people (and other addicts) lose sensitivity to dopamine, the "pleasure hormone." Meating lowers our dopamine levels, diminishing our ability to feel pleasure. Upping the dose is what addicts do when faced with diminishing returns. Parkinson's is a dopamine-deficiency and environmental contamination condition, as is obesity. We can think of both as mental disorders, brought on mainly by eating animals and junk.

Obesity can be thought of as the outcome of an underlying addiction to Meating and Junking: behavior we know to be harmful but which we can't control. Planting restores our dopamine sensitivity.

38. Inflammation

Inflammation, obesity, metabolic syndrome, heart "disease", and Meating and Junking all go together in one inseparable correlative, cause-and-effect mishmash. They're all the same thing, really. Whole plants, unlike low-carb diets, are anti-inflammatory. Whether it's inflammation, oxidation, obesity, atherosclerosis, diabetes, dementia, stroke or heart attacks, Planters get way less of it. These conditions and "disease" are elective.

39. Sugar and High Fructose Corn Syrup (HFCS)

Junk. I could have mentioned sweeteners earlier – for instance, when I mentioned vegetable oils, the other major form of plant junk – but I wanted to save them for near the end.

The fructose in figs and pears and peaches and plums is magnificent food, packaged as it is with fiber and other phytonutrients. People who eat the most fruits and vegetables have the best insulin sensitivity and the least diabetes. (We're also the happiest and 'most flourishing,' according to Conner et al, On carrots and curiosity. *Br J Health Psychol,* 2015.)

The fructose in table sugar and HFCS is disease- and obesity-causing poison, stripped of nutrients. We eat it at our peril. And we do, big time.

In the last century, we've upped our sugar intake from <2 kg to >45 kg (4 to 100 pounds) per person per year, and the added empty calories – which come mainly from guzzling super-sized portions of soda pop – definitely help cause obesity and insulin resistance. Refined sugar is ubiquitous in packaged items sold as food. We shouldn't touch any of it – it's not food.

As we see with gout, in which the purines in animals and the isolated fructose in junked plants both cause the "disease," it's the animals *and* the fractured plants that combine to make us fat and ill.

Junking contributes mightily to the diabetes epidemic, with the number of cases doubling in the last decade, up to a million new cases of diabetes each year now. Although some researchers, such as the inventor of 'biometrics' (the statistical analysis of biological data), John Komlos, thinks we've been becoming heavier for at least a hundred years, it's apparent that we've entered a geometric phase of obesity growth since the early 1970s, which corresponds roughly to the introduction of HFCS into the "food" chain.

Although LCBAs like to claim otherwise, we didn't eat less fat during the '70s, '80s and '90s - we ate more. But because we ate more of everything, the percentage of fat we ate went down. Fat consumption still went up.

It's a complicated issue, with good points being made for the various positions. My own opinion is that the consumption of two non-foods has reached a mutually reinforcing peak, and together they produce the hockey-stick graph typical of population and other geometric progressions.

We don't look at the sudden recent upturn of the world population graph and think that's when overpopulation started. The same with hyperinflation of currencies. We know that a constant 1 or 2% increase over many years eventually leads to a very short doubling time. Things look worse, but the same growth rate applies. As Albert Bartlett, the doyen of the subject, points out, our human brains are wired to recognize arithmetic growth, not geometric, so it's tempting to look at the obesity graph over time and blame everything on something that happened around the inflexion point, where a perfectly natural long-term process starts to cause extreme turbulence within a population. I'm not saying this to vindicate high-fructose corn syrup – it's not food and we shouldn't drink it.

A factor that few people consider is the exponentially greater contamination of our environment with alkylphenols and other chemicals since World War II. These animal-borne obesogens aren't recorded on obesity graphs along with processed sugars and animals, yet they may make account for a large proportion of animal fats' role in causing obesity. In effect, the number of animals we eat has risen fairly slowly, while their obesogenic effect has shot through the roof in the last few decades. Some researchers even speculate that almost all of the obesogenic and/or diabetogenic effects of animal fats are down to bio-magnified environmental toxins. In their view, fat people get more diabetes because their own body fat is so full of Meater poisons.

China has about 1/7th the obesity of the USA, and Japan has 1/8th. Yet the 3 nations have roughly equivalent diabetes rates. Something's going on besides the link between obesity and diabetes. Oriental people's fat may be more polluted with diabetogenic chemicals… Watch their diabetes rates rise rapidly in the future if they catch up with the US in the fat-wearing stakes.

Let me repeat: it's not just the animals that make us fat and diabetic, and it's not just the sugar. It's both, acting together, potentiating each other, so that Meating makes Junking even worse than Junking alone.

Most of the benefits of low-carbing and paleo'ing come from avoiding Junking, then letting the added Planting mask the damage caused by the über-Meating.

40. Artificial sweeteners

More junk, also obesogenic, and most of them carcinogenic into the bargain. Vile stuff; not food. It's ironic that products that are designed specifically to be devoid of calories can contribute to weight gain, mainly because people tend to eat more calories overall, thinking the low-cal nature of their sweetener cuts them slack to overindulge elsewhere.

41. Not breastfeeding ~ Infant formula

Breast milk is Nature's single perfect animal food for humans, high in nutrients and very low in protein. Kids who're raised on formula instead of being breastfed wind up being considerably heavier later in life; along with a host of other issues, including diabetes, asthma, cancer and several other inflammatory conditions.

Cow's milk fed to infants may in the future qualify as physical abuse or assault with a deadly weapon.

I second Dr. John McDougall: infant formula is a dangerous non-food, and should only be available on prescription to mothers unable to produce or obtain breast milk.

42. Alcohol

Alcohol, providing 7 calories per gram, is fattening until such time as it's not: when cirrhosis of the liver kicks in, at which time weight loss and death may follow, unless our transplant op is successful. Alcoholics tend to be emaciated. For the rest of us alcohol probably contributes more to weight gain by removing our inhibitions and making us more likely to eat stuff we might not when sober or to eat more than we might.

43. Intermittent fasting ~ Autophagy

Since relinquishing my Meater and Junker addictions, I find that fasting occasionally is much easier, and I find it beneficial. We regularly rest most of our muscles and organ systems, other than our cardiac and pulmonary systems which it's best to keep continually on the job, so why not give our digestive tracts time off for good behavior? I do, usually for a week at each solstice and equinox; for no particular reason except to connect to the cycle of seasons.

When we fast we burn up our glycogen stores of glucose in our muscles, then we start burning fat deposits, then we do quality control: we chuck anything we can lay our metabolic hands on into the mitochondrial boilers: broken mitochondria, broken proteins, broken gene strands, whatever's defective. Afterwards we're left with a lean, clean biting machine, with nothing but brand-new, authentic working parts. It feels great.

After day 3 or so, when we hit our peak of detox and our nadir of energy, it's a breeze. After two weeks, my longest stint, I felt refreshed, rejuvenated, full of energy and considerably lighter. Much of the weight comes back, being water that's associated with the glycogen stores we need to replenish in our muscles.

I'm going out on a limb here, but I've never heard of Meaters or Junkers being able to fast for long periods. I think their symptoms of detox are just too fierce, plus they miss their sugar and animal meal-time high too much.

Autophagy, besides being great for reducing body weight quickly, is one of the reasons why Planting confers greater longevity.

Enemas with body-temperature water – not coffee, which has killed some people, Gerson therapy notwithstanding – are a useful adjunct to fasting. The single-day transit time of Planter meals is conducive to easy enemas. Lord knows what happens with gunk that's been up between them thar hills for a week or more – my mind shies away, like a panicked horse.

(Please don't fast without supervision.)

(44.) The Dietary Guidelines of the USDA

The single greatest cause of obesity and degenerative "diseases" is probably what this US government department tells people is food. Short-sighted, venal and corrupt; controlled by Meater and Junker interests, the US Department of Agriculture is the clearest and most present danger to the nation and, by example and by trade diktat, to the rest of the world. Despite tens of thousands of studies in the last quarter century, amounting to near total consensus among the scientific community (in which obtaining consensus is like herding cats) about the dangers of Meating and the benefits of Planting, Meating has sat for decades atop the USDA's sickening "Food" Pyramid or upon their sickening My Plate, and receives 5 out of every 6 subsidy dollars.

Cui bono? That's a routine question to ask when a crime's been committed. Who profits? Corporations profit by feeding us rubbish that makes us fat and sick, then other corporations (owned by the same people), to deal with the disasters caused be eating non-foods, profit through selling us expensive insurance policies, pharmaceuticals and medical interventions; which are propagandized by giant advertising, marketing, public relations and media corporations, owned by the same people – all unnecessary for Planters. These gargantuan industries are all built on eating animals, or eating, drinking or smoking junk.

More than we know, we're a childish cowboy culture, still not weaned from our mother's titty; a consumer society programmed to consume the things that will create a market for other things that we're told will make us happy and fix the damage caused by the things we consumed in the first place. (Phew. Try that on one breath.)

Or we could just be true to our human nature, be Planters, and evade the clutches of the Meater oligarchs altogether.

The USDA is complicit in the deaths of millions of people each year, and it's a global disgrace.

(In *The Low-Carb Bullshit Artists Are Lying Us to Death*, I detail how LCBAs like Gary Taubes and his many plagiarists defame the late Senator George McGovern over his role in setting up the first US dietary guidelines.)

OK, let's move on… before I really start to speak my mind.

I've listed a collection of mechanisms by which Meating and Junking make us fat, and by which Planting makes us slender – more than one for each day and night Jesus spent fasting in the wilderness, before returning strong and lean, unmoved by his encounters with the tempting Meater devil.

I'm sure this isn't a complete list – that would take a book, all on its own. These are some of the more-than-plausible, proven biological mechanisms which confirm the epidemiological studies showing that Planters suffer from obesity to a negligible extent in comparison to Meaters and Junkers.

Weight management

As we can see, weight management isn't just a question of calories in = calories out. Plant energy is far more beneficial than animal energy, let alone junk energy.

This book isn't a weight loss manual. However, if we follow the science and eat nothing but whole plants, we're following the healthiest, most effective and safest weight loss program ever devised, and it's the only one that's permanent.

We're eating food.

Fat is a Meater and Junker issue.

Here are **the only ten words we need to know to manage our weight** in the best possible way, while also giving ourselves the best chance of living the longest, healthiest possible lives:

Eat a wide variety of whole plants. Add mushrooms, B_{12}.

That's all we need to know about nutrition.

If I were to expand slightly on this pithy weight-loss-guide-cum-healthcare-manual, I'd say:

To be slender and healthy, and to live a long life, we should eat plenty of whole fruits (especially berries), whole veggies (especially leafy greens, alliums and crucifers), whole grains (whichever we like or can tolerate), nuts (especially walnuts), seeds (especially flax, pumpkin, hemp, chia, sunflower and sesame seeds) and legumes (beans, peas, chickpeas and lentils). Add in mushrooms occasionally (especially white buttons) and drink clean water. Exercise moderately every day, preferably for an hour outdoors so we get enough sunlight on our skins to make vitamin D. Sleep enough, but not too much. Laugh, play, love, listen to music (especially Mozart), make music, sing, take part, join. And take a regular B_{12} supplement.

Before we leave obesity, I'd like to make one last observation. Have you ever noticed that we seem to find something when we're not looking for it, or perhaps when we've stopped looking? Looking for what? Oh, anything… small stuff like our car keys or… Enlightenment. Oh, there they are, under the sofa, or where William Carlos Williams found it, in the shape of a *red* wheel barrow:

"So much depends upon
a red wheel barrow
glazed with rain water
beside the white chickens."

The items we're missing are right there where we left them, or it's right there in front of us, in this very moment, where and when we're yet to notice it and claim it for our own.

When we're either vegans (who forego Meating on compassionate, ethical or spiritual grounds) who're eating a whole-food plant-based diet, or Planters who do the same for optimum health, ideal weight management just comes along for the ride. It's incidental. It's a freebie. If we're too skinny, we gain weight until we reach a new equilibrium. If we're overweight, the extra pounds melt away, with none of the low-carb side effects such as constipation, bad breath, atherosclerosis, increased colorectal cancer and decreased lifespan. Planting isn't necessarily about weight loss. It's about eating the healthiest possible diet, and perfect body weight is just one of a multitude of health benefits that accrue, from reversing arterial "disease" to preventing stroke and dementia… oh, the entire gamut of chronic Meater and Junker conditions I list in this book.

Weight loss? Meh. Low-Carb Bullshit Artists are big on weight loss because it's all they have to offer. Planting does it better, without trying.

That's it for obesity. We're now officially expert obesiologists, and none of us will ever eat another animal or piece of junk again. (My lips to God's ear.)

Let's take a closer look now at diabetes…

Diabetes

Let's lay the groundwork…

Planting always has two benefits. It gives us all the good stuff in plants and it has none of the bad stuff in animals and junk.

Meating always has the opposite double whammy: it's full of all the bad stuff in animals, with precious little of the good stuff from plants.

Our own eyes tell us that skinny vegans and vegetarians are the norm.

Population studies, such as the Adventist studies which started in 1974, confirm that our vision of obesity as a Meater and Junker issue is 20/20.

Migration studies confirm how genetically similar people have different health outcomes after migrating to new territories with new dietstyles. We can eat ourselves slender and healthy, or fat and sick – it's our choice.

I've listed 40 biological mechanisms of Meater/Junker obesity, and Planter leanness, which align with our own experience and the best epidemiology and migration studies (and also of studies of lapsed vegetarians.)

As a group, Planters are lean. Vegans can be overweight, usually when we're Junkers or sedentary, or both.

When we're Meaters and Junkers we're overweight, and our excess body fat is what sets us up for diabetes. However, it's not just our body fat that's linked to diabetes…

Again, the exceptional Meater low-carbers and paleofantasists may not be overweight, but they still tend to be diabetic. (Which is weird, because they're avoiding the carbs they say cause diabetes.) As we'll see, this is because they fill themselves with animal fat at each meal, instead of wearing an animal fat body suit full-time.

This is really important: Meaters who're overweight get more diabetes because (1) they carry **more body fat** made out of animal fat, and (2) animal fats are mega-polluted with **diabetes-causing chemicals**, and (3) there are **other diabetes-causing components of animals** that aren't in plants.

Meaters who're not overweight get more diabetes for reasons (2), constant exposure to toxic waste at mealtimes, and (3), the other obesogenic substances unique to, or concentrated in, animal flesh.

Continuing this important theme, **obese (Junker) vegans get half the diabetes of Meaters and Junkers of the same body weight**, because of (2), less exposure to diabetogenic environmental poisons, and no, or far less, exposure to (3). (NB. This is a key point to remember – while diabetes is connected to obesity, the connection to Meater obesity is twice as strong as that to Planter obesity.

Diabetes IS about Junking – eating processed sugars – but it's more about Meating.

We need to learn to count to two. Stopping at one and shouting eureka, it's the sugar! doesn't help us. It's not just sugar that causes diabetes, and it's not just animals. It's both, and, importantly, the addition of animals to sugars makes sugars more obesogenic and diabetogenic than sugars on their own.

Diabetes is about 'meat + sweet.'

Let's look now at the basics of glucose metabolism [the way the body uses digested nutrients for energy], to see why Meating and Junking make us so prone to diabetes, and why Planting is protective, even in overweight vegans.

Glucose metabolism

Glucose (sugar) is the substance that powers our cells, along with oxygen. In a healthy body, when we eat starch (carbohydrate) and digest it into glucose molecules, our pancreas releases a hormone called insulin, whose job it is to take the digested and absorbed glucose from our blood, ferry it through the outer membranes of our cells (particularly muscle cells) and, once inside the cells, to organelles called mitochondria, the cells' power plants, where the glucose is burned to produce energy.

We're sun- and oxygen- and sugar-powered beings. Sugar is so vital to our survival that, if we're deprived of sugar, our body has a fall-back mechanism called gluconeogenesis to create new glucose out of other nutrients, such as fats and proteins.

Now let's straighten out our terminology:

Diabetes

People with diabetes have unhealthily elevated blood sugar levels (and unhealthily depressed cellular glucose levels), which combine to produce a slew of unhealthy outcomes, or complications.

Type 1 diabetes

In type 1 diabetes, the insulin-producing beta cells within the islets of Langerhans in the pancreas have been destroyed, so the pancreas can't secrete enough (or any) insulin, so sugar builds up in the blood, where it can injure our arteries, system-wide.

Those of us with this condition need to take glucose-lowering medications or inject ourselves with insulin to manage our glucose. Accordingly, type 1 is also known as insulin-dependent diabetes. It's a life-long condition, and thought to be irreversible. (I'll come back to this.) It used to be called early- or juvenile-onset diabetes, because it was confined to childhood. Because of our modern meat + sweet, dairy-rich diet, this is no longer true, so... type 1.

Our later discussion of type 1 diabetes will focus on the multiple ingredients and mechanisms of Meating and Junking which degrade our pancreas's ability to produce insulin.

By definition, people with type 1 diabetes have hypoinsulinemia, low blood insulin levels.

Hyperglycemia
High blood sugar, or high blood glucose.

Type 2 diabetes
In type 2 diabetes, our pancreas secretes insulin but something blocks the insulin from bringing the glucose through the cell membranes, into the cells and to the mitochondria. Sugar builds up to dangerously high levels in the blood, with a concomitant overly high blood level of insulin, while energy production within cells is diminished.

Type 2 is usually a temporary, elective symptom of Meating and Junking, easily reversible within 3-4 weeks by pure Planting and exercise.

Type 2 used to be called adult- or late-onset diabetes, but now, because of massive Meating and Junking by juveniles, kids as young as 8 are developing it, so... type 2.

WARNING

Newbies to Planting, who're taking diabetes medications, should work with an understanding physician – in the majority of cases, on a pure Planter diet, *you will need to adjust your dosages,* or else you'll run the risk of dropping your blood sugar too low, before you come off your meds for good.

Our later discussion of type 2 diabetes will focus on animal fat and the multiple toxins within animal fat which combine to cause insulin resistance; heme iron and other animal peculiarities which do the same; plus the perils of fractionated plants.

Insulin resistance
Whatever's stopping insulin from performing its glucose-ferrying task is said to make our muscle cells resistant to insulin. The insulin is there but it doesn't work very well. Blood insulin may build up to dangerous levels.

The hyperglycemia of type 2 diabetes is caused by insulin resistance. (The high blood glucose levels of type 1 diabetes result from insulin insufficiency.)

As Dr. John McDougall says, besides facilitating the transport of glucose and proteins into muscle cells, another "important effect of insulin is to facilitate the storage of dietary fat into fat cells." So, when we're insulin resistant, not only can glucose not enter muscle cells; fats don't enter fat cells as easily, and the free fatty acids in our blood will rise. Fat will also accumulate ectopically, where it doesn't belong, within the muscle cells, where glucose is supposed to be. And the fat in the muscle cells creates free radicals and toxic fatty metabolites which impede insulin in its other role of attaching to insulin receptors and transporting glucose through the cell membrane. It's a circular mess.

John McDougall. Simple Care for Diabetes. The McDougall Newsletter December 2009.

Hyperinsulinemia

Dangerously high levels of insulin in the blood, secreted to try to deal with the high blood sugar level. Hyperinsulinemia can lead to cancer, insulin and insulin-like growth factor-1 (IGF-1) being similar in this regard.

Prediabetes

Types 1 and 2 diabetes may take many years to develop. Over the years our blood glucose levels rise higher and higher, as our pancreatic health declines and our insulin resistance increases.

Clinically, "People with a fasting glucose level of 100 to 125 mg/dL have impaired fasting glucose (IFG), or prediabetes. A level of 126 mg/dL or above, confirmed by repeating the test on another day, means a person has diabetes." (http://www.niddk.nih.gov/)

People with blood glucose below 100 mg/dL have healthy glucose metabolisms. (In other words, they're probably young or Planters.)

Gestational diabetes

A third form of diabetes – gestational diabetes – is the kind we give ourselves during pregnancy by eating Meater and Junker non-foods, even before we become pregnant.

Qiu et al concluded that "high egg and cholesterol intakes before and during pregnancy are associated with increased risk of gestational diabetes mellitus." Not just white sugar: animals.

Qiu C, Frederick IO, Zhang C, Sorensen TK, Enquobahrie DA, Williams MA. Risk of gestational diabetes mellitus in relation to maternal egg and cholesterol intake. *Am J Epidemiol.* 2011 Mar 15;173(6):649-58.

Type 1 ½ diabetes

In their paper, Type 1½ diabetes: myth or reality? *Autoimmunity.* 1999;29(1):65-83, R Juneja and JP Palmer talk about Type 1 ½ Diabetes: a mixture of type 1 because our pancreas is less able to secrete insulin, and type 2 because the insulin we do secrete is less effective.

Eatiological animal suspects include animal fats, cholesterol, glycotoxins, heme iron and nitrosamines from processed meats and eggs, in particular.

Type 1 ½ diabetes is a useful unofficial concept to describe the continuum between types 1 and 2 diabetes. As we'll see, types 1 and 2 have the same Meater and Junker Eatiology. Eating animals and junk cause beta cell damage and insulin resistance at the same time.

This is important to keep in mind. Meating and Junking, the two causes of diabetes (types 1 & 2), simultaneously damage our beta cells, thus limiting our ability to produce insulin, AND make us insulin resistant, thus increasing our need for the insulin we're less able to produce.

Think: Ouroboros, forever eating our own tail.

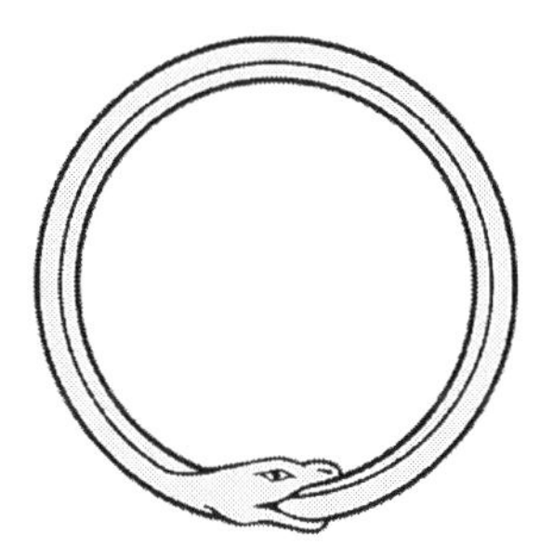

https://upload.wikimedia.org/wikipedia/commons/thumb/c/c8/Ouroboros-simple.svg/2000px-Ouroboros-simple.svg.png

Types 1 and 2 diabetes don't have separate causes and separate symptoms and separate treatments. They lie along a scale of same-ness. By the time we get a T2D diagnosis, we may already have lost half of our beta cells. This is in part because eating animal fats raises the level of free fats circulating in our blood – they're called NEFAs, or non-esterified fatty acids – and they are one of several animal agents that cause both insulin resistance and beta cell destruction, at the same time.

The causes of insulin resistance, prediabetes and all three forms of diabetes are Meating and Junking.

Their common symptom is high blood sugar, which results from a combination of insulin resistance AND beta cell destruction.

Their treatment is Planting, best done preventively, before the fact.

Diabetes in a nutshell

In a (large) nutshell, here's why Planters get a fraction of the diabetes we give ourselves with our knives and forks when we're Meaters and Junkers:

- Meaters and Junkers eat far more fat than Planters do
- Animal and junk fats are far more obesogenic and diabetogenic (diabetes-causing) than Planter fats
- Meaters and Junkers carry more body fat than Planters, some unhealthy low-carbers excepted
- Meaters have higher estrogen levels, and more estrogen-producing, diabetogenic bacteria in their gut flora
- Animal fats can contain more than a hundred thousand times as many diabetogenic environmental pollutants as plant fats do
- Meaters eat way more inflammatory AGEs than Planters (a.k.a. advanced glycation end-products, gerontotoxins or glycotoxins); think chickens, fishes and eggs.
- The hallmarks of animal and junk fats, and their contents, and other animal components such as heme iron, are that they're oxidizing and inflammatory, two processes which promote insulin resistance and diabetes
- Junkers eat far more high-glycemic carbs (sugar) than Planters do
- (No-glycemic) animal proteins provoke insulin secretion every bit as much as high-glycemic carbs (junk)
- Animals and sugars in combination are worse than their sum
- Meaters and Junkers secrete more insulin than Planters do
- Meaters and Junkers are far more insulin-resistant than Planters
- Planters have the best insulin sensitivity and the least diabetes.

The Adventist-2 study

That Planters get the least diabetes is beyond doubt.

Knowing this truth, Low-Carb Bullshit Artists and paleofantasists should all just STFU, because most of them base their idiotic claims on the evils of insulin resistance, and vegans are the least insulin-resistant people on the planet, with Planters the non-dairy cream of the crop. By the LCBAs' very own cherry-picked metric of ill-health – insulin resistance – no-animal eating annihilates high-animal eating. The extremely high whole-carb Planter diet obliterates low-carb.

What more needs to be said about the low-carb and paleo frauds?

Here's some more evidence. Take a look at the following graphic illustration of the results of a 2011 paper, by the same team from whom Neal Barnard got his 2009 obesity and diabetes data, above:

Tonstad S, et al., Vegetarian diets and incidence of diabetes in the Adventist Health Study-2, *Nutrition, Metabolism & Cardiovascular Diseases* (2011), page 7.

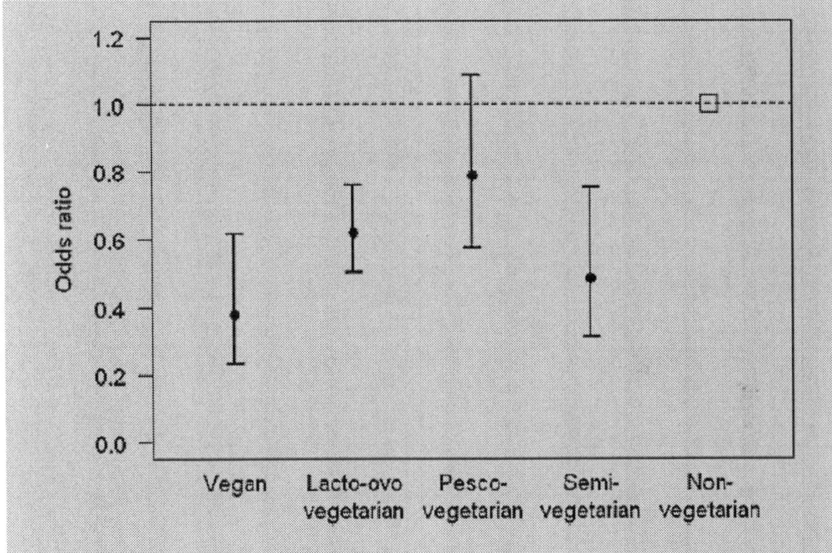

Figure 1 Odds ratios with 95% confidence intervals for incident diabetes by dietary group adjusted for age, BMI, ethnicity, gender, educational level, income, TV watching, sleep, alcohol, physical activity and cigarette smoking.

Meaters (nonvegetarians) are the sorry benchmark for ~~disease~~ in this study, because we humans give ourselves the most diabetes when we eat animals. Meaters are up at 1.0 (100%). In comparison, vegans average below 0.4 (40%). We're more than 2 ½ times more likely to get diabetes if we Meat.

Put another way, we can drop our risk of diabetes down a staircase as we remove from our plates the fishes, then the eggs and the dairy, and then all the animals.

It's up to us how healthy we want to be. Type 2 diabetes is an elective condition, brought on mainly by eating animals, while Junking contributes its share.

There is data to back up my claim that if the vegans in the Adventist-2 study became pure Planters, cutting out all junk, the risk of diabetes would plummet to 0.1 or less - 1/10th as much diabetes. 9 out of 10 cases prevented when we're Planters.

For example, the INTERHEART Study (*Lancet* 2004) shows that making 9 simple lifestyle changes can wipe out >90 % of our heart attacks, almost 80% of strokes and 91% of diabetes. Changes like not smoking, not using alcohol, getting enough exercise and not Meating or Junking.

Junked plants are responsible for most of the diabetes in vegans, who may still get diabetes even without eating animals. Low-carbers should resonate with my reasoning here: after all, they believe that high-glycemic carbs cause *all* diabetes. How wrong they are – Junking is the junior partner in the firm of Death, Meat and Junk, Inc.

As we can see, animals cause most of the Eatiology of diabetes. Dropping the animals from our diets removes 60% of the diabetes risk that Meaters face. Dropping the junk can remove much of the remaining 40%. All that would remain after that would be non-dietary environmental toxins, stress, normal oxidative and inflammatory wear-and-tear, and vitamin X deficiency – not enough exercise.

Here's what Tonstad and her team have to say about diet, body weight and diabetes:

"RESULTS— Mean BMI was lowest in vegans (23.6 kg/m^2) and incrementally higher in lacto-ovo-vegetarians (25.7 kg/m^2), pesco-vegetarians (26.3 kg/m^2), semi-vegetarians (27.3 kg/m^2), and nonvegetarians (28.8 kg/m^2). [<25 is healthy; >25 = overweight]

Prevalence of type 2 diabetes increased from 2.9% in vegans to 7.6% in nonvegetarians; the prevalence was intermediate in participants consuming lacto-ovo (3.2%), pesco (4.8%), or semi-vegetarian (6.1%) diets.

After adjustment for age, sex, ethnicity, education, income, physical activity, television watching, sleep habits, alcohol use, and BMI, vegans…, lacto-ovo vegetarians…, pescovegetarians…, and semi-vegetarians… had a lower risk of type 2 diabetes than nonvegetarians."

[Note: If the authors hadn't adjusted for BMI, the results would look even worse for the Meaters, because the Planters are so much skinnier than the Meaters. The authors were trying to account for why Meaters get so much more diabetes, and looking for reasons other than their body fat. That's like adding 40 pounds to a jockey (the average amount of extra weight Meaters carry, in comparison to vegans) and the vegan horse still wins, going away.]

"CONCLUSIONS— The 5-unit BMI difference between vegans and nonvegetarians indicates a substantial potential of vegetarianism to protect against obesity. Increased conformity to vegetarian diets protected against risk of type 2 diabetes after lifestyle characteristics and BMI were taken into account. Pesco- and semi-vegetarian diets afforded intermediate protection."

As a group, only vegans have ideal body weight, and vegans have the best insulin sensitivity and are least affected by diabetes. The more animals we add to our diet, the more diabetes we add. If vegetarians are content with "intermediate protection" against obesity and diabetes, so be it.

"Moderation kills," as Dr. Caldwell Esselstyn says.

Diabetes complications

At http://www.mayoclinic.org/diseases-conditions/type-2-diabetes/basics/complications/con-20031902, the Mayo Clinic says that

"Diabetes affects many major organs, including your heart, blood vessels, nerves, eyes and kidneys. Controlling your blood sugar levels can help prevent these complications.

Although long-term complications of diabetes develop gradually, they can eventually be disabling or even life-threatening."

In the USA, diabetes is the 7th leading cause of death, killing almost 69,000 Americans each year. Though the "disease" is called diabetes, what diabetics usually die of is cardiovascular complications such as stroke and heart "disease".

National Vital Statistics Reports, Vol. 60, No. 4, January 11, 2012 5

Table B. Deaths and death rates for 2010, and age-adjusted death rates and percent changes from 2009 to 2010, for the 15 leading causes of death: United States, final 2009 and preliminary 2010

[Data based on a continuous file of records received from the states. Rates are per 100,000 population. Rates are based on populations enumerated in the 2010 U.S. census as of April 1 for 2010 and estimated as of July 1 for 2009. Age-adjusted rates per 100,000 U.S. standard population are based on the year 2000 standard; see "Technical Notes." For explanation of asterisks (*) preceding cause-of-death codes, see "Technical Notes." Figures for 2010 are based on weighted data rounded to the nearest individual, so categories may not add to totals]

Rank[1]	Cause of death (based on the *International Classification of Diseases, Tenth Revision*, Second Edition, 2004)	Number	Death rate	Age-adjusted death rate		
				2010	2009[2]	Percent change
...	All causes	2,465,932	798.7	746.2	749.6	–0.5
1	Diseases of heart (I00–I09,I11,I13,I20–I51)	595,444	192.9	178.5	182.8	–2.4
2	Malignant neoplasms (C00–C97)	573,855	185.9	172.5	173.5	–0.6
3	Chronic lower respiratory diseases (J40–J47)	137,789	44.6	42.1	42.7	–1.4
4	Cerebrovascular diseases (I60–I69)	129,180	41.8	39.0	39.6	–1.5
5	Accidents (unintentional injuries) (V01–X59,Y85–Y86)[3]	118,043	38.2	37.1	37.5	–1.1
6	Alzheimer's disease (G30)	83,308	27.0	25.0	24.2	3.3
7	Diabetes mellitus (E10–E14)	68,905	22.3	20.8	21.0	–1.0
8	Nephritis, nephrotic syndrome and nephrosis (N00–N07,N17–N19,N25–N27)	50,472	16.3	15.3	15.1	1.3
9	Influenza and pneumonia (J09–J18)[4]	50,003	16.2	15.1	16.5	–8.5
10	Intentional self-harm (suicide) (X60–X84,Y87.0)[3]	37,793	12.2	11.9	11.8	0.8
11	Septicemia (A40–A41)	34,843	11.3	10.6	11.0	–3.6
12	Chronic liver disease and cirrhosis (K70,K73–K74)	31,802	10.3	9.4	9.1	3.3
13	Essential hypertension and hypertensive renal disease (I10,I12,I15)	26,577	8.6	7.9	7.8	1.3
14	Parkinson's disease (G20–G21)	21,963	7.1	6.8	6.5	4.6
15	Pneumonitis due to solids and liquids (J69)	17,001	5.5	5.1	4.9	4.1
...	All other causes (residual)	488,954	158.5	...	...	...

National Vital Statistics Reports Volume 60, number 4, January 11, 2012. Death, by Sherry L. Murphy, B.S.; Jiaquan Xu, M.D.; and Kenneth D. Kochanek, M.A.; Division of Vital Statistics, CDC, p. 5.

According to the Mayo Clinic, some of the potential complications of diabetes, besides death, include:

"• **Heart and blood vessel disease**. Diabetes dramatically increases the risk of various cardiovascular problems, including **coronary artery disease** with chest pain (**angina**), **heart attack**, **stroke**, narrowing of arteries (**atherosclerosis**) and **high blood pressure**. [Emphases added]

[Diabetes is a **coronary heart disease risk equivalent**, meaning that if we're diabetic with no diagnosis of heart "disease" then we're at the same risk of dying from heart "disease" as a non-diabetic person who's been diagnosed *with* heart "disease".]

• **Nerve damage (neuropathy).** Excess sugar can injure the walls of the tiny blood vessels (capillaries) that nourish your nerves, especially in the legs. This can cause **tingling, numbness, burning or pain** that usually begins at the tips of the toes or fingers and gradually spreads upward. Poorly controlled blood sugar can eventually cause you to **lose all sense of feeling** in the affected limbs. Damage to the nerves that control digestion can cause problems with **nausea, vomiting, diarrhea or constipation**. For men, **erectile dysfunction** may be an issue.

• **Kidney damage (nephropathy).** The kidneys contain millions of tiny blood vessel clusters that filter waste from your blood. Diabetes can damage this delicate filtering system. Severe damage can lead to **kidney failure or irreversible end-stage kidney disease**, which often eventually requires **dialysis or a kidney transplant**.

• **Eye damage**. Diabetes can damage the blood vessels of the retina (**diabetic retinopathy**), potentially leading to **blindness**. Diabetes also increases the risk of other serious vision conditions, such as **cataracts** and **glaucoma**.

• **Foot damage**. Nerve damage in the feet or poor blood flow to the feet increases the risk of various foot complications. Left untreated, cuts and blisters can become serious **infections**, which may heal poorly. Severe damage might require toe, foot or leg **amputation**.

• **Hearing impairment**. Hearing problems are more common in people with diabetes.

• **Skin conditions**. Diabetes may leave you more susceptible to skin problems, including **bacterial and fungal infections**.

• **Alzheimer's disease**. Type 2 diabetes may increase the risk of Alzheimer's disease. The poorer your blood sugar control, the greater the risk appears to be. The exact connection between these two conditions still remains unclear."

The connection between diabetes and Alzheimer's is unclear to the Mayo Clinic, perhaps; but it's not unclear to Eatiologists, who know that the same Meater and Junker diet's responsible for causing diabetes, Alzheimer's, coronary artery "disease", many cases of blindness besides diabetic retinopathy… and… and… and…

Risk factors for diabetes

Under "Risk Factors" for Type 2 Diabetes, the Mayo lists:

• Weight
• Fat distribution
• Inactivity
• Family history
• Race
• Age
• Prediabetes
• Gestational diabetes
• Polycystic ovary syndrome.

The Mayo scientists don't list • Meating and • Junking as risk factors for T2D, which is a shame, because **Meating and Junking are the biggest risk factors for diabetes**; types 1 and 2, and gestational diabetes.

Another risk factor the Mayo doesn't list is • Occupation. People who handle dead animals a lot in packing and slaughter factories get more diabetes, so it's posited that, as with obesity, there are **diabetogenic viruses** or other zoönotic infectious agents (prions?) in animals that are part of the cause of diabetes. The animal dose makes the poison, and these Meater professionals get far sicker than amateur Meaters, with a long list of conditions besides diabetes, because of their overdosing on animals.

Before I describe how Meating and Junking cause diabetes, how do we know if we have this dangerous "disease", or its fore-runner, prediabetes, the early condition of elevated-but-not-yet-critical blood sugar?

Symptoms of diabetes

The Mayo, at http://www.mayoclinic.org/diseases-conditions/type-2-diabetes/basics/symptoms/con-20031902, says that the symptoms of diabetes include:

"• **Increased thirst** and **frequent urination**. Excess sugar building up in your bloodstream causes fluid to be pulled from the tissues. This may leave you thirsty. As a result, you may drink — and urinate — more than usual.

• **Increased hunger**. Without enough insulin to move sugar into your cells, your muscles and organs become **depleted of energy**. This triggers intense hunger.

• **Weight loss**. Despite eating more than usual to relieve hunger, you may lose weight. Without the ability to metabolize glucose, the body uses alternative fuels stored in muscle and fat. Calories are lost as **excess glucose is released in the urine.**

• **Fatigue**. If your cells are deprived of sugar, you may become tired and **irritable**.

• **Blurred vision**. If your blood sugar is too high, fluid may be pulled from the lenses of your eyes. This may affect your ability to focus.

• **Slow-healing sores** or **frequent infections**. Type 2 diabetes affects your ability to heal and resist infections.

• **Areas of darkened skin**. Some people with type 2 diabetes have patches of dark, velvety skin in the folds and creases of their bodies — usually in the armpits and neck. This condition, called **acanthosis nigricans**, may be a sign of insulin resistance."

Sexual dysfunction in men and women is another common occurrence.

The Eatiology of Diabetes

Before I listed the symptoms of diabetes, I made a strong statement: that Meating and Junking are the biggest risk factors for all forms of diabetes. Let's see how.

Type 1 diabetes

Type 1 is the kind in which our pancreas can't produce insulin at all. To find out what causes type 1 diabetes, we need to find out what destroys our beta cells.

Type 1 diabetes is partly an auto-immune condition. One theory holds casein to blame. Apparently, a 17-amino acid chain in this cow's milk protein is identical to a similar chain in our pancreases, and casein's molecular mimicry of our pancreatic proteins confuses our immune systems into attacking ourselves.

It's more complicated than this: there may be a viral agent involved, we may need to be genetically predisposed, and there's a "probable link between mucosa-mediated immunoregulation" and type 1 diabetes… meaning that our intestinal bacteria are involved. [See Deranged gut flora, later, for an explanation of how Meating disrupts our gut flora.]

Leonard Harrison and Margo Honeyman. Cow's milk and Type 1 diabetes. The real debate is about mucosal immune function. *Diabetes* vol. 48 August1999; 1501-7.

But type 1 diabetes isn't just an auto-immune condition.

What else is toxic to pancreas cells? What kills them off?

Beta cell killers

There are a slew of ingredients in the Meater and Junker diet that can damage or destroy our beta cells, and prevent them from making insulin. Here's a list of the ones I know, with some cross-over between categories:

- Saturated fats
- Trans fats
- Omega-3 fats from fish oils (!) (via oxidation and elevated blood sugars)
- Partially hydrogenated vegetable oils
- Estrogens, and a corresponding lack of sex hormone-binding globulins
- Endocrine disruptors, or xeno-estrogens in environmental pollutants
- Persistent organic pollutants (POPs) such as dioxins, organochlorine pesticides, PCBs and DDT.
- Obesogens

- Diabetogens, chemical and possibly viral
- Cholesterol
- Heme iron
- Nitrites and nitrosamines
- Animal proteins
- Leucine, much of what we eat coming from animals. (Animal proteins, through the TOR pathway, can damage beta cells.)
- Heavy metals
- Oxidants or pro-oxidants – a general class of Meater and Junker items that produce free radicals, or oxidative stress, which can damage all our organs, including our pancreas
- Inflammation-causing substances (animals in general)

The Eatiology of diabetes shows it's a truly multi-, multi-factorial condition, far more complex than Low-Carb Bullshit Artists would have us believe.

We're not done with type 1 diabetes, but let's pick up the trail now that leads to type 2.

Hyperglycemia and hyperinsulinemia

Type 1 diabetes is a condition of **hyper**glycemia – having blood sugar levels that are too high. Type 1 is also a condition of **hypo**insulinemia, meaning very low insulin levels (which makes sense because the damaged pancreas can't make insulin).

Type 2 diabetes is a condition of **hyper**glycemia and **hyper**insulinemia. Our blood sugar levels are elevated, but so too are our insulin levels. Our (somewhat) healthy pancreases keep churning out more and more of the blasted stuff, but it just won't work.

This is a Meater and Junker condition known as

Insulin resistance

In a state of IR, our pancreatic beta cells are able to make enough insulin, the hormone that's responsible for transporting glucose out of the blood and into cells, where it's burned in the mitochondria to create ATP energy molecules. Something is stopping insulin from performing its glucose-ferrying task. Something is making us resistant to insulin. So, to combat the falling effectiveness of insulin, our pancreases overproduce insulin, leading to hyperinsulinemia, as mentioned above.

What causes insulin resistance? Certainly fractionated carbs can cause a very rapid spike in blood glucose, immediately followed by a rapid spike in insulin, secreted to deal with the glucose. This is how Junking causes IR. The low-carbers and the paleo crowd are right about this… but name me one nutritionist who ever said we should load up on processed junk like white bread and white sugar. Junking's not the end of the story.

The latest science shows that animal fat is the main cause of insulin resistance – animal fat, because of the effects of the fats themselves plus the environmental toxins that accumulate in fat.

Besides sludging our blood, animal fats prevent the insulin key from fitting into the cellular membrane lock, or insulin receptor site, thus preventing glucose from entering the cell. Once inside the cell, intramyocellular lipids (inside-muscle-cell-fats) impede glucose transport to and uptake by the mitochondria. (Are Meaters mitochondriacs?)

Hyperglycemia (excess blood sugar) is the result of insulin resistance, and diabetes may ensue, when our blood sugars stay too high, too long.

While diabetes is a condition OF high blood sugar, it's a condition that's caused mainly BY hyperlipidemia, excess FAT.

Lyudmila I. Rachek. Free fatty acids and skeletal muscle insulin resistance. *Progress in Molecular Biology and Translational Science* 2014, 121:267-292.

"Insulin resistance is now accepted to be closely associated with lipid [fat] accumulation in muscle cells…

Insulin resistance plays a key role in the development of type 2 diabetes mellitus and is also associated with several other diseases, such as obesity, hypertension, and cardiovascular diseases."

[This is a good use of the concept of "association." Type 2 diabetes is associated with obesity, and is caused in part by obesity. Type 2 diabetes is associated with cardiovascular "diseases", and helps cause them. Meanwhile, Meating and Junking underlie all three conditions, and help cause all of them.]

"Type 2 diabetes and obesity have become epidemic worldwide in the past few decades, and epidemiological and metabolic evidence indicates that the two conditions are linked closely through insulin resistance. The perturbation of free fatty acid (FFA) metabolism is now accepted to be a major factor contributing to whole-body insulin resistance, including that in skeletal muscle. **Acute exposure to FFAs and excess dietary lipid intake are strongly associated with the pathogenesis of muscle insulin resistance.**"

In other words, the fats we eat and fat accumulation in muscle cells and insulin resistance are inseparable. Their cause is Meating and Junking. Later we'll see that the fats we stored in our bellies and butts are as culpable as the fats we eat in causing insulin resistance, prediabetes and diabetes.

The process of insulin resistance develops over many years, slowly and insidiously, until, bang!, a tipping point is reached and our fasting blood sugars shoot through the roof. We felt ok, but we were gradually sickening. As with all geometric or compound growth rates, the same behavior (Meating and Junking) or growth rate that appeared benign suddenly results in a hockey-stick upward bend in the curve. Here's a graph from a Banting Memorial lecture – no, not William Banting the overweight 19th Century British undertaker, coffin-maker and diet pamphleteer – a Banting with something useful to say about diabetes, thank heavens.

R Taylor. Banting Memorial lecture 2012: reversing the twin cycles of type 2 diabetes. *Diabet Med.* 2013 Mar;30(3):267-75.

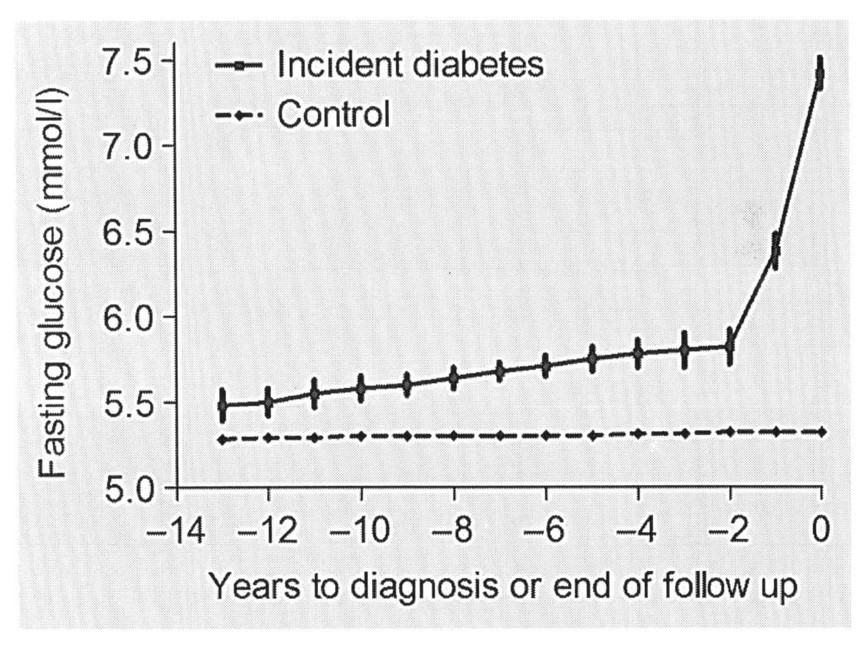

FIGURE 1 Change in fasting plasma glucose during the 13 years prior to onset of Type 2 diabetes.

Inchworm, inchworm, until inchworm morphs into insatiable dragon.

The beginning stage of diabetes is known as

Prediabetes

Prediabetes is the unhealthy state of having increased insulin resistance and elevated blood sugar levels, without having reached the somewhat arbitrarily defined clinical level at which we're diagnosed with diabetes, >125mg/dL.

More than 100 million Americans are prediabetic, and only 10 million of us know we are. That's more than 90 million Americans who're sick, but undiagnosed, with damage to hearts and arteries, kidneys and brains already happening because of insulin resistance and high blood sugars.

Still another 100 million Americans, because of being overweight, can be thought of as pre-prediabetic, with the risk factors of Meating and Junking firmly in places, while the accompanying-but-delayed blood sugar rise is still to manifest itself. And most of the remaining third of the population is not overweight but still at increased risk of insulin resistance because of animal fats (and their pollutants) and other animal components.

With prediabetes, if we don't control our blood sugars, either through unintended-consequence-laden drugs or through Planting and exercise, our condition may worsen until we give ourselves full-blown diabetes within ten years or so.

Adult onset diabetes

Adult onset diabetes is a term that's been replaced by type 2 diabetes. Adult onset is no longer used because our long-running epidemic of childhood obesity has led to kids as young as 8 developing diabetes. So prediabetes can be an issue in children very early in life, with consequent arterial damage, leading to eye, heart and kidney damage.

Childhood obesity has terrible consequences, which extend into adulthood, and should be nipped in the bud as early as possible. If a child is obese at the age of 6, they'll probably stay that way. Then, obese children – even if they later lose the weight – are far more likely to be sick as adults, and to die young… up to 20 years earlier.

Being obese in childhood is more predictive of inflammatory conditions in adulthood than the same kids' level of obesity in adulthood; conditions such as arthritis, cancer, gout and heart disease. Childhood obesity is like an iceberg: we see only fat children in the present, while submerged beneath the surface are (possibly slender) adults in the future who're cheated out of years of health and life.

Childhood obesity-related diabetes is the main reason that the latest generation of American children is the first ever who won't live longer than their parents. This is an outrageous situation, born out of our societal ignorance of what is and what isn't food.

Of course, the health issues these poor children face should be foremost in our minds, but the financial burden that present childhood obesity imposes on a future healthcare system is catastrophically high. A prudent government would subsidize the foods that have been shown to prevent childhood obesity, insulin resistance, prediabetes and diabetes – whole produce and fresh fruits, which currently receive less than 1% of the USDA's subsidies.

A prudent government would also eliminate or, at least, decrease their subsidization of non-foods shown to increase insulin resistance, such as animals and sugary junk, which currently receive more than 80% of subsidies. Most of the money goes to the politically powerful producers of high-fat, energy-dense, low-fiber, low-nutrient diabetogenic non-foods, instead of to the healthy low-fat, energy-spare, high-fiber, high nutrient, diabetes-preventing fruits, vegetables, beans, grains, nuts and seeds. Our government is using our money to fund the childhood obesity and diabetes epidemic.

This is the absurd situation: the agricultural arm of the US government fosters 'Meat + Sweet' by funneling hundreds of billions of dollars of free money to their cronies, and this will cost the medical arm of the government trillions of dollars to fight the future consequences of 'Meat + Sweet' – the sequelae of diabetes such as kidney disease, blindness, dementia and heart disease. Civilizations crumble for reasons exactly like this absurd misallocation of capital and resources. Will we go down in history as the empire that ate itself to death?

To take just one example: that the US government gives money to the producers of eggs, which one study has shown triple our risk of diabetes when we eat one a day, is bizarre, yet par for the course with the USDA. The bizarreness gets cranked up to another level when we find out that, because of federal 'truth in advertising' laws, the USDA can't allow egg producers to call their cholesterol hand grenades 'healthy' or 'nutritious.' Get this: they're not even allowed to call them 'safe.' Tell me: how can 'food disparagement' laws apply to non-foods that kill us?

People with diabetes who eat an egg a day double their risk of dying.

Animal flesh, milks and eggs are all obesogenic. So too are highly processed plant junk, with HFCS in sodas being one of the worst culprits in childhood obesity. We eat more than 20 times as much sugar now than we did a century ago, and our addiction is killing tens of thousands of us each year.

IT'S WHAT'S
OR DINNER.
American Egg Board
PORK & BOWLING
The US government
spends more than
$550 Million each year
to persuade Americans
to consume meat
and other animal products.
(and yet people complain about vegan propaganda)
Source: Meatonomics by David Robinson Simon
VeganStreet.com

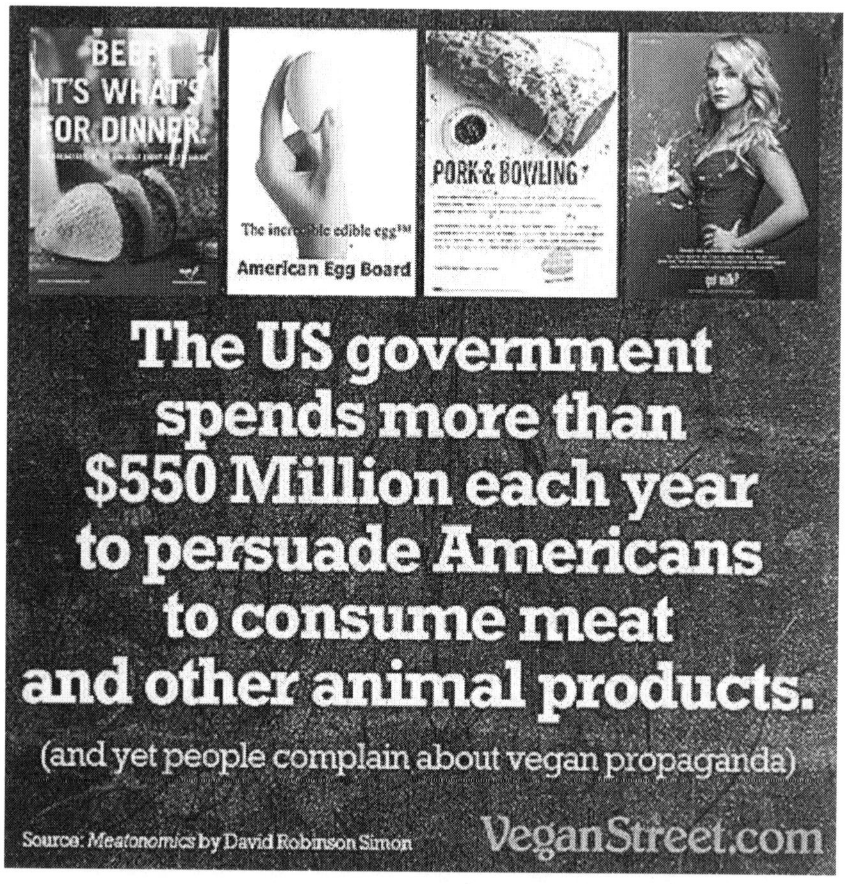

VeganStreet.com detailing the US government's role as a shill for Meating

(Propaganda is the right word: they're promoting harmful behavior.)

If I were Drug Czar for a day, I'd imprison the inventors of high fructose corn syrup and I'd slap huge taxes on sugar, a deadly drug at high dosages. At the very least, I'd stop funding the producers of sugar; the crack cocaine of non-foods. And I'd stop funding animal producers. Let's re-establish the price mechanism via supply and demand. I wonder how many burgers McDonald's would be able to push at $25 a pop, when deprived of their sickening, enabling subsidies. What's so special about the dealers of non-foods that their financial health takes precedence over the public's physical health? Surely a class action suit is in order?

Will it be the lawyers who save us?

To prevent childhood obesity and insulin resistance, Planting and exercise are best – low energy, high fiber and high nutrient intake allied with improved energy outgo. Plenty of sugar- and fiber-packed whole fruits and veggies, grains and beans. No high-calorie, low-fiber, low-nutrient junk (added sugars, HFCS, vegetable oils, fruit juices, white bread, white rice), and no high-calorie, low-fiber, low-nutrient animals (flesh, milk and eggs full of cholesterol, saturated and trans fats, and their inevitable toxic load of fat-loving environmental toxins). It's that simple.

Ground flax seeds are particularly beneficial, containing soluble fiber, omega-3 fatty acids and phytosterols, all promoters of insulin sensitivity. "Food is a package deal," so eating animals for omegas isn't smart.

We can think of this nutritional approach to preventing diabetes as whole-food vegan nutrition, or lifestyle medicine, or primordial prevention; primordial because it prevents the conditions that lead to ill-health from even arising. We heal ourselves, in advance, by not eating ourselves sick. Making simple lifestyle changes – Planting and exercise – can prevent >90% of diabetes. A single serving of animal a week raises our risk significantly, and we should eat as little high-glycemic junk as possible.

Okay, let's move on. Keeping in mind the overlap or continuum between types 1 and 2 diabetes, let's continue our examination of diabetes with…

"Diabesity" and Diabetes

There are several reasons why diabetes is so strongly linked to obesity:

1. Intramyocellular lipids

First, as Dr Neal Barnard has shown, the "intramyocellular lipids," a fancy way of saying "fats inside our muscle cells" (mainly the breakdown products of animal fats) prevent insulin from shepherding glucose through the outer cell membrane to the mitochondrial furnaces within the cells. Animal fat causes IR (insulin resistance) and our pancreas has to pump out more and more insulin to achieve the same result. We make plenty of insulin, even too much, but the fats are preventing the insulin from working properly.

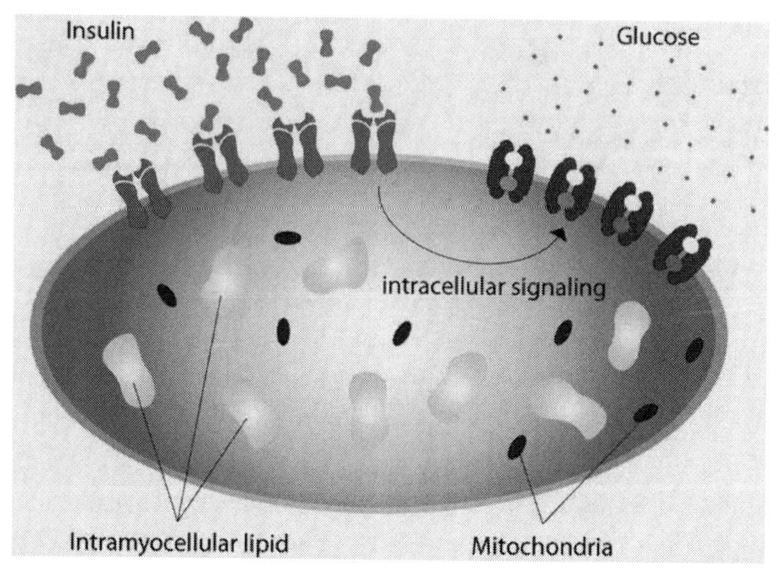

Intramyocellular lipids' ill-effects on glucose metabolism. Slide from a PowerPoint presentation by Dr. Neal Barnard: "Food for Life – Healthy Eating to Tackle Weight Problems, Cholesterol, and Diabetes."

For example, see: Neal D Barnard, Heather I Katcher, David JA Jenkins, Joshua Cohen, and Gabrielle Turner-McGrievy. Vegetarian and vegan diets in type 2 diabetes management. *Nutrition Reviews*® Vol. 67(5):255–263, which says:

"Vegetarian and vegan diets offer significant benefits for diabetes management. In observational studies, individuals following vegetarian diets are about half as likely to develop diabetes, compared with non-vegetarians. In clinical trials in individuals with type 2 diabetes, low-fat vegan diets improve glycemic control to a greater extent than conventional diabetes diets."

(The David JA Jenkins in this paper showing how it's best to manage T2D with an extremely high-carb Planter diet is the co-inventor of the Glycemic Index with which Low-Carb Bullshit Artists are besotted.)

The unhealthy build-up of fats in places where they're not supposed to be is called **ectopic fat accumulation**; ectopic as in an ectopic pregnancy, in which a fertilized egg may grow in a fallopian tube instead of the womb. This ectopic fat accumulation is driven by saturated fats from animals – lauric, myristic, palmitic and stearic fatty acids – and trans fats from animals and milk – and they're the ones that create muscular insulin resistance. Oleate, the fat from plants such as avos, nuts, seeds and olives provide improved blood sugar control and improved insulin sensitivity.

By the way, that fat is what immobilizes insulin and makes us insulin-resistant should have been the basis of diabetes research since the 1930s, following the work of Dr. H.P. Himsworth.

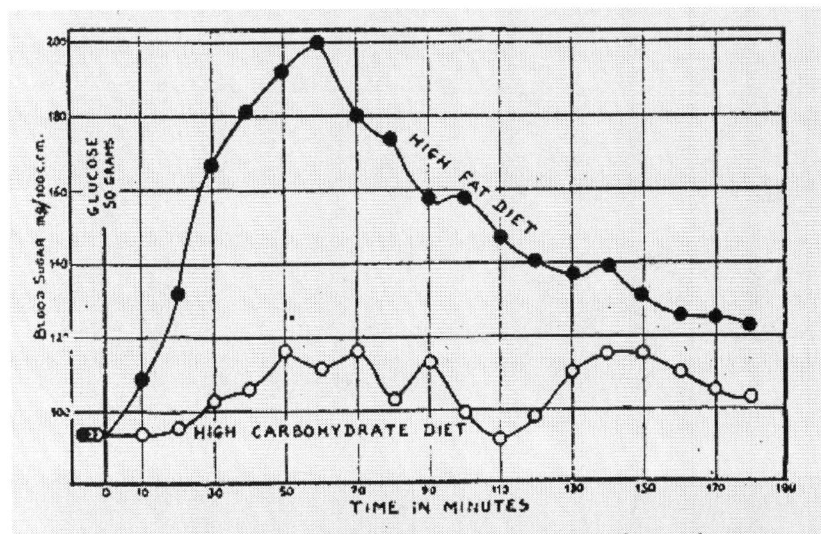

BRITISH MEDICAL JOURNAL

LONDON SATURDAY MAY 4 1940

INSULIN DEFICIENCY AND INSULIN INEFFICIENCY *

BY

H. P. HIMSWORTH, M.D., F.R.C.P.

Professor of Medicine in the University of London; Director of the Medical Unit, University College Hospital, London

FIG. 1.—Two blood glucose-tolerance curves from the same normal subject—one when taking a low carbohydrate–high fat diet and the other when taking an equicaloric high carbohydrate–low fat diet. On the former diet the glucose tolerance is impaired, on the latter it is improved (Himsworth, 1934b).

J.P. Himsworth. Insulin deficiency and insulin inefficiency. *BMJ* 4 May1940, 719-722.

In this paper from 1940, Himsworth did glucose tolerance tests with his subjects, feeding them either high-sugar or high-fat diets. The high-carbohydrate diet caused insulin levels to rise, which is what it's supposed to do. As Dr. John McDougall says: "That's why we eat… to raise our blood sugar."

John McDougall. Recorded Webinar 111215, How to Prevent and Treat Diabetes, Part 1.

But take a look at the massive insulin spike caused by the high-fat diet, which doesn't even come close to returning to baseline after three hours. How the medical community was able to forget this research, until Dr. Neal Barnard recently unearthed it, repeated it and confirmed it is almost a mystery, but not quite. Medical research is costly, and pharmaceutical companies expect a return on their investment from drug sales. Where's the money in telling people not to eat animals? (The same applies to the fiber in whole plants. Cui bono, telling people to eat whole plants? No one.)

Experimenters have nailed down the role of animal and junk fats in causing insulin resistance and diabetes, working both backwards and forwards. They add fat to the diet, and make people diabetic. They remove fat from the diet, and reverse diabetes. In one highly entertaining experiment, researchers used eggs to flick diabetes on and off like the proverbial light switch; on, off, on, off, over and again, just by adding and removing the incredible inedible egg. (In *The China Study*, Prof. T. Colin Campbell did something similar to poor lab rats, using casein (milk protein) to switch cancer on and off by varying the protein dose (which makes the poison).)

2. Nonalcoholic fatty liver "disease"

In the pre-diabetic stage, before our blood sugar rises very high, when we eat saturated and trans fats, we impede insulin's ability to activate the glucose transport receptors in our cell membranes.

We start the process of insulin resistance in our muscles, where 85% of the glucose we eat gets used. The locks in our muscle cell membranes become gummed up with fat, preventing the insulin key from working efficiently. With reduced ability to enter the muscle cells, the sugar begins to build up in our blood.

Our pancreas is forced to synthesize and release more insulin to deal with the excess glucose in our blood. Every meal, more animal fats sludge up our blood and gum up the insulin receptors in our muscle cells and, again, our pancreas has to work overtime to keep up. Year after year, every Meater meal.

After this sorry situation has persisted for a while, our livers get in on the act. One of our liver's many jobs is to supply our brains with glucose when we're not eating. Our brain has an insatiable, constant thirst for energy. When things are running smoothly, at mealtimes, insulin puts the liver's glucose-making engine into neutral, so that it idles when it's not needed.

But excess insulin in our blood, because of excess glucose in our blood, because of insulin resistance in our muscles, because of animal and junk fats in our diet, causes the beginnings of non-alcoholic liver disease. Fatty streaks start to appear in our livers, and liver function starts to decline.

After a while, if this continues, our livers may no longer switch off their glucose-making machine at mealtimes, and they may continue to flood our blood with glucose, even while we're eating glucose. This causes our pancreases to release even more insulin to deal with the extra extra glucose, which makes our livers more insulin resistant, and around and around. Poor snake, eternally eating its own tail.

3. Fatty pancreas

Our livers are quite extraordinary. They make thousands of different substances. They're our chemical factories and also our detoxifying organs, and they regenerate rapidly. Now, faced with an onslaught of animal fats (and cholesterol), our livers try to detoxify themselves. They expel fat into our blood in the form of VLDL triacylglycerol.

Sadly for us, VLDL now builds up in our pancreas, in our insulin-making cells in the islets of Langerhans. The pancreas now becomes less able to produce and secrete insulin.

In other words, the initial insulin resistance in our fatty muscles has caused insulin resistance in our fatty livers, which in turn is causing not just insulin resistance in our fatty pancreases (a feature of type 2 diabetes) but is also damaging and, in time, killing off the pancreas's irreplaceable beta cells, possibly permanently destroying our ability to produce any insulin at all (a feature of type 1 diabetes).

Our pancreas (that's been working overtime for years to produce insulin in an ever more insulin-resistant body) is now compromised, and insulin production declines. It's unable to secrete enough insulin at the very moment that insulin resistance requires it to secrete maximal amounts.

We're well on our way to having diabetes, which kicks in officially when our blood sugars exceed 125 mg/dL.

Saturated fat intake → fatty muscles → fatty liver → fatty pancreas → insulin resistance AND beta cell damage → type 1 ½ diabetes.

Really, types 1 and 2 differ only in degree. As long as we haven't killed off all our beta cells with animal fats, we have type 2. When they're all gone, then we have type 1. Type 1½ diabetes is an apt name.

That's how animal fats themselves help cause diabetes. There's more than just the intrinsically lethal qualities of the fats themselves…

4. Lipotoxicity

I'm sorry we're having this discussion of the role of fat poisoning in causing diabetes before we've had a chance to look at Part 3, which relates the dangers of persistent organic pollutants from the environment, or POPs.

Fats are where we store all the lipophilic, or fat-loving pollutants that we ingest. Animals store them in their fats. As human animals, Meaters have far higher concentrations of these damaging chemicals in their bodies than Planters, and these contaminants damage our pancreatic insulin-producing cells, diminishing or destroying our ability to make insulin.

When I say far more, I mean up to >100,000 times more. Not a hundred or a thousand – one hundred thousand times more.

Some scientists believe that most of animal fat's role in causing diabetes is down to the biomagnified pollutants within the animal fats we eat and the animal fats we tote around with us. That's how serious fat poisoning is.

Fortunately, lipotoxicity isn't a feature of the Planter diet.

At least 90% of our exposure to environmental toxins comes from eating animals, particularly animal fats. And the fatter we get, the more toxins we retain and the more lipotoxic we become. In other words, because of the pollutants in fat, the more overweight we become, the worse becomes the effects of our being overweight.

For example, according to the EPA, at http://www2.epa.gov/dioxin/learn-about-dioxin,

"• Dioxins are found throughout the world in the environment and they **accumulate in the food chain, mainly in the fatty tissue of animals.**

• More than **90% of human exposure** is through food, mainly **meat and dairy products, fish and shellfish.**

• Dioxins are highly toxic and can cause cancer, reproductive and developmental problems, damage to the immune system, and **can interfere with hormones**."

In other words, almost all persistent organic pollutants are found concentrated in the animals we eat, and (besides causing cancer and birth defects, et al) they seriously disrupt our endocrine systems, of which the insulin-producing pancreas is a vital part.

Additionally, in Michael Greger's words:

> "Fat cells filled with saturated fat activate an inflammatory response to a far greater extent. This increased inflammation, along with eating more saturated fat, has been demonstrated to raise insulin resistance through **free radical** and **ceramide** production." [Free radicals are what cause oxidation, and ceramide is a toxic fat metabolite, or breakdown product.]

There are multiple mechanisms via which Meating plays merry hell with our blood sugars.

> "Saturated fat also has been shown to have a direct effect on skeletal muscle insulin resistance. Accumulation of saturated far increases the amount of **diacyl-glycerol** in the muscles, which has been demonstrated to have a potent effect on muscle insulin resistance. It doesn't matter if the fat in our blood comes from our fat, or their fat.
>
> You can take muscle biopsies from people and correlate the saturated fat buildup in their muscles with insulin resistance.
>
> While monounsaturated fats are more likely to be detoxified or safely stored away, saturated fats create those toxic breakdown products like ceramide that causes lipotoxicity. Lipo meaning fat, as in liposuction, and toxicity. This fat toxicity in our muscles is a well-known concept in the explanation of the trigger for insulin resistance."

[See: http://nutritionfacts.org/video/lipotoxicity-how-saturated-fat-raises-blood-sugar/]

5. The Spillover Effect

In people who haven't been infected with obesogenic viruses from Meating chickens, the number of fat cells we have in our bodies stays constant throughout adulthood. Our level of obesity depends on how much fat we pack into our finite number of fat cells.

If we've filled all our fat cells to capacity, by becoming obese, some fat is constantly leaking out into our blood and circulating throughout our bodies, and this non-dietary fat causes insulin resistance in the same way as dietary fat, the fat we eat.

While in this obese state, we can even go on a fast and still be poisoning ourselves with fats and bioaccumulated lipotoxins, until such time as we've lost enough weight to stop the fat in our cells from slopping over.

Eating animal fat is one way to become diabetic; another way is to be a fat animal.

When our fat cells are constantly oozing out fat into our blood, a state of almost continuous oxidation and inflammation arises, and these are the pathological mechanisms that cause insulin resistance and beta cell death.

According to Michael Greger: "Being obese may result in as much insulin resistance as eating a high fat diet."

Put another way, a skinny person eating a high-animal, high-fat, high-protein, low-carb diet is the physiological equivalent of an obese individual who may be eating very little, but who's constantly spilling out fat from their fat cells and into their blood. That's why low-carbers can stay insulin resistant even when they're not overweight. They may look healthy from afar, but on the inside they're far from healthy.

As Michael Greger says, "If you put people on a low carb diet, fat builds up in their muscle within two hours, compared to a low fat diet, and insulin sensitivity drops. And the more fat in the muscle, the lower the ability to clear sugar from the blood. It doesn't take years for this to happen, just hours after these foods go into our mouths. A fat-rich diet can increase fat in the blood and this increase is accompanied by a decrease in insulin sensitivity."

Being fat and eating fat produce the same insulin resistance outcome. Saturated and trans fats from animals and hydrogenated vegetable oils have the same effect. Planters don't eat these, so we have the least diabetes.

[See: http://nutritionfacts.org/video/the-spillover-effect-links-obesity-to-diabetes/]

6. Diabetogens

Diabetogens are estrogens that help cause diabetes. They're produced by our gut bacteria when we feed them on animals and junk, high in fat, low in fiber. If excess estrogen from eating animals isn't bad enough; when we feed our gut flora animals, they create even more estrogen.

Our fat cells also make estrogens, so the obese are more affected.

We saw earlier that estrogen is implicated in causing cancer, particularly of the breast and prostate. Now we see it has a role in the Eatiology of diabetes too.

7. Increased sex-hormone binding globulin in Planters

Excessive amounts of circulating hormones such as estrogen can wreck our health, helping cause breast and prostate cancer and diabetes. A pure Planter diet produces more of a protein (called a sex-hormone binding globulin) which binds up and removes steroid hormones from circulation. How much more? More than 50% more in Planters than in Meaters. Fiber also clears out excess estrogens (bile acids and cholesterol, too). This is part of the reason why obese Planters have half the diabetes of obese Meaters of the same weight. It's definitely not just the sugar.

In the US, cattle are often injected with growth-promoting steroid hormones, both estrogens and androgens like testosterone, adding to their endogenous hormones.

Cows aren't food.

8. Endocrine disruptors

I've devoted an entire section of more than a hundred pages in this book to "food"-borne contaminants. Xenoestrogens, or foreign estrogens, are toxic chemicals which behave like our steroid sex hormones.

In describing "food"-borne contaminants, it took more than a page just to make an incomplete list of xenoestrogens that disrupt our hormonal or endocrine systems, of which the pancreas's beta cells are a part.

Included in that list of dozens of diabetes-causing chemicals (most of which are also carcinogenic, and some of which I referred to in Lipotoxicity, above) are such monstrosities as alkylphenols, BPA, cadmium, DDT, dieldrin, dioxins, parabens, phthalates, PAH, PCBs, PBDEs and tobacco smoke.

More than 90% of these poisons sneak into our body temples along with the animals we sacrifice.

Meaters with the highest concentrations of environmental pollutants in their blood get 38 times more diabetes than the least contaminated people, Planters. Not 38% more, i.e. 1.38 times as much – 38 times more, or 3800%.

That's huge.

And that's the main reason why losing weight the low-carb way is unhealthy, even deadly. Even though we may lose the weight by low-carbing, we can't lose *the effect of the weight*, which is the toxic dump of chemicals in the animal fats we eat. Plus the other free radicals and the inflammatories...

Fishes are the most contaminated things people eat, mistakenly believing they're food. Farmed Atlantic salmons are the worst of the worst.

9. Free radicals and inflammation

When we get down to the coal face of diabetes, the physiological processes of oxidation and inflammation in pathological amounts are the Meater miners digging away at our beta cells. Unless we prop them up with whole plants, our beta cell deposits will be undermined (over-mined?) to such an extent that they collapse in a deadly pile of diabetic rubble. We don't want to get stuck down that Meater shaft.

[A friend's comment after his divorce: "She got the mine, I got the shaft.]

Animal fats themselves cause oxidation and inflammation. Then they biomagnify pollutants to absurd concentrations, and they cause even more O+I.

10. Other pro-oxidants and inflammatory agents

Oxidation and inflammation (and resulting tissue damage) are signatures of Meating and Junking. Whole plants, which are foods, don't cause excess oxidation and inflammation. In net terms, plants are antioxidizing and anti-inflammatory.

Meater and Junker felons include:

- Advanced glycation end-products, or AGEs – think grilled pig flesh and chickens, in particular; all animals, in general
- Heme iron – all animals
- Nitrites and nitrosamines – think pigs again; all animals
- Cholesterol – brains and eggs, in particular; all animals
- Animal fats, already mentioned
- Animal proteins, ditto
- (Aspirin, or salicylic acid, found in many plants, is anti-inflammatory)

In Part 1B (Mechanisms), we saw how Meating-induced blood platelet hyperactivity is implicated in many inflammatory conditions. This is the case in diabetes. What lowers platelet activity? Planting – fruits (particularly berries) and veggies (particularly tomatoes, and mainly their pomace (the skin, juice and seeds). Whether a cause or an effect of diabetes, platelet activity is improved by plants, and made worse by animals.

11. Rapid uptake of glucose from high-glycemic junk

When we eat processed, fiber-depleted plants, there's very little digestion that needs to happen, and glucose enters our blood very quickly. This is followed by an equally rapid spike in insulin, to deal with the glucose, and our blood sugar can shoot way up, then crash way down, overshooting on the way down, so that we're left at a lower energy ebb than before the meal. Because we're energy-depleted a few hours after such a miserable meal, we'll probably repeat the process, again and again, putting long-term strain on our pancreas and laying down fat which leads to insulin resistance.

That's the gospel of type 2 diabetes according to most Meaters, except they don't usually pay us the courtesy of distinguishing between whole and fractionated carbs. They usually just say: because carbs cause a rapid insulin response, we should all eat lots of animals.

Unlike the fructose from whole fruits which is protective against diabetes, junk sugars such as sucrose and HFCS cause insulin resistance.

Less well known is that animal protein also elicits an insulin spike from our pancreas, even though there's no glucose in animals.

12. Potentiation of high-glycemic junk by animals
Low-fiber junk produces glucose and insulin spikes. Animals produce an insulin spike, in the absence of glucose. (Another role of insulin, besides ferrying glucose into muscle cells, is to ferry fats into fat cells.) If we put animals and junk together, watch out... The animals **potentiate** the sugar, meaning that they make its effect even worse. Potentiation is kind of like synergy, except it's on the dark side, because it makes our beta cells work twice as hard.

Modern Chinese people have become more diabetic in the last twenty years as they've eaten 30% *less* white rice, 40% more pigs and 20% more vegetable oils. The vegetable oil is a confounding factor: we can't say that the increase in diabetes is solely because of the increased pig consumption. What we can say is that diabetes in China has gone up as we've added more of one junk "food" (oil) and one animal (pigs), while reducing another junk "food" (white rice).

Two things are probably happening. The saturated fats in vegetable oil are contributing to diabetes, while the added animals are potentiating the (reduced) quantities of processed, high-glycemic rice.

Highly processed rice is bad for our pancreatic health. Processed rice + processed animals is even worse.

[See: http://nutritionfacts.org/video/if-white-rice-is-linked-to-diabetes-what-about-china/]

These are some of the reasons why Planters get so much less diabetes than Meaters and Junkers.

Type 2 diabetes
It's crucial to remember:

> **Type II Diabetes is a derangement *of* our sugar and insulin metabolism that's not primarily caused *by* eating sugar.**

Animal fat is the main problem when it comes to insulin resistance. Processed plants cause problems. Whole plants never do. Plants are at fault to the extent that the fiber and other nutrients are processed out of them, turning them from the healthiest of foods into non-foods. Of course, eating pure sugar, white flour and white bread isn't smart.

The Low-Carbers seem to have stubbed their heads on Dr. David Jenkins' and Dr. Thomas Wolever's Glycemic Index and either misunderstood it or not bothered to read any further. Or else they use it, knowing full well it doesn't support their case, because their core Meater audience will believe them if they just sound sciency enough. (Also known as baffling with bullshit.)

The Glycemic Index measures how much glucose is released after eating a food (or junk) that contains carbohydrates. Animals don't appear in GI tables, because they don't contain carbs. (That's not a plus. We're solar-powered beings, via sunlight and chlorophyll-produced sugar.)

Does this mean that animal eating doesn't cause an insulin response?

Categorically, no. It doesn't mean that at all. Because insulin ferries proteins into cells as well as glucose, animals, with their many proteins, can cause as much or more insulin release than processed plants. Things are slightly more complicated than the simple/simplistic/simple-minded low-carb explanation of glucose and insulin metabolism.

And some 'bad' carbs (such as the white rice on which hundreds of millions of oriental people have stayed diabetes-free for decades) are made twice as bad by the addition of animal proteins! If white rice is so bad, how come adding animals to it makes it worse. Especially fishes. Eating just 2 portions a week increases our risk of diabetes by 35%, more than the red flesh of animals does.

But, if we add beans to our rice instead, the glycemic response improves.

Dr. Jenkins himself is aware of the boundaries of his GI work. He advocates a Planter diet. Paleo is not his cene: he speaks of a "possible Myocene diet of leafy vegetables, fruit and nuts." In a paper called "The Garden of Eden—plant based diets, the genetic drive to conserve cholesterol and its implications for heart disease in the 21st century" (*Comparative Biochemistry and Physiology* Part A 136 (2003) 141–151), Jenkins and his team conclude that:

> "reintroduction of plant food components, which would have been present in large quantities in the plant based diets eaten throughout most of human evolution into modern diets can correct the lipid abnormalities associated with contemporary eating patterns [i.e. Meating and Junking] and reduce the need for pharmacological interventions [drugs]." Perfect.

Isn't it weird that paleonutters use Jenkins' work so much, to try to dupe people into believing that eating animals can be healthy, and yet the man himself disagrees with every word they say? Carbs are demons to them, and yet he advocates eating nothing but whole plants… mega-carbs.

The following graphic is easy to find on the web:

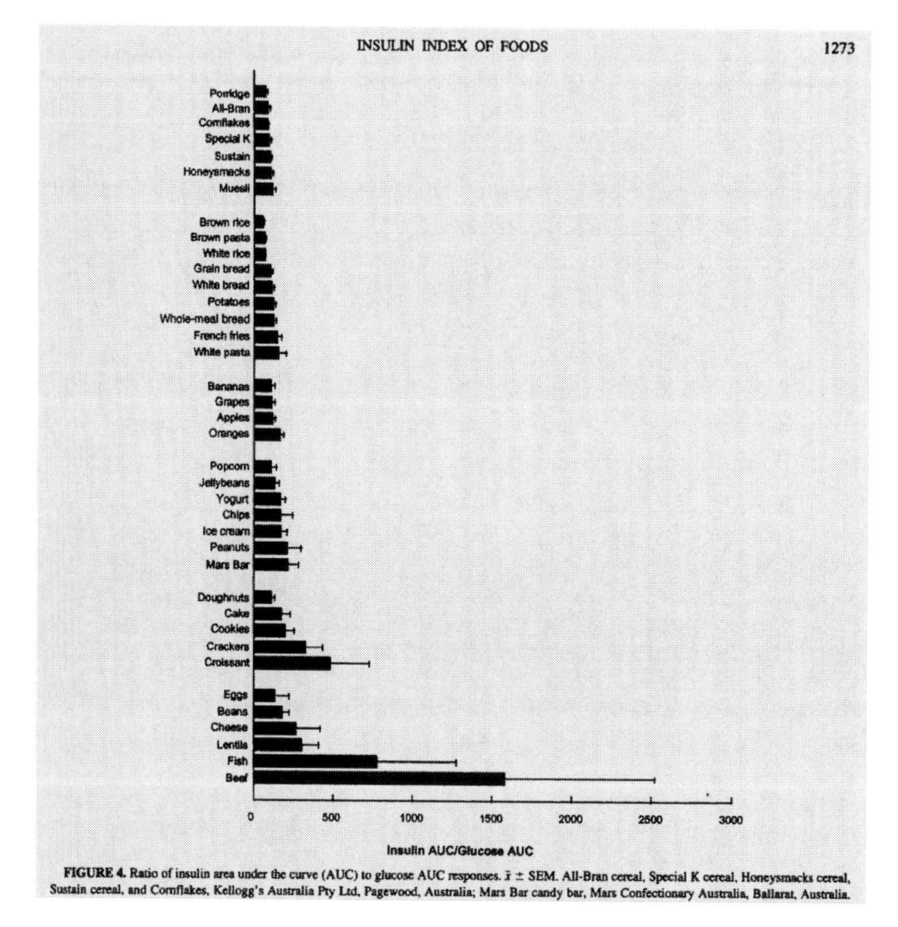

FIGURE 4. Ratio of insulin area under the curve (AUC) to glucose AUC responses. $\bar{x} \pm$ SEM. All-Bran cereal, Special K cereal, Honeysmacks cereal, Sustain cereal, and Cornflakes, Kellogg's Australia Pty Ltd, Pagewood, Australia; Mars Bar candy bar, Mars Confectionary Australia, Ballarat, Australia.

Holt et al. An insulin index of foods

It's in this paper: S H Holt, J C Miller, P Petocz. An insulin index of foods: the insulin demand generated by 1000-kJ portions of common foods. *Am J Clin Nutr* November 1997 vol. 66 no. 5 1264-1276.

This study contains information from *last century* that appears too obscure for Low-Carb Bullshit Artists to find, showing how animal proteins cause a large insulin spike, even though there's no glycemic (sugar) content in animals to show up on a Glycemic Index.

Let's take a look at this **Insulin Index of Foods**... Whoa, what's going on here? Looks like animals and junk are the clear losers. Just as we'd expect after dozens of clinical trials and intervention studies and case studies, all saying the same thing: insulin resistance is caused by eating animals and junk, and by being obese, as a result of eating animals and junk.

The authors have this to say about insulin and glucose: "...protein-rich foods and bakery products (rich in fat and refined carbohydrate) elicited insulin responses that were disproportionately higher than their glycemic responses."

Meaning, animals and junk are bad for us.

The authors sum up: "The results of this study confirm and also challenge some of our basic assumptions about the relation between food intake and insulinemia. Within each food group, there was a wide range of insulin responses, despite similarities in nutrient composition."

[In other words, a facile A-leads-to-B explanation won't suffice for glycemic load and insulin resistance.]

"The important Western staples, bread and potato, were among the most insulinogenic foods. Similarly, the highly refined bakery products and snack foods induced substantially more insulin secretion per kilojoule or per gram of food than did the other test foods. In contrast, pasta, oatmeal porridge, and All-Bran cereal produced relatively low insulin responses, despite their high carbohydrate contents. Carbohydrate was quantitatively the major macronutrient for most foods. Thus, it is not surprising that we observed a strong correlation between GSs [glucose scores] and Iss [insulin scores] ($r = 0.70$, $P < 0.001$)."

[Get that? Junk plants bad; whole plants good.]

"However, some protein and fat-rich foods (eggs, beef, fish, lentils, cheese, cake, and doughnuts) induced as much insulin secretion as did some carbohydrate-rich foods (e.g., beef was equal to brown rice and fish was equal to grain bread). As hypothesized, several foods with similar GSs had disparate Iss (e.g., ice cream and yogurt, brown rice and baked beans, cake and apples, and doughnuts and brown pasta). Overall, the fiber content did not predict the magnitude of the insulin response. Similar Iss were observed for white and brown pasta, white and brown rice, and white and wholemeal bread. All of these foods are relatively refined compared with their traditional counterparts.

"Collectively, the findings imply that **typical Western diets are likely to be significantly more insulinogenic than more traditional diets based on less refined foods**."

The take-home message should be that the two unfoods – animals and junk – are problematic for insulin metabolism, while foods – whole plants – are not.

Call me old-fashioned, but my heroes are stars like J. Shirley Sweeney, H.P. Himsworth, Walter Kempner, Nathan Pritikin, James Anderson, Neal Barnard, Brenda Davis, Gabriel Cousens, John McDougall, Caldwell Esselstyn Jr., Dean Ornish and Michael Klaper, all of whom have proven that type II diabetes isn't a disease; that it's an outward manifestation of the underlying causes I've chosen to call Meating and Junking; and who've cured tens of thousands of people.

My heroes all routinely reverse type 2 diabetes in less than a month with the same Planter diet: a naturally low-fat, high-fiber, no-animal, whole-truth-and-nothing-but-the-truth real food diet. According to Dr. John McDougall, 100% of cases of pure type 2 diabetes, caused by insulin resistance only, and with none of the "partial pancreatic insufficiency" typical of type 1, are reversible on a pure Planter diet.

Planting allows all people with pure type 2 diabetes to come off all their diabetes medications for good, usually in about a week. It's the exact same dietstyle that is most effective at preventing dementia and obesity: *Grain Brain* and *Wheat Belly*, my slender vegan ass! (I have a question for you, Dr. William Davis: how come your belly's so curvaceous? Perhaps you're eating too much meat and not enough whole wheat?)

Gestational diabetes

If pregnant women, or even women who're about to become pregnant, eat non-foods like processed animal flesh, fishes and eggs, then we're going to see lots of pregnancy-related, or gestational diabetes.

And those women will be about seven times more likely to go on to develop type 2 diabetes later on. (Gestational diabetes is a good wake-up call for Meater women, just as erectile dysfunction is for Meater men.) Affected women also run the risk of pre-eclampsia.

And her kids will be more likely to have birth defects, to be born pre-term and under-weight, or, sadly, to die.

For optimal health of both mother and child, wanna-be mothers should stop eating all animals at least a year before conceiving, the half-life of some heavy metals such as mercury allowing them to clear most of it out of their body before they share it with a vulnerable fetus.

Metabolic syndrome

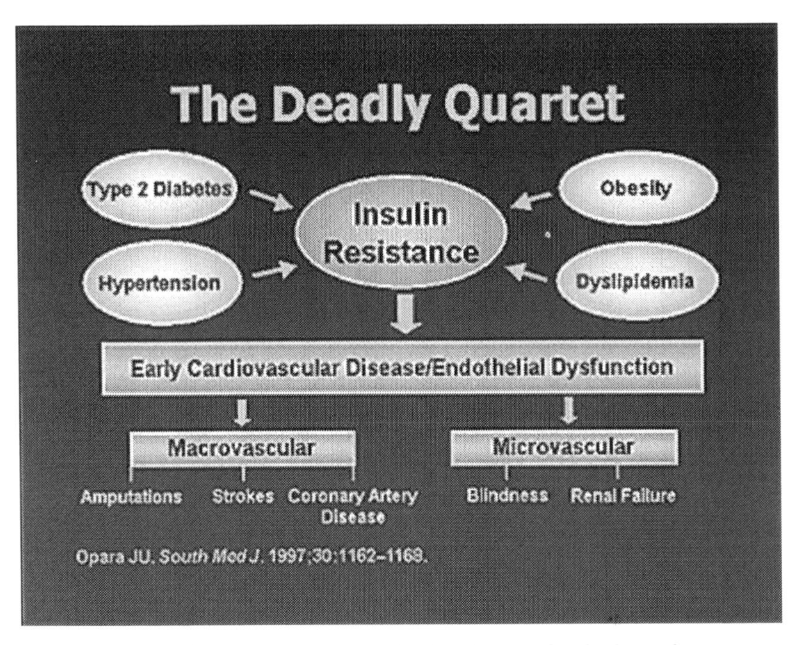

The Deadly Quartet of Metabolic Syndrome: faculty.ksu.edu.sa

The Deadly Quartet of metabolic syndrome, or syndrome X, are:

- Abdominal fat
- High blood sugars
- High blood fats (triglycerides)
- High blood pressure

Someone noticed that these four symptoms of Meating tend to go together. Good for them. But why stop there? Why not include some of the other symptoms of the Meater Eatiology such as

- High cholesterol
- High inflammatory markers
- Atherosclerosis
- Ischemia
- Hypoperfusion, et al,

all leading to the same endpoints for Meaters of coronary artery disease, strokes, amputations, blindness and renal failure, as well as auto-immune conditions etc.

My point is this: Linking everything to insulin resistance, as the above graphic appears to, is all well and good, but it doesn't address the real underlying causes of insulin resistance, Meating and Junking.

Meatobolic syndrome, as I call it, consists of a Deadly Century or more of Meater symptoms. No matter how many conditions of Meating we choose to lump together under a single umbrella term, Planting is what removes the underlying cause and makes it disappear like a rain squall.

Summary

Here's what we know about obesity, insulin resistance and diabetes:

- Planters have the least obesity.
- Planters eat slightly fewer calories than Meaters and Junkers.
- On isocaloric diets, Meaters put on more weight than Planters; roughly a pound a year. ("Controlling for calories")
- Obese vegans (i.e. Planter Junkers) get less diabetes than Meaters of the same body weight. ("Controlling for body weight") **Meaters can have up to 50% higher insulin levels at the same weight.** This is one of the most important points in the entire book. It's well worth pondering, particularly in view of low-carbers blaming diabetes on sugar, and nothing but the sugar. **People who eat the most sugar are protected in comparison to animal eaters.** NB.
- High-carbohydrate diets, up to 80%, create the best insulin sensitivity, and the least oxidation and inflammation, and therefore the least diabetes.
- Meating provides excess diabetogenic estrogens.

- Endocrine-disrupting persistent organic pollutants can harm or destroy the insulin-producing cells in our pancreases. These substances are in animals, not plants.
- Meating and Junking cause inflammation and oxidation, which promote diabetes. Plants are antioxidants and anti-inflammatories.

While obesity and insulin resistance go hand in hand in most cases, skinny low-carbers paradoxically continue to be insulin resistant because of their dietary intake of fats, lipotoxins and estrogens, and the overall oxidative and inflammatory nature of Meating.

The Unhealthy Low-Carb Weight Loss Paradox

Some people on some variant of a high-animal diet lose considerable amounts of weight. They do this by going short on one unhealthy non-food – junk – and going long on another – animals. They also usually go long on healthy whole plants, except starchy grains and vegetables.

Without ever admitting it, LCBAs smear ALL carbs as harmful, while encouraging us to eat antioxidant-rich whole plants, which mask the ill-effects of animals. In effect, Low-Carbers benefit from their sensible semi-Planting, while continuing their suicidal Meating.

Planting temporarily masks much of the injury low-carbers cause themselves. Not Junking is great, but the extra Meating's a killer.

As we saw with the research by Fleming and Noto et al above, low-carbers are unwittingly walking out on a disease gangplank while they contentedly admire their glorious weight loss ocean view. Narcissism and self-absorption rule. Low-carbing is all about weight loss and looking better; nothing about health and being well.

Here's the kicker: low-carbers often keep their diabetes even when they lose their obesity. Even obese Planters are protected against diabetes in comparison to Meaters. How now the obesity-diabetes connection?

It's simple. Slender low-carbers make their blood obese, and their muscle, liver and pancreas cells obese, with every bite of animal they take. They're slender on the outside, fat and diabetic on the in. Their diabesity is of an unseen, internal kind; as is their burgeoning heart "disease", liver and kidney "disease", vision loss and dementia.

Low-carbers are like guys 'n dolls who've jumped off a roof and who're singing the pleasures of flying (being slender) and who give us two thumbs up and yell "So far, so good" as they plummet past bemused Planters on the tenth floor (ten for the number of years of life low-carbers may be deprived of in comparison to the healthiest, exercising Planters).

To demonize whole carbs because processed carbs help cause diabetes is tantamount to throwing away all our birthday gifts because we don't like the paper they're wrapped in. To a large extent, the fiber wrapping of food is the food.

Low-carb = low-food = low-weight = low insulin sensitivity = high diabetes = low life expectancy = low intelligence.

Ultra-high carb = high-food = low weight = high insulin sensitivity = high life expectancy = high knowledge.

Low-carbing appeals strongly to manly Meaters of both genders, who want to lose weight by any means, as long as they can carry on Meating. Meaters allow themselves to be swayed by the silliest of Meater broscience, to cover themselves with the thinnest veneer of sciencyness to affirm a habit they don't want to change. Sadly, disbelieving the cholesterol theory has never saved a single Meater from a single heart attack or stroke.

There are many, many unhealthy ways to lose weight.

Weight loss techniques

Some Get Rich or Be Successful books tell us that the key to becoming rich or successful is to emulate the rich and successful. If we apply the same logic to weight loss, we should emulate the slender and healthy. There are many routes to slenderness, but in the long run there's only one way to be slender and healthy.

Here are some sad ways to waste away:

- AIDS
- Alcoholism
- Anorexia nervosa
- Atkins diet
- Banting
- Bulimia nervosa
- Calorie restriction diets
- Cancer
- Chemotherapy
- Cocaine addiction
- Crack whoring
- Dementia
- Dukan diet
- Dying
- Gastric band surgery
- Gastric bypass surgery
- Heroin addiction
- Hoax diet (inside joke for South Africans)
- Jaw wiring for weight loss by dentists
- Ketogenic diets
- Low-carb diets
- Orthorexia nervosa (about as common as unicorns)
- Paleo diets
- Extreme poverty
- Pre-frontal lobotomies performed by neurosurgeons
- Smoking
- Starvation
- Stomach stapling
- TB
- Unrequited love
- Vegetarianism
- Zone diet

I'm sure you can think of other life-shortening ways to lose weight. The only way to lose weight and keep it off permanently, while also adding years to our lives (and life to our years) is

- Planting (most of the weight loss effect & toxicity prevention), plus
- Exercise (a healthy, but junior contributor).

The other 'weight loss techniques' I mentioned above

1. Should lower insulin resistance – any weight loss should do this. In ketogenic diets, and high-animal diets in general, insulin doesn't work particularly well.
2. May not prevent diabetes, or may actually induce diabetes
3. May not lower our cholesterol levels significantly, or actually raise them
4. May cause cardiovascular disease
5. May raise our risk of multiple degenerative diseases, including blindness, kidney failure, fatty liver disease, colorectal cancer and Alzheimer's and… and… and…
6. May not be permanent, with the rebound making us fatter than before
7. Lower our life expectancy (Yes, death'll do that), or
8. A combination of any or all these risks

Only Planting

1. Gives us optimal insulin sensitivity
2. Reverses type 2 diabetes and lessens the impact of type 1
3. Lowers our cholesterol like a boom
4. Makes us 'heart attack-proof' and stroke-resistant
5. Heals multiple degenerative conditions, including atherosclerosis, hypertension, diverticulitis, rheumatoid arthritis and lupus and… and… and…
6. Lasts for life
7. Helps us live up to a decade longer, and
8. A combination of all these benefits.

I won't discuss all the life-shortening weight loss techniques. I'll just mention a few of my least favorite. I go to town on this subject in *The Low-Carb Bullshit Artists Are Lying Us to Death.*

William Banting, the 19th Century undertaker, coffin-maker and pamphleteer beloved of 21st Century low-carb broscientists, went from being obese to merely overweight, by adopting a slightly less foolish diet, which actually contained some fruits and vegetables, a.k.a. food.

Did his "Letter on Corpulence" in the 1860s add to his core business interests? The best modern evidence about high-animal diets says it did. Thomas Hobbes comes to mind when I think of Banting, because he was decidedly "nasty, British and short." Actually, no, Banting was a sweetheart, donating much of his pelf to charity. British and short, he was. And fat.

When Dr. Robert Atkins died, he was (un)well on his way to being morbidly obese and had a history of hypertension and heart disease, according to both his personal physician and his medical examiner/coroner.

According to NR Kleinfield, *New York Times* February 11, 2004:

"After Atkins' death in 2003, from brain injury following a fall, it was established that the six-foot-tall diet guru weighed 258 pounds.

Dr. Stuart Trager, chairman of the Atkins Physicians Council, a group of physicians who work as consultants to the Atkins organization, said… Dr. Atkins did not have a history of heart attack, nor was he obese. He said that Dr. Atkins weighed 195 pounds the day after he entered the hospital following his fall, and that **he gained 63 pounds from fluid retention during the nine days he was in a coma** before he died."

[Emphasis added, with difficulty, I was laughing so hard, and "laughter is the best medicine," so thank you, Dr. Trager.]

Whoops. Either the Atkins shill is telling a porky pie or the hospital staff accidentally hooked the poor doctor up to a fire hydrant instead of a drip.

And all the other ultra-high-animal, low-carb/paleo/ketogenic-type diets that have followed in Atkins' wake [funereal pun alert] have been shown to sicken us and kill us before our time.

Earlier I cited: H. Noto, A. Goto, T. Tsujimoto, M. Noda. Low-carbohydrate diets and all-cause mortality: A systematic review and meta-analysis of observational studies. PloS ONE 2013 8(1):e55030, and they told us how low-carbers live appreciably shorter lives.

If a diet is low in carbs, it has to be high in proteins and fats… what else is there? (And both are deadly in excess, particularly from animals.) Here's the conclusion of another study showing the destructive effects of a high-fat (HF), low-carb diet on multiple risk factors for death via heart "disease" –

Richard M. Fleming, MD. The Effect of High-, Moderate-, and Low-Fat Diets on Weight Loss and Cardiovascular Disease Risk Factors. *Preventive Cardiology* 2002;5:110–118:

> "Those following HF [high-fat, low-carb] diets may have lost weight, but at the price of **increased cardiovascular risk factors**, including increased LDL-C, increased TGs, increased TC, decreased HDL-C, increased TC/HDL ratios, and increased homocysteine, Lp(a), and fibrinogen levels."

[Translation: Low-carb diets raise our bad cholesterol, triglycerides (fats), total cholesterol, total-to-good-cholesterol ratio, inflammatory markers, lipoproteins and blood clotting factors, and lower our good cholesterol levels. Any one of those is dreadful. Low-carb flunks them all.]

> **"These increased risk factors not only increase the risk of heart disease, but also the risk of strokes, peripheral vascular disease, and blood clots."**

That's the kicker, right there. Those following low-carb diets may lose weight, "but at the price of increased cardiovascular risk factors" and death, and that's something the Low-Carb Bullshit Artists never tell their victims, desperate to lose weight by any means at all… as long as they can continue to eat animals:

> "We're going to make you sick and you're going to lose a lot of weight, but some of you are going to die. And we don't care. All we care is that you buy our nasty, lying little books before you shuffle off."

All low-carb and paleo diet books should carry black box or skull-and-crossed-bone warning labels, conspicuously displayed on their front covers. Half their profits should go into a fund set up to treat survivors or to pay restitution to bereaved family members. Hell, all their profits.

There's more, and it's not good for the LCBAs. **Everything that makes us lose weight should also lower our cholesterol**. It's almost impossible not to. Just about every one of the jokey weight loss techniques I listed above lowers our cholesterol when we lose weight… *except* the various manifestations of high animal diets: low-carb… paleo… ketogenic… Atkins… et slithering al.

Some raise our cholesterol levels, and that's why LCBAs devote so much of their time trying to demonize the cholesterol theory, or Diet-Heart, without mentioning any of the dozens of other ways eating animals kills us.

Exercise raises our HDL cholesterol levels, which is thought to be good. Strangely, one study shows a group of paleo dieters on a CrossFit exercise program who actually managed to lower their HDL levels while exercising strenuously. That's almost impossible to do – paleo manages it, while simultaneously wrecking other blood fat markers.

M M Smith, E T Trexler, A J Sommer, B E Starkoff, S T Devor. Unrestricted Paleolithic Diet is Associated with Unfavorable Changes to Blood Lipids in Healthy Subjects. *International Journal of Exercise Science* 7(2):128-139, 2014.

Even though the participants' body fat % came down significantly as a result of diet and exercise, their non-HDL (non-good), LDL and total cholesterol, and their triglycerides, all went up, while HDL went down.

(The triglyceride and HDL changes didn't meet the level of statistical significance.)

Exercise on its own would improve all these markers, as should weight loss. High-animal paleo is a sickening con job.

Low-Carb Bullshit Artists aren't good people. They don't have our best interests at heart. If there were nutritional Nuremberg trials for crimes against humanity, they'd all be in the dock.

So, stay safe, dear hearts, and don't listen to a word the LCBAs say.

(How can we tell when ex-journalist-turned-Low-Carb-Bullshit-Artist Gary Taubes is telling porky pies? His lips are moving. Or his pen.)

Stay safe, dear hearts. Eat plenty of whole plants. Eat an ultra-high-whole-carb diet. This way lies slenderness, insulin sensitivity, general good health and longevity.

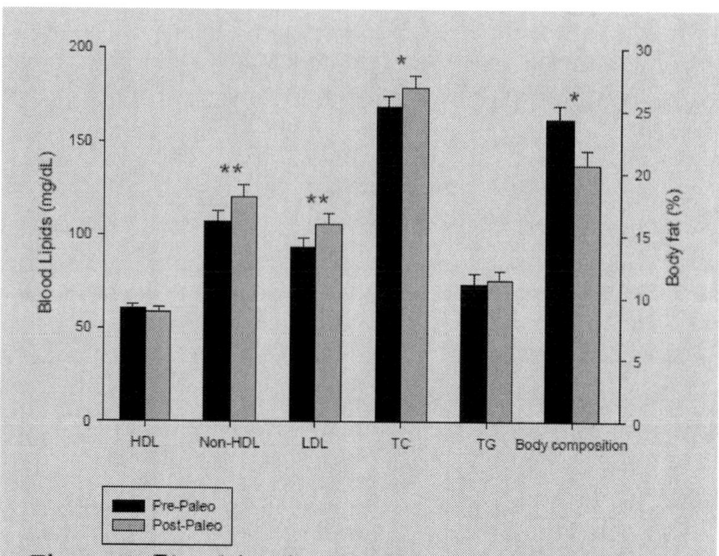

Figure 1. Blood lipids in healthy volunteer prior to and following a 10-week Paleolithic diet intervention. Non- high density lipoprotein (n-HDL), low density lipoprotein (LDL) and total cholesterol (TC) increased significantly from baseline, whereas no changes were observed with regard to high density lipoprotein (HDL) and triglycerides (TG). A significant decrease in body composition was observed compared to baseline. * $P < 0.05$; ** $P < 0.01$.

Smith et al, 2014. Unrestricted Paleolithic Diet is Associated with Unfavorable Changes to Blood Lipids in Healthy Subjects

'Pulses' and minuses

What should we eat if we don't want to give ourselves diabetes?

If we take the time to do a GoogleScholar search, typing in:

"Diabetes +…"

and then add in any of the following foods, we'll wade through a stream of peer-reviewed studies showing the benefits of eating:

- Pulses, which are dried beans, lentils and split peas
- Non-GM Soy (cuts our diabetes risk in half; slashes our odds of getting breast cancer too)
- Other beans; fabulously antidiabetogenic

- Whole grains, packed full of phytates, especially oats and barley; brown rice too; they're also cholesterol-lowering
- Nuts, high in magnesium and potassium
- Seeds, especially flax seeds, full of lignan precursors
- Green and white tea, with theanine and other phytonutrients
- Chamomile tea; an anti-inflammatory with multiple uses – pregnant women shouldn't drink it – it's too anti-inflammatory
- Hibiscus tea (what puts the red and the zing in Red Zinger)
- Coffee (yes, coffee, also protective against Parkinson's)
- Broccoli sprouts, very high in sulforaphane
- Cruciferous vegetables, high in sulforaphane
- Erythritol (an antioxidant-packed plant sweetener); xylitol may upset our stomachs – I eat it occasionally, without consequence
- Fruit (whole)
- Amla (Indian gooseberries)
- Cinnamon – the latest science tells us that Ceylon cinnamon doesn't lower blood sugars. Cassia – or Chinese cinnamon – does, but it can be toxic, so it's best not to rely on these plants for managing our blood sugars. Rather eat…
- A whole plant diet, in general

All of the antioxidant and anti-inflammatory foods in the Planter dietstyle have multiple health benefits besides preventing or healing diabetes. Oh, like preventing Parkinson's and cancers and heart "disease" and hypertension… and… and… and…

If on the other hand, during our scholarly search, we were to type in non-foods after 'Diabetes +…," we'd get slews of reports showing how they help cause diabetes and kill us. For example:

- Eggs
- Milk and other dairy products
- Meat (once a week → 74% increased risk)
- Processed flesh like bacon (Isn't it all processed?)
- Fishes, the most contaminated things we eat
- Baby formula
- Fruit juice, the totally fiber-free kind

- Sugar and HFCS
- Statin drugs, which raise our blood sugar levels (Planters don't eat drugs – we eat plants)

Of the non-foods, eggs and fishes are spectacularly diabetogenic. And the dose makes the poison: a study showed that über-Meaters who ate the most animal proteins were 73 times more likely to die from diabetes.

Another study showed that eating a single egg a week raises our diabetes risk about 75%. Two a week, 100%, and one a day, 200%, or three times as much. When we're already diabetic, an egg a day doubles our risk of death from all causes.

If our second weekly egg only increases our risk by 25%, as opposed to 75% for the first, perhaps we should skip the more lethal first egg and just eat the second one? Egg producers would probably tell us to eat more eggs, because the added risk of diabetes declines with each added egg: "More eggs, less risk." People who prefer no risk at all eat no eggs at all.

The damage done by animals in our diet is dose-dependent. There's no safe lower threshold of intake – the least little bit hurts (especially considering how long the ill-effects to our gut flora of a single animal meal persists).

Take this paper, for example: Spence JD, Jenkins DJ, Davignon, J. Dietary cholesterol and egg yolks: not for patients at risk of vascular disease. *Can J Cardiol.* 2010 Nov;26(9):e336-9.

Spence, Jenkins and Davignon conclude: "In our opinion, stopping egg consumption after a myocardial infarction or stroke would be like quitting smoking after lung cancer is diagnosed: a necessary act, but late." By the way, when they say that eggs aren't "for patients at risk of vascular disease," they mean anyone who's eating a SAD animal diet. Eggs aren't food, and they're diabetogenic, according to them. [Jenkins is the plant-strong co-inventor of the glycemic index, beloved of and abused by low-carbers.]

As I've mentioned and will mention often, fishes are the non-foods with the highest concentrations of endocrine-disrupting, diabetogenic chemicals, making heavy eaters 38 times more likely to make themselves diabetic.

Salmons and sardines are particularly contaminated with fat-soluble **hexachlorobenzene**, and salmons with **PCBs** – farmed are ten times worse than wild. Mercury is another concern the higher up the "food" chain we eat; and the cross-reactivity among different pollutants is considerable.

With animals, the subtraction of the whole is greater than the subtraction of the individual parts.

Even if not overweight, Meaters consume animal fats, contaminated with mass quantities of pancreas cell-killing industrial waste.

Other factors associated with more diabetes include:

- Paleo diets
- Low-carb diets in general
- Meater and Junker fats
- Heme iron – iron of animal origin
- Animal proteins
- Purines (animal protein breakdown products linked to gout)
- Omega-3 fats from Fishing, controversially and recently established
- Arsenic (found mainly in chickens; also in fishes)
- Amyloid (chickens; foie gras)
- BPA, dioxins and other pollutants, bioaccumulated in animals
- Endocrine disruptors such as pesticides, ditto
- Cadmium and other heavy metals, ditto
- Smoking
- Anything that causes inflammation, i.e. anything besides whole plants
- Endotoxins from bacteria, causing inflammation – dairy, eggs, flesh

When we live by the insulin resistance and diabetes sword, we die by the insulin resistance and diabetes sword. Low-Carb Bullshit Artists flunk out of diabetes gladiator school.

Planting is what prevents, stops and reverses diabetes. Nothing else comes close.

Some Planter anti-obesity and anti- diabetes greats:

Beans and other legumes

Eating beans is the best way to 'get' our plant protein, coming as it does in a package with lots of magnesium – protective against sudden cardiac death – and potassium – protective against stroke – our #1 and #4 killers; two nutrients in which Americans are severely deficient. (Probably all Meaters.)

Beans are a great weight management food, highly protective against diabetes. In fact, they're diabetes control superstars…

The fiber in beans is what our gut flora makes propionate and butyrate out of, and there are amylase-, or starch digestive enzyme-blocking substances in beans that ensure that some undigested starch reaches the gut flora in our colons, for them to snack on.

If we eat ≥3 servings of beans a week, we have a quarter of the risk of developing diabetes. Beans, peas, lentils and chickpeas drop our inflammatory markers such as C-reactive protein and vascular adhesion molecules like an elevator down a mine shaft.

To not eat beans regularly is to shorten our lives.

Nuts and seeds

Nuts and seeds are fatty and full of calories, but eating nuts has been found over and over again to be protective against weight gain, particularly the dangerous kind – abdominal obesity. They're also highly nutritious and satiating, so perhaps some of the lack of weight gain is because we eat less food overall. Nuts and seeds are the best source of arginine, above. An ounce a day is all we need - no need to consume mass quantities.

Flax seeds

Metabolic syndrome has four main features – abdominal fat, and high blood sugars, blood fats and blood pressure. Lignan-providing flaxseeds lower our fasting blood sugars, triglycerides, cholesterol and hemoglobin A1c levels (the conventional measure of diabetes). Ground flax is a great anti-diabetic food that damps down blood sugar spikes from high-glycemic plants.

(**Hemoglobin A1c** is a protein to which sugars attach and which they distort. The theory is that diabetics suffer ill-health and low energy because their proteins are distorted by the sugars on them. Planters have optimum A1c levels.)

To *not* eat nuts and seeds regularly is to live shorter lives.

Whole grains

Oatmeal for breakfast is a great way to start the day, especially if we add berries. A great anti-diabetes food, oats are also a great cholesterol lowerer. All whole grains are fabulous for diabetes prevention or maintenance.

Celiac and gluten exceptions should take care. Otherwise, everyone should eat plenty of whole grains, especially in combination with legumes, even if Frances Moore Lappé did create an enduring nutritional muddle when she got it all wrong about incomplete proteins in her *Diet for a Small Planet* back in 1971. She corrected this error later, and, to her everlasting credit, hers was the first major book that alerted us to the environmental devastation wrought by Meating.

Of course, highly processed grains such as white rice, and highly sugared breakfast cereals are a no-no for everyone, but particularly for diabetics.

Amla (Chinese gooseberries)

Amla is also a marvelous anti-diabetic food: it lowers our blood sugars, LDL- cholesterol and triglycerides, and raises HDL or good cholesterol. It's one of the most antioxidant foods available. Very bitter – must be good.

Green tea

Green tea helps prevent obesity, with theanine just one of its many phytonutrients. White tea with lemon is even higher in antioxidants.

Fruit

Fruits are wonderful foods, ideal for countering obesity and diabetes. We shouldn't let high fructose corn syrup and processed sugars like sucrose tarnish fruit's reputation. The people who eat the most fresh fruit have the least obesity and diabetes. Berries such as blueberries are spectacular at blunting the effects of other high glycemic foods, so if we're going to indulge in pancakes made out of crummy flour, we should eat them with plenty of high-antioxidant, anti-inflammatory berries.

The gigantic Global Burden of Disease Study tells us that about 4.9 million deaths each year can be attributed to low fruit consumption. More than 100,000 Americans die each year because we're not meeting even the pathetically low national dietary guidelines for fruit and veg.

To not eat plenty of fruit every day is to shorten our lives.

Important note: If you're overweight or diabetic, please work with a nutrition expert if you're going to adopt a Planter diet, preferably a Planter nutritionist or a lifestyle physician. You should know that plants are powerful healing drugs which may interfere with any pharmaceutical drugs you're taking. (Especially grapefruit.) Anyone taking diabetes medications should be particularly careful because whole plants will improve your insulin sensitivity enormously, lowering your need for metformin et al, within days, and putting you at risk of hypoglycemia, or low blood sugar. You will need to adjust your dosage, until, depending on the functioning of your pancreas's beta cells, medications become entirely unnecessary. In what percentage of cases of pure type 2 diabetes, with sufficient pancreatic function? According to Dr. John McDougall: 100%.

A final word about type 1 diabetes

A long time ago, at the beginning of this discussion of diabetes, I hinted that type 1 may be improvable, if not reversible. That's true.

If all our beta cells are gone, then there's nothing we can do. Beta cells are like teeth – we can't grow new ones in adulthood – and without beta cells we're truly insulin-dependent, permanently.

If, however, our mix of type 1 and type 2 has led to a situation where our insulin resistance is so high that our few remaining beta cells are effectively powerless against overwhelming odds, then there's hope.

As Dr. Neal Barnard, Dr. Gabriel Cousens, Dr. John McDougall and others have shown, when we go on a pure Planter diet and we improve our insulin sensitivity out of sight, it often becomes possible to lower the insulin needs of type 1 patients, and, rarely, it's possible for diagnosed type 1'ers to come off all their insulin, their suppressed few beta cells once again able to carry the glucose load. They weren't true type 1s.

In effect, there are people who've been diagnosed with type 1 who actually have a bad case of type 1½. And when we remove all insulin resistance, it's found that their type 1 condition isn't total – and may be reversed. Even in the absence of a complete reversal of type 1, a lowered insulin requirement is a great health benefit.

All told, the best way to cure diabetes of any stripe is to not give it to ourselves in the first place. The best remedy for our future diabetes diagnosis is to start Planting, right now, because we already have, at best, undiagnosed pre-prediabetes.

Armed with Planter insight, our present selves become capable of compassion for our future selves. Let's not, years from now, look back at our present selves and ask why we didn't love ourselves (or other animals) enough to have acted when we had the Planter fulcrum in our hands, and the place to stand, which would have allowed us to move our entire world.

Diabetic retinopathy
One of five animal-borne causes of vision damage and blindness.

Here's a breaking news flash: if we elect to stop having type II diabetes, our diabetic retinopathy disappears. Who'd'a thunk it?

So how do we do that? Let's map it out: As we've just seen in the Eatiology of T2D, Meating and Junking → Insulin Resistance → Type II Diabetes → Diabetic Retinopathy.

While Meating and Junking cause diabetic retinopathy, Planting reverses it.

OK, moving on from diabetes…

Diarrhea
In the developed world, diarrhea comes mainly from eating animals, due to their near-universal contamination with fecal bacteria.

Another recurring cause is the consumption of non-human milk by those lucky enough to be lactose intolerant, but who don't take the hint.

In the third world, contaminated water supplies kill I-don't-know-how-many-thousands of kids each day.

For more, see Part 2 (~~Food~~borne Pathogens); diarrheagenic pathogens

Disc degeneration & herniation
Atherosclerosis – a Meater affliction – causes the degeneration of the discs in our spines, via diminished blood and oxygen supply. As our vertebral arteries shut down, particularly the ones supplying the lumbar and sacral (lower) spine, less blood can perfuse into the cartilage pads that are intercalated between our backbones, like little shock absorbers.

Our spinal discs have no blood vessels in them, so they receive their nutrition from blood that perfuses in from the outside. They're particularly vulnerable to mal-nutrition. Diseased Meater arteries lead to diseased Meater vertebrae and diseased Meater spinal discs.

Disc herniation also occurs in a high-cholesterol milieu.

For more, see under: Lower back pain

Diverticulosis and Diverticulitis
Diverticulitis is one of the "pressure diseases" promoted by low-fiber Meating and Junking.

Diverticulitis ("inflammation of a diverticulum, especially in the colon, causing pain and disturbance of bowel function," per Wikipedia) and

Diverticulosis ("a condition in which diverticula are present in the intestine without signs of inflammation") are both symptoms of the disease known as "not eating whole plants." There, I just coined a new word: **Aphytophagy**. A-phyto-phagy – not plant eating.

Diverticulitis is a **fiber-deficiency disease**, according to Drs Hugh Trowell, A.G. Shaper, Neil Painter and Denis Burkitt and other physicians who spent decades practicing in central Africa, and who noticed that rural Africans eating a traditional low-animal high-plant diet had few of the "Diseases" of Civilization that are epidemic in the westernized world. In fact, not even a few; none at all of some conditions.

They include all the pressure "disease" symptoms of Meating: constipation, hemorrhoids, hiatal hernia, varicose veins and diverticulosis/-itis; related digestive tract conditions such as appendicitis, gall bladder disease, gallstones, peptic ulcers, gastro-intestinal reflux disease and colorectal cancer; obesity, diabetes, hypertension and ischemic heart disease; and an almost total absence of auto-immune conditions.

(Aren't we the smart ones? We noticed that auto-immune conditions increase with greater latitude: the further we move from the equator the more arthritis and MS and lupus we get. So, it must be the vitamin D, we shouted; we're getting less and less sun the further north (or south) we go. Well, vitamin D is important but, no, it's not the panacea. The panacea is Planting. The further we travel from the equator the more animals people eat. Get lots of sun, sure, but just say no to the animals. That's the solution to auto-immunity.)

This is really important:

The conditions listed above are all "food"-borne, elective "diseases". They're cases of Affluenza.

When we choose Meating and Junking we will develop some of these symptoms. When we choose Planting we remain free of them.

When we don't know how to eat, we don't know how to poop.

And when we don't eat or poop properly, we become fat and diabetic and heart-diseased.

I recall a ditty from childhood that goes like this:

> "For the want of a nail the shoe was lost;
> For the want of the shoe the horse was lost;
> For the want of the horse the rider was lost;
> For the want of the rider the battle was lost;
> For the want of the battle the kingdom was lost;
> All for the want of a horse shoe nail."

Little things add up. Moderation sucks. That's how it is in nutrition. If we eat unfoods, we lose a nail, and then a shoe, and then a horse, then a rider, then a battle, until finally we lose the kingdom, all for the want of an apple or a mess of pottage, a dinner of herbs or some sprigs of kale.

Diverticulitis and all the other maladies just listed are merely symptoms of the underlying mal-nutrition of Meating and Junking, which rapidly disappear on a Planter diet.

Without fiber in the diet – and there's no fiber in animals, and precious little in junk – a slew of bad things happen.

Firstly, fiber is what our healthy gut bacteria feed on, and they in turn feed us their byproducts – health-promoting, inflammation-preventing, immune system-modulating short-chain fatty acids like butyrate and propionate.

Secondly, there's not enough material in our intestines to bulk out our stools and cause peristaltic waves of muscle contraction that push our poop towards the exit. This means increased transit times. That is, it takes much longer for Meaters' poop to transit our 30-odd-feet of digestive tract than Planters. Increased transit time means more exposure to carcinogenic bile acids, which are made of excess cholesterol, and decreased stool bulk means even more exposure to these carcinogens, because they're more concentrated. The result: more colon cancer and, as we've seen, more breast cancer… because bile acids get recycled and then concentrated in breast tissue.

Without fiber to bulk out stools, they become hard and impacted and difficult to move. Remember, waste products in out intestines are moved by muscular contractions segmenting our bowels and pushing poop ahead of them, and then the next ring of muscles contracts. Hard, dehydrated poop that stays in our guts for days (instead of the hours which is all it takes to clear vegans' bowels) means that the muscles of our colons have to strain really hard to move things along, and the high pressure can lead to the formation of diverticula – little out-pocketings or balloonings in the intestinal wall. If these get some poop or bacteria in them, then infection can set in, and the result sometimes is surgery, sometimes is… death.

Closely associated is the way some old people die, from a brain aneurysm caused by sitting on the loo, rocking backwards and forwards, "straining at stool," clenching their abdominal muscles to try and dislodge a difficult stool.

This may be more than you care to know about me, but I mention this as being representative of whole-food vegans: I poop more than once a day and it never takes me more than a single minute at a time. When the 'defecation reflex' kicks in, I head for the head; lid up; drop me trews; sit; poop; wipe; wash; dry; trousers up; flush; seat down; wash handies; dry; boom. One minute; two at the max.

That's how healthy intestines are supposed to work. If we're not pooping at least every day, we're sick, and we're making ourselves sicker.

A short note on the Fiber Theory

It turns out that Denis Burkitt and his peers were wrong about fiber. Oh, they were right in one sense (the important macro-sense) but they were wrong in a strict nitpicky sense.

As reductionists in service of Meating love to point out, adding fiber supplements to the diet does diddly to lower our risk of, say, colorectal cancer. Therefore, they claim the fiber theory is wrong.

What Burkitt, and Trowell should have had in mind, though, wasn't fiber supplements: they should have stuck to African diets that are high in fiber, not fiber taken out of plants, isolated and stuffed back in again. And then they were right, because, when it comes to providing optimum bowel and total systemic health, a lot of fiber's heavy lifting is done by phytates and other phytonutrients that are tightly bound to fiber, or by short-chain fatty acids like butyrate which feed our gut flora, who then feed our gut lining in return. Burkitt et al got the epidemiology right; not the nutrition science.

So, yes to high fiber foods. Sorry, that's a tautology. So, yes to foods (which, being whole plants, are fiber-filled) and no to fiber additives, and no to anything else like animals (with zero fiber and next-to-zero phytonutrients) or junk (which seconds that emotion).

Drug resistance

After Alexander Fleming discovered penicillin back in 1928, some public health officials thought we'd erased infectious diseases altogether and for all time. Fleming himself, though, warned against the overuse of antibiotics, saying that bacteria would adapt to the drugs, become resistant and make the drugs useless.

Bacteria have been around for billions of years. They come into existence, reproduce and die in the matter of days. A human generation is about 25 years. During that time, thousands of bacterial generations come and go. So, in human terms, bacteria can select for traits very quickly.

When we use antibiotics, some bacteria will survive and pass on their genetic material. In effect, using antibiotics selects for bacteria that aren't affected by the drugs. Very rapidly, we can produce a generation of bacteria that are entirely resistant to our most powerful antibiotics. Two example of such 'superbugs' are Methicillin- (or Multi-drug-) Resistant *Staphylococcus aureus* (MRSA) and *Clostridium difficile* (better known as *C. diff.*), both now common in the unfood supply.

Fleming's prediction appears to be coming true. While doctors overprescribe antibiotics, often for viral infections (for which they're useless) or as placebos, the main overuse of antibiotics comes from industrial animal farming. The conditions in modern feedlots and CAFOs (Concentrated Animal Feeding Operations) are so overcrowded and unhealthy, antibiotics are used prophylactically to prevent illness among entire herds rather than to treat individual sick animals. Stock raising requires antibiotics on a vast scale, else the whole system would collapse.

Though the animal industry has been warned about the dangers of the superbugs they're creating, they're unwilling or unable to stop their mega-usage of antibiotics, and our government is unwilling to say boo to them. Dr Margaret Chan, head of the World Health Organization, has warned that we're facing a future in which these wonder drugs may no longer be part of the medical armamentarium. Cuts and scrapes may once again be death sentences from tetanus, and bacterial infection from animal fecal bacteria may also kill many more than they already do… future dead loved ones will become collateral damage of our present Meating habit.

For more, see Part 2 (~~Food~~borne Pathogens) – A Word on Meating and Antibiotic Resistance

Dry eye "disease"

As we've already seen, animal diets are particularly dehydrating. Dry eye disease – ok, you caught me; it's not a disease – having dry eyes affects millions of people, and billions of dollars are spent trying to remedy the situation.

Again, it's not a disease; it's a symptom of the initiating behavior. I'll give you a clue what that behavior is by telling you that dry eyes are easily remedied by (1) drinking lots of water (duh) and (2) eating a wide variety of whole plants (ditto).

Chronic dyspepsia (indigestion)

Would it surprise us if our beautiful rocket ship were to pink and shudder or even conk out if we were to fill its tank with diesel, and high-sulfur diesel at that?

So why would it surprise us if the non-foods known as animals were to cause us indigestion? Besides what's bred in the bone of animals, they're the carriers of infectious *Salmonella* and *E. coli* and *Campylobacter* and the other bugs that upset our stomachs. We should be grateful if we're not among the 10% of those infected who graduate from dyspepsia to a worse Meater malady, irritable bowel syndrome.

See also: Irritable bowel syndrome

Elective "diseases"

'Elective surgery' is an established medical term for surgical procedures that aren't obligatory, which may still be beneficial to the patient, either functionally, psychologically or cosmetically.

Elective ailments such as diabetes, heart disease, hypertension, Alzheimer's and auto-immune conditions such as rheumatoid arthritis are ones we elect to have by electing to eat animals and junk.

Eczema

See under: Atopic diseases

Embolism

See Embolism, under the Mechanisms of Meating

Emphysema

See under: COPD - Chronic obstructive pulmonary disease

Endometriosis

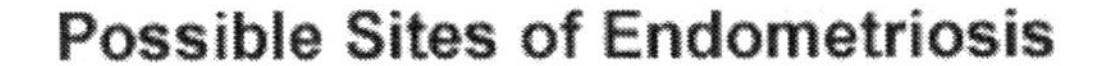

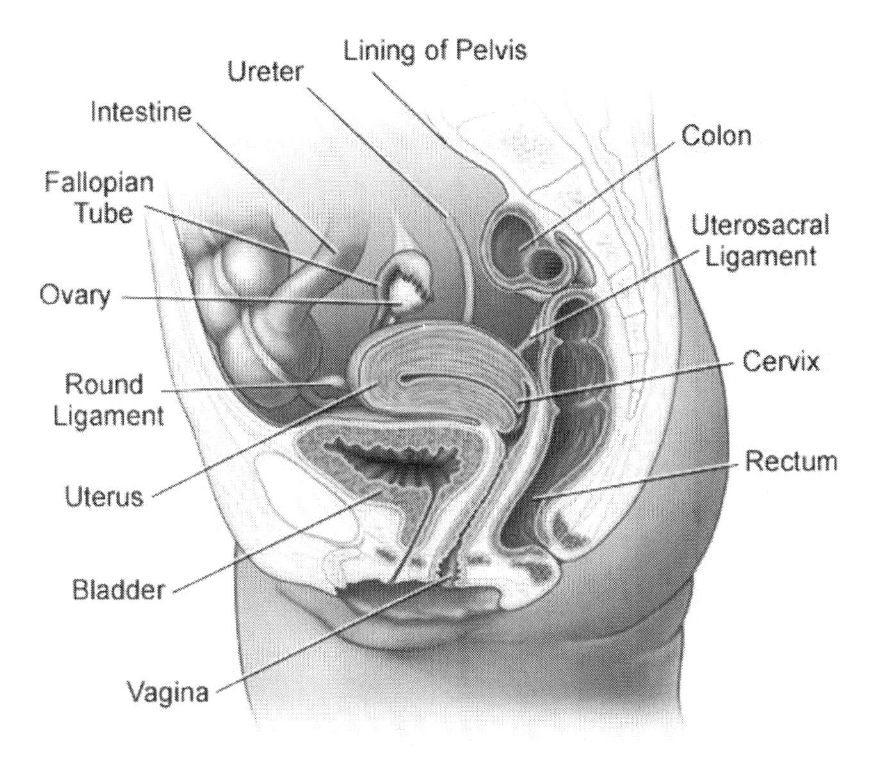

http://healthcare.utah.edu/healthlibrary/health-lib-image.php?imageid=142103

The "Possible Sites of Endometriosis" diagram above shows where endometrial cells may grow in inappropriate sites outside the uterus in the lower abdomen.

According to PubMedHealth, "Endometriosis is one of the most common medical conditions affecting the lower abdomen (lower belly) in women. In endometriosis, the kind of tissue that normally lines the inside of the womb (endometrial tissue) also grows outside of it. This can happen without the woman being aware of it. But in other women endometriosis is a chronic disease, associated with severe pain and fertility problems.

It often takes years for endometriosis to be diagnosed as the cause of these problems. Until the diagnosis is made, many women try to cope with their pain somehow. They believe that the pain — even really bad pain — is a normal part of their menstrual period.

There is currently no cure for endometriosis. But there are many things that can be done to relieve the symptoms. And if treatment is adapted to suit women's personal circumstances and the severity of their endometriosis, many can cope quite well with the disease."

MedlinePlus says: "Endometriosis is a problem affecting a woman's uterus – the place where a baby grows when she's pregnant. Endometriosis is when the kind of tissue that normally lines the uterus grows somewhere else. It can grow on the ovaries, behind the uterus or on the bowels or bladder. Rarely, it grows in other parts of the body.

This "misplaced" tissue can cause pain, infertility, and very heavy periods. The pain is usually in the abdomen, lower back or pelvic areas. Some women have no symptoms at all. Having trouble getting pregnant may be the first sign.

The cause of endometriosis is not known. Pain medicines and hormones often help. Severe cases may need surgery. There are also treatments to improve fertility in women with endometriosis."

These two health authorities tell us: we don't know what causes it, and we don't know how to reverse it. Take two aspirin and don't call me in the morning.

Well, I think we can do better than that. Endo is strongly linked to POPs – persistent organic pollutants – in the environment. The strongest link is to Dioxin, "the most toxic compound synthesized by man." (I guess no women work over there at Monsanto. Well, good for you.)

The FDA says that "over 95% [of dioxin exposure is] coming through dietary intake of animal fats."

Er, where are animals fats found? In animals.

So: Meating → high animal fat intake → high POP contamination via biomagnification → increased risk of endometriosis.

Endo-meat-riosis?

Suggestively, the symptoms of endometriosis, such as painful periods, pelvic pain and infertility, all improve or disappear on a Planter diet. Maybe that's as a result of other Planter benefits, but maybe it's also because of reduced incidence of Endo. Planting certainly minimizes our risk of dioxin contamination. (Did I say thank you, Monsanto?)

With endometrial cancer, epidemiology shows that a more plant-based diet is protective: Indians have 1/9th as much EC as Americans. Pigs and chickens (nitrosamines) and cow milk products (casein?) seem to be the worst Meater culprits; crispy carbs the worst Junk villains, because of acrylamide.

[See: http://nutritionfacts.org/2012/01/05/epa-dioxin-limit-has-national-chicken-council-worried-products-could-be-declared-unfit-for-consumption/]

Epilepsy

According to Michael Greger:

> "Neurocysticercosis is the infection of the human central nervous system by pork tapeworm larvae. It is the most common parasitic disease of the human brain. Little, baby pork tapeworms invading one's brain has become an increasingly important emerging infection in the United States, and it is the #1 cause of epilepsy in the world."

[See: http://nutritionfacts.org/video/chronic-headaches-and-pork-tapeworms/]

Fishes are highly contaminated with heavy metals and PCBs. Women eating them may give birth to children with epilepsy.

Speaking personally, I used to suffer from almost daily seizures, the result of a trauma-induced benign meningioma. After its surgical removal, I was told that I'd have to take a drug called epilim for the rest of my life. I wasn't willing to do that, so – foolishly – I would stick a tablet under my tongue each time I felt a fit coming on. The fit would come… and then pass.

I put the passing of the seizure down to the rapid action of the drug. My doctor laughed when I told him this, saying it takes hours for the drug to get to where it's got to go to do its work. Ok, then, I said: maybe it's acting as a placebo. Or, my doc said, the seizure would have passed anyway, drug or no.

Which told me something inconvenient: the only way to find out would be not to take the drug the next time I felt a seizure coming on.

That scared me, but the next time I got a signal saying "Stop what you're doing and lie down," I offered up a fervent little animist prayer and hoped for the best. And nothing. The seizure came and went, just as it always did. And in the days and months that followed, seizures came and went, some more violent than others, sometimes leaving me feeling like the breath was being crushed out of me, until now, five years later, months go by sometimes without a twinge, and the twinges are much milder than they once were. Some I even ignore, just carry on doing what I'm doing.

I'm not saying this proves anything about my vegan diet. What I am saying is that I believe that, by eating nothing but food, I'm doing the absolute maximum of which I'm capable to prevent another brain tumor and to minimize the electrical disturbances that still arise from the original tumor and the trauma of brain surgery. My phyto-food is my medicine; medicine, my phood.

I don't give a thought to my brain – or any aspect of my health – because Planting is making my body and mind and spirit, not perfect, but the best I can be. Planting and country living.

For what it's worth, my experience, submitted for your consideration… segueing neatly into another Meater malady to which I give no thought:

Erectile dysfunction

ED or impotence, in both men and women, in whom it's more commonly referred to as "Clitoral Insufficiency," is a symptom of a Meaterialist lifestyle.

The animals we eat get their post-mortem revenge on us by hardening our heart vessels – our hearts are already hard – and setting us up for cardiac or cardiovascular disease and death – heart attacks and strokes, our #1 and #2 killers.

But our #1 and our #2 killers aren't two different things: they're the same thing, they just look different. They're different outcomes of the same underlying cause: Meating and Junking. It's just a matter of chance which explodes first – the damaged arteries in our hearts or the atherosclerotic arteries in our brains. So if we go down in the death records as "myocardial infarction" it's only because our stroke was taking longer to arrive.

Heart disease = stroke = hypertension = intermittent claudication = lower back pain = … erectile dysfunction.

They look different but they're all the same. They could all be called foodborne illnesses if the stuff we eat that causes them could be called food. (The fact that animals and junk causes atherosclerosis is all the proof we should need that they're not food. And, the fact that whole plants were shown 25 years ago [21 July 1990] by Dean Ornish to reverse heart disease is all the proof we should need to know that plants are food.] Better yet, heart disease and stroke et al can be called symptoms of mal-nutrition. They're outcomes of an eating disorder. They're manifestations of Meating.

Penile arteries are slenderer than coronary arteries, so they get blocked sooner. This may be a very good thing, if understood properly. Taking the ridiculous drug named viagra® only suppresses the symptoms and doesn't remove the root cause (pun alert) of one's failure to achieve tumescence. Temporarily improving the blood flow through diseased, crippled arteries so that one can maintain a 12-hour tower of power isn't my idea of good medicine (or fun sex).

Men with erectile dysfunction and women with clitoral insufficiency should say a prayer of gratitude for the gift of being told that our entire arterial trees are gunged up with atheromas – not just our nether regions; everywhere – and that we need to make significant lifestyle changes if we don't want to go from alive and kicking to – Bang! – stone cold dead from Sudden Cardiac Death (SCD), which is what happens to more than half of first time heart attack victims. No warning… just: Bang! Dead.

Except we *were* given warnings, and plenty of them too. We "couldn't get it up," as the saying goes, though it would be more accurate to say that "it wouldn't get up." We couldn't get wood.

Or we were suffering from lower back pain. Or sciatica. Or high blood pressure. Or hypertensive retinopathy (damage to our eyes caused by long-term high blood pressure). These are not just aches and pains associated with getting old. These are all warnings about the same thing: the underlying atherosclerosis, caused by the Meating that underlies that.

OK, so now we know. We should be thankful when we suffer a "failure to launch." And do something about it. Stop eating the animals, already. (How manly is it to eat animals now, o manly men? Meaters make lousy lovers.)

Essential tremor

ET is the most common form of neurological disorder, affecting more than 4% of people over 40; those who eat animals, that is. Harmane is the neurotoxic β-carboline alkaloid that causes this brain disease which manifests in uncontrollable hand tremors. Harmane is found in cooked animal muscles, particularly those of chickens.

Heavy Meaters have 21 times the odds of developing this condition. Thus, Essential Tremor is essentially caused by the eating disorder called Meating. It can be reversed by eating a whole plant diet.

Eye "disease"

Whenever I hear the words 'eye disease' I think of 'I disease,' as if it's a form of egocentrism. Eye disease *is* usually the outcome of nutritional 'self-centeredness.' It stems from putting our eating desires before our health, and our eating pleasure before animals' hopes to "live long and prosper."

The five common forms of non-trauma-induced eye "disease" all turn out to be, at least, ameliorated by Planting and harmed by Meating. At worst, they're direct symptoms of or caused by Meating.

They are: diabetic and hypertensive retinopathy; cataracts; glaucoma; and 'age-related' macular degeneration.

Each of these Meater symptoms is covered more fully under their separate headings.

Fatty liver "disease"

Fatty liver "disease" comes in two varieties: alcoholic and non-alcoholic. In other words, a fatty liver is caused by Junking (alcoholic) and Meating + Junking (nonalcoholic, caused by fructose from Junk, and animal cholesterol and animal fats).

Again, it's not a disease: it's a symptom of our eating disorder.

Fibrosis

The title of this paper says a mouthful about fibrosis, and nutrition in general:

S Petta et al. Industrial, not fruit fructose intake is associated with the severity of liver fibrosis in genotype 1 chronic hepatitis C patients. *J Hepatol.* 2013 Dec;59(6):1169-76.

We see this time and again; studies that show that HFCS (high fructose corn syrup) and other processed Junk forms of fructose are harmful, while fructose from whole fruit is beneficial.

Fibrosis and liver disease are strongly linked to POPs or persistent organic pollutants, which bioaccumulate in animals, making them dangerous to eat.

Small wonder that these mutagens would affect our livers, our bodies' main detox and recycling centers. POPs include such lovelies as DDT, DDE and dieldrin; substances banned decades ago, yet still rife in the world.

As expected, liver fibrosis improves on a Planter diet.

Fibromyalgia

According to MedlinePlus at the NIH: "Fibromyalgia is a disorder that causes muscle pain and fatigue. People with fibromyalgia have "tender points" on the body. Tender points are specific places on the neck, shoulders, back, hips, arms, and legs. These points hurt when pressure is put on them.

People with fibromyalgia may also have other symptoms, such as

- Trouble sleeping
- Morning stiffness
- Headaches
- Painful menstrual periods
- Tingling or numbness in hands and feet
- Problems with thinking and memory (sometimes called "fibro fog")

No one knows what causes fibromyalgia. Anyone can get it, but it is most common in **middle-aged women**. People with **rheumatoid arthritis** and **other autoimmune diseases** are particularly likely to develop fibromyalgia. There is **no cure** for fibromyalgia, but medicine can help you manage your symptoms. Getting enough sleep, exercising, and **eating well may also help**."

I've highlighted some interesting points. No known cause… no cure… women particularly vulnerable… rheumatoid arthritis connection… auto-immunity.

From Healthline: "According to the Arthritis Foundation, about 1.3 million American adults have RA [rheumatoid arthritis], and three times as many women as men are affected by the disease."

RA and fibromyalgia have much in common, and we know that RA is a symptom of Meating; an auto-immune response to dead animals and animal-borne endotoxins and bacteria sloshing around in our bloodstream.

Trials have shown that fibromyalgia responds well, just the way RA does, to a high-antioxidant Planter diet, the purer the better, which may or may not be what MedlinePlus means by "eating well." Animal-free diets free of animal proteins, animal fats, and inflammatory arachidonic acid, heme iron and Neu5Gc are just what the healer ordered for fibromyalgia.

The many other symptoms of fibromyalgia listed above are common among Meaters, unusual among Planters. Just feeling better all-round on a Planter diet boosts the morale of fibromyalgians considerably.

Junk (especially anything containing aspartame) should also be shunned, along with the frumious bandersnatch.

Prestigious health organizations may claim that the etiology of this *disease* is unknown and that no cure is available, but the Eatiology of this animal-borne condition is well-known; as such, it reverses very nicely on a diet of pure plants. I wonder how many decades will pass before the NIH awakens to the best nutrition science.

Flatulence

The reason why Meaters think that baked beans cause *all of us* to fart is because baked beans make *them* fart like the cowpokes round the campfire in *Blazing Saddles*. Why? Because they routinely feed their gut flora on animals, so they've selected for animal-eating gut flora, not bean-eating bacteria. Within a month or so of Pure Planting, flatulence evaporates… because our now-bean-eating bacteria are loving the food.

Adding an Indian spice called hing to the cooking beans takes things down a notch on the Beaufort Scale. It's also called asafoetida, which I remember 'cos it makes yer ass a less fetid place.

"Food" poisoning

An entire section of this book shows that "food" poisoning is largely an issue for Meaters and for innocent bystanders caught in the crossfire, whose food has been cross-contaminated with animal fecal bacteria.

Gallstones

According to Healthline:

"Gallstones are hard deposits in your gallbladder, a small organ that stores bile, a digestive fluid made in the liver. Gallstones may consist of cholesterol, [bile] salt[s], or bilirubin, which are discarded red blood cells. Stones can range in size, from tiny sand grains to large ones the size of golf balls.

[Which becomes problematic when we try to squeeze them down a bile duct that's a quarter the diameter of a pencil.]

What Causes Gallstones?

Gallstones may develop when there is **too much cholesterol** in the bile secreted by your liver. Bile usually dissolves or breaks down cholesterol. But if your liver makes more cholesterol than your bile can dissolve, hard stones may develop.

Other causes include the following:

Bilirubin

Bilirubin is a chemical produced when your liver destroys old red blood cells. Some conditions such as cirrhosis of the liver and certain blood disorders cause your liver to produce more bilirubin than it should. Stones form when your gallbladder cannot break down the excess bilirubin. These hard substances are also called pigmented stones.

Concentrated Bile

Your gallbladder needs to empty bile in order to be healthy and function properly. If it fails to empty its bile content, the bile becomes overly concentrated, which causes stones to form."

If gallstones are made out of crystallized cholesterol (and they are, 8 or 9 times out of 10), and cholesterol comes either from eating animal cholesterol, or from eating animal fats that provoke cholesterol production, who would we logically expect to suffer more from gallstones – Meaters or Planters? More than a million Americans get gallstones each year, 90% of them omnivores, and about 20 million Americans have gallstones.

The gallbladder is a muscular little sack that contracts to churn bile (gall) and to pump it down the bile duct and into the duodenum. This pumping action can cause excruciating pain when solid, jagged crystals are what's being pumped, instead of liquid bile.

Gallstones are also made out of bilirubin (from dead red blood cells) and bile salts (which is what cholesterol is turned into for (1) excreting cholesterol from the body and (2) for secretion into the duodenum to emulsify and digest fats).

About 700,000 Americans have their gallbladders removed each year. I guess they prefer to have the op rather than stop eating animals. Now that's what I call elective surgery! I doubt if their physicians tell them about the free and painless nutrition option. For one, they probably don't know. And, two, it's not a particularly lucrative treatment.

Gallstones are almost impossible to create on an animal-free diet. I think that's something that surgeons should be compelled to tell their patients, before they chop out their gallbladders... something that happens 2,000 times a day in the USA.

[See: http://nutritionfacts.org/video/cholesterol-gallstones/]

Gangrene

Gangrene is one of the pernicious side-effects of the elective Meater and Junker condition known as type II diabetes. Others are dementia, kidney "disease", cardiovascular "disease" and blindness.

See under: Diabetes

GERD (Gastro-esophageal reflux disease)

Because of increased abdominal pressure and because of constipation-caused straining at stool, Meaters are far more likely to have hiatus hernia, the condition which causes the ring of smooth muscle making up the gastroesophageal [stomach/esophagus] sphincter to be pushed up above the diaphragm. This makes acid reflux more likely, and GERD may follow, as may Barrett's esophagus.

Another reason why Meaters have more GERD is that something in animals, particularly egg yolks, increases the secretion of **cholecystokinin,** the hormone that makes the gallbladder contract, and this hormone causes the GE sphincter to slacken too much.

Planting alleviates both these problems and makes Planters generally GERD-free, though coffee may cause reflux in some.

Glaucoma

Our optic nerves link our eyeballs to our brains, and glaucoma is their gradual deterioration.

We met our phyto-friends, the yellow-orange pigments lutein and zeaxanthin earlier while visiting with Cataracts, the world's #1 cause of blindness. Glaucoma is #2 and, while we don't know its etiology or its Eatiology, I've got my suspicions, because eating lots of (L+X-containing) leafy green vegetables works famously to combat glaucoma. So, it's my opinion that glaucoma is caused EITHER by a surfeit of animals in the diet OR by a deficiency of plants OR both.

Plant nutrients are so powerful that just one serving of kale A MONTH reduces glaucoma risk by 69%. Surely we can all manage one serving of leafy greens a month: spinach or collard greens or arugula or Swiss chard?

Some of us might even be adventurous and bump it up to two servings a month. Hail, let's go out on a limb then saw if off and say: some of us might even eat leafy greens every day. Why not? They're the healthiest, most nutrient-packed foods on the planet, with multiple health benefits besides saving our sight. What's stopping us? Fear of fabulous good health? Black currants and berries are also great anti-glaucoma foods. To NOT eat leafy greens every day is to shorten our lives. Same with nuts. Same with beans. Use your bean - eat real food.

We should all phyte the good phyte every day, every meal.

Gout

There are three main mal-nutritional causes of gout: alcohol, the purines in animals (not legumes or cauliflower) and the fructose in junk (HFCS) not the fructose in high-fiber, whole fruits and veg, which are protective.

In acid conditions (i.e. Meating), purines form uric acid, which can also crystallize into excruciating kidney stones. Gout is the painful inflammatory condition caused by jagged uric acid crystals in our joints. It's elective.

For more, see under: Purines; Kidney stones

Guillain-Barré syndrome

This paralyzing condition is also called "acute inflammatory demyelinating polyneuropathy," and it comes mainly from eating *Campylobacter*-contaminated chickens.

After a bout of *Campylobacter* "food" poisoning, an unlucky small percentage of people develop an incredibly fast-acting auto-immune condition which attacks the myelin sheaths of our nerves. We land up unable to move, unable to breathe without the assistance of a respirator, in a matter of days!

According to Michael Greger:

> "With the virtual elimination of polio, the most common cause of **neuromuscular paralysis** in the United States now comes from **eating chicken**." [emphasis added]

[See: http://nutritionfacts.org/video/fecal-bacteria-survey/]

So, if this dreadful paralysis is caused by eating chickens, is the paralysis the disease? Or is the eating of chickens the disease?

Halitosis

A Meater affliction. For more, see under: Bad breath

Hay fever

Also known as allergic rhinitis. (Did you know 'rhino-' is Latin for 'nose'?)

The general rule pertains: Planters suffer from hay fever far less than Meaters. It's believed that high antioxidant levels are protective. Animals are low in antioxidants, and also cause oxidative stress themselves.

See under: Atopic diseases

Heart "disease"

See under: Cardiac "disease"; cardiovascular "disease"; Sudden Cardiac Death

Heiner syndrome

Milk is a pediatrician's cash cow. I've come to the conclusion that when infants fall ill, if we stop feeding them cows' milk, in most cases they'll get better, almost immediately, almost no matter what ails them. Take this paper, for example, detailing severe lung (and other) problems in 8 kids:

Moissidis I, Chaidaroon D, Vichyanond P, Bahna SL. Milk-induced pulmonary disease in infants (Heiner syndrome). *Pediatr Allergy Immunol.* 2005 Sep;16(6):545-52.

"Heiner syndrome is a food hypersensitivity pulmonary disease that affects primarily infants, and is mostly caused by cow's milk (CM). They were fed CM from birth and their **chronic respiratory symptoms** began at age 1-9 months. The symptoms were in the form of **cough** in seven, **wheezing** in three, **hemoptysis** [coughing up of blood] in two, **nasal congestion** in three, **dyspnea** [difficult or labored breathing] in one, recurrent **otitis media** (OM) [middle ear inflammation] in three, recurrent **fever** in four, **anorexia**, **vomiting**, **colic** or **diarrhea** in five, **hematochezia** [blood in the feces] in one, and **failure to thrive** (FTT) in two. All had radiologic evidence of **pulmonary infiltrates** [blood, pus or protein in the lungs]…

Milk elimination resulted in remarkable improvement in symptoms within days and clearing of the pulmonary infiltrate within weeks."

Come on, dear hearts, cows' milk is *not* food for beloved human infants.

Hemorrhoids

Hemorrhoids or piles fall under the heading of pressure "disease".

Hemorrhoids are enflamed anal veins resulting from the high abdominal pressure attendant upon low-fiber animal and junk diets.

Not having to strain while pooping, and having soft bulky stools that are easily moved by waves of bowel muscle peristalsis, high-fiber Planters tend not to become constipated or get piles. Meaters aren't so lucky.

Hiatus hernia

Another of the pressure "diseases", hiatus hernia is when increased abdominal pressure forces the esophageal sphincter up above the diaphragm. Acid reflux, gastro-intestinal reflux disease (GERD), Barrett's esophagus or esophageal cancer may result from hiatal hernia.

High blood pressure

There are several causes of high blood pressure, both Meater and Junker.

High sodium intake is one. Just cutting down on salt could save tens of thousands of lives every year. As if chickens weren't bad enough as is, most retail chickens are plumped up for sale with salt water, causing a single chicken breast to exceed our daily limit for sodium intake.

Independent of its role in fluid and electrolyte balance, sodium contributes to hypertension by damaging our arteries. Additives aside, animals are generally high in sodium. A single rasher of bacon exceeds our daily sodium limit (>1500mg). Pretty rash.

Atherosclerosis, a Meater malady, leads to stiffening and narrowing of the arteries, the main contributor to high blood pressure.

Nitrates in plants are converted into nitric oxide, the signaling molecule that allows our arteries to dilate. Animals lack nitrates. Animals are also pro-oxidant and pro-inflammatory. High uric acid levels (from the purines in animals and the fructose in junk) add to the vasoconstrictive effect of Meating.

Essential hypertension is a strictly Meater affliction; when we're Pure Planters we simply don't give it to ourselves.

Hormonal dysfunction

Eating animal hormones and eating endocrine-disrupting xenoestrogens that are magnified in animal flesh leads Meaters to have unsatisfactory endocrine function.

For more, see under: Estrogen; Hormones

Hyperactivity

Food dyes, preservatives like sodium benzoate and HFCS (high fructose corn syrup, sometimes with a sprinkle of mercury in it) in junk (like sodas) can take the lion's share of the blame, but some can also go to eggs (with their high phthalate contaminant levels).

See also: ADHD (Attention deficit hyperactivity disorder)

Hypertension

High blood pressure may be an acute, temporary condition. Hypertension is the chronic, long-term condition of having constantly high blood pressure.

For all the same reasons that Meaters have acute high blood pressure, Meaters also have chronic hypertension: a diet that is high in sodium, devoid of fiber, devoid of phytonutrients, devoid of nitrates, oxidizing, inflammatory and ischemic. (Otherwise, it's fine.) In Michael Greger's words: "High blood pressure is just a symptom of diseased dysfunctional arteries," and that's just what Meating and Junking cause: diseased, dysfunctional arteries.

[See: http://nutritionfacts.org/video/lifestyle-medicine-treating-the-causes-of-disease/]

Low-fat, low-sodium, high-fiber, high-nitrate whole plant foods are powerful preventers and removers of hypertension, with whole grains particularly effective at lowering blood pressure.

Hypertensive retinopathy

HR is one of the top five causes of non-trauma blindness or vision loss.

According to this online post by Franklin W. Lusby, MD at MedlinePlus:

High blood pressure and eye disease

"Hypertensive retinopathy is damage to the retina from high blood pressure. The retina is the layer of tissue at the back part of the eye. It changes light and images that enter the eye into nerve signals that are sent to the brain.

Causes

High blood pressure can damage blood vessels in the retina. The higher the blood pressure and the longer it has been high, the more severe the damage is likely to be.

You have a higher risk of damage and vision loss when you have diabetes, high cholesterol level, or you smoke."

[https://www.nlm.nih.gov/medlineplus/ency/article/000999.htm]

Would you believe, if our hypertension goes away, then our hypertensive retinopathy gets better too? Well, what's stopping us? Why are we choosing to keep our elective non-disease?

Let's map this out:

Meating → Atherosclerosis → Hypertension → Hypertensive retinopathy.

So, if we stop with the animal eating already, we may not go blind. Planting prevents diabetic retinopathy too.

Diabetes and high cholesterol are also implicated: get rid of those two Meater symptoms and our eyesight improves. As for smoking, the Platters told us "Smoke gets in your eyes," so we can carry on smoking, as long as we stay out of the wind. Not so such.

Hypertensive retinopathy is a symptom of animal eating which improves on a whole plant diet.

Hypospadias

Hypospadias is a condition in which one is born with a smaller penis. Chickens are particularly implicated, in part because of their high phthalate content. How's that for an unwanted side-effect of Meating?

Iatrogenic deaths

'Iatros' is Greek for doctor. Iatrogenic means 'caused by doctors or medical treatment.' If one takes the (more than 100,000) deaths each year in America from ADRs (adverse drug reactions) which are "side effects" of taking normal prescription medications, and adds in doctor errors, wrong prescriptions and hospital-acquired infections (thanks mainly to industrial animal agriculture and industrial medicine's overuse of antibiotics), then modern allopathic medicine is the third leading cause of death in the USA.

The American medical system kills almost a quarter of a million people every year.

So why is that in this list? Because most doctors are Meaters, so not only are doctors killing us through best practice, they're killing us by not recommending a whole plant diet, which is far more powerful in combatting chronic "disease" – which is what kills most of us – than all their drugs and procedures and radiation and surgeries combined. (I blame not the doctors, but an out-of-touch medical system.)

For acute, short-term, life-threatening situations – as with trauma and infection – modern ER medicine is absolutely brilliant; the best ever (in-hospital infection and sepsis, aside.)

For chronic, long-term, lifestyle situations, Western medicine is worse than useless: it's a very big part of the problem, exacerbated by near-total ignorance of nutrition.

A good way to stay healthy is to stay healthy enough not to fall into their clutches. We don't want to go to hospital… people die there.

Whole Planters need to take far fewer medications (for a wide spectrum of conditions), take far fewer sick days and go to hospitals far less often. Small wonder we live longer than when we're Meaters.

Impotence

A Meater "failure to launch," reversible on a whole plant diet.

For more, see under: Erectile Dysfunction

Infectious diseases

Once thought to be totally under control, infectious diseases are on the rise worldwide. Why? For one, climate change is changing the range of disease vectors, e.g. allowing mosquitoes to live at greater altitudes, meaning they can go further up mountain slopes where previously unaffected people live.

The second reason has more to do with nutrition. Meater animal farmers are feeding antibiotics to the animals they raise, in squalid, overcrowded conditions, in such eye-watering quantities that we're developing superbugs that are resistant to cocktails of our most powerful drugs.

We're genetically modifying the microbiome so that we have no remedy for infections they may cause. We select for mutations that quickly become established in new generations of bacteria. CAFOs are perfect breeding grounds for such bacteria.

There are much smarter people than me who think that this Meater irresponsibility may prove lethal to many millions of us in the future.

Infectobesity

Obesity of infectious origin as a result of Meating! Yipes.

See under: Obesity

Infertility

Not only do Meater men of a certain age suffer more impotence (erectile dysfunction, ED) and Meater women of a certain age suffer more clitoral insufficiency, with decreased lubrication and arousal, but Meater couples have far more difficulty becoming pregnant as well.

Why?

D'ya think it could be the hormones? That'd be my guess. Sexual reproduction, with human sex hormones and animal sex hormones and animal reproductive fluids – milk – all mixed together in one full catastrophe.

Did you know, for instance, that human estrogen – our girly hormone – is indistinguishable from chicken girly hormone estrogen? The word is: identical. Should we be surprised then that eating chickens is strongly linked to "anovulatory infertility." Because our endocrine systems get so discombobulated by extra chicken estrogen, women stop making their own eggs or ova; they stop ovulating… which makes impregnation kinda difficult.

(Endocrine disruption is also what makes twin births 5 or 6 times more common among Meaters than Planters.)

And it's not just chickens, though they're the worst. There are sex steroid hormones in all the animals we eat, whether as chunks or as liquids. Understandably, animal milks are chockablock with hormones, including growth hormones, ready for transmission to a cow baby. Who thinks that's a good idea, drinking that stuff when we're thinking of creating and growing a human baby?

In his video, "Meat Hormones and Female Infertility," Michael Greger sums up the difficulty of conceiving while Meating:

> "Eat a single serving of any meat and you increase your infertility risk 30%, and red meat increases risk 40%, but just a single serving of chicken, half a chicken breast a day, and women increase their infertility risk more than 50%—more than bacon and hot dogs!"

Animals, particularly aquatic creatures, also concentrate environmental xenoestrogens, but Meaters shouldn't give them a first, second or third thought. Planters should though; would-be Planter mums should eat only organic fruit and veg, to avoid these fertility-reducing substances.

Why shouldn't Meaters worry about them? Because real animal estrogens such as estradiol are about 4 orders of magnitude more damaging. To worry about xenoestrogens when one drinks cow's milk would be like worrying about getting run over by a Mack truck's paint job, instead of being concerned about the 10 tons of steel under the duco.

Another contributory factor to female infertility is obesity, a condition far more germane to Meaters than Planters.

In men, via the same hormones and endocrine disruptors, and also via animal fats, Meating causes reduced sperm counts, decreased sperm motility and deformed sperm shape… poor semen quality.

Here's an interesting study for Meaters: J. A. Attaman, T. L. Toth, J. Furtado, H. Campos, R. Hauser, J. E. Chavarro. Dietary fat and semen quality among men attending a fertility clinic. *Hum. Reprod.* 2012 27(5):1466 – 1474.

They conclude:

"The associations of total fat intake with lower sperm count and concentration appeared to be primarily driven by intake of saturated fat… **Increasing saturated fat intake by 5%** of total calories at the expense of carbohydrates was associated with **a 38%... lower total count**, whereas the same 5% intake increase from monounsaturated fat … or polyunsaturated fat… at the expense of carbohydrates was unrelated to the total sperm count."

So, a 5% increase in Meater or Junker fat intake leads to a 38% lower sperm count in Meater men. (I'd hate to see what a 15% fat increase causes. What would a 114% decrease in sperm count look like? Would we go back in time?)

Plant fats have no effect on our sperm count.

Sperm cells are very vulnerable to oxidation, that is, damage by free radicals, so our testicles have ten times the amount of vitamin C in them than any other part of our bodies. That's because vit. C is a powerful antioxidant and it protects our semen from oxidative stress. Plants are a great source of vitamin C; animals and junk have none.

Fellers, Meating's mangling our little swimmers! What will it take for us to get angry about the bullshit line we've been fed about meat and masculinity?

Plant or phytoestrogens like those found in soy aren't just protective against cancer; they don't cause male infertility the way that animal estrogens do. And plants high in vitamin C, like peppers and citrus fruits, put our testicles into ideal shape for sperm production.

[See: http://nutritionfacts.org/video/male-fertility-and-diet/]

See also under: Birth defects

Inflammatory bowel "diseases"

The IBDs include Crohn's "disease" and ulcerative colitis. They're exacerbated by eating animals in general, in particular animal fats, animal proteins and arachidonic acid, and improved by eating plants, especially high-fiber-content veggies and fruit.

For more, see under: Crohn's "disease"; Ulcerative colitis

Insulin resistance

See under: Diabetes ~ Diabesity ~ Obesity

Lower IQ

Why are vegan kids smarter than their Meater peers? Do smarter kids choose to be vegans? Or is it the other way round; does veganism make kids smarter? Or both? Or does Meating make kids dumber?

A: All of the above, probably. And it's true, Planterlets are smarter than Meaterlets; slenderer and slightly taller, too. *Femina et Homo sapienter.*

As usual, the benefits of Planting are a combination of the pluses of whole plants plus the absence of Meater drawbacks.

Fishes are often touted as "brain food," probably because the presence of long-chain omega 3 fatty acids is supposed to improve arterial health and thus improve blood supply to the brain. Well, "food is a package deal," so I don't see the benefit of eating one beneficial-in-moderation ingredient if it's accompanied by animal fats, animal cholesterol, arachidonic acid and… drum roll… neurotoxic pollutants such as PCBs and mercury.

(Also, as we'll see later, high intake of long-chain omega 3 fats from fishes – DHA and EPA – increases our risk of cancer, especially prostate cancer.)

Among the dozens of contaminants in all fishes (who swim in humanity's sewers, a.k.a. our oceans), mercury is the zinger for brain health, stunting the brain development of infants. In fact, the best way for a Meater mother to detoxify herself from mercury and other heavy metals – heavy meatals! –

is to pass them on to the fetus developing in her womb and then expel them during childbirth.

Planting carries the least toxic burden of environmental contaminants and pathogens. Planting achieves the greatest artery health and supplies natural human neurotransmitters in the best possible way. These are ideal conditions for optimum brain development.

Can anyone imagine an "indigo child" eating animals or other junk? Not all Planter kids are indigos; I can't imagine that any indigos aren't Planters.

Irritable bowel syndrome

"An estimated 10-20% of the general population suffers from irritable bowel syndrome (IBS), which accounts for about 4 million doctors' visits a year," according to Michael Greger. That's somewhere between about 30 and 60 million Americans. What are all these people eating that's hyper-sensitizing the linings of their digestive tracts?

[See: http://nutritionfacts.org/video/kiwifruit-for-irritable-bowel-syndrome/]

One major cause of IBS is infection by bacteria such as *Campylobacter*, *E. coli* and *Salmonella*, all animal-borne fecal pathogens. One in ten "food" poisoning recoverees suffers a long-term, even permanent "post-infectious functional gastrointestinal disorder" like chronic indigestion (functional dyspepsia) or IBS. Inflammation of the bowel while infected can lead to permanent debility, so-called **spastic colon**.

Jaundice

The NIH's MedlinePlus summarizes Jaundice as follows:

"Jaundice causes your skin and the whites of your eyes to turn yellow. Too much bilirubin causes jaundice. Bilirubin is a yellow chemical in hemoglobin, the substance that carries oxygen in your red blood cells. As red blood cells break down, your body builds new cells to replace them. The old ones are processed by the liver. If the liver cannot handle the blood cells as they break down, bilirubin builds up in the body and your skin may look yellow. [Bilirubin is also the constituent of some gallstones, which may form under conditions of excess bilirubin.]

Many healthy babies have some jaundice during the first week of life. It usually goes away. However, jaundice can happen at any age and may be a sign of a problem. Jaundice can happen for many reasons, such as

- Blood diseases
- Genetic syndromes
- Liver diseases, such as hepatitis or cirrhosis
- Blockage of bile ducts
- Infections
- Medicines"

Decline in liver function has several causes, but Meating is the most controllable, nutritional cause. Genetics aside, even Medicines in the above list is more relevant to Meaters than to Planters, Meaters being more likely to be on medications. With cirrhosis, Junker alcohol is to blame. With other liver diseases, the Hep E from pigs is the factor most responsible.

Pure Planting provides optimal liver (and blood) health, and the best immunity against infection.

For some of the ways Meating compromises liver and gallbladder health, please see under: Liver "disease" and Gallstones.

By the way, dear NIH. "Jaundice [DOES NOT] cause your skin and the whites of your eyes to turn yellow."

Naming something a disease doesn't explain anything. Eatiology explains jaundice.

Jaundice (from the French word for yellow, 'jaune') is the condition of yellow eyes and skin caused by Meating.

Kidney failure

What are the kidneys and what do they do?

According to the NIH website: "The kidneys are two bean-shaped organs, each about the size of a fist. They are located just below the rib cage, one on each side of the spine. Every day, the two kidneys filter about 120 to 150 quarts of blood to produce about 1 to 2 quarts of urine, composed of wastes and extra fluid. The urine flows from the kidneys to the bladder through two thin tubes of muscle called ureters, one on each side of the bladder. The bladder stores urine... When the bladder empties, urine flows out of the body through a tube called the urethra, located at the bottom of the bladder."

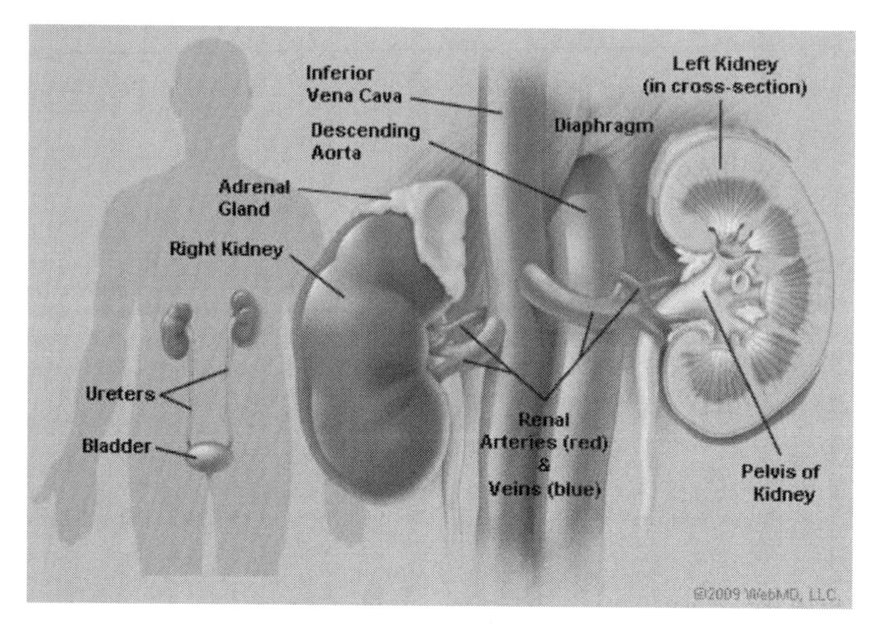

Kidneys. Image by WebMD, LLC.

That's a lot of blood to filter. So it shouldn't surprise us that the same dietstyle that causes general damage to our arteries also damages our kidneys' arteries. Meating brings cholesterol and animal proteins and fats into our bodies, which aren't capable of detoxing them, leading to atherosclerosis, system-wide, and raised blood pressure.

When proteins stop being retained by our kidneys and start appearing in our urine, particularly albumin – a condition known as microalbuminurea – we know our kidneys are packing up. If our kidneys are throwing in the towel, we know our arteries are diseased, that we're at increased risk of heart "disease" and stroke, and that we're destined to live shorter lives.

Animal proteins cause inflammation, hyper-filtration and protein leakage. Industrial sugars cause increased uric acid levels, and contribute to hypertension, both injurious to our kidneys.

Meating and Junking cause kidney "disease".

Planting is protective against atherosclerosis, acidosis and inflammation and, therefore, maintains healthy kidney function – no hyper-filtration, no proteins leaking into our urine.

Meaters with type II diabetes (another elective condition caused by electing to eat animals) are also electing to destroy their kidneys. Kidney failure, blindness (diabetic retinopathy), limb amputations due to gangrene, cardiovascular "disease" and dementia are common complications of diabetes, i.e. common complications of Meating.

These conditions are all avoidable on a Planter diet.

For more, see under: Animal proteins; Hyper-filtration and Protein leakage

Kidney stones

Most kidney or renal stones are built out of substances known as oxalates (which sound like they come from bovines), compounded with calcium. Beets are particularly high in oxalates, as are beet greens, Swiss chard, cinnamon, spinach and turmeric, but Planting leads to less oxalate stone formation, while Meating leads to more. This is because oxalate stones form in an acidic environment, which is what Meating provides. A Planter diet is alkalizing.

It would be a mistake to look at the oxalate content of the things we eat and make the assumption that high oxalate content translates into high oxalate stone formation. It does in Meaters but it doesn't in Planters, so when we're Planters we can eat all the beets we want without problems (barring a rare genetic predisposition to oxalate over-absorption). When we're Meaters we should probably cut back on high-oxalate foods, if we can't cut back on animals.

Meating causes the acidosis that turns neutral plant oxalates into unhealthy Meater kidney stones. This acidosis is also causative of muscle wasting (via calcium from the muscles being used to buffer systemic acid) and the inflammatory arthritic condition known as gout.

Meating also causes a less prevalent form of kidney stone that's made out of uric acid. Animals are high in substances called purines, and they wreak their particular havoc on our kidneys through their breakdown product, uric acid, high concentrations of which can crystallize into solid, jagged kidney stones. Gout is the outcome of uric acid crystals in our joints.

For more, see under: Gout

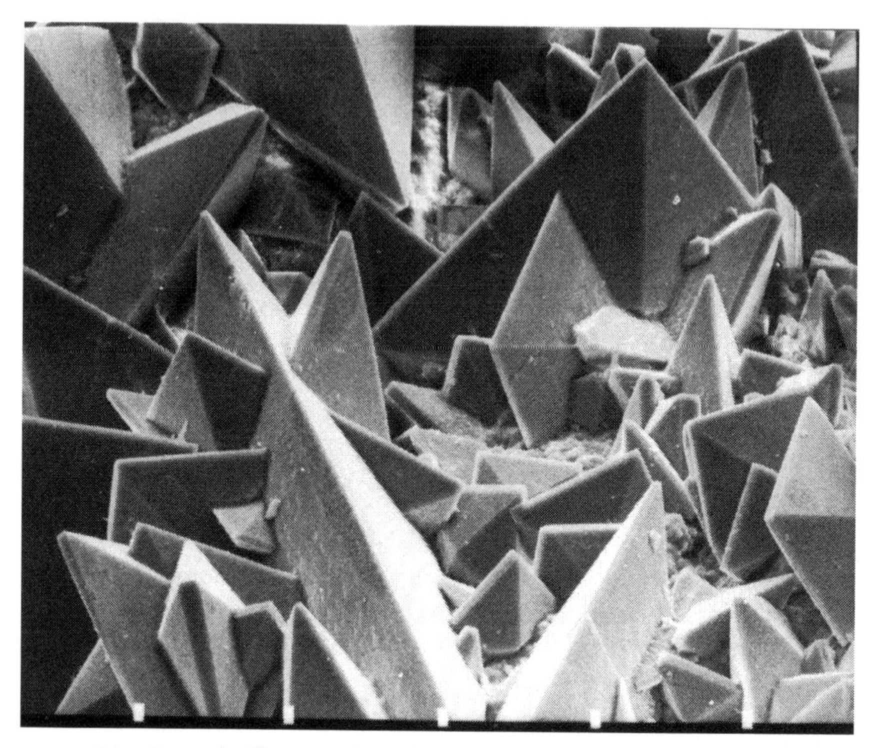

en.wikipedia.org/ - Close-up view of a kidney stone. No wonder that hurts…

Leukemias

Leukocytes are white blood cells. Leukemias are blood cancers.

"According to MedlinePlus at the NIH: "Leukemia is cancer of the white blood cells. White blood cells help your body fight infection. Your blood cells form in your bone marrow. In leukemia, the bone marrow produces abnormal white blood cells. These cells crowd out the healthy blood cells, making it hard for blood to do its work.

There are different types of leukemia, including

• Acute lymphocytic leukemia
• Acute myeloid leukemia
• Chronic lymphocytic leukemia
• Chronic myeloid leukemia."

Regardless of the sub-type of leukemia, all are caused predominantly by eating animals and smoking cigarettes, two easily identified, if not easily eradicated lifestyle choices. The carcinogenic nitrosamines in animals makes one hot dog as cancer-causing as five cigarettes.

(But let's face it, if an addictive personality such as me can quit Meating, Smoking and Drinking and Other Drugging, then anyone can. Giving up the animals first makes the rest far easier, because of what we take up instead and the multiple blessings we receive as Planters.)

For more, see under: Blood cancers; Lymphomas; Multiple myeloma

Liver "disease"

Population studies show that the correlation between alcohol usage and liver disease isn't as strong as that between Pigging Out – eating pigs – and liver disease. Meating causes more liver "disease" than alcoholism.

As agin Meating as I am, I didn't see that one coming. That's a gobsmacker. What causes that?

Other than the full catastrophe of Meater hyperlipidemia, atherosclerosis, ischemia, oxidation and inflammation? Infectious *Hepatitis E* viruses in pigs, with which Meaters can then infect other humans.

As if Planters needed another reason to seek a mate among fellow Planters besides Meaters' lack of consciousness, lower IQ, rank body odor, bad breath, obesity, fish-borne STDs, erectile dysfunction, et bloomin' cetera. Infectious liver "disease". Dang.

Longevity

Planters live longer, and have fewer health challenges in old age.

See under: Mortality

Lou Gehrig's disease

See under: ALS

Lower back pain

Lower back pain that doesn't stem from physical injury is usually the result of the Meater eating disorder.

Back pain is a symptom of atherosclerosis, one of the prime Meater mechanisms of bodily harm. What happens is that the small lumbar and cervical arteries supplying our vertebrae stenose or close down, reducing the blood supply to and damaging our spine. The pain is a result of this; also a result of lactic acid build-up due to inefficient garbage disposal.

Back pain, like erectile dysfunction, is a notable early warning of heart "disease". Atherosclerosis affects all our arteries, not just the central ones, and our penile and back arteries are smaller than our coronary arteries, so they close down first, in effect saying, "Please change your diet; you're killing us!"

American pre-teens eating SADly already manifest disc degeneration.

Lupus erythematosus

Here's the NIH's take on lupus:

"Systemic lupus erythematosus (SLE) is an autoimmune disease in which the body's immune system mistakenly attacks healthy tissue. It can affect the skin, joints, kidneys, brain, and other organs."

Under Causes, they say:

"The underlying cause of autoimmune diseases is not fully known."

But then they give us a hint by saying: "SLE is much more common in women than men. It may occur at any age, but appears most often in people between the ages of 10 and 50. African Americans and Asians are affected more often than people from other races. SLE may also be caused by certain drugs."

Rheumatoid arthritis is a related auto-immune condition, caused by Meating, and… guess what? It too is more common in women than men. Why might that be? Besides having different endocrine systems, which give women a ten-year advantage over men with respect to heart "disease", and therefore longer lives, women eat differently. Western women tend to eat more dairy products and poultry than men.

One of the many downsides of eating chickens is amyloidosis, the creation of misfolded animal proteins which are involved in dementia, diabetes and atherosclerosis.

Lupus isn't a disease. Lupus is an auto-immune response to Meating. The evidence for this is that lupus – like insulin resistance and coronary artery "disease" and… and… and… - is best treated with a diet of pure plants. If we stop wolfing down animals, then the wolf stops eating us.

Under Symptoms, the Meater scientists over at the NIH say: "Symptoms vary from person to person, and may come and go. Almost everyone with SLE has joint pain and swelling. Some develop arthritis. The joints of the fingers, hands, wrists, and knees are often affected.

Other common symptoms include:

• Chest pain when taking a deep breath
• Fatigue
• Fever with no other cause
• General discomfort, uneasiness, or ill feeling (malaise)
• Hair loss
• Mouth sores
• Sensitivity to sunlight
• Skin rash – a "butterfly" rash in about half people with SLE. The rash is most often seen over the cheeks and bridge of the nose, but can be widespread. It gets worse in sunlight.
• Swollen lymph nodes.

Other symptoms depend on which part of the body is affected:

• Brain and nervous system: headaches, numbness, tingling, seizures, vision problems, personality changes
• Digestive tract: abdominal pain, nausea, and vomiting
• Heart: abnormal heart rhythms (arrhythmias)
• Lung: coughing up blood and difficulty breathing
• Skin: patchy skin color, fingers that change color when cold (Raynaud's phenomenon)
• Kidney: swelling in the legs, weight gain

Some people have only skin symptoms. This is called **discoid lupus**."

Under Treatment, the NIH (mistakenly) says: "There is no cure for SLE. The goal of treatment is to control symptoms. Severe symptoms that involve the heart, lungs, kidneys, and other organs often need treatment from specialists."

I beg to differ. We don't need specialists to treat lupus; we need a generalist known as a plant-based nutritionist.

The symptoms listed above are symptoms of the symptom known as lupus, and lupus is a symptom of the elective disease known as eating animals.

When we become Planters, we elect not to have lupus, and we elect not to damage ourselves further with the drugs the NIH recommends for its treatment: NSAIDs, corticosteroids, hydroxychloroquine - cytotoxic (or cell-poisoning) drugs. They really don't have a clue. They say: "Side effects from these drugs can be severe, so you need to be monitored closely if you take them."

Or we could simply stop eating the animals.

Again, according to the NIH: "If you have SLE, it is also important to:

- Wear protective clothing, sunglasses, and sunscreen when in the sun
- Get preventive heart care
- Stay up-to-date with immunizations
- Have tests to screen for thinning of the bones (osteoporosis)."

Planters have the least heart "disease" and the least osteoporosis, two other symptoms of Meating.

Under Possible Complications, the NIH says: "Some people with SLE have abnormal deposits in the kidney cells. This leads to a condition called lupus nephritis. Patients with this problem may go on to develop kidney failure and need dialysis or a kidney transplant.

SLE can cause damage in many different parts of the body, including:

- Blood clots in the legs or lungs
- Destruction of red blood cells or anemia of chronic disease
- Fluid around the heart endocarditis, or inflammation of the heart (myocarditis)
- Fluid around the lungs and damage to lung tissue
- Pregnancy problems, including miscarriage
- Stroke
- Severely low blood platelet count (platelets are needed to stop any bleeding)
- Inflammation of the blood vessels."

These aren't separate symptoms confined to lupus; these are symptoms of Meating, one of whose mechanisms is molecular mimicry (laying the table for an auto-immune response), and the others are the result of other Meating mechanisms, such as atherosclerosis (another immune response!), ischemia, inflammation and oxidation. When we eat animals all these things happen at once. When we stop eating animals, all the Meater mechanisms stop. And then Planter healing begins.

When to Contact a Medical Professional? According to the NIH, "Call your health care provider if you have symptoms of SLE. Call your health care provider if you have this disease and your symptoms get worse or a new symptom occurs."

Better yet, if our HCP is a Meater, don't call them at all. Find a lifestyle medicine practitioner who knows about food's power to heal and food's ability to maximize our own bodies' incredible powers of self-healing.

We can eat ourselves healthy on a diet of pure plants.

Here's what this eating disorder looks like:

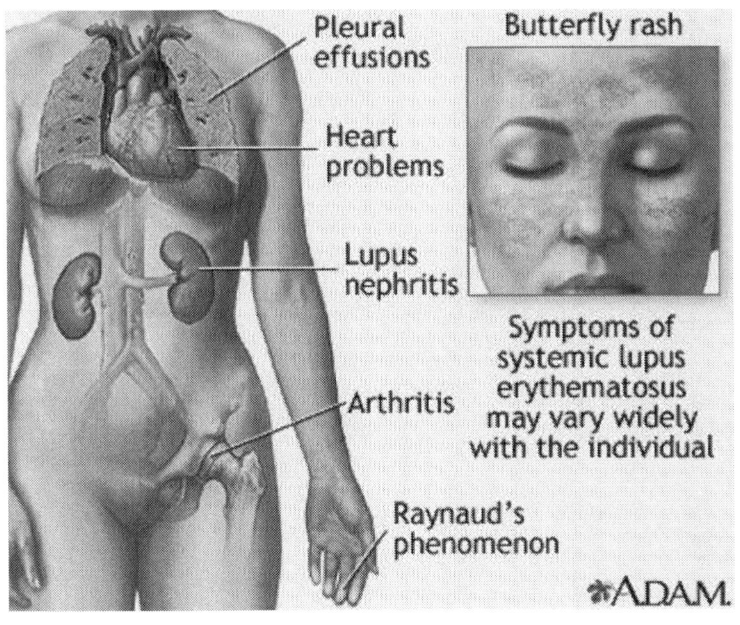

Systemic lupus erythematosus (SLE)
https://www.nlm.nih.gov/medlineplus/ency/images/ency/fullsize/17134.jpg

PS. The NIH gave another clue to the Eatiology of Lupus above: not only does it affect women more than men, it affects "African Americans and Asians… more often than people from other races." Now isn't that interesting? By Asians, they mean Asians living (and eating) in America. If there are two groups of humans in which lupus has never, ever appeared among those eating their traditional high-starch, low-animal diet, it is African Africans and Asian Asians.

With the single minor exception of celiac/gluten/wheat immune response, the same applies to all the major auto-immune conditions: they're symptoms of the 1st World eating disorder known as Meating.

Lymphomas

MedlinePlus says: "Lymphoma is a cancer of a part of the immune system called the lymph system. There are many types of lymphoma. One type is Hodgkin disease. The rest are called non-Hodgkin lymphomas.

Non-Hodgkin lymphomas begin when a type of white blood cell, called a T cell or B cell, becomes abnormal. The cell divides again and again, making more and more abnormal cells. These abnormal cells can spread to almost any other part of the body. Most of the time, doctors don't know why a person gets non-Hodgkin lymphoma. You are at increased risk if you have a weakened immune system or have certain types of infections."

As seen under Blood cancers, above, the main contributors to lymphoma formation are smoking cigarettes and eating animals, two easily preventable lifestyle choices.

Meaters have four times the risk of lymphoma than Planters. (I'm surprised it's not higher; perhaps some of the Planters thought cigarettes were a good idea because they're vegan…)

Macular degeneration

Age-related macular degeneration is "the leading cause of legal blindness in older men and women, affecting more than 10 million Americans," according to Michael Greger.

[See: http://nutritionfacts.org/2015/01/01/foods-for-macular-degeneration/]

The retina is the screen at the back of the eyeball movie house on which the lens projects an (upside-down) image of the outside world. It's protected against UV radiation damage by a cell layer known as the retinal pigment epithelium.

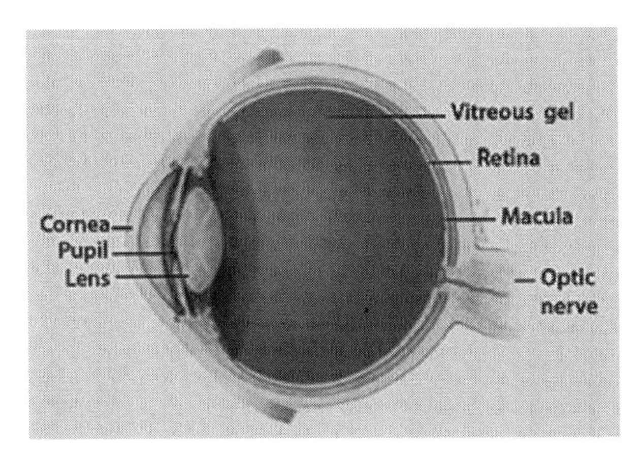

The eye. https://nei.nih.gov/sites/default/files/health-images/macular.jpg

There are pigments in plants that protect plants from radiation damage. These same plant pigments make up the retinal pigment epithelium: we eat them and they go straight to our eyeballs and take up residence there – we incorporate them; they become us. Two yellow phyto-pigments in particular: lutein and zeaxanthin.

As we saw under Cataracts, the top sources of lutein+zeaxanthin (measured together) are kale, spinach, turnip greens, Swiss chard, collards, mustard greens and cress. Leafy greens, in other words. Our retinas are best built out of leafy green veggies. Shouldn't we all be eating them every day, knowing that?

Animals are rubbish at providing L+Z. Animals contain L+Z to the extent they've eaten or been fed L+Z, leading, as we saw with eggs to miniscule concentrations. And then, "food being a package deal," the L+Z comes packaged with the full catastrophe of animal this, that and the other thing.

The Wikipedia-definition of the "*macula* or *macula lutea* (from Latin macula, "spot" + lutea, "yellow") is an oval-shaped pigmented area near the center of the retina of the human eye." It's the area of our keenest vision. It's next to the fovea, in case you get lost and need to ask directions.

L+Z protect our maculae by best absorbing the sky blue part of the electromagnetic spectrum, so preventing oxidative stress.

Macular degeneration has two components:

- Build-up of rubble known as Drusen or Drusen bodies
- Loss of pigmentation over time

One druse; several drusen. They're made out of lipids and proteins and, while they may not cause ARMD, they're a sign of it. My entirely unjustified opinion is that Meater atherosclerosis, which is after all a systemic condition, impairs arterial blood flow to and, especially, venous return from the eyes, and this reduced efficiency in waste removal leads to the build-up of this soft drusen dross in our retinas over time. That's my conjecture, and I'm willing to be schooled on this topic. It seems logical to me.

The best way to prevent pigmentation loss is to eat plenty of pigments in the form of leafy green vegetables (which are the most nutrient-packed, healthiest foods anyway, with multiple health benefits.)

Macular degeneration can be deferred and even prevented by not eating animals, and by eating plenty of plants, especially leafy green ones.

Cyclical Mastalgia

Cyclical mastalgia is the breast pain that some women experience during their periods. Elevated **prolactin** hormone levels appear to cause it. So what causes high prolactin levels? Eating animals. Women with breast pain who go vegan usually become symptom-free very rapidly.

Early Menarche/Menses

See under: Premature puberty

Mental health

Many suicides are diet-related. Why? Is it because Meaters suddenly think "Oh, my God, what have I done?" and decide to off themselves? No, we tend to try to atone for past mistakes by becoming Planters before we haul out the shotgun. Though I have met one 3rd generation vegan, whose mother never wittingly ate a single animal, almost all Planters like me were once Meaters like me. There's no Us and Them; there's only We.

No. Firstly, Meating causes inflammation in our brains via high homocysteine levels; homocysteine being the sulfur-containing metabolite of the sulfur-containing amino acid, methionine, present at low levels in plants, but high levels in animals.

Secondly, there are anti-inflammatory compounds in plants, phytochemicals such as salicylic acid – better known as aspirin – that counter Meater brain inflammation.

Thirdly, plants make human neurotransmitters, oh yes, they do. Including dopamine, melatonin, tryptophan and the "happiness hormone," serotonin.

And who wouldn't be happier and less suicidal with more of the happiness hormone coursing through our brains?

It turns out serotonin can't get into our brains because it can't cross the blood-brain barrier.

Aaaaaaaaaahhh. Boo hoo.

But its precursor, tryptophan can.

Yay! Then we make serotonin from tryptophan in our brains.

Here's Michael Greger on the subject:

> "Contrary to popular belief, the consumption of animal foods may actually decrease tryptophan levels in the brain. Carbohydrates, on the other hand, can boost transport across the blood-brain barrier, which has been used to explain premenstrual cravings.
>
> Tryptophan is one amino among many found in proteins, and they compete with one another for transport across the blood-brain barrier into the brain. And since tryptophan is present in most animal proteins in relatively small quantities it gets muscled out of the way. If you eat plant foods, though, the carbohydrates cause a release of insulin, which causes your muscles to take up the non-tryptophan amino acids as fuel, and so your tryptophan can be first in line for brain access.
>
> Animal foods can even make things worse: "When tryptophan is ingested as part of a protein meal, serum tryptophan levels rise but brain tryptophan levels decline (Fernstrom and Faller 1978) due to the mechanism of transport used by tryptophan to cross the blood–brain barrier.""

[See: http://nutritionfacts.org/video/a-better-way-to-boost-serotonin/]

What's the best source of tryptophan? Seeds like pumpkin, sesame and sunflower, which have high carbohydrate content and high tryptophan-to-total-protein ratios, and whose tryptophan thus out-competes other amino acids for transport through the blood-brain barrier.

(Isn't it great that eating seeds makes us less nuts?)

High antioxidant levels in food confer protection against depression. In other words, fruits, legumes and vegetables, especially leafy greens.

All animals are bad, but eating fishes causes depression, big time (despite high long-chain DHA and EPA omega-3 fatty acid levels), because of contamination with mercury et al. Fishes are, after all, swimming in humanity's cesspits 24/7 and are thus the most polluted animals on Earth.

By every metric of mood and mental health, vegans are better off than animal eaters:

- Less depression
- Less pre-menstrual depression
- Less social anxiety disorder (shyness?)
- Less aggression (duh)
- Better sleep patterns
- Better "global mood."

QED, lower rates of suicide for vegans, and better mental health altogether… even though faced with the never-ending heartache of bearing witness to institutionalized cruelty in animal agriculture.

Metabolic syndrome

Although it usually includes the "Deadly Quartet," Wikipedia describes metabolic syndrome as: "a collection of five of the following medical conditions: abdominal (central) obesity, elevated blood pressure, elevated fasting plasma glucose, high serum triglycerides, and low high-density lipoprotein (HDL) levels.

Metabolic syndrome is associated with the risk of developing cardiovascular "disease" and diabetes. Some studies have shown the prevalence in the USA to be an estimated 34% of the adult population, and the prevalence increases with age.

Metabolic syndrome is also known as metabolic syndrome X, cardiometabolic syndrome, syndrome X, insulin resistance syndrome, Reaven's syndrome (named for the "Father of Insulin Resistance," Dr. Gerald Reaven), and CHAOS (in Australia = Coronary artery disease, Hypertension, Adult onset diabetes, Obesity, and Stroke).

Metabolic syndrome and prediabetes may be the same disorder, just diagnosed by a different set of biomarkers."

Interesting… but as a whole food vegan, I could care less about low HDL cholesterol. It's irrelevant to me, only possibly protective in someone with elevated LDL, though I wouldn't count on it. The equation of metabolic syndrome with prediabetes shows at least an inkling of awareness about reality.

The Mayo Clinic has this to say: "Metabolic syndrome is a cluster of conditions — increased blood pressure, a high blood sugar level, excess body fat around the waist and abnormal cholesterol levels — that occur together, increasing your risk of heart disease, stroke and diabetes.

Having just one of these conditions doesn't mean you have metabolic syndrome. However, any of these conditions increase your risk of serious disease. If more than one of these conditions occur in combination, your risk is even greater."

As the prison warden told Cool Hand Luke, "What we have here is a failure to communicate."

While I agree with both these sources about the symptomology of metabolic syndrome, and its connection to diabetes and heart "disease", there's a simple, unspoken cause behind all these listed symptoms, plus the ones these experts say they cause: Meating does it.

Animal fat causes central/abdominal obesity. Meating and Junking cause insulin resistance and high blood sugars. Meating whacks our cholesterol and blood pressure. Meating causes atherosclerosis and cardiovascular "disease".

Everything's connected.

Why not include diabetes and heart "disease" and stroke in a more meaningful "cluster of conditions?"

Metabolic syndrome exists only as a grab bag of symptoms that people have noticed occur together. Well, if we broaden our vision, we'll notice that abdominal fat, elevated cholesterol and elevated blood sugars and hypertension, and elevated insulin resistance and heart "disease" and stroke all form a far more relevant cluster of symptoms than metabolic syndrome: the consequences of Meating, the single underlying condition that's responsible for all of them. With some Junking on the side.

To say, as the Mayo Clinic does, "If you have metabolic syndrome or any of the components of metabolic syndrome, aggressive lifestyle changes can delay or even prevent the development of serious health problems" is to totally misunderstand what's going on.

They're saying that one group of things can lead to another. That's just plain wrong. They're all the same thing; they're all the same serious health problem. Some symptoms just appear before others, quite logically, like prediabetes not coming after diabetes. "Aggressive lifestyle changes"... well, actually, quite gentle lifestyle changes... including not eating animals prevents the full catastrophe, even reverses the full catastrophe.

A simple way to think of Meating is this:

Meating → abdominal fat = insulin resistance = elevated blood sugars = elevated cholesterol = elevated blood pressure = diabetes = ischemic heart "disease" = hemorrhagic stroke= constipation = breast cancer = prostate cancer = kidney "disease"... and on and on... They're all the same thing. By that, I mean they're all apparently different, but they have the same Eatiology: they're products or symptoms of eating animals and junk.

Let's call this expanded concept MEATABOLIC SYNDROME, because that's what it is: a giant syndrome made up of a "Deadly Century," not a deadly quartet or quintet.

As you can probably tell, the concept of metabolic syndrome pisses me off. It's a useful partway step towards seeing the big picture, but, because it stops there, it seems to prevent people from going beyond it and reaching the proper archetype – seeing that metabolic syndrome is only a subset of the meatabolic disturbances caused by a pre-existing malady: our cultural inability to distinguish food from non-food.

Naming things seems to cut off thought. OK, now we've named this group of symptoms, that's it, we can put it in a box and forget about it. That's sad. Armed with the understanding that animals aren't food, the label 'metabolic syndrome' is seen as the laughably inadequate pastiche that it is.

Call it what we will – I'm not ego-bound to the term – the concept of Meating (or meat eating or eating animals or zoöphagy or carnivorism or Carnism or omnivoraciousness or meatabolic syndrome, whatever) explains chronic "disease" like no other forensic tool.

When we get it or grok it in its fullness, it's as if a rebus or picture puzzle suddenly shakes into focus. It's as if we can suddenly see after years of blindness. A great Aha! moment. And once we see the truth about the centrality of eating animals in the Eatiology of degenerative conditions, there's no possible way to unsee it. Clunk. It explains so much that's otherwise obscure.

(Alas, we'll never again be able to watch friends and loved ones undergoing useless, damaging, symptom-treating surgeries, poisonings and radiations (while continuing their symptom-producing Meating!) without feeling overwhelmingly sad.)

My wish for this book is that it will help just one person see the world of nutrition and health as it truly is, and then I'll be content, job done. May that person be you…

MGUS

Monoclonal gammopathy of undetermined significance (MGUS) is the condition that precedes multiple myeloma, a cancer of the blood. Planters get about a quarter as much MGUS as Meaters.

For more, see under: Multiple myeloma

Microalbuminuria

Protein in the urine is a warning signal of declining kidney function, and a good biomarker of future heart "disease" and mortality. Hands up any of us who thinks that Meaters have more albumin seeping out into their urine than Planters? We'd be right.

For more, see under: Kidney failure

Milk Apnea

Milk-induced CNS (central nervous system) respiration center suppression in infants that may lead to SIDS/crib death.

See: Crib death

Molecular mimicry

MM is what happens when we eat non-human animals, whose proteins mimic human animal proteins: the ensuing 'friendly fire' from our immune system damages or destroys our own tissues.

See under: Auto-immune conditions

Mood

Despite all the shit we have to put up with from mindless Meaters (in other words, ourselves – the people we used to be); despite the terrible cruelty we see being perpetrated on defenseless animals to provide nonfoods that sicken their eaters; despite seeing that many of the world's intractable problems are caused by the senselessness of Meating… Despite all the psychological burdens, Planters are happier than Meaters, for physiological reasons, as well as the psychological one that stems from knowing one's "doing unto others."

There is a strong Eatiological basis for the better mood states of non-animal eaters.

For more, see under: Mental health

Mortality

When we're Meaters we're better at dying than Planters: we get more practice.

Considering all the Meater mechanisms that are attacking our bodies simultaneously, our bodies are incredibly resilient. It's amazing that our motors can run fairly well on such poor fuel, so well, in fact, that the owners of the motors don't even realize that what they've got isn't the best there is.

It's also a shame that we're so resilient. If we were to collapse writhing on the ground after eating just one fast "food" burger – which would be lucky for us if we did – instead of their damage being so slow and incremental, untold billions of animals would be spared unspeakable lives and deaths, and our world could truly be heaven on earth.

I digress.

The longest-lived people on Earth are the residents of the Blue Zones, most of whom eat animals, but in amounts that approach zero, getting only 10% of calories from proteins, and <1% from animals. The 2nd best-studied and 2nd longest-lived people used to be the traditional Okinawans (who've sadly started Meating and Junking). They had more centenarians than any other population. They ate maybe 6 eggs a year, and perhaps a dollar coin-sized piece of fish once a month.

The best-studied and longest-lived people are the vegan portion of the 7th Day Adventist population centered around Loma Linda, California. They eat no animals at all.

The Adventist studies show that vegan SDAs outlive lesser mortals by about a decade.

These studies compare vegan SDAs to vegetarians and flexitarians and omnivores. In the case of longevity, BMI (body mass index, a reasonably good indicator of obesity), hypertension, type II diabetes and cardiovascular "disease", there's a stepwise improvement in every condition measured as animals disappear from the diet. The more animals we eat; the worse our long-term health outcome.

And small wonder: why would the conditions caused by animals not disappear from the population as they stopped eating the animals that caused the conditions?

I know that sounds kind of circular, but, really, if we understand that eating animals is what causes chronic ailments, it's hard to understand how other people don't/can't/won't see this glaring truth: adding animals to one's diet brings nothing but misery, "disease" and premature death.

In the Adventist studies, Planting brings longer life and less obesity, diabetes, hypertension, heart attack and stroke. Of course it does, because obesity = diabetes = hypertension = heart attack = stroke. They're all the same thing! It wouldn't be possible to increase diabetes, say, and to decrease stroke. The same diet – Meating – that causes heart "disease", also causes diabetes, also causes stroke…

And the same sane diet, Planting, that leads whole plant vegans to be the only sector of society with a "normal" BMI (<25), also leads vegans to be heart attack-proof, and normotensive and to have optimal glucose sensitivity, and to die far less often from stroke.

Heart surgeons and oncologists and kidney pros and all the other medical specialists need not apply: Planting prevents the ailments that are their stock-in-trade, because their ailments are produced by Planting's antithesis: Meating.

Got Meat? Got Milk? Got Death. Got it?

Mucus production

Yes, the latest studies show that consuming dairy products does lead to the formation of more mucus and increased nasal and sinus congestion.

Got milk? Got mucus.

Extra snot. Yum.

Multiple myeloma

According to the Mayo Clinic website: "Multiple myeloma is a cancer that forms in a type of white blood cell called a plasma cell. Plasma cells help you fight infections by making antibodies that recognize and attack germs.

Multiple myeloma causes cancer cells to accumulate in the bone marrow, where they crowd out healthy blood cells. Rather than produce helpful antibodies, the cancer cells produce abnormal proteins that can cause kidney problems."

It's ironic that one of the "germs" that plasma cells make antibodies to "recognize and attack" is animal protein. Meaters have four times the incidence of multiple myeloma as Planters. Why do Planters get so much, if it's Meating that causes MM? These Planters are probably also Junkers: aspartame in diet sodas and acrylamide in crispy carbs are also suspects in MM.

The time from diagnosis with multiple myeloma to death is about four years. Rather than trying to reverse this blood cancer after getting it, perhaps we should have compassion on our future selves and practice Planter prevention.

Multiple sclerosis

In Michael Greger's words:

> "Multiple sclerosis is an unpredictable and frightening degenerative autoimmune inflammatory disease of the central nervous system in which our body attacks our own nerves. It often strikes in the prime of life and can cause symptoms in the brain, such as cognitive impairment; in the eye, such as painful loss of vision; as well as tremors, weakness, loss of bladder control, pain, and fatigue."

[See: http://nutritionfacts.org/2014/07/22/how-to-treat-multiple-sclerosis-with-diet/]

MS is horrendous. And yet there's hope…

With auto-immune conditions, the exceptions to the rule of Meater Eatiology are unusual: celiac disease as a response to proteins in wheat and other grains, and rheumatic fever caused by molecular mimicry of proteins in heart muscle by *Streptococcus* bacteria being two examples.

The majority of auto-immune responses are reactions to the introduction into our bloodstreams of animal proteins or, at least, fragments of proteins called peptides.

We've seen that cholesterol provokes an immune response in us: cholesterol is thus an antigen, and macrophages are the antibodies that gobble up cholesterol and attempt to remove it. Not being well adapted to handle cholesterol, our bodies incorporate it into foam cells instead of excreting it, and the cascade known as atherosclerosis begins.

Similarly, animal proteins are antigens. Our immune systems recognize them as foreigners and attempt to destroy them, sending antibodies to do the wet work. Sadly, our antibodies can't tell the difference between identical peptide sequences. Our immune systems aren't speciesist: they can't distinguish between animals. (If animals aren't food, we shouldn't expect them to be able to do so! Follow the logic wherever it leads, my friend.) We're animals; they're animals; our immune systems can't tell the difference. Therefore, QED, ergo, thus... we shouldn't eat them.

And now, getting to the good news. Pure Planting stops the thrice-daily mealtime aggravation of MS and, at least, prevents progression of this symptom of Meating. No, it's not a disease; it's yet another symptom of Meating. If we stop the Meating, the symptom is ameliorated and may even disappear, depending on how advanced the condition is and how much irreversible damage we've done to ourselves with our knives and forks.

MS, like type I diabetes, like rheumatoid arthritis, like lupus, is an elective undisease. Selecting to eat plants reverses autoimmune conditions, stopping inflammation and swelling, and deleting pain.

It's our choice. We just have to ask ourselves which we prefer: the pain of auto-immunity or the pleasure of Meating.

Muscular atony

When infants are fed cows' milk, SIDS/crib death may be one outcome. A **blue baby** or a **floppy baby** are others. The latter condition is known as muscular atony.

For more, see under: SIDS

Myocardial Infarction

On the WebMD site, we read the following under "What Is a Heart Attack?":

"The heart requires its own constant supply of oxygen and nutrients, like any muscle in the body. Two large, branching coronary arteries deliver oxygenated blood to the heart muscle. If one of these arteries or branches becomes blocked suddenly, a portion of the heart is starved of oxygen, a condition called "cardiac ischemia."

If cardiac ischemia lasts too long, the starved heart tissue dies. This is a heart attack, otherwise known as a myocardial infarction – literally, "death of heart muscle.""

Dr. William Castelli is worth quoting again here. During the 60-odd years of the Framingham Heart Study, he says they have never seen a heart attack in anyone with a total cholesterol score lower than 150 [3.9 in the units used by the UK and colonies].

This is the safe level that all health authorities should set so that people can make themselves "heart attack-proof," in Caldwell Esselstyn's words.

Instead, each year hundreds of thousands of people who've been told that their cholesterol level is safe at 170 or 180, even 200 for crying out loud, end up clutching at their chests in agony and gasping like beached fishes, while their heart muscles die inside them.

The reason why we aren't told to get our cholesterol down to 150 is that, without drugs, which come with their own problems, it's not possible to eat animals and to get one's cholesterol down into the safe zone.

It's one or the other: Meating or a healthy heart.

So much for "Real food for real people." (RIP, James Garner.) In Dr Neal Barnard's words: "The beef industry has contributed to more American deaths than all the wars of this century, all natural disasters, and all automobile accidents combined. If beef is your idea of "real food for real people" you'd better live real close to a real good hospital."

Nonalcoholic fatty liver "disease"

Fatty liver "disease" used to be caused mainly by alcohol causing fatty deposits in the liver, leading to inflammation, liver disease and, possibly, cirrhosis or cancer, liver failure and death.

That was then. Now, nonalcoholic fatty liver "disease" is more common than alcoholic. What's to blame? Animals and junk.

The fructose and hydrogenated fats in junk and the cholesterol and saturated fats in animals. (Yet another case of our two unfoods – animals and junk – behaving in the same way, even though processed junk may be entirely vegan. Their Eatiology is the same.)

Less saturated fat → less insulin production → less fat deposition → less fatty liver "disease".

Autopsies show that 9 out of 10 obese people have a degree of N-A FLD.

As with insulin resistance… as with atherosclerosis… as with hypertension, fatty livers return to normal functioning on a Planter diet.

Non-Hodgkin's lymphoma

Non-Hodgkin's lymphoma is a blood cancer that's lethal about a third of the time. 75% of those who get it have been infected with **bovine leukemia virus**. The chances are good that avoiding eating animals will greatly increase our chances of avoiding this dread condition.

For more, see under: Lymphomas

Obesity

Obesity is a cause and an effect. It's caused by Meating and Junking, not by eating whole plants. Then, once we're obese, it helps cause an array of further problems, ranging from insulin resistance to diabetes to heart "disease" and cancer. The effects of obesity stem both from the types of fats Meaters and Junkers eat, and from the hyper-magnified levels of pollutants contained within animal fats.

Planters are the slenderest, least polluted people in the world. Planting roots out obesity. (Because "food is a package deal," losing weight via low-carb, high animal diets cannot be safely recommended.)

For a more detailed discussion, see: Diabetes ~ Diabesity ~ Obesity, earlier in this section.

Oral lichen planus

OLP is an auto-immune condition that affects the mucosal lining of our mouths, causing painful pre-cancerous lesions. It affects about 2% of us and there hasn't been a remedy until now: purslane, a common plant.

Now… I have no evidence for this, but my vegan gut tells me that if a plant fixes this auto-immune condition, then it's probably not a plant that causes it. My money's on animals, but hey! I'm biased. It's worth a try, giving up animals to see if it helps. While Planting is free, possible side-effects include lower cholesterol, lower blood pressure, less insulin resistance and a longer life. So sue me.

Osteoarthritis

Osteoarthritis is a degenerative joint condition caused in part by "mechanical wear and tear." It's also an "active joint disease" with inflammation and oxidation leading to cell death and cartilage damage.

Planting may only *soothe* the physical abrasion in our joints, but it certainly reverses the inflammatory and oxidative stress caused by Meating, as shown by a decline in tumor necrosis factors (TNFs), a marker for inflammation.

"Tumor necrosis factor is a powerful inflammatory cytokine, infamous for the role it plays in autoimmune attacks like inflammatory bowel disease," says Michael Greger. It seems likely that a diet that lowers TNF activity will be useful in combating osteoarthritis.

Plants that have proven especially beneficial to osteoarthritis sufferers include turmeric, rosehips, and soy.

Osteoporosis

Brittle bone "disease". A complicated condition, made more mysterious by the recent reversal of the long-held doctrine that animal protein causes calcium to be leached from bones to counter systemic acidosis. Very irritating. The old theory fit my vegan confirmation bias perfectly, and now I've had to give it up. Dang.

So what causes it? I don't think anyone knows exactly, but Meating and Junking make it worse and Planting makes it better. (Anyone seeing a pattern developing here?) And the regions with the highest dairy consumption have the brittlest bones: USA, UK, Netherlands, New Zealand, Scandinavia… must be the television sets. (Get some exercise, couch potato.)

Glycotoxins (AGEs) make it worse; animals are by far the most relevant source of glycotoxins.

Phosphorus injected into animals and used as a preservative in junk makes it worse by "disrupting hormonal regulation." Phytic acid in plants is less absorbable and therefore less harmful.

And dairy? Here's the result of one study, in the words of Michael Greger:

> "A hundred thousand men and women followed for up to 20 years; what did they find? Milk drinking women had higher rates of death, more heart disease, and significantly more cancer for each glass of milk. Three glasses a day was associated with nearly twice the risk of death. And they had significantly more bone and hip fractures too."

[See: http://nutritionfacts.org/video/is-milk-good-for-our-bones/][No.]

Got milk? Got early death, and brittle bones too, to add injury to injury.

Planters eating lots of phytates, found in beans, grains, nuts and seeds, have optimal bone density.

For more, see under: Bone fractures

Ovarian cancer

Ovarian cancer is one of the estrogen-dependent malignant conditions, others being uterine cancer, breast cancer, testicular cancer and prostate cancer.

Low-fat Planting is how we avoid high estrogen levels.

Cocky vegans should stop eating french fries and potato chips – the acrylamide produced by cooking carbs at high temperatures is carcinogenic, and may cause ovarian cancer.

Pancreatic cancer

Our pancreas is a terrible place for cancer to take hold. The prognosis is poor, with many dying within six months of diagnosis, and >95% dying within 5 years. It's very quick.

Meating – particularly chickens and pigs – doubles our risk of this cancer. Is it the IGF-1? Is it the nitrosamines and nitrosamides? Is it the industrial pollutants in the saturated fats? Is it the saturated fats themselves? Is it lactose? Is it animal proteins? It turns out that all of these are involved.

Thankfully, we don't need to dot our tees and cross our eyes before taking animals off the menu. It takes a special kind of insanity *not* to stop eating animals until we achieve Perfect Nutrition Knowledge about the exact Eatiology of ill-health. That's like thinking bullets aren't dangerous if we don't know the rifle's muzzle velocity. (Picture a small kid with her hands over her eyes, saying: "You can't see me.")

What's the opposite of *Orthorexia nervosa*, the supposed nervous disorder related to compulsive healthy eating? I suggest that *Pararexia* or *Heterorexia nervosa* is the omnipresent Meater reality: a well-demonstrated nervous disorder related to obsessively eating animals and other unhealthy junk.

Just because a majority of Westerners eat animals, doesn't mean it's not a mental illness. As compassionate eater Jiddhu Krishnamurti said: "It is no measure of health to be well adjusted to a profoundly sick society."

Dr. Geoffrey Rose finishes his famous paper called "Sick Individuals and Sick Populations" with these words: "…priority of concern should always be the discovery and control of the causes of incidence." Meating.

Paralysis

In the words of Michael Greger:

> "A neuropathic strain of the fecal bacterium *Campylobacter* found in poultry can trigger Guillain-Barré syndrome, a rapid and life-threatening paralysis… Now that polio is largely a thing of the past, the most common cause of acute paralysis in the United States is, ultimately, chicken consumption."

[See: http://nutritionfacts.org/video/poultry-and-paralysis/]

For more, see Part 2 (~~Food~~borne Pathogens)

Parkinson's "disease"

Dairy products are the best understood cause of Parkinson's. Contamination with neurotoxic chemicals like PCBs and tetrahydroisoqinoline (common in cheese) and pesticides may be to blame.

As mentioned before, fishes bioaccumulate a neurotoxic amino acid called BMAA (β-Methylamino-L-alanine), made by blue-green algae, which we then consume in high concentrations when eating the animals. BMAA is often found in the brains of Parkinson's sufferers; also in the brains of Alzheimer's and ALS sufferers.

Whole plants, exercise and coffee are protective against Parkinson's. Trauma, pesticides, animals in general, aquatic creatures and dairy products promote Parkinson's. Animal amino acids out-compete L-dopa for uptake into the brain… and Parkinson's is a dopamine-deficiency condition.

Lifestyle modification to maximize Planting and exercise is the best way to avoid Parkinson's, and the best way to deal with it if one already has it.

Diminished penis size

Sorry to tell you this, guys. If your mom ate chicken during her pregnancy with you, the chances are that you were born with a penis about a centimeter shorter than it would otherwise have been. Now I know we've been told that it's not the size of the boat that counts; it's the motion in the ocean. But can't bigger boats cause more motion in the ocean?

(If you decide to sue, please don't involve me. And maybe it's the USDA you should be suing, because of the criminal nutrition advice they give, not your sainted mother.)

For more, see under: Hypospadias

Peptic ulcer

Peptic ulcers are between rare and non-existent in whole plant-eating cultures.

What causes them?

Helicobacter pylori bacteria and NSAID drugs, for the most part. Planters get only about 1/10th of the bacterial infections Meaters get so often from fecal bacteria in animals, and Planters' diets generally provide enough anti-inflammatory compounds to make 'non-steroidal anti-inflammatory drugs' superfluous.

Peripheral artery "disease"

If we remember that "atherosclerosis is an omnipresent pathology," then it makes sense that the arteries furthest from our hearts will be particularly damaged. They're the end-of-the-line blood vessels, downstream from all the atherosclerotic plaques and lesions, and they cause problems in the tissues they serve, particularly poor oxygenation of our calves and lower legs.

See also: Claudication

PITS (Perpetration-Induced Traumatic Stress)

Sometimes also called Participation-Induced Traumatic Stress, PITS is a mental condition akin to PTSD, or Posttraumatic Stress Disorder, in which perpetrators become severely unstable emotionally as a result of the killing or other violence in which they take part.

Slaughterhouse and other Meater workers are prone to this debilitating mental condition. Amateur Meaters must be affected to some extent. In effect, Meating makes us all 'combat veterans,' whether we know it or not.

Polyps

Polyps are the lumpy precursors to colorectal cancer that form from endothelial cells lining our colons, and they're caused by eating animals. Polyamines such as spermine, putrescine and cadaverine are strongly implicated. Polyps are different to diverticula, which are pressure-related balloonings of the gut wall, also caused by Meating.

Diets high in fiber and antioxidants, low in fat prevent polyps. In other words, Planting. Fruits, especially berries, and veggies are great. Phytate-packed beans are the best.

For more, see under: Colorectal cancer

Pre-diabetes

Just about everyone eating a First World diet is pre-diabetic. That is, of course, if we aren't already diabetic, which a growing number are. Pre-diabetes is characterized by insulin resistance and high blood glucose.

As we saw under Type II diabetes above, it's caused by Meating and Junking, and if this combined form of mal-nutrition continues, it will probably evolve into full-blown diabetes. The "cure" is relatively simple: lots of exercise and a whole plant diet with plenty of and a wide variety of fruits and vegetables, nuts, seeds and legumes. In other words, the same diet that reverses every other chronic condition: the very high-carb diet.

Pre-eclampsia

According to MedicineNet.com, pre-eclampsia is a "condition in pregnancy, also known as [toxemia] … characterized by abrupt hypertension (a sharp rise in blood pressure), albuminuria (leakage of large amounts of the protein albumin into the urine) and edema (swelling) of the hands, feet, and face. Pre-eclampsia is the most common complication of pregnancy. It affects about 5% of pregnancies. It occurs in the third trimester (the last third) of pregnancy.

Pre-eclampsia occurs most frequently in first pregnancies. It is more common in women who have diabetes or who are carrying twins."

As noted in the diabetes and twin birth sections, these are Meater anomalies. Pre-eclampsia is part of the same concatenation of causes and effects; gestational diabetes, in particular. Without knowing which animal culprit is responsible (or needing to know) – glycotoxins, heme iron, nitrosamines, etc. – pure Planting minimizes the risk of type II diabetes, gestational diabetes, pre-eclampsia and twin births. Also minimizes the risk of infant mortality and birth defects.

Not only do we have it within our power to eat ourselves healthy; when eating for two, we have the power to eat them healthy too.

Pre-hypertension

Just about everyone eating a First World diet is pre-hypertensive. That is, of course, if we aren't already hypertensive, which a growing number are. Blood pressure is defined by two readings, the systolic and the diastolic pressures – and is spoken as, for example, 120 over 80, which is considered normal. 120 here measures systole – when one's heart contracts – and 80 measures diastole – when the heart muscle relaxes.

Hypertension is chronic, persistent elevated blood pressure, and, by convention, begins at 140 over 90. All pressures in between are considered to reflect pre-hypertension. It's a state that says, hey, you're not really sick yet, but you're on your way.

Mapped, the Eatiology of hypertension looks like this: Meating and Junking → atherosclerosis → hypertension. So pre- and malignant hypertension are fairly easily preventable, stoppable and reversible. One just has to stop beating one's alimentary canal against a Meater wall three times a day. Dr Walter Kempner of Duke University famously first demonstrated this using a diet of rice and fruit more than 50 years ago.

Premature puberty

Premature puberty in girls is largely a result of hormone overload from drinking cows' milk. Besides the psycho-social aspects of starting one's period or growing breasts at the age of 8, the added years of lifetime exposure to estrogen sets up these unfortunates for cancers of breast, uterus and ovary.

Thanks to the growth hormone IGF-1, all animal eating leads to more rapid growth and earlier menarche. Endocrine disrupting chemicals that bio-accumulate in animals are also implicated. Got milk? Got early teenage pregnancies and abortions. Milk isn't food, unless it's our mother's breast milk.

Pressure "diseases"

Pressure diseases aren't. They're symptoms of fiber-depleted diets, meaning Meating and Junking.

Meating + Junking → low fiber → constipation → increased abdominal pressure → hemorrhoids; hiatus hernia; varicose veins; diverticulosis

Pressure symptoms such as these are rampant in SAD eaters; almost non-existent in traditional and vegan cultures. Pressure "diseases" increase in direct proportion to the amount of Meating and straining we do.

Prion "disease"

See: Bovine spongiform encephalopathy (BSE) in Pt. 2C (Other Pathogens)

Prostate cancer

One of the estrogen-dependent malignancies; a Meater affliction, with the lowest fat milks being the most dangerous (because of increased hormone concentration).

For more, see under: Breast cancer; Testicular cancer

Psoriasis

According to the NIH's MedlinePlus webpage, "Psoriasis is a skin disease that causes itchy or sore patches of thick, red skin with silvery scales. You usually get the patches on your elbows, knees, scalp, back, face, palms and feet, but they can show up on other parts of your body. Some people who have psoriasis also get a **form of arthritis** called **psoriatic arthritis**.

A **problem with your immune system** causes psoriasis. In a process called cell turnover, skin cells that grow deep in your skin rise to the surface. Normally, this takes a month. In psoriasis, it happens in just days because your cells rise too fast.

Psoriasis can last a long time, even a lifetime. Symptoms come and go. Things that make them worse include • Infections • Stress • Dry skin • Certain medicines."

But not, apparently, diet, in their opinion.

Continuing, "Psoriasis usually occurs in adults. It sometimes runs in families. Treatments include creams, medicines, and light therapy."

I think we can do better than that. In fact, I know we can.

If psoriasis "runs in families," it practically gallops in Meater families. It's an outcome of families sharing menus, not genes. It's an elective condition brought on by the non-foods we elect to eat.

Psoriasis is an inflammatory, auto-immune "disease"; it's related to arthritis, and they both come to a shuddering halt when we remove the fauna from our plates.

Planting is generally anti-inflammatory; Meating is generally inflammatory. One of the Planter anti-inflammatory pathways is this one:

Planting → high potassium intake → increased adrenal gland function → increased production of anti-inflammatory glucocorticoid steroid hormones → less inflammation.

As we see from the Top of the Pops Potassium list below, courtesy of the USDA's National Nutrient Database for Standard Reference Release 27, plants are packed with potassium. Animals have little, and what little they have comes coupled with multiple 'ingredients' that cause inflammation.

I've highlighted the three animal products that appear in the top 25 potassium-containing consumables. Note that the pig and the turkey only make the top 25 because they appear in enormous portions of over a kilo (2.2 pounds) each; not a fair contest. And who, in their right mind, would consume whey after they've been weaned from the teat?

NDB_No	Description	Weight(g)	Measure	Potassium, K (mg) Per Measure
19304	Molasses	337	1.0 cup	4934
11432	Radishes, oriental, dried	116	1.0 cup	4053
11382	Potatoes, mashed, dehydrated, granules with ~~milk,~~ dry form	200	1.0 cup	3696
16049	Beans, white, mature seeds, raw	202	1.0 cup	3626
16108	Soybeans, mature seeds, raw	186	1.0 cup	3342
16045	Beans, small white, mature seeds, raw	215	1.0 cup	3315
19355	Syrups, sorghum	330	1.0 cup	3300
12005	Seeds, breadnut tree seeds, dried	160	1.0 cup	3218
16040	Beans, pink, mature seeds, raw	210	1.0 cup	3074
16071	Lima beans, large, mature seeds, raw	178	1.0 cup	3069
16419	Soy meal, defatted, raw, crude protein basis (N x 6.25)	122	1.0 cup	3038
16119	Soy meal, defatted, raw	122	1.0 cup	3038
1115	Whey, sweet, dried	145	1.0 cup	3016
16014	Beans, black, mature seeds, raw	194	1.0 cup	2877
10980	Pork loin, fresh, backribs, bone-in, raw, lean only	1071	1.0 ribs	2870
16101	Pigeon peas (red gram), mature seeds, raw	205	1.0 cup	2854
16074	Lima beans, thin seeded (baby), mature seeds, raw	202	1.0 cup	2834
5708	Turkey, retail parts, enhanced, breast, meat only, raw	1171	1.0 breast	2775
16016	Beans, black turtle, mature seeds, raw	184	1.0 cup	2760
16030	Beans, kidney, california red, mature seeds, raw	184	1.0 cup	2742
16042	Beans, pinto, mature seeds, raw	193	1.0 cup	2688
16019	Beans, cranberry (roman), mature seeds, raw	195	1.0 cup	2597
16067	Hyacinth beans, mature seeds, raw	210	1.0 cup	2594
16027	Beans, kidney, all types, mature seeds, raw	184	1.0 cup	2587
16080	Mung beans, mature seeds, raw	207	1.0 cup	2579

USDA National Nutrient Database for Standard Reference Release 27: potassium.

I also wouldn't consume molasses by the cup, so I think that's a false winner, and I wouldn't swallow sorghum syrup at all. Otherwise, it's nothing but beans, beans, beans.

Psoriasis is the result of an animal-borne eating disorder, a case of friendly fire exacerbated by zoö-inflammation. Like rheumatoid arthritis, psoriasis doesn't exist in the world's Blue Zones or among 3rd Worlders following their traditional no-junk, minimal-animal, mega-plant, high-phosphorus diets.

Psoriasis sufferers find relief from their mal-de-merde within weeks of switching to a shit-free Planter diet.

Psychopathy and Sociopathy

In "How to Tell a Sociopath from a Psychopath," Scott A. Bonn, PhD, tells us that these terms shouldn't be used interchangeably. While they're both Antisocial Personality Disorders (ASPDs), they have separate listings in the *American Psychiatric Association's Statistical Manual of Mental Disorders* (DSM-5), fifth edition, 2013.

(https://www.psychologytoday.com/blog/wicked-deeds/201401/how-tell-sociopath-psychopath)

Here's what Bonn says psychos and socios have in common:

- A disregard for laws and social mores
- A disregard for the rights of others
- A failure to feel remorse or guilt
- A tendency to display violent behavior

I'd like you to consider those four traits in the light of the reality that animals aren't food. If, because they're not food, all animals were to enter into our sphere of compassion, and, if society thus expanded beyond its current narrow speciesist definition of humans only and included all sentient life forms, then do Meaters not satisfy all four 'pathic' criteria at every meal? There's no blame here – this is what we've been indoctrinated to be by loving parents and responsible educators and irresponsible industrialists and corrupt government departments.

Here follows an extended quote from Bonn, describing the differences between these two Meater conditions:

> "Sociopaths tend to be nervous and easily agitated. They are volatile and prone to emotional outbursts, including fits of rage. They are likely to be uneducated and live on the fringes of society, unable to hold down a steady job or stay in one place for very long. It is difficult but not impossible for sociopaths to form attachments with others. Many sociopaths are able to form an attachment to a particular individual or group, although they have no regard for society in general or its rules. In the eyes of others, sociopaths will appear to be very disturbed. Any crimes committed by a sociopath, including murder, will tend to be haphazard, disorganized and spontaneous rather than planned.
>
> Psychopaths, on the other hand, are unable to form emotional attachments or feel real empathy with others, although they often have disarming or even charming personalities. Psychopaths are very

> manipulative and can easily gain people's trust. They learn to mimic emotions, despite their inability to actually feel them, and will appear normal to unsuspecting people. Psychopaths are often well educated and hold steady jobs. Some are so good at manipulation and mimicry that they have families and other long-term relationships without those around them ever suspecting their true nature.
>
> When committing crimes, psychopaths carefully plan out every detail in advance and often have contingency plans in place. Unlike their sociopathic counterparts, psychopathic criminals are cool, calm, and meticulous. Their crimes, whether violent or non-violent, will be highly organized and generally offer few clues for authorities to pursue. Intelligent psychopaths make excellent white-collar criminals and "con artists" due to their calm and charismatic natures."

Bonn thinks that psychopaths are born and that sociopaths are made. I disagree. I think Meating makes both, and that empathy, socio- and psychopathy lie on a continuum, predicated upon what we've been told to eat.

Children have to be trained to eat animals, instead of food. Indoctrinated. Aberrant childhood behaviors of psychopaths often include arson and animal abuse. If you just thought "BBQ," I wouldn't be surprised.

If we consider that the general public laps up the antics of fictional serial killers such as Hannibal Lecter and Dexter Morgan [a name formed by concatenating the names of two large animal breeds], we shouldn't be surprised that eating animals – even human flesh – plays a large role in their behavior. "A census taker once tried to test me. I ate his liver with some fava beans and a nice chianti," says Hannibal the Cannibal, and "I'm having an old friend for dinner."

To be able to think that we love animals while also being eaters of animals, without any apparent cognitive dissonance, is an indicator of how far out of alignment we are with our own psyches; our own true natures.

Junking contributes its share to these mental conditions. For example, real life serial killer and cannibal, Jeffrey Dahmer kept severed heads in the same fridge as the candy he brought home from his job at the Ambrose Chocolate Factory in Milwaukee, WI. Dean Corll, "The Candy Man," used bonbons to lure dozens of young boys to their deaths in Houston, TX, in the early '70s. And, notoriously, Dan White, the killer of The Castro's openly gay supervisor Harvey Milk, used what's now known as the "Twinkie Defense" to claim that he wasn't *compos mentis* at the time.

And that about sums up the situation: none of us who're eating animals and junk is in our right minds.

Rheumatoid arthritis

Rheumatoid arthritis is a chronic, systemic, inflammatory auto-immune response brought on by eating animals. When our immune systems detect animal protein antigens, they produce antibodies to attack and dispose of them.

Then either the antigen/antibody combinations move into our joints or the antibodies mistakenly engage similar proteins to the antigens within our joint cartilage… either way causing inflammation, pain and disfigurement as the cartilage and bone of our joints are progressively destroyed. 4 out of 5 RA sufferers will become disabled.

As with other auto-immune conditions, RA isn't the disease: it's a symptom of the underlying cause – introduction of toxic animal fragments… Meating.

(If animals cause immune responses in us, can they be considered food? If animals cause immune responses in us, are they not 'evolutionarily novel?')

A whole-food vegan diet stops rheumatoid arthritis from progressing, ending the inflammation and the pain, though it may not be able to reverse permanent disfigurement. Veganism benefits RA sufferers via multiple mechanisms. It removes inflammation-causing, animal-borne substances like arachidonic acid and Neu5Gc from the food supply, and because it's high in potassium, it ramps up adrenal function, thereby increasing circulation of steroid hormones like cortisol which activate anti-stress and anti-inflammatory pathways.

Planting fixes what Meating causes: less pain and stiffness in RA sufferers, in a matter of weeks.

For a variety of reasons, women are far more likely to get RA and, when they do, are more likely to self-report worse symptoms. Besides differences in genetics and endocrine function, this may be in part because women are more inclined to urinary tract infections.

In Michael Greger's words:

> "Rheumatoid arthritis may be triggered by autoimmune friendly fire against a urinary tract infection bacteria called *Proteus mirabilis*, which could help explain why sufferers randomized to a plant-based diet experience such remarkable benefit."

As usual, Planting mends what Meating makes worse.

[See: http://nutritionfacts.org/video/why-do-plant-based-diets-help-rheumatoid-arthritis/]

Sarcoidosis
See under: Amyloidosis, a Meater condition

Sciatica
Meating → atherosclerosis → stenosis (narrowing) of all arteries, including the lumbar and sacral arteries supplying the lower spine → hypoperfusion of tissues → disc degeneration + lower back pain.

Via a similar cascade of ill-effects Meating may narrow the arteries and veins that feed the sciatic nerve, the thick one that runs down our legs from our lower spine. Lack of perfusion to the nerve itself, plus a build-up of cholesterol and metabolic waste products such as lactic acid because of inadequate venous drainage, can irritate the nerves and lead to sciatica, a condition in which we suffer pain in the back that may also send stabs of pain shooting down our legs.

Planters with cholesterol levels below 150 total [3.9 in old money] don't get sciatica. It comes from eating animals. Sciatica, like gout and kidney stones, is a "Disease" of Affluence.

Scurvy
Scurvy is the result of Vitamin C deficiency. A Meater and Junker malady, surely? Whole plants are packed full of Vitamin C and there's precious little in animals.

Seizures
See under: Epilepsy; Neurocysticercosis

Sexual dysfunction
The inability to achieve or maintain an erection, in men; in women, also known as clitoral insufficiency, which may be accompanied by vaginal dryness… for both genders, an entirely Meater malady.

See under: Erectile Dysfunction

SIDS

Sudden Infant Death Syndrome; caused by feeding milk to helpless infant victims.

For more, see under: Crib Death

Sociopathy

See under: Psychopathy and Sociopathy

Lower sperm counts & poor semen quality

Animal fat, particularly saturated fat, significantly lowers the sperm count of Meaters; a 5% increase in saturated fats causes a 38% decrease in sperm count. (Attaman et al. Dietary fat and semen quality among men attending a fertility clinic, 2012, op. cit.) Meating and Junking Manly Men should take note.

Then, if we consider that sperm count and longevity are positively correlated, the declining sperm counts of Meaters are a biomarker for their increased risk of death.

Some of the reasons saturated fats depress sperm counts include steroid hormones and bio-accumulated dioxins and heavy metals, all of which act as endocrine-disrupting xenoestrogens.

See also: Infertility

Spina bifida

In the words of John McDougall, MD, "Spina bifida… is a birth defect where the backbone and spinal canal do not close before birth, producing an often-serious abnormality. This sometimes-fatal condition is due to a diet deficient in the plant-derived nutrients, most importantly folate..."

Small stool size

Small dense dry stools are an unhealthy byproduct of eating animals and junk. Meaters can be thought of as suffering from the effects of stool deficiency, the consequences of which may be constipation, diverticular "disease", polyps or colorectal cancer.

It's safer and healthier to bulk up with plants.

Straining at Stool

Putting great effort into defecating when constipated, raising abdominal pressure so high that a brain aneurysm may form or even burst, causing a possibly lethal hemorrhagic stroke (the kind which accounts for about 15% of strokes.)

One thing leads to another… It's all connected. Sadly, I've lost two elderly friends who've died this way, found dead or dying in the loo.

Other "pressure non-diseases" include **diverticulosis** (herniations of the colon wall), **hemorrhoids** (swellings of the veins around the anus), **hiatus hernia** (in which the esophageal sphincter is forced up above the diaphragm), **varicose veins** (caused by reverse pressure in the legs).

Meating → constipation → straining at stool → diverticula + hemorrhoids + hiatal hernia + varicose veins (+ possible aneurysm) → premature death

For more, see under: Constipation; Diverticulitis and Diverticulosis; Hemorrhoids; Hiatus hernia; Varicose veins

Stroke (Cerebrovascular "disease")

In *Mafeking Road*, Herman Charles Bosman writes, with ponderous wit: "Leopards? – Oom [Uncle] Schalk Lourens said – Oh, yes, there are two varieties on this side of the Limpopo. The chief difference between them is that the one kind of leopard has got a few more spots on it than the other kind. But when you meet a leopard in the veld, unexpectedly, you seldom trouble to find out what kind he belongs to. That is unnecessary. Because, whatever kind of leopard it is that you come across in this way, you only do one kind of running. And that is the fastest kind."

That's how I feel about the two kinds of stroke, hemorrhagic and ischemic: I plan to run as fast away from them as I can, without stopping to tell them apart. Suffering as I do from occasional epileptic seizures, the aftermath of a successfully removed benign brain tumor, I know what it's like to suffer a (temporary) brain attack. Anything it takes, I'll do, just to avoid a more permanent brain attack. (We who've survived serious physical setbacks are the lucky ones, I think. We're given time and motive to review our life situations and make beneficial changes.)

Strokes fall into the medical category of cardiovascular disease. As you'd expect from me by now, I beg to differ. I see these heart and related artery conditions as symptomatic of the underlying Meater eating disorder. Which, if discontinued, removes the risk of the overlying symptom: stroke.

According to the American Heart Association, in a piece entitled "What is Cardiovascular Disease?" (which I quoted from earlier under CVD):

http://www.heart.org/HEARTORG/Caregiver/Resources/WhatisCardiovascularDisease/What-is-Cardiovascular-Disease_UCM_301852_Article.jsp#

"An **ischemic stroke** (the most common type, ~90%) happens when a blood vessel that feeds the brain gets blocked, usually from a **blood clot**. When the blood supply to a part of the brain is shut off, brain cells will die. The result will be the inability to carry out some of the previous functions as before like walking or talking."

[In-digestion can cause serious damage.]

"A **hemorrhagic stroke** (~10%) occurs when a blood vessel within the brain bursts. The most likely cause is **uncontrolled hypertension**.

Some effects of stroke are permanent if too many brain cells die after a stroke due to lack of blood and oxygen to the brain. These cells are never replaced. The good news is that some brain cells don't die — they're only temporarily out of order. Injured cells can repair themselves. Over time, as the repair takes place, some body functioning improves. Also, other brain cells may take control of those areas that were injured. In this way, strength may improve, speech may get better and memory may improve. This recovery process is what rehabilitation is all about."

Well, I don't fancy the AHA's version of good news. I prefer my own: Planting can prevent most cases of both ischemic and hemorrhagic stroke, so we needn't run the risk of brain damage from cell death. I believe not in rehabilitation, but **prehabilitation**. Make it safe to live in. Fix it before it gets broke. As Scipio Africanus did with Carthage, tear down the city walls and sow the fields with salt so nothing will grow there. Practice primordial prevention.

As seen earlier, Planting reverses atherosclerosis, the major cause of ischemic stroke, and also prevents hypertension, the proximate cause of hemorrhagic stroke, both by removing animal fats and junk oils and animal cholesterol from the fuel supply.

No dead animals for me, thank you. I value my consciousness too much.

Sudden Cardiac Death

SCD is "defined as the sudden, unexpected natural death from a cardiac cause a short time (generally < an hour) after the onset of symptoms in a person without any known previous condition."

In my worldview, heart disease is a symptom, not a disease… a symptom of the underlying cause which I've chosen to call Meating… Eating flesh… Eating animals.

If we don't eat animals, and if we don't eat junk, then it's impossible to have enough cholesterol out of which to build atheromas and cause coronary or arterial "disease". That's how plant diets reverse atherosclerosis: they starve the body of cholesterol and cholesterol stimulators like sat fats and trans fats and hydrogenated vegetable oils, so there's nothing to build with.

So, if cardiac disease is a symptom… then so too is SCD. I know this is just semantics, but I think it helps to look at reality and call it what it is. In this case, a quick, excruciating death is a symptom of mal-nutrition.

Chiuve SE, Korngold EC, Januzzi JL Jr, Gantzer ML, Albert CM. Plasma and dietary magnesium and risk of sudden cardiac death in women. *Am J Clin Nutr.* 2011 Feb; 93(2):253-60.

"Most patients who suffer sudden cardiac death are not considered at high risk on the basis of established criteria, and **up to 55% of men and 68% of women have no clinically recognized heart disease before sudden death**." (Are the people who're dying wrong to die, or are the established criteria wrong?)

55% and 68%. In other words, most people who die of heart attacks get it right at the very first try. Our odds of surviving a suicide attempt are far better. For more than half of men, and more than 2/3 of women, the first symptom of heart "disease" we experience is... death. No second chances, no lifestyle changes, no dietary modifications… Just, dead.

And we die with so-called normal cholesterol levels. This happens because only vegans have optimal cholesterol levels without resorting to drugs (Total below 150 and 70-75 LDL). No Meater can hope to bring their cholesterol level down into this safe range. SCD victims die thinking their cholesterol levels are ok. Dietary guidelines from the USDA, lack of guidance from the CDC and inertia from the medical establishment have enshrined fatally high cholesterol levels as 'normal.'

Well, hundreds of thousands of people die each year – bang, dead! – from SCD with normal cholesterol. This is nothing less than scandalous.

Meating is a lifestyle and a deathstyle choice.

Sudden Infant Death Syndrome

How feeding cows' milk to human babies can be fatal.

See under: SIDS; Crib death

Suicide

See under: Mental health

Surgery, chemotherapy and radiation

In "Teachers," Mr. Sardonic, Leonard Cohen sings: "Some girls wander by mistake into the mess that scalpels make…" That's what Meaters do, because their diet puts them far more in need of radical interventions like surgery or other "palliative care." And then, when diagnosed with an eating disorder like heart "disease", they ignore the best treatment, which is Planting. The same goes for cancer, with chemo and radiation.

In a paper by Dr. Caldwell Esselstyn Jr (Updating a 12-year experience with arrest and reversal therapy for coronary heart disease (an overdue requiem for palliative cardiology). *Am J Cardiol.* 1999;84:339–341) we read:

"Modern cardiology has given up on curing heart disease. Its aggressive interventions – coronary artery bypass graft, atherectomy, angioplasty, and stenting – do not reduce the frequency of new heart attacks or prolong survival except in small subsets of patients."

Heart surgeries are useless in the long run, especially if we carry on Meating. They're temporary local fixes for permanent systemic problems. Yes, they can be beneficial in emergencies, but why not just eat properly and make ourselves "heart attack-proof," as Esselstyn says, with a total cholesterol reading of under 150mg/dl [3.879 mmol/l]?

"Coronary artery disease is essentially nonexistent in cultures whose nutrition assures cholesterol levels <150 mg/dL. Patients with advanced coronary artery disease may abolish disease progression through a plant-based diet and cholesterol-lowering medication to achieve and maintain a total cholesterol <150 mg/dL."

Well, if we act soon enough… if we use primordial prevention to prevent even the risk factors for "disease", way before primary prevention (which starts with the first symptoms), then we won't have to take statin drugs to help bring our cholesterol down. This is good, because statins have serious (side-) effects, and in a majority of cases, the first symptom of heart "disease" is called… Death (via Sudden Cardiac Death).

Testicular cancer
Endocrine-disrupting chemicals that bio-accumulate in animals are implicated in the growing incidence of testicular cancer. Also breast cancer, prostate cancer and birth defects.

Bio-magnification is often the reason why Meating is so harmful compared to Planting.

Dairy products are another cause of testicular cancer. Of Parkinson's "disease" too. There're more estrogens and progesterone in commercial milk today; hence the "dramatic increase in estrogen-dependent malignant diseases, such as ovarian cancer, uterine cancer, breast cancer, testicular cancer and prostate cancer."

[See: http://nutritionfacts.org/video/dairy-sexual-precocity/]

"From a massive new study in Canada last year, total meat consumption was directly related to the risk of not only stomach cancer, but colon cancer, and rectal cancer, and pancreatic cancer, and lung cancer, and breast cancer, and prostate cancer, and testicular cancer, and kidney cancer, and bladder cancer, and more leukemia as well."

[See: http://nutritionfacts.org/video/hot-dogs-leukemia/]

If animals were food, they wouldn't cause us so much harm.

Transit time
The amount of time it takes food (or Undigestible Foodlike Objects) to travel from one's mouth, through one's gastro-intestinal tract and out one's anus. Transit times can be many days longer for Meaters than Planters, as is the time between bowel movements. Not a healthy state of affairs...

See under: Constipation

Twin births
Twin births are the result of a maternal eating disorder. Yes, you heard me right. Meaters have five times as many twins as Planters. Why? Because of all the hormones in the animals we eat. Giving birth to twins is a dangerous anomaly brought about by Meating. (To all you twins out there... I'm glad you're here. Hi, Nicky. Hi, Zandy.)

Ulcerative colitis
An inflammatory bowel "disease", ulcerative colitis is made worse by Meating; improved by Planting.

Meating does some of its wrecking via arachidonic acid… four times the risk of this IBD with a high-animal diet. This condition, and other inflammatory conditions like rheumatoid arthritis, all improve on an arachidonic acid-free vegan diet. Plants contain numerous anti-inflammatory substances too. UC is a whole-fiber deficiency symptom.

For more, see under: Colorectal cancer; Inflammatory bowel "disease"; Deranged Gut Flora

Urinary tract infections

Most women will experience a urinary tract infection at some stage. It turns out that eating chickens is the major cause of UTIs. Ground-up cows are another source. Here's how it works:

Diarrheagenic strains of *E. coli* bacteria live in the animals that go to slaughter. On the disassembly line at the killing house, shit splatters everywhere and contaminates everything. The bacteria transfer to the packaged animal parts that go to grace our supermarket display cases, then cross-contaminate shopping carts and check-out counters, and then kitchen counters at home.

People eat the shit-daubed carcasses, which still contain bajillions of fecal bacteria despite the cooking process.

Or we can just touch them, without eating them.

The bacteria enter our colons and take up residence, wrecking the balance of our intestinal flora. Some of the bacteria then crawl from the anus across our perineum and then into our urethra, and behold! A urinary tract infection; its Eatiology traced from animal factory farm to human bladder.

According to www.dummies.com/how-to/content/the-anatomy-of-the-perineum.html: "The female urogenital triangle is home to the opening of the vagina, the urethra, and the clitoris." This is where we self-infect ourselves with potentially deadly chicken-borne UTIs.

In the words of Michael Greger:

> "Millions of women get extra-intestinal *E. coli* infections every year—urinary tract infections with the potential to invade the bloodstream and cause **fatal sepsis**, or **blood poisoning**. The strains of *E. coli* that cause extra-intestinal infection are an increasingly important endemic problem and underappreciated "killers". Billions of health care dollars,

millions of work days, and hundreds of thousands of lives are lost [worldwide] each year to extra-intestinal infections due to *E. coli*."

[See: http://nutritionfacts.org/video/chicken-out-of-utis/]

All for the love of eating chickens…

See also: Bladder infections; Part 3 (~~Food~~borne contaminants)

Uterine cancer

One of the estrogen-dependent malignancies; a Meater affliction.

If we avoid dairy products, we remove most of our risk of uterine cancer.

For more, see under: Breast cancer; Testicular cancer

Vaginosis

See under: Bacterial vaginosis

Varicose veins

One of the pressure "diseases".

Meating-induced constipation causes back pressure in the veins of our legs, causing them to become permanently distended, or varicose.

The consequences of the very high pressure achieved by 'straining at stool' can include hiatal hernia, hemorrhoids, diverticula in the colon and varicose veins. Varicose veins hardly hever happen in healthy whole Planters; they're far more common among Meaters.

For more, see under: Constipation, Diverticulosis, Hemorrhoids, Hiatal hernia, Straining at stool

Venous thromboses

See under: Blood clots

Wheeze

A symptom of a symptom, whether hay fever or asthma, which can be alleviated by a whole plant diet. The most common Meater cause is cow's milk, a.k.a. 'liquid meat.'

Wrinkles

Too much sun; smoking; eating too many animals (any at all), because of hypoperfusion and the protein-tangling glycotoxins; eating too few plants – not enough antioxidants; time; repetition.

Yeast infections

See under: Candida

Zoönotic diseases

Animal-borne diseases are treated in Part 2 (~~Food~~borne Pathogens), but only in so far as they relate to nutrition. So, for example, mosquito-borne malaria isn't an eating disorder, while *Campylobacter* infection is, because it comes from eating animal fecal bacteria.

~

Summary of Animals, Themselves

There, that's it: a short Meater Eatiology from A to Z.

A seriously well-trained Planter physician or nutritionist could double what I've written about the Meater causes of degenerative ailments. But enough is enough: we've seen ample to draw the conclusion that animals and junk aren't food. We've seen, almost invariably, that Planting sets right what Meating and Junking set wrong.

We've also seen that Planting confers a double benefit: It benefits us with all the wonderful healing properties of Planting, while being absolutely free of all the harmful properties of Meating and Junking.

Conversely, every mouthful of Meating and Junking we take is a harm inflicted PLUS a missed opportunity of healing gained.

It's my estimate that 90% of all the Western "diseases" of affluence are merely symptoms of Meating. Lifestyle changes – most particularly Planter dietstyle changes – but also including cutting out smoking and booze, increasing exercise, meditating and resting and sleeping enough – can cut our risk of dying from degenerative "diseases" by 90%.

For example, the INTERHEART study (*Lancet*, 2004) showed that lifestyle modification can prevent >90% of heart "disease". (So, real diseases and genes, not Meating and Junking and lifestyle issues, account for less than 10% of our problems. Isn't it strange that almost all our research funding, medical interventions and charitable donations go to fixing the 10%?)

S Yusuf, S Hawken, S Ounpuu, T Dans, A Avezum, F Lanas, M McQueen, A Budaj, P Pais, J Varigos, L Lisheng; INTERHEART Study Investigators. Effect of potentially modifiable risk factors associated with myocardial infarction in 52 countries (the INTERHEART study): case-control study. *Lancet.* 2004 Sep 11-17;364(9438):937-52.

And it's all connected. Heart "disease" = dementia = auto-immune conditions = stroke = diabetes = hypertension = Meating. Meating helps cause 90% of all deaths from chronic, long-term degenerative conditions. Planting drops our risks considerably or removes them altogether.

Now let's take a look at Part 2, in which I introduce the pathogens which Meating supplies in quantities at least ten times greater than Planting…

Part 2 (~~Food~~borne Pathogens)

EPI Rankings of the top 50 pathogen-food combinations

Appendix A: Rankings of top 50 pathogen-food combinations
From: Batz et al - Ranking the Risks: The 10 Pathogen-Food Combinations with the Greatest Burden on Public Health
(Emerging Pathogens Institute 2011)
Table A-1: Top 50 pathogen-food combinations, by combined QALY/$Rank

Rank	Pathogen	Food	QALY loss	Cost of illness ($ mil.)	Illnesses	Hospitalizations	Deaths
1	*Campylobacter*	Poultry	9,541	1,257	608,231	6,091	55
2	*Toxoplasma*	Pork	4,495	1,219	35,537	1,815	134
3	*L. monocytogenes*	Deli Meats	3,948	1,086	651	595	104
4	*Salmonella*	Poultry	3,610	712	221,045	4,159	81
5	*L. monocytogenes*	Dairy	2,632	724	434	397	70
6	*Salmonella*	Complex foods	3,195	630	195,655	3,682	72
7	*Norovirus*	Complex foods	2,294	914	2,494,222	6,696	68
8	*Salmonella*	Produce	2,781	548	170,264	3,204	63
9	*Toxoplasma*	Beef	2,541	689	20,086	1,026	76
10	*Salmonella*	Eggs	1,878	370	115,003	2,164	42
11	*L. monocytogenes*	Complex foods	1,316	362	217	198	35
12	*Salmonella*	Beef	1,073	212	65,716	1,237	24
13	*Salmonella*	Pork	1,073	212	65,716	1,237	24
14	*Norovirus*	Produce	779	311	847,184	2,274	23
15	*Salmonella*	Dairy	1,000	197	61,235	1,152	23
16	*Yersinia enterocolitica*	Pork	1,013	180	69,889	381	21
17	*Toxoplasma*	Produce	772	209	6,104	312	23
18	*Salmonella*	Seafood	854	168	52,274	984	19
19	*Campylobacter*	Dairy	1,034	136	65,886	660	6
20	*Vibrio vulnificus*	Seafood	541	282	93	90	35
21	*E. coli O157*	Beef	828	144	33,410	1,131	11
22	*Norovirus*	Seafood	461	184	501,684	1,347	14
23	*Salmonella*	Breads and Bakery	585	115	35,845	675	13
24	*L. monocytogenes*	Pork	439	121	72	66	12
25	*L. monocytogenes*	Poultry	439	121	72	66	12
26	*L. monocytogenes*	Produce	439	121	72	66	12
27	*L. monocytogenes*	Seafood	439	121	72	66	12
28	*Campylobacter*	Produce	693	91	44,178	442	4
29	*Norovirus*	Breads and Bakery	392	156	425,958	1,144	12
30	*Salmonella*	Deli/Other Meats	561	111	34,352	646	13
31	*Norovirus*	Poultry	387	154	421,225	1,131	11
32	*Campylobacter*	Pork	584	77	37,215	373	3
33	*Campylobacter*	Beef	580	76	36,952	370	3
34	*Toxoplasma*	Poultry	410	111	3,242	166	12
35	*C. perfringens*	Beef	285	101	314,612	143	8
36	*C. perfringens*	Poultry	234	83	258,080	117	7
37	*Toxoplasma*	Dairy	261	71	2,062	105	8
38	*Norovirus*	Beef	205	82	222,445	597	6
39	*C. perfringens*	Complex foods	212	75	233,501	106	6
40	*Campylobacter*	Eggs	341	45	21,749	218	2
41	*E. coli O157*	Produce	283	49	11,408	386	4
42	*Shigella*	Complex foods	245	54	58,930	654	4
43	*Toxoplasma*	Deli/Other Meats	188	51	1,490	76	6
44	*Norovirus*	Pork	144	57	156,185	419	4
45	*E. coli O157*	Complex foods	232	40	9,371	317	3
46	*Norovirus*	Deli/Other Meats	113	45	123,055	330	3
47	*Cryptosporidium*	Produce	203	28	34,286	125	2
48	*Yersinia enterocolitica*	Dairy	173	31	11,917	65	4
49	*Salmonella*	Beverages	171	34	10,455	197	4
50	*Norovirus*	Dairy	109	43	118,322	318	3
		Totals	57,006	13,010	8,257,659	50,216	1,216

Batz et al - Ranking the Risks: The 10 Pathogen-Food Combinations with the Greatest Burden on Public Health, Appendix A: Rankings of top 50 pathogen-food combinations (The Emerging Pathogens Institute, 2011), pp. 63-4.
(QALY = quality-adjusted life-years, a measure of 'stolen health.)

Although I'm going to be referring mainly to government sources in this section, I'll be citing this data often here and in Part 2B (~~Food~~borne Pathogens – The EPI).

Part 2A (~~Food~~borne Pathogens: the CDC's Top 31)

Jean Anthelme Brillat-Savarin: "Tell me what you eat, and I'll tell you what you are."

Pathogens defined

What is a pathogen? For our purposes, a pathogen is any biological agent that causes disease in its human host. The infectious agent may be a parasite, a virus, a bacterium, a prion, a fungus or viroid.

Parasites include protozoa (single-celled organisms) and worms.

Foodborne pathogens are those that enter our systems via what we eat. In reality, we'll see that 'foodborne' in this case is a misnomer: more than 90% of all foodborne illnesses – maybe as many as 99%, if we eat properly – come from the animals we eat (or from plants that have been contaminated with animal feces). As we've already seen in Part 1 (Animals, Themselves), animals aren't food, and pathogens serve to drive this point home.

The vast majority of food poisoning comes from eating animals. Specifically, with some insignificant exceptions, food poisoning comes from swallowing animal parasites and animal fecal bacteria. "Food" poisoning is a zoönosis – an animal disease that infects humans.

The CDC

The Centers for Disease Control and Prevention (CDC) is the USA's leading public health organization. "CDC works 24/7 to protect America from health, safety and security threats." As the word 'Centers' implies, the single organization is made up of separate specialized centers of expertise. While outstanding in many ways, the CDC has two serious flaws:

1. There is no nutrition center at the CDC. This is more than unfortunate, because Planter nutrition and lifestyle medicine are now controlling and preventing more illness than all the other branches of medicine put together.
2. Most of the scientists working at the CDC are Meaters, so they're unable to see their own bias when it comes to the Eatiology of "disease". Ignorance of what is and what isn't food is the norm.

What the CDC does well is supply statistical information. We'll take a look at their list of 31 "pathogens causing US foodborne illnesses, hospitalizations and deaths," before checking in with the Emerging Pathogens Institute to study their top 50 pathogen-food combinations, as listed on page 345, after which we'll branch out and study another 30-odd Meater pathogens that are sickening, institutionalizing and killing us.

Pathogens causing US foodborne illnesses, hospitalizations, and deaths, 2000–2008							
Adapted from:							
Nat. Center for Emerging & Zoonotic Infectious Diseases Div. of Foodborne, Waterborne & Environmental Diseases, CDC							
Pathogen type	**Pathogen**	**Est. annual illnesses**	**Est. annual hospitalizations**	**Est. annual deaths**	**Hospitalization Rate (%)**	**Death Rate (%) (hospitalized)**	**Death Rate (%) (infected)**
Viruses	Astrovirus	15,000	87	0	0.58	0.00	0.00
Viruses	Hepatitis A virus	1,600	99	8	6.19	8.08	0.50
Viruses	Norovirus	5,500,000	15,000	150	0.27	1.00	0.003
Viruses	Rotavirus	15,000	350	0	2.33	0.00	0.00
Viruses	Sapovirus	15,000	87	0	0.53	0.00	0.00
Bacteria	*Bacillus cereus,* foodborne	63,000	20	0	0.03	0.00	0.00
Bacteria	*Brucella* spp.	840	55	1	6.55	1.82	0.12
Bacteria	*Campylobacter* spp.	850,000	8,500	76	1.00	0.89	0.01
Bacteria	*Clostridium botulinum* , foodborne	55	42	9	76.36	21.43	16.36
Bacteria	*Clostridium perfringens* , foodborne	970,000	440	26	0.05	5.91	0.003
Bacteria	*Escherichia coli* (STEC) O157	63,000	2,100	20	3.33	0.95	0.03
Bacteria	*Escherichia coli (STEC) non-O157*	110,000	270	1	0.25	0.37	0.001
Bacteria	Enterotoxigenic *E. coli (ETEC)*	18,000	12	0	0.07	0.00	0.00
Bacteria	Diarrheagenic *E. coli* other than STEC & ETEC	12,000	8	0	0.07	0.00	0.00
Bacteria	*Listeria monocytogenes*	1,600	1,500	250	93.75	16.67	15.63
Bacteria	*Mycobacterium bovis*	60	31	3	51.67	9.68	5.00
Bacteria	*Salmonella spp* ., nontyphoidal	1,000,000	19,000	380	1.90	2.00	0.04
Bacteria	*Salmonella enterica* serotype Typhi	1,800	200	0	11.11	0.00	0.00
Bacteria	*Shigella* spp.	130,000	150	0	0.12	0.00	0.00
Bacteria	*Streptococcus* spp. Group A, foodborne	240,000	1,100	6	0.46	0.55	0.003
Bacteria	*Streptococcus*	11,000	1	0	0.01	0.00	0.00
Bacteria	*Vibrio cholerae* , toxigenic	84	2	0	2.38	0.00	0.00
Bacteria	*Vibrio vulnificus*	96	93	36	96.88	38.71	37.50
Bacteria	*Vibrio parahaemolyticus*	35,000	100	4	0.29	4.00	0.01
Bacteria	*Vibrio spp* ., other	18,000	83	8	0.46	9.64	0.04
Bacteria	*Yersinia enterocolitica*	98,000	530	29	0.54	5.47	0.03
Parasites	*Cryptosporidium* spp.	58,000	210	4	0.36	1.90	0.01
Parasites	*Cyclospora cayetanensis*	11,000	11	0	0.10	0.00	0.00
Parasites	*Giardia intestinalis*	77,000	230	2	0.30	0.87	0.00
Parasites	*Toxoplasma gondii*	87,000	4,400	330	5.06	7.50	0.38
Parasites	*Trichinella* spp.	160	6	0	3.75	0.00	0.00
	TOTALS	9,402,295	54,717	1,343	0.58	2.45	0.014

Pathogens causing US foodborne illnesses, hospitalizations & deaths, 2000-2008 (CDC, 2012)

[Adapted from a pdf file available at www.cdc.gov/foodborneburden]
[Note: by the CDC's own admission, these numbers are serious under-estimates.]

According to the above table, the CDC shows that 31 pathogens – 5 viruses, 21 bacteria and 5 parasites – are responsible for most foodborne illnesses in the USA, totaling almost 10 million illnesses, 55 thousand hospitalizations and 1,343 deaths annually.

However, the CDC says elsewhere that these figures are under-estimations. For example, their publication "CDC Estimates of Foodborne Illness in the United States," available at www.cdc.gov/foodborneburden, says:

"CDC 2011 Estimates… of Foodborne Illness in the United States: CDC estimates that each year roughly 1 in 6 Americans (or 48 million people) gets sick, 128,000 are hospitalized, and 3,000 die of foodborne diseases."

Table: Comparison of 31 known vs. unspecified agents…

Table 1. Estimated annual number of domestically acquired foodborne illnesses, hospitalizations, and deaths due to 31 pathogens and unspecified agents transmitted through food, United States

Foodborne agents	Estimated annual number of **illnesses** (90% credible interval)	%	Estimated annual number of **hospitalizations** (90% credible interval)	%	Estimated annual number of **deaths** (90% credible interval)	%
31 known pathogens	9.4 million (6.6–12.7 million)	20	55,961 (39,534–75,741)	44	1,351 (712–2,268)	44
Unspecified agents	38.4 million (19.8–61.2 million)	80	71,878 (9,924–157,340)	56	1,686 (369–3,338)	56
Total	47.8 million (28.7–71.1 million)	100	127,839 (62,529–215,562)	100	3,037 (1,492–4,983)	100

www.cdc.gov/foodborneburden/PDFs/FACTSHEET_A_FINDINGS.pdf

In this table, the CDC lists the damage caused by our 31 known pathogens, but then asserts that they account for only 20% of the food poisoning illnesses caused each year, and 44% of the hospitalizations and deaths. Other "unspecified agents" account for the rest.

"CDC has estimates for two major groups of foodborne illnesses:

Known foodborne pathogens— 31 pathogens known to cause foodborne illness. Many of these pathogens are tracked by public health systems that track diseases and outbreaks.

*Unspecified agents— Agents with insufficient data to estimate agent-specific burden; known agents not yet identified as causing foodborne illness; microbes, chemicals, or other substances known to be in food whose ability to cause illness is unproven; and agents not yet identified. Because you can't "track" what isn't yet identified, estimates for this group of agents started with the health effects or symptoms that they are most likely to cause—acute gastroenteritis."

The 31 "known foodborne pathogens" we're about to study come mainly from Meating, an Eatiology unknown to the CDC. Even when it does say that eating specific animals is the cause of a particular "food"-borne "disease", the CDC never counsels us not to eat animals: instead, it delivers long instructions on how to decontaminate them and make them safer to eat. I'll provide strong evidence that Meating is responsible for the lion's share of the 20% of known foodborne pathogens, plus we'll see plenty of evidence showing why Meating is responsible for most of the 80% of foodborne acute gastroenteritis caused by "unspecified agents." I'll specify even more Meater agents in Part 3 (~~Food~~borne contaminants).

There are about 50 million cases of foodborne illness each year; almost 130,000 hospitalizations and more than 3,000 resulting deaths, according to the CDC. Later in the same publication, the CDC says that "Reducing foodborne illness by 10% would keep about 5 million Americans from getting sick each year."

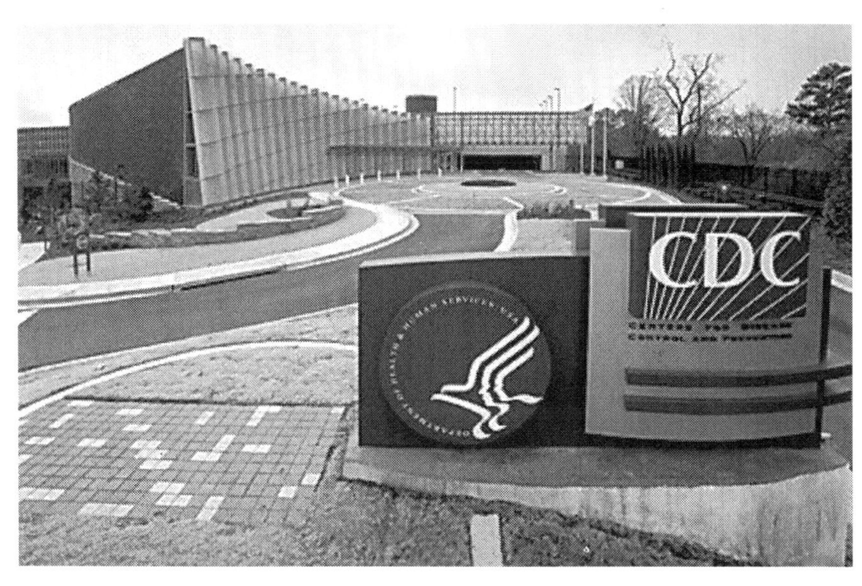

www.cdc.gov – CDC Roybal Campus Building 19.

In another publication, *CDC and Food Safety*, the CDC says:

"Food borne illness is a common, costly–yet preventable–public health problem. Each year, one in six Americans get sick from contaminated foods or beverages; 3,000 die. *Salmonella*, a bacteria [sic] that commonly causes foodborne illnesses, results in more hospitalizations and deaths than any other bacteria found in food and incurs $365 million in direct medical costs annually.

Reducing foodborne illness by 10% would keep five million Americans from getting sick each year."

The US population is roughly 320 million people in 2015. 1/6th of 320 million is about 53 million people, 10% of which is the roughly five million people the CDC mentions above.

These are things to keep in mind while we go through the CDC's table of 31 Pathogens causing US foodborne illnesses, hospitalizations & deaths, 2000-2008. This table lists fewer than 10 million cases of food poisoning, about 1 in 5. And it lists less than half the hospitalizations and deaths. Even so, it's the best information we have…

(Later on, we're going to see that even the upwardly revised numbers provided by the CDC may be wildly under-estimated, and the butcher's bill from Meater pathogens may be an order of magnitude higher, with up to tens of thousands of deaths.)

Now let's take a closer look at each one of the CDC'S top 31 food poisoning pathogens. Once we know them a bit better, we can discuss and summarize them.

Viruses (5)

Astrovirus

Estimated annual number of Americans infected: **15,000**
Estimated number of hospitalizations caused: **87**
Estimated number of annual deaths caused: **0**

"Astroviruses cause gastroenteritis, predominantly **diarrhea**, mainly in children under five years old although it has been reported in adults. Astroviruses are a leading cause of infantile viral gastroenteritis worldwide... Second only to Rotovirus as a cause of childhood diarrhea. Underreported; usually mild illness. Also affects the elderly and the otherwise immune-compromised. **Avian and ovine** sources; **fecal-oral** transmission." – CDC

Astrovirus is relatively benign. Its main reservoir is birds, but it's found in many mammals.

We get it from eating contaminated food and drinking contaminated water.

The CDC says: "Fecal-oral transmission." Please note this in all future cases of pathogen infection, when the words "fecal-oral transmission" occur: the pathogen has gone from shit to mouth – transmission from animal shit (fecal) to human mouths (oral).

Symptoms include malaise, abdominal pain, fever, nausea and vomiting.

Hepatitis A virus

Estimated annual number of Americans infected: **1,600**
Estimated number of hospitalizations caused: **99**
Estimated number of annual deaths caused: **8**

"Hepatitis A is a liver infection caused by the *Hepatitis A* virus (HAV). Hepatitis A is highly contagious. It is usually transmitted by the **fecal-oral route**, either through **person-to-person contact or consumption of contaminated food or water**."

http://www.cdc.gov/hepatitis/HAV/index.htm

Norovirus

Estimated annual number of Americans infected: **5,500,000**
Estimated number of hospitalizations caused: **15,000**
Estimated number of annual deaths caused: **150**

"Norovirus is a very contagious virus. You can get norovirus from an **infected person, contaminated food or water, or by touching contaminated surfaces**. The virus causes your stomach or intestines or both to get inflamed (acute gastroenteritis). This leads you to have stomach pain, nausea, and diarrhea and to throw up.

Norovirus is the **most common cause of acute gastroenteritis** in the United States. Each year, it causes **19-21 million illnesses** and contributes to **56,000-71,000 hospitalizations** and **570-800 deaths.**"

[Note: These figures are far higher than the CDC's own estimates in the Table of 31 Pathogens, above.]

Norovirus is also the most common cause of foodborne-disease outbreaks in the United States.

The best way to help prevent *norovirus* is to practice proper hand washing and general cleanliness."

Source: http://www.cdc.gov/norovirus/about/overview.html

Norovirus and food

"Norovirus is the **leading cause of illness and outbreaks from contaminated food** in the United States. Most of these outbreaks occur in the **food service settings like restaurants**. Infected food workers are frequently the source of the outbreaks, often by touching ready-to-eat foods, such as raw fruits and vegetables, with their bare hands before serving them. However, any food served raw or handled after being cooked can get contaminated with norovirus.

Norovirus outbreaks can also occur from foods, such as **oysters**, **fruits, and vegetables that are contaminated at their source**."

Source: http://www.cdc.gov/norovirus/about/transmission.html

This virus is spread via the fecal-oral route. It's a virus that comes with animal shit, and sometimes the animal is human.

To say, as the CDC does that the "best way to help prevent norovirus is to practice proper hand washing and general cleanliness" is disingenuous at best. It would only be true if "general cleanliness" applied to farmers. If farmers didn't use animal shit-contaminated water in their pesticide and other sprays, then we wouldn't get "fruits and vegetables… contaminated at their source." How else can it get there? Fruits and vegetables lack anuses and don't excrete feces.

If plants are contaminated, as the CDC says, the only source of pathogenic contamination is animals, with farmed animals supplying nearly all of it. (A US government department called Wildlife Services has been eradicating wildlife for decades on behalf of animal agriculture interests.)

Any time plants are cited as sources of fecal pathogens, it's because of Meater cross-contamination. Food – whole plants – is made dangerous to eat by Meater farmers, Meaters even if they're practicing plant agriculture, when they cross-contaminate food with animal shit.

Contamination with pathogens such as deadly *norovirus* and, as we'll see later, a relatively low but still significant amount of industrial chemicals such as chemical fertilizers, is why we should all try to eat organic produce as much as we can. If we take the added expense out of our medical budget, we're way ahead of the game.

To augment the CDC's suggestion: the best way to prevent *norovirus* is, most importantly, to adopt safe, organic (preferably veganic) sustainable agriculture, avoiding tainting plants with animal waste and its accompanying pathogens; avoid eating items that are sourced from defecators (animals); and we should wash your hands, stay clean and stay away from low-budget restaurants. (And touch as little paper money as possible.)

And, as Michael Greger says: "we should always wash all fruits and veggies under running water, as one solution to pollution is dilution." A dilute vinegar solution works very well.

[See: http://nutritionfacts.org/video/norovirus-food-poisoning-from-pesticides/]

Millions of illnesses, tens of thousands of hospital visits and hundreds of deaths could be avoided each year if Meaters just kept their shit to themselves. It's galling to me that even pure Planters are at risk of contracting and dying from Meaters' animal-shit-borne pathogenic "diseases" – it's not fair… and we vegans prize universal fairness.

Rotavirus

Estimated annual number of Americans infected: **15,000**
Estimated number of hospitalizations caused: **350**
Estimated number of annual deaths caused: **0**

"Rotavirus (worldwide)

- First identified as cause of diarrhea in 1973
- Most common cause of severe gastroenteritis in infants and children
- Nearly universal infection by age 5 years
- Responsible for up to 500,000 diarrheal deaths each year worldwide

Rotavirus Complications

- Severe diarrhea
- Dehydration
- Electrolyte imbalance
- Metabolic acidosis

Immunodeficient children may have more severe or persistent disease

Epidemiology

Occurrence

Rotavirus occurs throughout the world. The incidence of rotavirus is similar in developed and developing countries, suggesting that improved sanitation alone is not sufficient to prevent the infection. The prevalence of specific rotavirus strains varies by geographic area.

Reservoir

The reservoir of rotavirus is the **gastrointestinal tract and stool of infected humans**.

Rotavirus Disease in the United States

Estimated 3 million cases per year
95% of children infected by 5 years of age
Annually responsible for:

- more than 400,000 physician visits
- more than 200,000 emergency dept. visits

- 55,000 to 70,000 hospitalizations
- 20 to 60 deaths
- Annual direct and indirect costs are estimated at approximately $1 billion
- Highest incidence among children 3 to 35 months of age."

Source: www.cdc.gov/vaccines/pubs/pinkbook/downloads/rota.pdf

In the case of *rotavirus*, humans are the animal reservoir of this **fecally transmitted virus**. Planters and Meaters are at equal risk of contamination.

Sapovirus

Estimated annual number of Americans infected: **15,000**
Estimated number of hospitalizations caused: **87**
Estimated number of annual deaths caused: **0**

Sapovirus is a member of the same virus family as *Norovirus*: *Caliciviridae*. It has a similar diarrhea-causing effect.

Source: www.cdc.gov/eid-static/powerpoint/1805-sapovirus-otbreaks.pptx

Viruses – Summary

Estimated annual number of Americans infected: **5,546,600**
Estimated number of hospitalizations caused: **15,623**
Estimated number of annual deaths caused: **158**

As mentioned above under Norovirus, the CDC says that their own figures are greatly underestimated.

Table: Pathogens causing US foodborne illness, hospitalizations, and deaths

(By pathogen type – viruses)

Pathogens causing US foodborne illnesses, hospitalizations, and deaths, 2000–2008						
Pathogen type	Est. annual illnesses	%	Est. annual hospitalizations	%	Est. annual deaths	%
Viruses	5,546,600	58.99%	15,623	28.55%	158	11.76%
Bacteria	3,622,535	38.53%	34,237	62.57%	849	63.22%
Parasites	233,160	2.48%	4,857	8.88%	336	25.02%
Total	9,402,295	100.00%	54,717	100.00%	1,343	100.00%

Viruses account for almost 60% of infections, yet we may be better off being infected by a virus than a bacterium or a worm. Viruses account for fewer than 30% of hospitalizations and fewer than 12% of deaths from foodborne illness.

Of the five viruses that cause "food" poisoning, *norovirus* is by far the most relevant, accounting for almost all the viral illnesses (99%), hospitalizations (96%) and deaths (95%), according to the CDC's self-admittedly underestimated data.

On a population level, *astrovirus*, *Hep A*, *rotavirus* and *sapovirus* are almost irrelevant. Every year about 2.5 million Americans die; 8 deaths are attributed to these four viruses.

Whether the host is a human or a non-human animal, the five most relevant "food" poisoning causes are spread by the fecal-oral route.

Animal shit is what carries these pathogenic causes of "food" poisoning. Steering clear of animals and their shit at mealtimes leads to fewer viral infections, hospitalizations and deaths.

We saw earlier that norovirus may kill as many as 800 Americans each year, so the estimated number of annual deaths is probably in the order of a thousand, not the 158 cited above. If 2½ million Americans die each year, that means viruses are responsible for only one in 2,500 deaths, a low number. Still, each death mattered to the individuals and their families, and Meating was responsible for most of them.

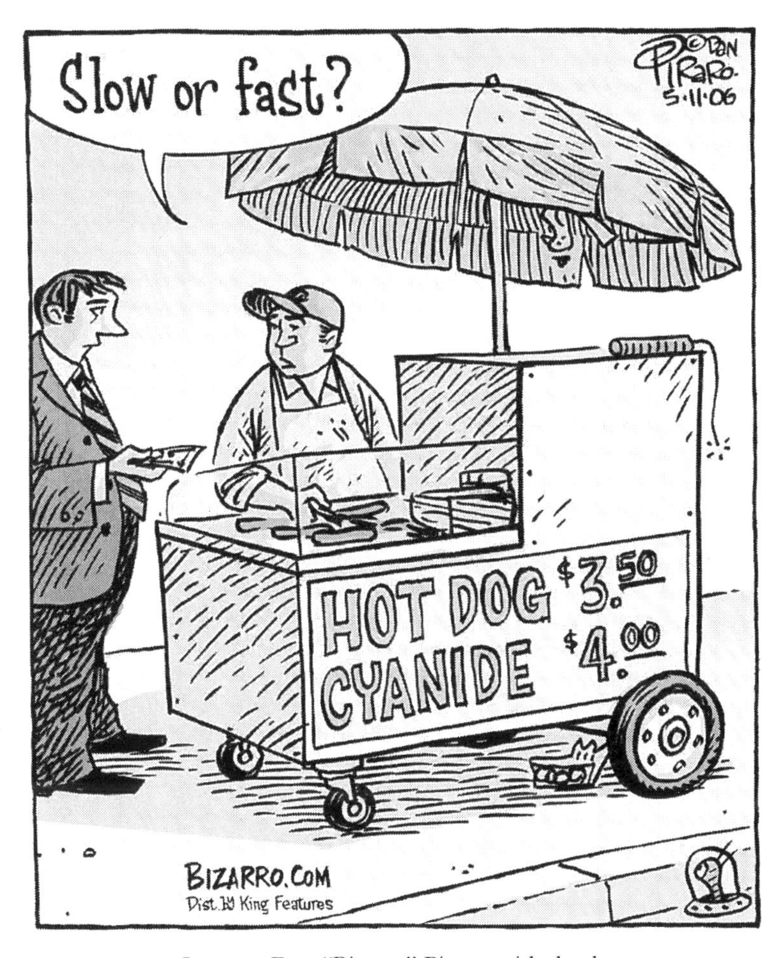

Cartoon: Dan "Bizarro" Piraro, with thanks

Bacteria (21)

The 21 bacteria the CDC lists among the 31 pathogens that cause the majority of the burden of illness, hospitalization and death in the USA are as follows:

- *Bacillus cereus*, foodborne
- *Brucella* spp.
- *Campylobacter* spp.
- *Clostridium botulinum*, foodborne
- *Clostridium perfringens*, foodborne
- Diarrheagenic *E. coli* other than STEC & ETEC
- Enterotoxigenic *E. coli* (ETEC)
- *Escherichia coli* (STEC) non-O157
- *Escherichia coli* (STEC) O157
- *Listeria monocytogenes*
- *Mycobacterium bovis*
- *Salmonella enterica* serotype Typhi
- *Salmonella* spp., nontyphoidal
- *Shigella* spp.
- *Streptococcus*
- *Streptococcus* spp. Group A, foodborne
- *Vibrio cholerae*, toxigenic
- *Vibrio parahaemolyticus*
- *Vibrio* spp., other
- *Vibrio vulnificus*
- *Yersinia enterocolitica*

(The abbreviation 'spp.' stands for species.)

Let's take a look at each of these species now.

The CDC website at http://www.cdc.gov/ is my prime source for most of the following.

***Bacillus cereus*, foodborne**

Estimated annual number of Americans infected: 63,000
Estimated number of hospitalizations caused: 20
Estimated number of annual deaths caused: 0

Wikipedia says: "Some strains [of *Bacillus cereus*] are harmful to humans and cause foodborne illness, while other strains can be beneficial as probiotics for animals. It is the cause of "**fried rice syndrome**", as the bacteria are classically contracted from fried rice dishes that have been sitting at room temperature for hours (such as at a buffet)."

In terms of its burden of health impact, *Bacillus cereus* is of minor importance. (*Cereus* isn't so serious.) When it comes to food, fresh is best, so we should be safe and not leave it lying around. Planters can avoid "fried rice syndrome" by not eating fried rice in the first place: veggie oil isn't a whole food.

***Brucella* spp.**

Estimated annual number of Americans infected: **840**
Estimated number of hospitalizations caused: **55**
Estimated number of annual deaths caused: **1**

According to www.cdc.gov/brucellosis/index.html:
'Brucellosis is an infectious disease caused by bacteria. People can get the disease when they are in contact with **infected animals** or **animal products** contaminated with the bacteria. Animals that are most commonly infected include **sheep, cattle, goats, pigs, and dogs**, among others.

Humans are generally infected with brucellosis in one of three ways:

- **...undercooked meat** or **unpasteurized/raw dairy products**
- **Breathing in the bacteria** that cause brucellosis (inhalation)
- Bacteria entering the body **through skin wounds or mucous membranes**

Bacteria can also enter wounds in the skin/mucous membranes through contact with infected animals. This poses a problem for workers who have close contact with animals or animal excretions (newborn animals, fetuses, and excretions that may result from birth). Such workers may include:

- **slaughterhouse workers**
- **meat-packing plant employees**
- **veterinarians**

People who hunt animals may also be at risk."

There's a special "CDC Feature – Hunters: Protect Yourself from Brucellosis"

[Er… Don't hunt?

Don't eat animals?]

"Person-to-person spread of brucellosis is extremely rare. **Infected mothers** who are breast-feeding may transmit the infection to their **infants**. **Sexual transmission** has been rarely reported. While uncommon, transmission may also occur via tissue transplantation or blood transfusions."

Campylobacter **spp.**

Estimated annual number of Americans infected: **850,000**
Estimated number of hospitalizations caused: **85,000**
Estimated number of annual deaths caused: **76**

I'm going to quote the CDC at length in this section on *Campylobacter*, because their attitude towards this public health menace is representative of their responses to all the other pathogens.

It's difficult, especially for Meater readers, to understand how biased and unscientific the CDC is when it comes to dealing with fecally transmitted pathogens. The scientists are Meaters working within the Meatrix. Planters, unfettered with attachments to the zeitgeist of animal agriculture, would make far different (and far more scientific evidence-based) recommendations than the Meaters at the CDC.

I'll draw attention to my comments. Otherwise the text (with my emphases) is from:
http://www.cdc.gov/nczved/divisions/dfbmd/diseases/campylobacter/.

"What is campylobacteriosis?

Campylobacteriosis is an infectious disease caused by bacteria of the genus *Campylobacter.* Most people who become ill with campylobacteriosis get diarrhea, cramping, abdominal pain, and fever within two to five days after exposure to the organism. The **diarrhea may be bloody** and can be accompanied by nausea and vomiting. The illness typically lasts about one week. Some infected persons do not have any symptoms. In persons with compromised immune systems, *Campylobacter* occasionally spreads to the bloodstream and causes a serious **life-threatening infection.**

How common is *Campylobacter*?

Campylobacter is **one of the most common causes of diarrheal illness** in the United States. Most cases occur as isolated, sporadic events, not as part of recognized outbreaks. ...about 14 cases are diagnosed each year for each 100,000 persons in the population. Many more cases go undiagnosed or unreported, and campylobacteriosis is estimated to affect over **1.3 million persons every year** [1 in 250 Americans]. Although *Campylobacter* infection does not commonly cause death, it has been estimated that approximately 76 persons with *Campylobacter* infections die each year.

What sort of germ is *Campylobacter*?

***Campylobacter jejuni* grows best at 37°C to 42°C, the approximate body temperature of a bird (41°C to 42°C), and seems to be well adapted to birds, who carry it without becoming ill.**

Are there long-term consequences?

Most people who get campylobacteriosis recover completely within two to five days, although sometimes recovery can take up to 10 days. Rarely, *Campylobacter* infection results in long-term consequences. Some people develop **arthritis**. Others may develop a rare disease called **Guillain-Barré syndrome** that affects the nerves of the body beginning several weeks after the diarrheal illness. This occurs when a person's **immune** system is "triggered" to attack the body's own nerves resulting in **paralysis**. The paralysis usually lasts several weeks and requires intensive medical care. It is estimated that **approximately one in every 1,000 reported**

Campylobacter **illnesses leads to Guillain-Barré syndrome**. As many as 40% of Guillain-Barré syndrome cases in this country may be triggered by campylobacteriosis."

Commentary

Eating chickens is now the most common cause of neuromuscular paralysis in the USA. People with Guillain-Barré syndrome stay conscious and alert while they lose all muscle control, their breathing done for them by ventilator machines. It didn't matter whether it was white meat or dark, drumstick or breast.

Such appalling "sequels" to pathogenic infection are called 'sequelae.' (One sequela, two sequelae.)

"How do people get infected with this germ?

Campylobacteriosis usually occurs in single, sporadic cases, but it can also occur in outbreaks, when two or more people become ill from the same source. **Most cases of campylobacteriosis** are associated with **eating raw or undercooked poultry meat or from cross-contamination of other foods by these items**. Outbreaks of *Campylobacter* have most often been associated with **unpasteurized dairy products, contaminated water, poultry, and produce.** Animals can also be infected, and some people get infected from contact with the stool of an ill dog or cat. The organism is not usually spread from one person to another, but this can happen if the infected person is producing a large volume of diarrhea.

It only takes a very few *Campylobacter* organisms (fewer than 500) to make a person sick. Even one drop of **juice** [juice?] from raw chicken meat can have enough *Campylobacter* in it to infect a person! One way to become infected is to cut poultry meat on a cutting board, and then use the unwashed cutting board or utensil to prepare vegetables or other raw or lightly cooked foods. The *Campylobacter* organisms from the raw meat can get onto the other foods."

Commentary

Another common source of cross-contamination is the leaked "juice" from chickens in shopping trollies and on check-out counters.

"How does food or water get contaminated with *Campylobacter*?

Many **chicken flocks are infected with *Campylobacter*** but show no signs of illness. *Campylobacter* can be easily spread from bird to bird through a common water source or through contact with infected feces.

When an infected bird is slaughtered, *Campylobacter* organisms can be transferred from the intestines to the meat. In 2011, *Campylobacter* was found on **47% of raw chicken samples bought in grocery stores** and tested through the National Antimicrobial Resistance Monitoring System (NARMS). *Campylobacter* can also be present in the giblets, especially the liver.

Unpasteurized milk can become contaminated if the cow has an infection with *Campylobacter* in her udder or if the milk is contaminated with manure. Surface water and mountain streams can become contaminated from **infected feces from cows or wild birds**...

What can be done to prevent *Campylobacter* infection?

Some simple food handling practices can help prevent *Campylobacter* infections.

- Cook all poultry products thoroughly. Make sure that the meat is cooked throughout (no longer pink) and any juices run clear. All poultry should be cooked to reach a minimum internal temperature of 165°F.
- If you are served undercooked poultry in a restaurant, send it back for further cooking.
- Wash hands with soap before preparing food
- Wash hands with soap after handling raw foods of animal origin and before touching anything else.
- Prevent cross-contamination in the kitchen by using separate cutting boards for foods of animal origin and other foods and by thoroughly cleaning all cutting boards, countertops, and utensils with soap and hot water after preparing raw food of animal origin.
- Do not drink unpasteurized milk or untreated surface water.

- Make sure that persons with diarrhea, especially children, wash their hands carefully and frequently with soap to reduce the risk of spreading the infection.
- Wash hands with soap after contact with pet feces."

Commentary

Considering how widespread and how dangerous *Campylobacter* infection is and can be, surely the top recommendation for its prevention should be to avoid eating animals?

Meater scientists haven't the first idea that Meating on the scale we do it is an aberration. It's only very recently become the norm in newly industrialized countries. Meating is an occupational hazard of Western civilization; an historical anomaly.

If alien scientists came to earth, and let's say they ate soil, not plants or animals, then they'd be free of bias when it came to looking at our so-called food supply. If one of them got a job at the CDC, she'd immediately see what the Meaters can't see: that it's the Meating that's causing the "food" poisoning. She'd say, quite rightly:

We need to tell everyone that the most dangerous thing we're routinely doing is eating animals, and, if we stop eating animals, our risk of infecting ourselves and others (even those not eating animals) plummets to near zero.

That's how evidence-based science would work, if it were practiced at the CDC. Unfortunately, Meater scientists can't follow the evidence to its logical conclusion of Planting, only.

According to the Emerging Pathogens Institute, *Campylobacter* in Poultry is the #1 worst pathogen-food combination, accounting for the loss of 9,541 QALY (Quality-adjusted life years) in the US population, costing $1.257 billion annually, sickening 608,231 people, hospitalizing 6,091 but, surprisingly, killing only 55.

That's some butcher's bill. As Everett Dirksen said: "A billion here, a billion there, and pretty soon you're talking about real money." Here's what it looks like when we add in the other top 50 pathogen-food combinations these fecal bacteria infest:

Campylobacter **pathogen-food combinations, according to the EPI**

From: Batz et al - Ranking the Risks: The 10 Pathogen-Food Combinations with the Greatest Burden on Public Health (Emerging Pathogens Institute 2011)

Table A-1: Top 50 pathogen-food combinations, by combined QALY/$Rank

Pathogen	Rank	Food	QALY loss	Cost of illness ($ mil.)	Illnesses	Hospitalizations	Deaths
Campylobacter	1	Poultry	9,541	1,257	608,231	6,091	55
Campylobacter	19	Dairy	1,034	136	65,886	660	6
Campylobacter	28	Produce	693	91	44,178	442	4
Campylobacter	32	Pork	584	77	37,215	373	3
Campylobacter	33	Beef	580	76	36,952	370	3
Campylobacter	40	Eggs	341	45	21,749	218	2
Campylobacter **(total)**			**12,773**	**1,682**	**814,211**	**8,154**	**73**

Chickens are the main source of *Campylobacter* infection – while 90% of chickens are contaminated with fecal matter (shit), half of all poultry bought in supermarkets is crawling with *Campylobacter.*

Unmentioned by the CDC is that one in ten people infected with *Campylobacter* gets irritable bowel syndrome. (Same with *Salmonella* and *E. coli.*) Having bought a few raffle and lottery tickets in my time, I'm not tempted to risk the 1-in-10 odds of irritable bowel, let alone the 1-in-1,000 odds of *Campylobacter* turning into Guillain-Barré syndrome.

If veggies and fruits are infected with *Campylobacter,* the source of the fecal contamination is obviously from animal agriculture.

***Clostridium botulinum*, foodborne**

Estimated annual number of Americans infected: **55**
Estimated number of hospitalizations caused: **42**
Estimated number of annual deaths caused: **9**

Facts about Botulism

(Source: http://emergency.cdc.gov/agent/botulism/factsheet.asp)

Botulism is a muscle-paralyzing disease caused by a toxin made by a bacterium called *Clostridium botulinum.*

Foodborne botulism is usually caused by eating improperly home-canned goods. (Wound botulism is a separate entity caused by infection of cuts.)

This is one kind of food poisoning that's really food poisoning, home canners getting it wrong when laying up the beans and other veggies.

Botulism is pretty rare. However, if it gets us, we're gonna be pretty sick – 4 out of 5 will be hospitalized – and once we're there we've got worse than Russian Roulette chances of survival. (We should avoid hospitals *and* the plague: iatrogenic deaths *and* hospital-acquired infections happen in hospitals.)

***Clostridium perfringens*, foodborne**

Estimated annual number of Americans infected: **970,000**
Estimated number of hospitalizations caused: **440**
Estimated number of annual deaths caused: **26**

At the CDC website (http://www.cdc.gov/foodsafety/clostridium-perfingens.html), there's a banner shouting: "NEW! Tips to Prevent Illness from *Clostridium Perfringens*.) I'll leave you to decide whether the word "vegan" appears among their tips.

"What is *Clostridium perfringens*?
Clostridium perfringens (*C. perfringens*) is a spore-forming gram-positive bacterium that is found in many environmental sources as well as in the **intestines of humans and animals**. *C. perfringens* is commonly found on **raw meat and poultry**. It prefers to grow in conditions with very little or

no oxygen, and under ideal conditions can multiply very rapidly. Some strains of *C. perfringens* produce a toxin in the intestine that causes illness.

How common is *C. perfringens* food poisoning?
C. perfringens is one of the most common causes of foodborne illness in the United States. It is estimated that it causes nearly a **million cases of foodborne illness** each year."

Commentary
As you're aware, my definition of food differs considerably from the CDC's. They claim there are "nearly a million cases of foodborne illness each year" due to *C. perfringens*. I claim there are none, though there are indeed a million cases of animal-borne illness each year. Food doesn't carry animal-shit pathogens, unless it's been cross-contaminated.

"What are the symptoms of *C. perfringens* food poisoning?
Persons infected with *C. perfringens* develop **diarrhea and abdominal cramps** within 6 to 24 hours (typically 8-12). The illness usually begins suddenly and lasts for less than 24 hours. Persons infected with *C. perfringens* usually do not have fever or vomiting. The illness is not passed from one person to another.

Who is at risk of *C. perfringens* food poisoning?
Everyone [?] is susceptible to food poisoning from *C. perfringens*. The very young and elderly are most at risk of *C. perfringens* infection and can experience more severe symptoms that may last for 1-2 weeks. Complications including dehydration may occur in severe cases."

Commentary
Everyone is susceptible to food poisoning from *C. perfringens*? Everyone? I beg to differ. Surely those that don't take part in high-risk behavior, such as eating *C. perfringens*-contaminated animals, are at lower risk?

"What are common food sources of *C. perfringens*?
Beef, poultry, gravies, and dried or pre-cooked foods are common sources of *C. perfringens* infections. *C. perfringens* infection often occurs when foods are prepared in large quantities and kept warm for a long time before serving. Outbreaks often happen in institutions such as hospitals, school cafeterias, prisons, and nursing homes, or at events with catered food.

How can *C. perfringens* food poisoning be prevented?

To prevent the growth of *C. perfringens* spores that might be in food after cooking, foods such as beef, poultry, gravies, and other foods commonly associated with *C. perfringens* infections should be cooked thoroughly to recommended temperatures, and then kept at a temperature that is either warmer than 140°F (60°C) or cooler than 41°F (5°C); these temperatures prevent the growth of *C. perfringens* spores that might have survived the initial cooking process. Meat dishes should be served hot right after cooking.

Leftover foods should be refrigerated at 40°F or below as soon as possible and within two hours of preparation. It is okay to put hot foods directly into the refrigerator. Large pots of food like soup or stew or large cuts of meats like roasts or whole poultry should be divided into small quantities for refrigeration. Foods should be covered to retain moisture and prevent them from picking up smells from other foods. Leftovers should be reheated to at least 165°F (74°C) before serving. Foods that have dangerous bacteria in them may not taste, smell, or look different. Any food that has been left out too long may be dangerous to eat, even if it looks okay."

Commentary

What a Meater rigmarole! That's a long and complicated list of things to do to decontaminate animals, and then we're still at risk. Alternatively, we could avoid risk by simply not eating animals. They aren't any good for us anyway, with or without the *C. perf.* Real foods don't harbor animal shit bacteria, unless they get put there.

I quoted that long paragraph on prevention from the CDC to show how chaos theory works. Sensitive dependence on initial conditions can cause wildly different outcomes. For Meaters, the fact that animals are contaminated with shit and bacteria means we have to do all sorts of stuff to make the animals safe to eat (and they still never are).

Planters simply don't eat the animals, and are thus safe from *C. perfringens* infection, unless… Meater cross-contamination.

Final Comments

According to the CDC, *Clostridium perfringens*-contaminated "foods" sicken 970,000 people, hospitalize 440, and kill 26 each year.

Appendix A: Rankings of top 50 pathogen-food combinations
From: Batz et al - Ranking the Risks: The 10 Pathogen-Food Combinations with the Greatest Burden on Public Health
(Emerging Pathogens Institute 2011)
Table A-1: Top 50 pathogen-food combinations, by combined QALY/$Rank

Pathogen	Rank	Food	QALY loss	Cost of illness ($ mil.)	Illnesses	Hospitalizations	Deaths
C. perfringens	35	Beef	285	101	314,612	143	8
C. perfringens	36	Poultry	234	83	258,080	117	7
C. perfringens	39	Complex foods	212	75	233,501	106	6
***C. perfringens* (total)**			**731**	**259**	**806,193**	**366**	**21**

According to the Emerging Pathogens Institute, which lists only the top 50 worst pathogen-food combinations, *Clostridium perfringens* subtracts 731 years of life from Americans each year, while costing more than a quarter billion dollars, sickening more than 800,000, hospitalizing 366 and killing 21. The most infested things we eat? Cows and chickens.

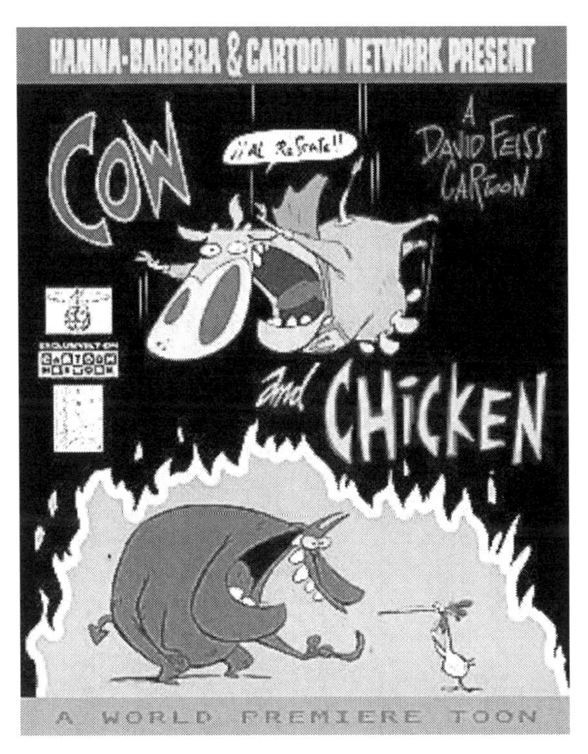

"Cow and Chicken No Smoking Poster" by Source. Licensed under Fair use via Wikipedia – https://en.wikipedia.org/wiki/File:Cow_and_Chicken_No_Smoking_Poster.jpg.

***Escherichia coli* (*E. coli*)**

E. coli are complicated.

Here are the numbers for the four classes of *E. coli* named by the CDC in my table of Pathogens causing US foodborne illnesses, hospitalizations & deaths, 2000 – 2008:

***Escherichia coli* (STEC) O157**

Estimated annual number of Americans infected: **63,000**
Estimated number of hospitalizations caused: **2,100**
Estimated number of annual deaths caused: **20**

***Escherichia coli* (STEC) non-O157**

Estimated annual number of Americans infected: **110,000**
Estimated number of hospitalizations caused: **270**
Estimated number of annual deaths caused: **1**

Enterotoxigenic *Escherichia coli* (ETEC)

Estimated annual number of Americans infected: **18,000**
Estimated number of hospitalizations caused: **12**
Estimated number of annual deaths caused: **0**

Diarrheagenic *E. coli* other than STEC & ETEC

Estimated annual number of Americans infected: **12,000**
Estimated number of hospitalizations caused: **8**
Estimated number of annual deaths caused: **0**

***Escherichia coli* (total)**

Estimated annual number of Americans infected: **203,000**
Estimated number of hospitalizations caused: **2,390**
Estimated number of annual deaths caused: **21**

That doesn't look too bad, does it? 1 death per 10,000 infections. Chewing gum's probably more dangerous.

Covering *E. coli* in depth is beyond my expertise, so I'm just going to attempt a brief simplification of what STEC and ETEC et al are all about, before making some general comments about *E. coli*.

Those who lose the will to live when faced with microscopic detail can skip over this intro and meet up with the rest of us again later.

Intro to *E. coli*

Some strains of *E. coli* are benign members of our beneficial gut flora; others are pathogenic, meaning they cause "disease".

The ones that reside in our intestines are enteric or **intestinal *E. coli***; those that leave the gastrointestinal tract are called systemic or extraintestinal *E. coli*.

The pathogenic ones that stay in our guts are **diarrheagenic *E. coli***. They cause diarrhea. (Not all intestinal *E. coli* are pathogenic.)

Of the diarrheagenic *E. coli*, some secrete Shiga toxins, so they're called **STEC** (Shiga toxin-producing *E. coli*); others don't.

Of the STECs, some belong to a pathotype (disease-causing group) called *E. coli* O157; others don't.

Those that do are called *E. coli* (STEC) O157 and, predictably, those that don't are called *E. coli* (STEC) non-O157.

The **non-STEC** *E. coli* are called Enterotoxigenic *E. coli* (ETEC). (Entero- = gut; toxigenic = poisoning; so they still cause diarrhea, just without the Shiga toxins. (Their toxins "stimulate the lining of the intestines causing them to secrete excessive fluid, thus producing diarrhea.")

Lastly, "Diarrheagenic *E. coli* **other** than STEC & ETEC" is a grab-bag category of *E. coli* bacteria that do what it says on the label: they cause diarrhea, but they're not STECs or ETECs.

It's actually more complicated than this, with six diarrheagenic pathotypes, but some of us may be suicidal at this point, so I'll call a halt.

Discussion

Here's the CDC's list of four *E. coli* categories again:

- *E. coli* (STEC) O157
- *E. coli* (STEC) non-O157
- Enterotoxigenic *E. coli* (ETEC)
- Diarrheagenic *E. coli* other than STEC & ETEC

NB

It's important to note well that the CDC's four groups of pathogenic *E. coli* are all intestinal, diarrheagenic bacteria that misbehave within our intestines to cause diarrhea.

But what about the extraintestinal *E. coli*; those that leave the safe-ish confines of our intestines to work their mischief in other body sites, potentially far more harmfully, causing urinary tract and other infections, possibly causing blood poisoning/sepsis and death? As we'll see later, this is a crucial limitation of the CDC pathogen list.

How do we become polluted with *E. coli* bacteria?

According to the CDC at http://www.cdc.gov/ecoli/general/index.html:

"*Escherichia coli* (*E. coli*) bacteria normally **live in the intestines of people and animals**. Most *E. coli* are **harmless** and actually are an important part of a healthy human intestinal tract. However, some *E. coli* are pathogenic, meaning they can cause illness, either diarrhea or **illness outside of the intestinal tract.** The types of *E. coli* that can cause diarrhea can be transmitted through **contaminated water or food**, or through **contact with animals or persons**."

Commentary

That's what we get when we hire Meater cowboys to do a Planter woman's job: vague bullshit.

E. coli infestation comes overwhelmingly from eating animals, whose secretions and dead bodies are awash with these fecal bacteria. *E. coli* contamination comes from the bacteria in the animal shit in the animals we eat; also from animal shit cross-contaminating innocent plant bystanders.

E. coli is a good biomarker for animal shit in general, on animal "foods". Retail turkeys, chickens and ground-up cows are all 80% or more adulterated with feces; plus almost half of all pigs.

About 1.1% of hamburgers are contaminated with the well-known *E. coli* O157:H7, an intestinal diarrheagenic bacterium. If a fast "food" outlet serves 1000 burgers a day, 11 people will be infected with this potentially lethal pathogen. **Hemolytic-uremic syndrome** is what causes some kids' livers to fail after *E. coli* O157:H7 infection. (Still like those chances?)

While O157:H7 is an 'adulterant,' illegal to sell, profit trumps public health and Big Animal is still allowed to sell the "Big Six," a group of Shiga-toxin-producing *E. coli* that are known to sicken twice as many people as O157.

The Big Six are:

- *E. coli* O26
- *E. coli* O45

- *E. coli* O103
- *E. coli* O111
- *E. coli* O121
- *E. coli* O145

In Africa, the Big Five are the Cape buffalo, the African elephant, the African leopard, the African lion and the rhinoceros. When it comes to killing us, the Big Five animals have nothing on the Big Six in the animals we eat.

Cross-contamination

Anus-free alfalfa sprouts are more contaminated with shit-borne O157:H7 than hamburgers: about 1.5% of sprout containers are contaminated with fecal bacteria. Fortunately, or unfortunately, depending on one's view, a tiny fraction of the population knowingly, willingly eats sprouts.

Money can't buy me love, but it sure can buy me *E. Coli*

One benefit of QE (Quantitative Easing) may be that the trillions of dollars the Fed dreams into existence may actually one day trickle down the banksters' legs and seep out into general circulation, at which point the USA may lose its #1 status of having the world's most *E. coli*-contaminated banknotes (55%). "Dilution is the solution to pollution." Speaking public health-wise, if not economically, US currency is the world's shittiest. The world's central banks' drive towards a cashless society may have unintended public health benefits.

Antibiotic resistance

Many multi-drug resistant species of *E. coli*, *Salmonella*, *Enterococcus* and *Campylobacter* are now common in the animals we eat, thanks to the profligate use of antibiotics in animal aggroculture.

Extraintestinal *E. coli*

Earlier, the CDC said that "some *E. coli* are pathogenic, meaning they can cause illness, either diarrhea or **illness outside of the intestinal tract**."

OK, so the CDC knows about extraintestinal *E. coli*. So why include only the diarrhea-causing ones in their list of 31 pathogens? Aren't the illnesses, hospitalizations and deaths caused by extraintestinal *E. coli* important?

[Could it be that announcing that Meating kills (possibly) tens of thousands of us via *E. coli* would outrage (awaken?) the public? Or damage Big Animal's business? Or make the CDC appear incompetent? I don't like being cynical, but I don't know what else to think.]

Far and away the biggest sources of extraintestinal *E. coli* are the bacteria we swallow along with shit-smeared animals – they're intestinal *E. coli* for a while, and then they migrate out of our tripes and into our blood and other organs, becoming extraintestinal pathogenic *E. coli* (ExPECs) of dietary origin.

For example…

Urinary Tract Infection as a symptom of Meating
E. coli O11/O77/O17/O73:K52:H18-ST69 is one of several strains in a class of *E. coli* that causes urinary tract infections. They're in half the chickens and turkeys sold in the USA. They should be far more famous than they are; far more famous than their lethal cousin O157:H7. While deadly, O157:H7 is to ST69 as the school bully is to Vlad the Impaler.

Using genetic fingerprinting, ST69 has been tracked from farm animals in slaughterhouses to retail outlets to women's mouths to their bowels to their urinary tracts. The chain of evidence is unbroken: after we've eaten them, ST69s travel from the feces in our anuses over our perineums to our urethras and, from there, to our bladders. Voila, UTI! From their shit to our shit to our bladders.

Chicken Meaters are the main cause of millions of UTIs, both their own and also of those in people they cross-contaminate. Just touching a dead chicken or her "juice" is enough.

Unlike *E. coli* O157, these UTI-causing bacteria switch from being intestinal bacteria to being extraintestinal bacteria. They creep out of the intestinal tract (where they may have behaved as inoffensive commensals) and invade other body systems, where they may cause infection (as in the urinary tract). Often infection leads to sepsis (blood poisoning) and, often, death.

As Michael Greger says:

> "The strains of *E. coli* that cause extra-intestinal infection are an increasingly important endemic problem and underappreciated "killers". Billions of health care dollars, millions of work days, and **hundreds of thousands of lives are lost** each year to extra-intestinal infections due to *E. coli*."

Wait a moment. "Hundreds of thousands of lives… lost… to *E. coli*?" That makes no sense. The CDC says all pathotypes of *E. coli* cause only **21 deaths** each year in America.

That's because our health authorities list death by septicemia in a different category than death by pathogen, even if the pathogen causes the fatal septicemia. It's a bit like crediting the bowling ball when the pins go flying, instead of the bowler.

According to the most up-to-date-at-the-time-of-writing mortality information, the "CDC's National Vital Statistics Reports Volume 60, Number 4, 11 January 2012: Death," by Sherry L. Murphy et al:

Septicemia is our no. 11 cause of death in America, claiming 34,843 lives annually.

National Vital Statistics Reports, Vol. 60, No. 4, January 11, 2012 5

Table B. Deaths and death rates for 2010, and age-adjusted death rates and percent changes from 2009 to 2010, for the 15 leading causes of death: United States, final 2009 and preliminary 2010

[Data based on a continuous file of records received from the states. Rates are per 100,000 population. Rates are based on populations enumerated in the 2010 U.S. census as of April 1 for 2010 and estimated as of July 1 for 2009. Age-adjusted rates per 100,000 U.S. standard population are based on the year 2000 standard; see "Technical Notes." For explanation of asterisks (*) preceding cause-of-death codes, see "Technical Notes." Figures for 2010 are based on weighted data rounded to the nearest individual, so categories may not add to totals]

Rank[1]	Cause of death (based on the *International Classification of Diseases, Tenth Revision*, Second Edition, 2004)	Number	Death rate	Age-adjusted death rate		
				2010	2009[2]	Percent change
...	All causes	2,465,932	798.7	746.2	749.6	−0.5
1	Diseases of heart (I00–I09,I11,I13,I20–I51)	595,444	192.9	178.5	182.8	−2.4
2	Malignant neoplasms (C00–C97)	573,855	185.9	172.5	173.5	−0.6
3	Chronic lower respiratory diseases (J40–J47)	137,789	44.6	42.1	42.7	−1.4
4	Cerebrovascular diseases (I60–I69)	129,180	41.8	39.0	39.6	−1.5
5	Accidents (unintentional injuries) (V01–X59,Y85–Y86)[3]	118,043	38.2	37.1	37.5	−1.1
6	Alzheimer's disease (G30)	83,308	27.0	25.0	24.2	3.3
7	Diabetes mellitus (E10–E14)	68,905	22.3	20.8	21.0	−1.0
8	Nephritis, nephrotic syndrome and nephrosis (N00–N07,N17–N19,N25–N27)	50,472	16.3	15.3	15.1	1.3
9	Influenza and pneumonia (J09–J18)[4]	50,003	16.2	15.1	16.5	−8.5
10	Intentional self-harm (suicide) (X60–X84,Y87.0)[3]	37,793	12.2	11.9	11.8	0.8
11	Septicemia (A40–A41)	34,843	11.3	10.6	11.0	−3.6
12	Chronic liver disease and cirrhosis (K70,K73–K74)	31,802	10.3	9.4	9.1	3.3
13	Essential hypertension and hypertensive renal disease (I10,I12,I15)	26,577	8.6	7.9	7.8	1.3
14	Parkinson's disease (G20–G21)	21,963	7.1	6.8	6.5	4.6
15	Pneumonitis due to solids and liquids (J69)	17,001	5.5	5.1	4.9	4.1
...	All other causes (residual)	488,954	158.5	...	...	...

National Vital Statistics Reports, Vol. 60, No. 4, January 11, 2012

34,843 is a far cry from hundreds of thousands of deaths, so I'll assume Dr. Greger means worldwide. His "hundreds of thousands" quote comes from this paper:

T.A. Russo & J.R. Johnson. Medical and economic impact of extraintestinal infections due to *Escherichia coli*: focus on an increasingly important endemic problem. *Microbes Infect*, 5(5):449-456, 2003. (http://www.ncbi.nlm.nih.gov/pubmed/12738001.)

Russo and Johnson say:

> "...under-appreciation and misunderstandings exist among medical professionals and the lay public alike regarding *E. coli* as an extraintestinal pathogen. Underappreciated features include (i) the wide

> variety of extraintestinal infections *E. coli* can cause, (ii) the high incidence and associated morbidity, mortality, and costs of these diverse clinical syndromes, (iii) the pathogenic potential of different groups of *E. coli* strains for causing intestinal versus extraintestinal disease, and (iv) increasing antimicrobial resistance.
>
> In this era in which health news often sensationalizes uncommon infection syndromes or pathogens, **the strains of *E. coli* that cause extraintestinal infection are an increasingly important endemic problem and underappreciated "killers." Billions of health care dollars, millions of work days, and hundreds of thousands of lives are lost each year to extraintestinal infections due to *E. coli*.**"

Wow. It works like this:

Eating chickens → infection with *E. coli* O11/O77/O17/O73:K52:H18-ST69 et al → extraintestinal infections (including UTIs) → septicemia → at least 34,843 dead people in the US, each year.

Though to a lesser extent than chickens, other beings such as cows and pigs are also reservoirs of UTI-causing bacteria.

Now, let's be clear: I'm not claiming that all cases of fatal septicemia are caused by pathogenic strains of *E. coli*. Other mostly-Meater-ingested pathogens and pollutants are also causing sepsis.

For the sake of argument, let's make a conservative guess that *E. coli* O11… ST69 causes just 10% of the annual septicemia deaths.

That's about 3,500; and that's almost three times the number of deaths the CDC claims for all 31 of our most egregious pathogens combined; 167 times the number of deaths they attribute to intestinal *E. coli*.

Hell, even 1% of septicemia deaths via extraintestinals is 350 deaths; 16 times the CDC's intestinal diarrheagenics.

No wonder extraintestinal infections by *E. coli* are "underappreciated" killers: the CDC's not counting them. They're only counting the comparatively insignificant intestinal infections, two orders of magnitude smaller.

At the other end of the scale, the possibility exists that chickens are killing ten thousand or more Americans each year via a shit storm of extraintestinal *E. coli* species that infest every second dead chicken sold to the public. Many of these bacteria are antibiotic-resistant.

Why is the CDC's definition of food poisoning so narrow that they only recognize *E. coli*-induced diarrhea, which kills 21 people, while ignoring *E. coli*-induced septicemia, which may be killing up to a thousand times as many?

Urinary tract infections and fatal septicemia are chicken-borne "diseases", sickening millions, and, possibly, killing thousands.

Here are the EPI's numbers, just for *E. coli* O157 in the 50 worst food/pathogen combinations:

Appendix A: Rankings of top 50 pathogen-food combinations
From: Batz et al - Ranking the Risks: The 10 Pathogen-Food Combinations with the Greatest Burden on Public Health (Emerging Pathogens Institute 2011)
Table A-1: Top 50 pathogen-food combinations, by combined QALY/$Rank

Pathogen	Rank	Food	QALY loss	Cost of illness ($ mil.)	Illnesses	Hospitalizations	Deaths
E. coli O157	21	Beef	828	144	33,410	1,131	11
E. coli O157	41	Produce	283	49	11,408	386	4
E. coli O157	45	Complex foods	232	40	9,371	317	3
***E. coli O157* (total)**			**1,343**	**233**	**54,189**	**1,834**	**18**

QALY = quality adjusted life years

The Emerging Pathogens Institute appears equally "under-appreciative" of the public health burden of extraintestinal *E. coli* – O157 is the only strain of *E. coli* they mention in their list of the worst 50 pathogen-food combinations. Their estimate of the dollar cost of O157 is roughly a quarter of a billion dollars.

According to this paper by Asima Banu, Jyoti S Kabbin and Mridu Anand – Extraintestinal Infections due to *Escherichia Coli*: An Emerging Issue. *Journal of Clinical and Diagnostic Research*. 2011 June, Vol-5(3): 486-490:

"*Escherichia coli* is an important nosocomial and community acquired pathogen and one of the commensals of the human intestinal tract. The pathogenic strains of *Escherichia coli* have long been recognized as the agents of foodborne diarrhea. **It is not always appreciated that *E. coli* is an important cause of extraintestinal diseases – "diseases" that occur in bodily sites outside the gastrointestinal tract.**

These include **the urinary tract, the central nervous system, the circulatory system, and the respiratory system…** E. coli strains that induce extraintestinal diseases are termed as extraintestinal pathogenic *E. coli* (ExPEC). **In terms of morbidity and mortality, ExPEC has a great impact on public health,** with an **economic cost of several billion dollars annually.**"

Underestimation of *E. coli* (and the extraintestinal effects of bacteria, in general) is probably the main reason why the CDC estimates that their own numbers reflect only 20% of bacterial illnesses.

Listeria monocytogenes

Estimated annual number of Americans infected: **1,600**
Estimated number of hospitalizations caused: **1,500**
Estimated number of annual deaths caused: **250**

According to Dr. Michael Greger:

> "The third leading cause of foodborne disease related death in the United States— after [chicken-borne] Salmonella, and the meatborne brain parasite toxoplasma, is **Listeria**, a type of foodborne bacteria that has the rare ability to survive and thrive in cold, acidic, salty environments, otherwise known as deli meats, hot dogs, and refrigerated ready-to-eat chicken and turkey products. The fatality rate of infection is 20-30%, making it the most dangerous foodborne bacteria in the U.S. meat supply."

[See: http://nutritionfacts.org/video/viral-meat-spray/]

According to Wikipedia (https://en.Wikipedia.org/Wikipedia/Listeria):

"The two main clinical manifestations [of listeriosis] are **sepsis** and **meningitis**. Meningitis is often complicated by **encephalitis**, when it is known as meningoencephalitis, a pathology that is unusual for bacterial infections."

According to the CDC (http://www.cdc.gov/listeria/sources.html):

"How does someone get listeriosis?
People get listeriosis by eating food contaminated with *L. monocytogenes.* Babies can be born with listeriosis if their mothers eat contaminated food during pregnancy. ...healthy people may consume contaminated foods without becoming ill. People at risk can prevent listeriosis by **avoiding certain higher-risk foods** and by handling and storing food properly."

Commentary: A Planter translates

People "can prevent listeriosis by avoiding certain higher-risk" non-foods (animals; the highest risk) "and by handling and storing" animals not at all."

(But at least the CDC says to avoid certain foods, and later names and shames sprouts + the animal culprits.)

The CDC makes no mention of the sequelae such as sepsis or meningitis that the Wikipedia stub talks about. I guess those are caused by extraintestinal bacteria which don't give us the runs, so they don't count.

"**Reservoir**
Listeria monocytogenes is **commonly found in soil and water**. Animals can carry the bacterium without appearing ill and can contaminate **foods of animal origin, such as meats and dairy products.**

Transmission
Most human infections follow consumption of **contaminated food**…

When *Listeria* bacteria get into a food processing factory, they can live there for years, sometimes contaminating food products. The bacterium has been found in a variety of foods, such as:

- **Uncooked meats and vegetables**
- **Unpasteurized (raw) milk and cheeses** as well as other foods made from unpasteurized milk
- Cooked or processed foods, including certain **soft cheeses, processed (or ready-to-eat) meats, and smoked seafood**

Listeria are killed by cooking and pasteurization. However, in some ready-to-eat meats, such as **hot dogs and deli meats**, contamination may occur after factory cooking but before packaging or even at the deli counter…

Unlike most bacteria, *Listeria* can grow and multiply in some foods in the refrigerator."

Commentary
Here follows a little graphic from the CDC showing where *Listeria* hides in foods. You know me by now, so I only see one food – sprouts.

Now, we in the West tend to read from left to right, so, sure, let's list sprouts first, seeing as they contribute about a zillionth of the *Listeria*-related illness as deli meats, hot dogs, fishes and cow products.

Vital Signs Graphic: *Listeria* hides in many foods

Listeria hides in many foods
Sprouts
Deli meats &
Hot dogs
Smoked seafood
Soft cheeses
Raw milk
CDC
Vitalsigns
www.cdc.gov/vitalsigns
CDC

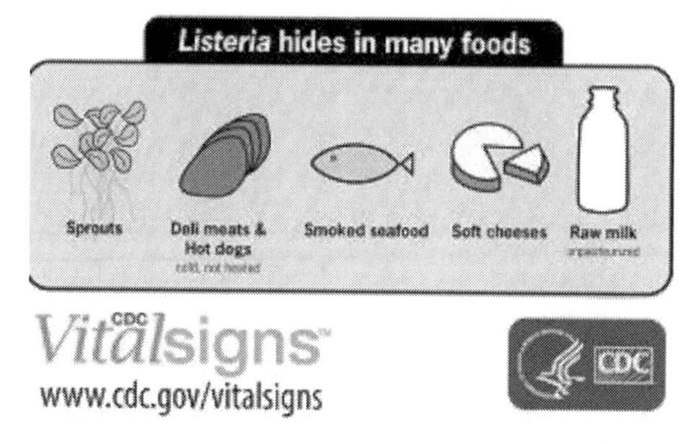

http://www.cdc.gov/listeria/sources.html

Although *Listeria* bacteria are found in soil and water, it gets into us mainly via the animals we eat, and plants which are contaminated with animal shit.

Listeriosis isn't usually a foodborne illness; it's usually an animal-borne illness.

Listeria doesn't affect that many people. According to the above [under-reported] CDC information, only 1,600 Americans come down with listeriosis each year. But, if we do get it, watch out!

1,500 of the 1,600 who're infected land up in hospital (93.75%), and if we do end up in hospital we have exactly the same odds of dying as when playing Russian roulette: 1 in 6, or 16.67%. (Do Russians play Russian roulette, or is this a case of slanging foreigners, in much the way syphilis used to be called the English Disease or French Pox, depending on which side of the English Channel or La Manche we lived?)

With 255 annual deaths (per another CDC table (see: Pathogens causing the most illnesses, hospitalizations & deaths each year)), *Listeria* is the third leading pathogenic killer, after *Salmonella* and *Toxoplasma*, causing 19% of "food"-borne deaths.

According to the Emerging Pathogens Institute, *Listeria* accounts for 2 of the Top 5 worst pathogen-food combinations that kill us: #3, *Listeria* in Deli Meats, accounting for 104 deaths annually, and #5, *Listeria* in Dairy, killing 70 people a year.

Here's a summary of the burden of *Listeria* in 6 animal and 1 plant categories.

(Emerging Pathogens Institute 2011) Table A-1: Top 50 pathogen-food combinations, by combined QALY/$Rank							
Pathogen	Rank	Food	QALY loss	Cost of illness ($ mil.)	Illnesses	Hospitalizations	Deaths
L. monocytogenes	3	Deli Meats	3,948	1,086	651	595	104
L. monocytogenes	5	Dairy	2,632	724	434	397	70
L. monocytogenes	11	Complex foods	1,316	362	217	198	35
L. monocytogenes	24	Pork	439	121	72	66	12
L. monocytogenes	25	Poultry	439	121	72	66	12
L. monocytogenes	26	Produce	439	121	72	66	12
L. monocytogenes	27	Seafood	439	121	72	66	12
***L. monocytogenes* (total)**			**9,652**	**2,656**	**1,590**	**1,454**	**257**

Here's what contamination with *Listeria* does to normally pathogen-free produce, followed by the percentage of Planter burden:

Food	QALY loss	Cost ($ mil.)	Illnesses	Hospitalizations	Deaths
Produce	439	121	72	66	12
Percentage	5%	5%	5%	5%	5%

According to the EPI, one in twenty cases of listeriosis comes from eating plants, with the rest from animals. Which is what we should expect when comparing foods to non-foods.

I've got to say though: the regularity of the numbers in the above table looks pretty hinkey to me, almost as if they're guessing that 20% should be equally shared out between pigs, chickens, veggies and sea creatures.

While *Listeria* bacteria do exist in the soil, most *Listeria* contamination of produce comes from the same source as the fecal cross-contamination of produce: animal agriculture. Animal agriculture may not just kill people eating animal products. Even the healthiest foods may be cross-contaminated with fecal and other bacteria.

Mycobacterium bovis

Estimated annual number of Americans infected: **60**
Estimated number of hospitalizations caused: **31**
Estimated number of annual deaths caused: **3**

Commentary

Bovine Tuberculosis is a rare condition in humans brought about mainly by consumption of raw cow's milk and other animal products. Perhaps Meaters are comfortable eating the flesh of animals who may have had TB.

Salmonella spp., nontyphoidal

Estimated annual number of Americans infected: **1,000,000**
Estimated number of hospitalizations caused: **19,000**
Estimated number of annual deaths caused: **380**

Salmonella enterica serotype Typhi

Estimated annual number of Americans infected: **1,800**
Estimated number of hospitalizations caused: **200**
Estimated number of annual deaths caused: **0**

Salmonella bacteria come in two broad categories. The first, the non-typhoidal group of species, infects a million Americans each year, sending about 2% of those to the hospital, and killing about 2% of those who're hospitalized.

The second type, serotype Typhi, are much rarer and much less destructive. They only cause 1,800 cases and 200 hospitalizations per year, with no deaths attributed to them.

Salmonellosis

Salmonella poisoning is a good time to settle the age-old debate: "Which came first, the chickens or the eggs?"

Appendix A: Rankings of top 50 pathogen-food combinations
From: Batz et al - Ranking the Risks: The 10 Pathogen-Food Combinations with the Greatest Burden on Public Health
(Emerging Pathogens Institute 2011)
Table A-1: Top 50 pathogen-food combinations, by combined QALY/$Rank

Pathogen	Rank	Food	QALY loss	Cost of illness ($ mil.)	Illnesses	Hospitalizations	Deaths
Salmonella	4	Poultry	3,610	712	221,045	4,159	81
Salmonella	8	Produce	2,781	548	170,264	3,204	63
Salmonella	10	Eggs	1,878	370	115,003	2,164	42
Salmonella	12	Beef	1,073	212	65,716	1,237	24
Salmonella	13	Pork	1,073	212	65,716	1,237	24
Salmonella	15	Dairy	1,000	197	61,235	1,152	23
Salmonella	18	Seafood	854	168	52,274	984	19
Salmonella	23	Breads and Bakery	585	115	35,845	675	13
Salmonella	30	Deli/Other Meats	561	111	34,352	646	13
Salmonella	49	Beverages	171	34	10,455	197	4
Salmonella (total)			**13,586**	**2,679**	**831,905**	**15,655**	**306**
Produce %			20%	20%	20%	20%	21%

And the answer, according to the EPI, is... Chickens come first by a long shot. Compared to eggs, chickens out-debilitate, out-cost, out-sicken, out-hospitalize and out-kill us by factors of 2-to-1 in each category.

That 20% of cases come from plants, cross-contaminated with animal shit, is an indictment of the foolish way we practice agriculture.

According to the CDC (http://www.cdc.gov/nczved/divisions/dfbmd/diseases/salmonellosis/):

"What is salmonellosis?
Salmonellosis is an infection with bacteria called *Salmonella.* Most persons infected with *Salmonella* develop **diarrhea, fever, and abdominal cramps** 12 to 72 hours after infection. The illness usually lasts 4 to 7 days, and most persons recover without treatment.

However, in some persons, the diarrhea may be so severe that the patient needs to be hospitalized. In these patients, the ***Salmonella* infection may spread from the intestines to the blood stream [septicemia]**, and then to other body sites and can cause death unless the person is treated promptly with antibiotics. The elderly, infants, and those with impaired immune systems are more likely to have a severe illness.

What sort of germ is *Salmonella*?
Salmonella is actually a group of bacteria that can cause diarrheal illness in humans. They are microscopic living creatures that pass from the **feces of people or animals** to other people or other animals. There are many different kinds of *Salmonella* bacteria. *Salmonella* serotype Typhimurium and *Salmonella* serotype Enteritidis are the most common in the United States. *Salmonella* germs have been known to cause illness for over 100 years. They

were discovered by an American scientist named Salmon, for whom they are named.

How can *Salmonella* infections be treated?
Salmonella infections usually resolve in 5-7 days and often do not require treatment other than oral fluids. Persons with severe diarrhea may require rehydration with intravenous fluids. Antibiotics, such as ampicillin, trimethoprim-sulfamethoxazole, or ciprofloxacin, are not usually necessary unless the infection spreads from the intestines. **Some *Salmonella* bacteria have become resistant to antibiotics, largely as a result of the use of antibiotics to promote the growth of food animals.**

Are there long term consequences to a *Salmonella* infection?
Persons with diarrhea usually recover completely, although it may be several months before their bowel habits are entirely normal. A small number of persons with *Salmonella* develop **pain in their joints, irritation of the eyes, and painful urination**. This is called **Reiter's syndrome**. It can last for months or years, and can lead to **chronic arthritis** which is difficult to treat. Antibiotic treatment does not make a difference in whether or not the person develops arthritis."

Commentary
Though one's salmonellosis may be cured, one can still be left with permanent sequelae such as chronic arthritis, eye damage and Reiter's syndrome.

"How do people catch *Salmonella*?
Salmonella live in the intestinal tracts of humans and other animals, including birds. *Salmonella* are usually transmitted to humans by **eating foods contaminated with animal feces**. Contaminated foods usually look and smell normal. **Contaminated foods are often of animal origin, such as beef, poultry, milk, or eggs, but any food, including vegetables, may become contaminated.** Thorough cooking kills *Salmonella*. Food may also become contaminated by the hands of an infected food handler who did not wash hands with soap after using the bathroom.

What can a person do to prevent this illness?
There is no vaccine to prevent salmonellosis. Because **foods of animal origin** may be contaminated with *Salmonella*, people should **not eat raw or undercooked eggs, poultry, or meat.** Raw eggs may be unrecognized in some foods, such as homemade Hollandaise sauce, Caesar and other

homemade salad dressings, tiramisu, homemade ice cream, homemade mayonnaise, cookie dough, and frostings. Poultry and meat, including hamburgers, should be well-cooked, not pink in the middle. Persons also should not consume raw or unpasteurized milk or other dairy products. **Produce should be thoroughly washed.**

Cross-contamination of foods should be avoided. Uncooked meats should be kept separate from produce, cooked foods, and ready-to-eat foods. Hands, cutting boards, counters, knives, and other utensils should be washed thoroughly after touching uncooked foods. Hand should be washed before handling food, and between handling different food items...

How common is salmonellosis?
Every year, approximately 40,000 cases of salmonellosis are reported in the United States. Because many milder cases are not diagnosed or reported, **the actual number of infections may be thirty or more times greater**. Salmonellosis is more common in the summer than winter.

Children are the most likely to get salmonellosis. The rate of diagnosed infections in children less than five years old is about five times higher than the rate in all other persons. Young children, the elderly, and the immunocompromised are the most likely to have severe infections. It is estimated that approximately **400 persons die** each year with acute salmonellosis.

What can I do to prevent salmonellosis? [the CDC paraphrased]

- Cook poultry, ground beef, and eggs thoroughly.
- Send back undercooked meat, poultry or eggs in a restaurant
- Wash hands, kitchen work surfaces, and utensils with soap and water
- Be particularly careful with foods prepared for infants, the elderly, and the immunocompromised.
- Wash hands with soap after handling reptiles, birds, or baby chicks, and after contact with pet feces.
- Avoid direct or even indirect contact between reptiles (turtles, iguanas, other lizards, snakes) and infants or immunocompromised persons.
- Don't work with raw poultry or meat, and an infant (e.g., feed, change diaper) at the same time.
- Mother's milk is the safest food for young infants. Breastfeeding prevents salmonellosis and many other health problems.

Commentary

These are the best recommendations our top disease control and prevention organization has to offer. The problem with the CDC, the Centers for Disease Control and Prevention, is that because there is no Nutrition Center at the CDC(&P), there is very little understanding of how prevention is achieved. We've known for a quarter-century (Ornish, 1990) that Planting prevents heart "disease"; an outcome confirmed multiple times by other researchers and healers. (If eating properly cures the "disease", how big a leap is it to grok that eating badly is the disease?)

We know Planting reverses atherosclerosis, hypertension, type II diabetes, breast and prostate cancer, and prevents them too. The medical literature is bristling with the works of the lifestyle physicians, showing how to prevent chronic, degenerative, non-infectious "diseases" through Planting.

How difficult would it be for just one Meater expert of infectious diseases over at the CDC to finally get the 25-year-old news that Meating underlies most causes of death and disability in the West, and for that scientist to say: "Enough already. Should we go on telling people to cook animals thoroughly, else they may die, and wash their hands, utensils and counters, and other bullshit like that?"

We need to hear from the CDC that the best way to prevent salmonellosis (and most other pathogenic diseases) is to stop or limit our eating of the animals that host the pathogens. (At least they could sneak that suggestion into their inadequate list of recommendations.) We know animals aren't food, because they're intrinsically lethal (Part 1 of this book). Contamination with pathogens adds to their lethality (Part 2). Contamination with industrial pollutants makes them even more deadly (Part 3). And their severe deficiencies put the final boot in (Part 4).

Eggs cause more than 140,000 cases of salmonellosis a year. Animal shit-infested sprouts cause 100, and animal shit-coated melons cause another 50. Retail turkeys and chickens are extremely contaminated. Two out of every ten people who're poisoned with *Salmonella* are being infected by Meaters when they tuck into their produce.

By the way, *Salmonella* bacteria are incredibly difficult to get rid of in the kitchen, just using soap and water. The best way to get rid of them is not to bring them in in the first place OR to burn the house down: our choice.

Later, under Drug Resistance, we'll see that *Salmonella* is one of the pathogens that's becoming increasingly resistant to multiple classes of antibiotics. The CDC had the good grace to mention this above. They said: "Some *Salmonella* bacteria have become resistant to antibiotics, largely as a result of the use of **antibiotics to promote the growth of food animals**."

They know it, so why don't they act on it and ban their use, like other countries have done? Why? Because animal agriculture in the US is way too rich and powerful. The Meaters run the show at the CDC, the FDA, the USDA and in congress.

Salmonellosis is an elective Meater "disease", which Meaters elect to share with others.

According to the body count for *Salmonella* infections, which we saw in the Emerging Pathogens Institute's ranking of the Top 50 worst Pathogen-Food Combinations above:

Salmonella, a fecal bacterium inserted into the "food" chain via animal agriculture, accounts for 11 of the top 50 worst pathogen-food combos, including the cross-contamination of produce, leading to 170,264 illnesses, 3,204 hospital stays and 63 deaths per year from eating *Salmonella*-infected produce, and racking up more than half a billion dollars annually in healthcare costs.

The total bill for *Salmonella*:

Each year, via *Salmonella*, Meater agriculture causes more than a million illnesses, hospitalizes almost 20,000 people, kills 378, causes the loss of 16,781 years of life, and costs $3.3 billion.

(And, remember, the number of illnesses is vastly understated; by a factor of 5, according to the CDC themselves.)

Shigella spp.

Estimated annual number of Americans infected: **130,000**
Estimated number of hospitalizations caused: **150**
Estimated number of annual deaths caused: **0**

According to the CDC (http://www.cdc.gov/shigella/index.html):
"Shigella – Shigellosis
Shigellosis is an infectious disease caused by a group of bacteria called *Shigella* (shih-GEHL-uh). Most who are infected with *Shigella* develop **diarrhea, fever, and stomach cramps** starting a day or two after they are exposed to the bacteria. Shigellosis usually resolves in 5 to 7 days. Some people who are infected may have no symptoms at all, but may still pass the *Shigella* bacteria to others. The spread of *Shigella* can be stopped by frequent and careful handwashing with soap and taking other hygiene measures.

What is *Shigella*?
Shigellosis is a diarrheal disease caused by a group of bacteria called *Shigella*. Shigella causes about **500,000 cases** of diarrhea in the United States annually.

What are the symptoms of *Shigella*?
Symptoms of shigellosis typically start 1–2 days after exposure and include:

- Diarrhea (sometimes bloody)
- Fever
- Abdominal pain
- Tenesmus (a painful sensation of needing to pass stools even when bowels are empty)

Can there be any complications from *Shigella* infections?
Possible complications from Shigella infections include:

- Post-infectious arthritis.
- Blood stream infections.
- Seizures.
- Hemolytic-uremic syndrome or HUS.

***Shigella* is often resistant to antibiotics.**
How is *Shigella* spread?
Shigella germs are present **in the stools of infected persons** while they have diarrhea and for up to a week or two after the diarrhea has gone away.

Shigella is very contagious; exposure to even a tiny amount of contaminated **fecal matter**—too small to see–can cause infection.

How can I reduce my risk of getting shigellosis?
[Basically: Avoid swallowing animal shit. With *Shigella*, the animal is human.]

Streptococcus spp. Group A, foodborne

Estimated annual number of Americans infected: **240,000**
Estimated number of hospitalizations caused: **1,100**
Estimated number of annual deaths caused: **6**

Streptococcus

Estimated annual number of Americans infected: **11,000**
Estimated number of hospitalizations caused: **1**
Estimated number of annual deaths caused: **0**

Strep infections are also via person-to-person transmission, are relatively un-burdensome in health terms (with few hospitalizations and deaths) and aren't a big factor in terms of foodborne illness, except in cases of food prep by infected people. This may change if animal agriculture continues its hyper-use of antibiotic-resistance-creating antibiotics.

That is, right now…

As I mentioned briefly on page 277, and as I'll discuss at greater length on pages 446-9, Dr. Margaret Chan, Director General of the WHO, warned in 2013 that animal agriculture's hyper-use of antibiotics and, to a far lesser extent, the medical community's overuse of antibiotics, may make strep throat a lethal condition in the near future because of the antibiotic resistance these two industries are creating in bacteria.

***Vibrio cholerae*, toxigenic**

Estimated annual number of Americans infected: **84**
Estimated number of hospitalizations caused: **2**
Estimated number of annual deaths caused: **0**

Sources of Infection & Risk Factors

[Source: http://www.cdc.gov/cholera/infection-sources.html]

"Cholera is an acute intestinal infection causing profuse watery diarrhea, vomiting, circulatory collapse and shock. Many infections are associated with milder diarrhea or have no symptoms at all. If left untreated, 25-50% of severe cholera cases can be fatal.

Who gets cholera?
A person can get cholera by **drinking water or eating food contaminated** with the cholera bacterium. Large epidemics are often related to **fecal contamination of water supplies** or **street vended foods**. The disease is occasionally spread through eating raw or undercooked shellfish that are naturally contaminated.

Environmental Source
Brackish and marine waters are a natural environment for the etiologic agents of cholera, *Vibrio cholerae* serogroup O1 or O139. There are **no known animal hosts** for *Vibrio cholerae*, however, the bacteria attach themselves easily to the chitin-containing shells of **crabs, shrimps, and other shellfish**, which can be a source for human infections when eaten raw or undercooked.

Global Cholera Epidemics
Cholera is a major cause of epidemic diarrhea throughout the developing world. There has been an ongoing global pandemic in Asia, Africa and Latin America for the last four decades. In 2011, a total of 58 countries reported a cumulative total of 589,854 cases including 7,816 deaths (case fatality rate of 1.3%) to the World Health Organization (WHO). "

Commentary
Cholera is mainly a public health issue: uncommon within developed water supply infrastructures. It kills thousands of people annually in the Third World. The United States is thus protected against cholera, so long as Third World conditions don't return to the country as a result of severe economic

dislocation. At present, little is being spent on the US's crumbling infrastructure. By one estimate, the shortfall exceeds one trillion dollars. As a result, roads, bridges and, of particular importance, dams are falling into a state of disrepair. This may have severe public health implications in the near future, when cholera may make a return.

Vibrio vulnificus – the "flesh-eating bacterium"

Estimated annual number of Americans infected: **96**
Estimated number of hospitalizations caused: **93**
Estimated number of annual deaths caused: **36**

Happily uncommon, this "flesh eating-bacterium" is definitely something we don't want to encounter outside our nightmares. Almost everyone who gets infected with it lands up in hospital, fighting necrotizing ("flesh-eating") wounds, undergoing amputations, and still 4 out of every 10 patients die.

By way of comparison, *Yersinia enterocolitica* from eating pigs infects more than a thousand times as many people as *V. vulnificus*, yet it kills fewer people.

According to the CDC (http://www.cdc.gov/vibrio/vibriov.html):

"*Vibrio vulnificus* is a bacterium in the same family as those that cause cholera and *Vibrio parahaemolyticus*. It normally lives in warm seawater and is part of a group of *vibrios* that are called "halophilic" because they require salt.

V. vulnificus can cause disease in those who eat **contaminated seafood** or have **an open wound that is exposed to seawater**. Among healthy people, ingestion of *V. vulnificus* can cause **vomiting, diarrhea, and abdominal pain**. In immunocompromised persons, particularly those with chronic liver disease, *V. vulnificus* can **infect the bloodstream**, causing a severe and life-threatening illness characterized by fever and chills, decreased blood pressure (septic shock), and blistering skin lesions. *V. vulnificus* bloodstream infections are fatal about 50% of the time. [That is incredibly high.]

V. vulnificus can cause an infection of the skin when open wounds are exposed to **warm seawater**; these infections may lead to skin breakdown and ulceration. Persons who are immunocompromised are at higher risk for invasion of the organism into the bloodstream and potentially fatal complications."

[I don't know the answer to this question: Will we see an explosion in *V. vulnificus* infections as seawater becomes a degree or two warmer?]

"How common is *V. vulnificus* infection?
V. vulnificus is a **rare** cause of disease, but it is also **underreported**. Between 1988 and 2006, CDC received reports of **more than 900 *V. vulnificus* infections from the Gulf Coast states**, where most cases occur.

How do persons get infected with *V. vulnificus*?
Persons who are immunocompromised, especially those with chronic liver disease, are at risk for *V. vulnificus* when they **eat raw seafood, particularly oysters.**

How can *V. vulnificus* infection be diagnosed?
Doctors should have a high suspicion for this organism when patients present with **gastrointestinal illness, fever, or shock following the ingestion of raw seafood, especially oysters, or with a wound infection after exposure to seawater**.

Under **Treatment**: "Necrotic tissue should be debrided; severe cases may require fasciotomy or limb amputation."

What can be done to improve the safety of oysters?"
Commentary
The CDC, when faced with this flesh-eating bacterium in animals, then takes 135 words to tell us how to improve the safety of oysters. This is truly weird (to a scientist or a Planter). Instead of saying, as an evidence-based nutrition scientist might, "Possible infection with *V. vulnificus* is yet another reason why shellfish should not be eaten at all," they act like a PR firm for this non-food. Almost as if their constituency is the animal industry and not the general public…

"**Some tips for preventing *V. vulnificus* infections**, particularly among immunocompromised patients, including those with underlying liver disease:

- Do not eat raw oysters or other raw shellfish. [At last, something we agree on.]
- Cook shellfish (oysters, clams, mussels) thoroughly.
- For shellfish in the shell, either a) boil until the shells open and continue boiling for 5 more minutes, or b) steam until the shells open and then continue cooking for 9 more minutes. Do not eat those shellfish that do not open during cooking. Boil shucked oysters at least 3 minutes, or fry them in oil at least 10 minutes at 375°F.
- Avoid cross-contamination of cooked seafood and other foods with raw seafood and juices from raw seafood.
- Eat shellfish promptly after cooking and refrigerate leftovers.
- Avoid exposure of open wounds or broken skin to warm salt or brackish water, or to raw shellfish harvested from such waters.
- **Wear protective clothing (e.g., gloves) when handling raw shellfish.**"

Again, weird: Do all people who're immunocompromised know that they are? What does it say about a supposed food that immunocompromised people shouldn't eat it? As a Planter nutrition counselor I recommend whole plants to people on the basis that they strengthen immunity.

Oh, and the last suggestion really cracked me up: raw shellfishes are so potentially lethal, we'd better wear protective clothing when we touch them. What do they mean by: e.g. gloves? What else? We may need respirators too? Should we use autoclaves? Sulfurous acid?

All that fuss and bother to defuse a Meater "food" bomb… I'd rather just eat… food.

The people at the CDC need to wake the hell up and employ some lifestyle physicians or, at least, someone who's taken a class in Planter nutrition – that would put the Prevention in CDC&P.

Vibrio parahaemolyticus

Estimated annual number of Americans infected: **35,000**
Estimated number of hospitalizations caused: **100**
Estimated number of annual deaths caused: **4**

Another *Vibrio* that infects seafood, particularly raw bivalves. Far more common than its *V. vulnificus* cousin, *V. parahaemolyticus* infects thousands of times more people but kills only a handful. Those of us who *love* eating oysters should pray this is the *Vibrio* infection we get.

Vibrio spp., other

Estimated annual number of Americans infected: **18,000**
Estimated number of hospitalizations caused: **83**
Estimated number of annual deaths caused: **8**

According to Wikipedia, there are 77 strains of *Vibrio* bacteria, from *V. adaptatus* to V. xuii. Not all of them are pathogenic – disease-causing – in humans. However, those that are, mostly share the same etiology, provenance and symptomology as the 2 less dangerous *Vibrios* we've dealt with above – *cholerae* and *parahaemolyticus*:

- They're found in salt or brackish water.
- When conditions of temperature and salinity are right, they infect sea life such as prawns, shrimps, clams and oysters, causing zoonoses that may kill these creatures.
- When infected after eating infected sea creatures, humans develop gastroenteritis, with watery diarrhea, cramping, nausea or vomiting. (Sepsis may occur in exposed wounds.)
- The CDC will tell you to cook your "food" well to prevent infection.

And someone not wedded to the concept of eating animals as a sane health strategy might suggest one eat nothing but whole plants.

Yersinia enterocolitica

Estimated annual number of Americans infected: **98,000**
Estimated number of hospitalizations caused: **530**
Estimated number of annual deaths caused: **29**

According to the CDC (http://www.cdc.gov/nczved/divisions/dfbmd/diseases/yersinia/):

"Yersiniosis is an infectious disease caused by a bacterium of the genus *Yersinia*. In the United States, most human illness is caused by one species, *Y. enterocolitica*. Infection with *Y. enterocolitica* can cause a variety of symptoms depending on the age of the person infected. Infection with *Y. enterocolitica* occurs most often in young children. Common symptoms in children are **fever, abdominal pain, and diarrhea, which is often bloody**. Symptoms typically develop 4 to 7 days after exposure and may last 1 to 3 weeks or longer. In older children and adults, right-sided abdominal pain and fever may be the predominant symptoms, and may be confused with appendicitis. In a small proportion of cases, complications such as **skin rash, joint pains, or spread of bacteria to the bloodstream** can occur.

What sort of germ is *Y. enterocolitica*?
The **major animal reservoir** for *Y. enterocolitica* strains that cause human illness is **pigs**, but other strains are also found in many other animals including rodents, rabbits, sheep, cattle, horses, dogs, and cats. In pigs, the bacteria are most likely to be found on the tonsils.

How do people get infected with *Y. enterocolitica*?
Infection is most often acquired by eating contaminated food, especially **raw or undercooked pork products**. The preparation of raw pork intestines (chitterlings) may be particularly risky. Infants can be infected if their caretakers handle raw chitterlings and then do not adequately clean their hands before handling the infant or the infant's toys, bottles, or pacifiers. Drinking contaminated **unpasteurized milk or untreated water** can also transmit the infection. Occasionally *Y. enterocolitica* infection occurs after contact with infected animals. On rare occasions, it can be transmitted as a result of the bacterium passing from the stools or soiled fingers of one person to the mouth of another **person**. This may happen when basic

hygiene and handwashing habits are inadequate. Rarely, the organism is transmitted through contaminated blood during a transfusion.

How common is infection with *Y. enterocolitica*?

Y. enterocolitica is a relatively infrequent cause of diarrhea and abdominal pain. Based on data from the Foodborne Diseases Active Surveillance Network (FoodNet), which measures the burden and sources of specific diseases over time, approximately one culture-confirmed *Y. enterocolitica* infection per 100,000 persons occurs each year. Children are infected more often than adults, and the infection is more common in the winter."

[The above prevalence of 1 in 100,000 translates into 3,200 cases in a population of 320 million people. Elsewhere, the CDC estimated the annual number of Americans infected to be 98,000.]

"What can be done to prevent the infection?

1. Avoid eating raw or undercooked **pork**.
2. Consume only pasteurized milk or **milk products**.
3. Wash hands with soap and water before eating and preparing food, after contact with animals, and after handling raw meat.
4. After handling raw chitterlings, clean hands and fingernails scrupulously with soap and water before touching infants or their toys, bottles, or pacifiers. Someone other than the foodhandler should care for children while chitterlings are being prepared. [Really? Are we all hicks now?]
5. Prevent cross-contamination in the kitchen:
   - **Use separate cutting boards for meat and other foods**
   - Carefully clean all cutting boards, counter-tops, and utensils with soap and hot water after preparing raw meat.
6. Dispose of **animal feces** in a sanitary manner."

Commentary

If the CDC were a product safety organization… but, wait a moment, they are. And the products they're passing as safe for our health (via "disease" control and prevention) are animal non-foods… They keep giving lethal products a clean bill of health. They keep telling us how to try to decontaminate them with heat and cold and chemical cleaners.

It's as if a car safety watchdog were to say: This car may blow up if you drive it faster than 30 mph. This car has a tendency to veer suddenly to the left. This car may flip over like a tortoise in a mild breeze. What can be done to make this car safer? Don't drive the car faster than 30 mph. Don't drive routes that require right turns. Stay home on windy days.

What they should be saying is: this car is a deathtrap and it shouldn't even be allowed on the road. It's a nutritional Chevy Corvair. It flips over like a Suzuki Samurai. (*Consumer Reports* should also not be giving animals a passing grade as food.)

Instead of saying, as recommendation #1 for prevention of infection, every time, "As far as possible avoid eating animals, because they harbor pathogenic life forms," the CDC speaks of not 'handlin' raw chitlins' and, preciously, "disposing of animal feces in a sanitary manner." Yes, by all means let's dispose of the animal feces, but how do we do that when the animal feces and their accompanying bacteria are IN the animals the CDC says are safe to eat? Hello, is anyone awake over there?

If we have to use "separate cutting boards for meats and other foods" because meats are so potentially dangerous, then meats aren't foods, and the word 'other' is hopelessly inappropriate. By all means, let Meaters use separate cutting boards: one for animals and one for foods. Planters need only a single board on which to prepare food.

So where is *Yersinia*?

About 70% of all retail pigs in the US is contaminated with *Yersinia*, 90% of which are multi-drug resistant strains. Eating pigs is helping create a potentially antibiotic-free future for humanity.

Sequelae of *Yersinia* infection, unmentioned by the CDC on their web page I'm quoting from, include almost 50 times greater odds of autoimmune arthritis, and Graves' "disease", a thyroid autoimmune condition, among many others.

Surely these are "diseases" that can be better controlled and prevented by not eating pigs than by washing one's hands after handling raw chitterlings while someone else cares for the children?

Bacteria – Summary

Estimated annual number of Americans **infected** by bacteria annually:
3,622,535
(out of 9,402,295 total sicknesses caused by pathogens) *
= **38.53% of illnesses** caused by pathogens

Estimated number of **hospitalizations** caused: **34,237**
(out of 54,717 total hospitalizations caused by pathogens)
= **62.57% of hospitalizations** caused by pathogens

Estimated number of annual **deaths** caused: **849**
(out of 1,343 total deaths caused by pathogens)
= **63.22% of total deaths** caused by pathogens

* According to the CDC itself, this number represents 20% of the total real number of sicknesses, about 50 million a year.

Bacteria account for almost 40% of infections, but more than 60% of both hospitalizations and deaths.

~

Parasites (5)

Note: Much of the information in this section comes from the CDC website at http://www.cdc.gov/parasites/.

Protozoa

Protozoa are single-celled organisms with animal-like behaviors that can be pathogenic parasites in humans.

Cryptosporidium parvum

Estimated annual number of Americans infected: **58,000**
Estimated number of hospitalizations caused: **210**
Estimated number of annual deaths caused: **4**

"Cryptosporidiosis is a diarrheal disease caused by **microscopic parasites**, *Cryptosporidium*, that can live in the intestine of **humans and animals** and is **passed in the stool** of an infected person or animal. Both the disease and the parasite are commonly known as "Crypto."

The parasite is protected by an outer shell that allows it to survive outside the body for long periods of time and makes it **very resistant to chlorine-based disinfectants**.

During the past 2 decades, Crypto has become recognized as one of the most common causes of **waterborne disease** (recreational water and drinking water) in humans in the United States.

The parasite is found in every region of the United States and throughout the world."

Crypto may be found in soil, food, water, or surfaces that have been contaminated with the feces from infected humans or animals. (www.cdc.gov/parasites/food.html)

The most common symptom of cryptosporidiosis is **watery diarrhea**.

Other symptoms include:

- Stomach cramps or pain
- Dehydration
- Nausea
- Vomiting
- Fever
- Weight loss

Crypto is an animal feces public health issue more connected to our water supply than our food supply. Fewer than 100,000 Americans are infected with *Crypto* annually, and relatively few are hospitalized or die.

Cyclospora cayetanensis

Estimated annual number of Americans infected: **11,000**
Estimated number of hospitalizations caused annually: **11**
Estimated annual number of deaths caused: **0**

"Cyclosporiasis is an intestinal illness caused by the microscopic parasite *Cyclospora cayetanensis*. People can become infected with *Cyclospora* by consuming **food or water** contaminated with the parasite."

"Symptoms may include the following:

- Frequent bouts of watery diarrhea
- Loss of appetite and weight
- Cramping, bloating, and/or increased gas
- Nausea (vomiting is less common)
- Fatigue
- Low-grade fever"

Cyclospora life cycle (per the CDC):

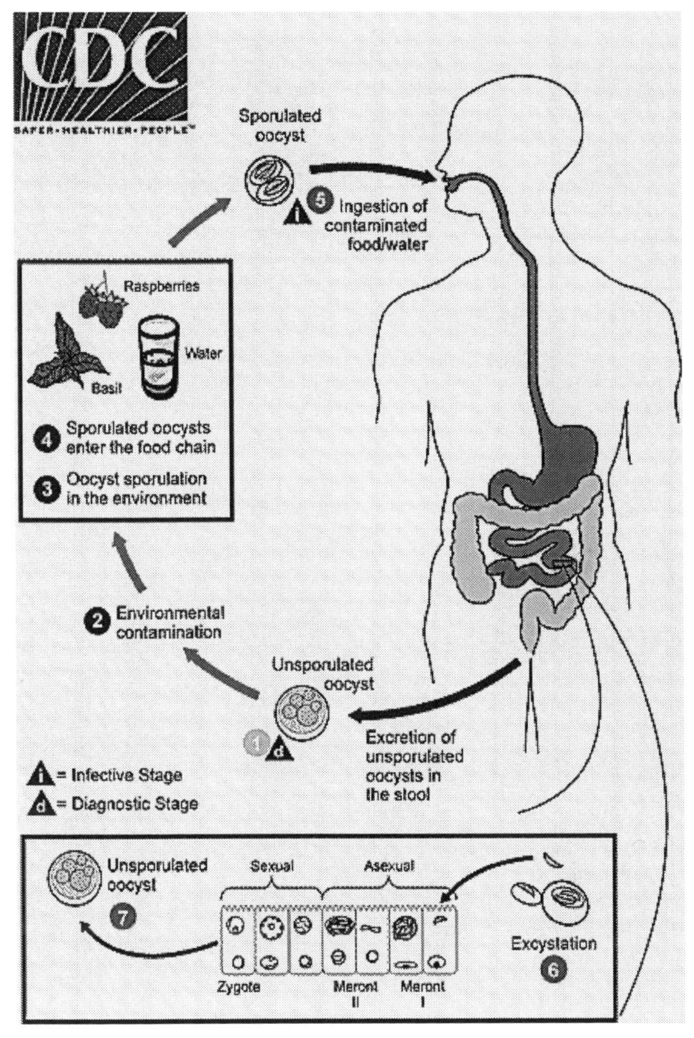

Cyclospora life cycle
http://www.cdc.gov/parasites/cyclosporiasis/biology.html

Raspberries and basil. Not an animal in sight.

Also worth looking at is the CDC's **Cyclosporiasis Fact Sheet** available for download at:
http://www.cdc.gov/parasites/cyclosporiasis/resources/pdf/cyclosporiasis_general-public_061214.pdf

This is what we see at the top of the page:

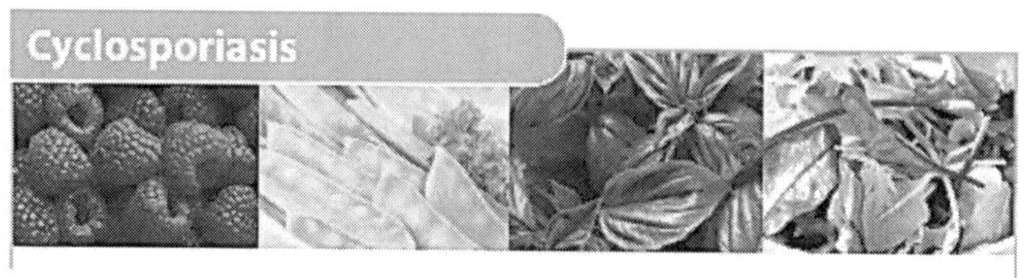

CDC. Cyclosporiasis

Raspberries, sugar peas, basil and leafy greens. Not an animal in sight. Berries are the most nutritious of all fruits, and leafy greens are the most nutrient-dense vegetables… in other words, our best possible foods.

Then we go on to read:

"How is it spread?

People can become infected by consuming food or water **contaminated with feces** (stool) that contains the parasite."

Now let's ask a question or two:

Q1: How much feces (shit) is generated by berries, peas, basil and lettuce? (See the life cycle diagram above, too, for indictment of raspberries and basil.)

Q2: How likely is it that this so-called Fact Sheet was written by a vegan?

This parasitic infection is caused by eating **foods contaminated with animal shit**, yet the bullshitters at the CDC want us to think we should be more scared of eating fruit and vegetables than dead chickens and cows?

It's clear that this parasitic "disease" affects vegetable foods only insofar as they've been cross-contaminated with excreta from animals, both human and other species. We shouldn't hold our breath waiting for the CDC to say so. Instead of blaming the contaminant – the root cause – they affix blame to the produce which is contaminated with shit. In other words, mainly cross-contaminated by animal agriculture.

Cyclospora is almost irrelevant to the burden of illness in the USA, causing illness in 0.0034% (34 in a million), hospitalizing 0.0000034% of the population (34 in a billion, if there were that many of us) and killing none. The only reason I've given it so much space is that it clearly demonstrates the CDC's unconscious, built-in pro-Meater, un-Planter bias.

Giardia intestinalis

Estimated annual number of Americans infected: **77,000**
Estimated number of hospitalizations caused annually: **230**
Estimated annual number of deaths caused: **2**

"*Giardia* is a microscopic parasite that causes the **diarrheal illness** known as giardiasis. *Giardia*… is found on surfaces or in soil, food, or water that has been **contaminated with feces** from **infected humans or animals.**

Giardia is protected by an outer shell that allows it to survive outside the body for long periods of time and makes it tolerant to chlorine disinfection. While the parasite can be spread in different ways, water (**drinking water and recreational water**) is the most common mode of transmission."

"Giardiasis is the most frequently diagnosed intestinal parasitic disease in the United States and among travelers with chronic diarrhea. Signs and symptoms may vary and can last for 1 to 2 weeks or longer. In some cases, people infected with Giardia have no symptoms.

Acute symptoms include:

- Diarrhea
- Gas
- Greasy stools that tend to float
- Stomach or abdominal cramps
- Upset stomach or nausea/vomiting
- Dehydration (loss of fluids).

This animal-shit-borne pathogen affects our water more than our food, and is almost irrelevant nutritionally except to say: the fewer animals we eat, the less shit we eat, the less often we'll be contaminated. In places where *giardia* is endemic in the water, washing food – plants – with un-boiled water probably isn't helpful. Eating plants with removable peels like pineapples, bananas and citrus fruit is protective for travelers in the tropics.

Summary: *Cryptosporidium parvum, Cyclospora cayetanensis, Giardia intestinalis*

Estimated annual number of Americans infected: **145,000**
Estimated number of hospitalizations caused annually: **451**
Estimated annual number of deaths caused: **6**

These three relatively benign parasitic infections are estimated to cause the deaths of 6 unlucky Americans each year. About 1 death every two months. Compare this to the one-a-minute death rate from animal-borne heart attacks.

What these infections have in common is:

- They're all caused by parasitic protozoa that are excreted in animal feces
- Unsurprisingly, they all cause diarrhea.
- They are caused primarily by exposure to contaminated water (either drunk or swum in) rather than by food poisoning.
- Although many are infected by these parasites, they bear little of the burden of hospitalizations and deaths from food poisoning.

Toxoplasma gondii

Estimated annual number of Americans infected: **87,000**
Estimated number of hospitalizations caused annually: **4,400**
Estimated annual number of deaths caused: **330**

According to the CDC at http://www.cdc.gov/parasites/:

"Toxoplasmosis is considered to be a **leading cause of death attributed to foodborne illness** in the United States. **More than 60 million** men, women, and children in the U.S. carry the *Toxoplasma* parasite, but very few have symptoms because the immune system usually keeps the parasite from causing illness.

However, women newly infected with *Toxoplasma* during pregnancy and anyone with a compromised immune system should be aware that toxoplasmosis can have severe consequences."

Comment:
That's the CDC's version of who's at risk. Here's a better version. Meaters are most at risk of toxoplasmosis because Meaters (1) eat animals which contain *T. gondii* and (2) are immunocompromised by eating animals. Planters who don't chow down on old kitty litter, or soil contaminated with *T. gondii*, have a fraction of the exposure to these protozoa.

"Toxoplasmosis is considered **one of the Neglected Parasitic Infections, a group of five parasitic diseases that have been targeted by CDC for public health action**."

Per the CDC's Neglected Parasitic Infections in the United States:

"Toxoplasmosis is a preventable disease caused by the parasite *Toxoplasma gondii*. An infected individual can experience fever, malaise, and swollen lymph nodes, but can also show no signs or symptoms. A small number of infected persons may experience **eye disease**, and infection during pregnancy can lead to **miscarriage** or **severe disease in the newborn**, including **developmental delays, blindness, and epilepsy**.

Once infected with *T. gondii*, people are generally **infected for life**. As a result, infected individuals with weakened immune systems — such as in the case of advanced HIV disease, during cancer treatment, or after organ transplant—can experience disease reactivation, which can result in severe illness or even death. In persons with advanced HIV disease, inflammation of the brain (**encephalitis**) due to toxoplasmosis is common unless long-term preventive medication is taken. Researchers have also found an association of T. gondii infection with the risk for mental illness, though this requires further study.

Although *T. gondii* can infect most **warm-blooded animals**, **cats** are the only host that shed an environmentally resistant form of the organism (oocyst) in their feces. Once a person or another warm-blooded animal ingests the parasite, it becomes infectious and travels through the wall of the intestine. Then the parasite is carried by blood to other tissues including the muscles and central nervous system."

***T. Gondii* Life Cycle:**

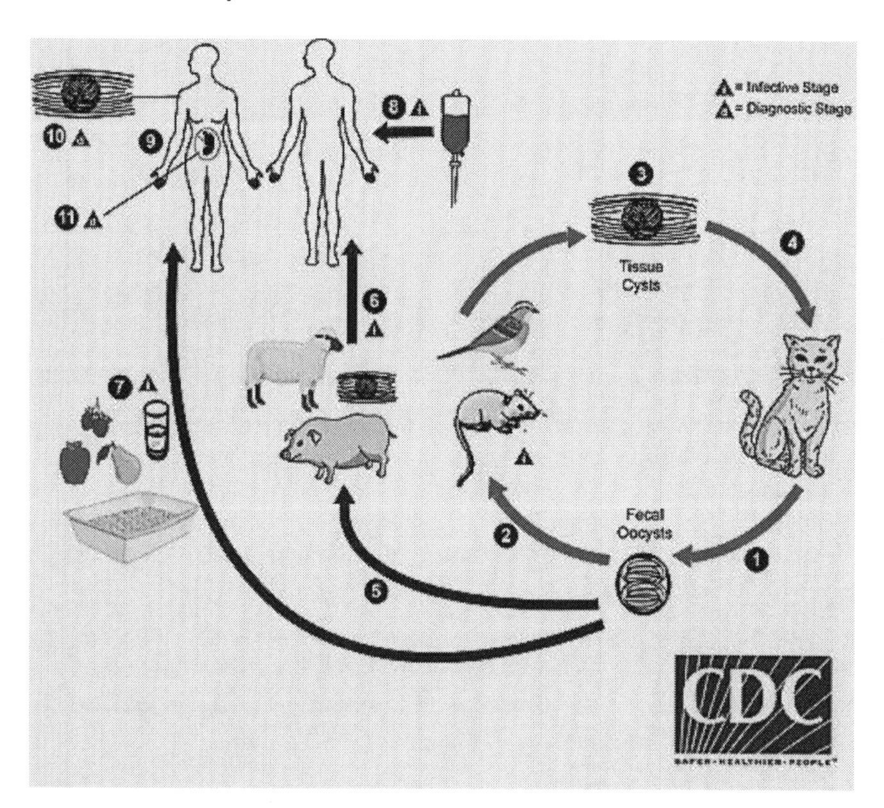

Toxoplasmosis. http://www.cdc.gov/parasites/toxoplasmosis/biology.html

"Why be concerned about toxoplasmosis in the United States?

- Toxoplasmosis is a leading cause of foodborne illness-related death and hospitalization in the U.S. — causing an estimated **327 deaths and 4,428 hospitalizations each year**.
- The *T. gondii* parasite infects over 1 million persons each year in the United States. An estimated 4,800 individuals each year develop **symptomatic eye disease** from *T. gondii* infection leading to vision loss.
- There are approximately 400 – 4,000 cases of **congenital (mother-to-child) toxoplasmosis** each year.
- Individuals whose immune systems are severely compromised can develop **encephalitis**, or have further spread of disease, which can be fatal."

Comment

By far the greatest source of human contamination with *T. gondii* comes from the central route shown in the life cycle graphic above: via eating animals. Plants and water infected with kitty litter, or cat shit itself, play a negligible role. The CDC could create more "safer, healthier people," as their logo touts, if they were to accentuate the major cause of bacterial transmission: Meating. Instead, they bang on about how to make animals safe to eat and whether or not we should keep cats as companions. It's as if I were to write a treatise on automobiles and spoke only of convertibles: they're nice and all, but the overwhelming majority of vehicles have solid roofs. As with bio-magnified industrial pollutants, the animals we eat are far more polluted than plants with bio-accumulated pathogenic life forms such as *T. gondii.*

"The only known definitive hosts for *Toxoplasma gondii* are members of family *Felidae* (domestic cats and their relatives)... **Animals bred for human consumption and wild game** may also become infected with tissue cysts after ingestion of sporulated oocysts in the environment.

Humans can become infected by any of several routes:

- **eating undercooked meat of animals harboring tissue cysts.**
- consuming food or water contaminated with cat feces or by contaminated environmental samples (such as fecal-contaminated soil or changing the litter box of a pet cat).
- blood transfusion or organ transplantation.
- transplacentally from mother to fetus.

In the human host, the parasites form tissue cysts, most commonly in skeletal muscle, myocardium, brain, and eyes; these cysts may remain throughout the life of the host."

Comment

OK, if cats are the reservoir of *T. gondii*, it's best not to eat them. We should also handle with care kitty litter trays and kitty poop. Domestic cats aren't the problem – Meating is.

Toxoplasma parasites really hit us where it hurts: our muscles, hearts, eyes and brain. Most cases of toxoplasmosis can be avoided by not eating the 'intermediary hosts' of the parasite: the infected animals we eat.

In the US "food" supply, a high percentage of lambs are en-toxoplasma-cated. According to this paper (J. P. Dubey, N. Sundar, D. Hill, G. V. Velmurugan, L. A. Bandini, O. C. H. Kwok, D. Majumdar, and C. Su. High prevalence and abundant atypical genotypes of toxoplasma gondii isolated from lambs destined for human consumption in the USA. *Int. J. Parasitol.*, 38(8 – 9):999-1006, 2008): "Antibodies… to *T. gondii* were found in 27.1% of… lambs… 15.7% [of] strains belong to the Type III lineage."

"These results indicate high parasite prevalence and high genetic diversity of *T. gondii* in lambs, which has **important implications in public health**." I'll say.

The same lead researcher led a team that later did a study on goats.

J.P. Dubey, C. Rajendran, L.R. Ferreira, J. Martins, O.C.H. Kwok, D.E. Hill, I. Villena, H. Zhou, C. Su, J.L. Jones. High prevalence and genotypes of Toxoplasma gondii isolated from goats, from a retail meat store, destined for human consumption in the USA. *International Journal for Parasitology* 41 (2011) 827–833.

And what did they find? "Antibodies to *T. gondii* were found in… 53.4%... of… goats [tested]."

They conclude: "Taken together, these results indicate high parasite prevalence and moderate genetic diversity of *T. gondii* in goats, which have **important implications in public health**."

By the way, when scientists speak in measured tones, saying stuff like "this has important implications in public health," it's the same as regular people jumping up and down, shouting: "Holy cannelloni, check this out!"

Farmed and wild animals are highly contaminated with *T. gondii. T. gondii* aren't only in lambs and goats. They're in a large percentage of all the animals we buy or shoot to eat, particularly pigs. Not all the cleaning and separating and cooking and chilling of dead animal parts the CDC recommends is going to change that.

Sadly, one in ten of us Americans already has *toxoplasma* parasites in our brains. Sequelae of infection include bipolar disorder, Parkinson's and schizophrenia, so we'd better boost our immune function (by eating lots of plants) to prevent *T. gondii* causing the toxoplasmosis which chews up our brains, hearts, eyes and muscles.

Here's the butcher's bill for *Toxoplasma*, according to the Top 50 pathogen-food combinations, from the 2011 Emerging Pathogens Institute report:

(Emerging Pathogens Institute 2011)
Table A-1: Top 50 pathogen-food combinations, by combined QALY/$Rank

Rank	Pathogen	Food	QALY loss	Cost of illness ($ mil.)	Illnesses	Hospitalizations	Deaths
2	*Toxoplasma*	Pork	4,495	1,219	35,537	1,815	134
9	*Toxoplasma*	Beef	2,541	689	20,086	1,026	76
17	*Toxoplasma*	Produce	772	209	6,104	312	23
34	*Toxoplasma*	Poultry	410	111	3,242	166	12
37	*Toxoplasma*	Dairy	261	71	2,062	105	8
43	*Toxoplasma*	Deli/Other Meats	188	51	1,490	76	6
		Totals	8,667	2,350	68,521	3,500	259

We have a fraction of the risk of giving ourselves toxoplasmosis when we're Planters. 8.9% of the quality-adjusted life year loss, 8.9% of the cost, 8.9% of the illnesses, 8.9% of the hospitalizations and 8.9% of the deaths, according to these weirdly consistent EPI figures.

If we avoid cross-contamination with animal shit by eating veganically grown fruits and veg, we drop our risk even further towards zero.

For the fifth and last parasite – and the 31st and last pathogen – on the CDC's list of pathogens causing the most illnesses, hospitalizations and death in the USA, we have a worm.

Roundworms [nematodes] – *Trichinella* spp. (species)

Estimated annual number of Americans infected: **160**
Estimated number of hospitalizations caused annually: **6**
Estimated annual number of deaths caused: **0**

According to the CDC, "**Trichinellosis**, also called **trichinosis**, is a disease that people can get by **eating raw or undercooked meat** from animals infected with the microscopic parasite *Trichinella*…

Pigs, feral hogs, cougars and black bears can all harbor *Trichinella* infection. Successful trichinae control programs by the U.S. pork industry have nearly eliminated the disease in domestic swine raised in confinement, but hogs raised outdoors in close contact with rodents and other wildlife have an increased chance of acquiring *Trichinella* infection…

Worldwide, an estimated 10,000 cases of trichinellosis occur every year. Several different species of *Trichinella* can cause human disease; the most common species is *Trichinella spiralis*, which has a global distribution and is the species most commonly found in pigs."

Trichinosis is no longer a great threat to public health in the USA, thanks, apparently, to the good work of CAFO piggery operations. Success! The poor pigs are now much safer for Meaters to eat.

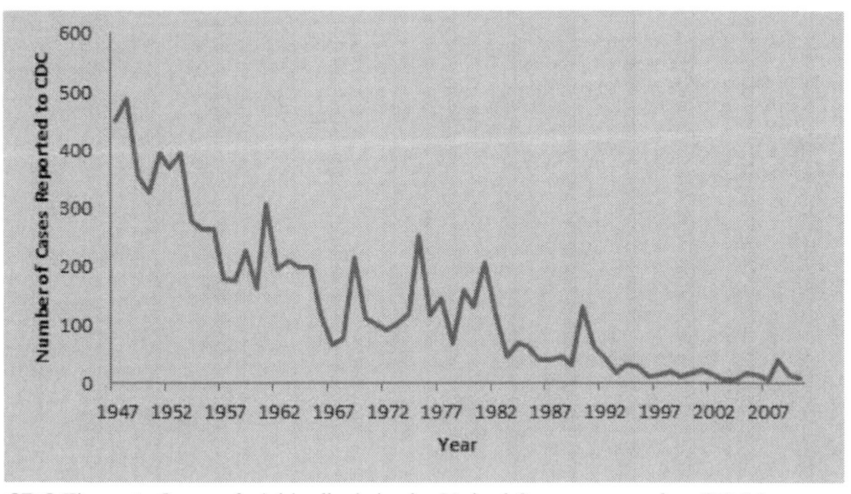

CDC Figure 1. Cases of trichinellosis in the United States reported to CDC by year, 1947-2010

Pathogens – Summary

Viruses – Summary

Estimated annual number of Americans infected: **5,546,600**
Estimated number of hospitalizations caused: **15,623**
Estimated number of annual deaths caused: **158**

Bacteria – Summary

Estimated annual number of Americans infected: **3,622,535**
Estimated number of hospitalizations caused: **34,237**
Estimated number of annual deaths caused: **849**

Parasites – Summary

Estimated annual number of Americans infected: **233,160**
Estimated number of hospitalizations caused: **4,857**
Estimated number of annual deaths caused: **336**

Viruses account for almost 60% of infections, yet we may be better off being infected by a virus than a bacterium or a worm. Viruses account for less than 30% of hospitalizations and less than 12% of deaths from foodborne illness.

Bacteria account for almost 40% of infections, but more than 60% of both hospitalizations and deaths.

Parasites are what we should really avoid: only 2.5% (one in forty) illnesses cause almost 10% of hospitalizations and 25% (one in four) deaths from food poisoning.

It seems that as infectious organisms become more complex, their virulence increases. Parasites box far above their weight. Meating too: it accounts for at least 90% of the "food"-borne burden of infection. Now let's hear from the Emerging Pathogens Institute…

EPI Rankings of the top 50 pathogen-food combinations

Appendix A: Rankings of top 50 pathogen-food combinations
From: Batz et al - Ranking the Risks: The 10 Pathogen-Food Combinations with the Greatest Burden on Public Health
(Emerging Pathogens Institute 2011)
Table A-1: Top 50 pathogen-food combinations, by combined QALY/$Rank

Rank	Pathogen	Food	QALY loss	Cost of illness ($ mil.)	Illnesses	Hospitalizations	Deaths
1	*Campylobacter*	Poultry	9,541	1,257	608,231	6,091	55
2	*Toxoplasma*	Pork	4,495	1,219	35,537	1,815	134
3	*L. monocytogenes*	Deli Meats	3,948	1,086	651	595	104
4	*Salmonella*	Poultry	3,610	712	221,045	4,159	81
5	*L. monocytogenes*	Dairy	2,632	724	434	397	70
6	*Salmonella*	Complex foods	3,195	630	195,655	3,682	72
7	*Norovirus*	Complex foods	2,294	914	2,494,222	6,696	68
8	*Salmonella*	Produce	2,781	548	170,264	3,204	63
9	*Toxoplasma*	Beef	2,541	689	20,086	1,026	76
10	*Salmonella*	Eggs	1,878	370	115,003	2,164	42
11	*L. monocytogenes*	Complex foods	1,316	362	217	198	35
12	*Salmonella*	Beef	1,073	212	65,716	1,237	24
13	*Salmonella*	Pork	1,073	212	65,716	1,237	24
14	*Norovirus*	Produce	779	311	847,184	2,274	23
15	*Salmonella*	Dairy	1,000	197	61,235	1,152	23
16	*Yersinia enterocolitica*	Pork	1,013	180	69,889	381	21
17	*Toxoplasma*	Produce	772	209	6,104	312	23
18	*Salmonella*	Seafood	854	168	52,274	984	19
19	*Campylobacter*	Dairy	1,034	136	65,886	660	6
20	*Vibrio vulnificus*	Seafood	541	282	93	90	35
21	*E. coli O157*	Beef	828	144	33,410	1,131	11
22	*Norovirus*	Seafood	461	184	501,684	1,347	14
23	*Salmonella*	Breads and Bakery	585	115	35,845	675	13
24	*L. monocytogenes*	Pork	439	121	72	66	12
25	*L. monocytogenes*	Poultry	439	121	72	66	12
26	*L. monocytogenes*	Produce	439	121	72	66	12
27	*L. monocytogenes*	Seafood	439	121	72	66	12
28	*Campylobacter*	Produce	693	91	44,178	442	4
29	*Norovirus*	Breads and Bakery	392	156	425,958	1,144	12
30	*Salmonella*	Deli/Other Meats	561	111	34,352	646	13
31	*Norovirus*	Poultry	387	154	421,225	1,131	11
32	*Campylobacter*	Pork	584	77	37,215	373	3
33	*Campylobacter*	Beef	580	76	36,952	370	3
34	*Toxoplasma*	Poultry	410	111	3,242	166	12
35	*C. perfringens*	Beef	285	101	314,612	143	8
36	*C. perfringens*	Poultry	234	83	258,080	117	7
37	*Toxoplasma*	Dairy	261	71	2,062	105	8
38	*Norovirus*	Beef	205	82	222,445	597	6
39	*C. perfringens*	Complex foods	212	75	233,501	106	6
40	*Campylobacter*	Eggs	341	45	21,749	218	2
41	*E. coli O157*	Produce	283	49	11,408	386	4
42	*Shigella*	Complex foods	245	54	58,930	654	4
43	*Toxoplasma*	Deli/Other Meats	188	51	1,490	76	6
44	*Norovirus*	Pork	144	57	156,185	419	4
45	*E. coli O157*	Complex foods	232	40	9,371	317	3
46	*Norovirus*	Deli/Other Meats	113	45	123,055	330	3
47	*Cryptosporidium*	Produce	203	28	34,286	125	2
48	*Yersinia enterocolitica*	Dairy	173	31	11,917	65	4
49	*Salmonella*	Beverages	171	34	10,455	197	4
50	*Norovirus*	Dairy	109	43	118,322	318	3
		Totals	57,006	13,010	8,257,659	50,216	1,216

Batz et al - Ranking the Risks: The 10 Pathogen-Food Combinations with the Greatest Burden on Public Health, Appendix A: Rankings of top 50 pathogen-food combinations.

Here's that EPI data again, which we're now going to study in more depth.

Part 2B (~~Food~~borne Pathogens: the EPI)

Introduction

Okay, so we've looked at the 31 "food"-borne pathogens the CDC deems most relevant to "food" poisoning. As we saw, while plant foods [tautology alert] *are affected* by pathogens that appear naturally in the environment, I'm now going to demonstrate that Planting can remove at least 90% of our risk of "food" poisoning; and even more when we eat plants uncontaminated with animal shit. Germs aren't usually in food - animals carry them.

Here I'd like to introduce the paper from the Emerging Pathogens Institute at the University of Florida which I've already referred to a few times in passing:

Michael B. Batz, Sandra Hoffmann and J. Glenn Morris, Jr. Ranking the Risks: The 10 Pathogen-Food Combinations With the Greatest Burden on Public Health. *EPI* 2011.

We first saw the table above at the beginning of Part 2A (~~Food~~borne Pathogens: The CDC). It's Table A-1: Top 50 pathogen-food combinations, by Combined QALY /$ Rank, as found in Batz et al's APPENDIX A: Rankings of Top 50 Pathogen-Food Combinations, on pp. 63-4.

(Quality-Adjusted Life Years (QALYs) are "a measure of health-related quality of life," and their loss is a measure of the damage done by pathogen-laden "foods"... pathogens being living, infectious disease-causing contaminants, like viruses, bacteria or parasites, such as worms and protozoa.)

Because – to repeat one of Michael Greger's mantras – "Food is a package deal" – each mouthful we eat carries the risk of contamination, illness, hospitalization and death in the form not only of chemicals, but invisible toxic or toxin-producing life forms, it's best to eat the least contamination we can. We do this by eating plants and avoiding eating animals.

Table A-1 lists the top 50 "pathogen-food combinations" and the damage that they do. These are the foods and un-foods most likely to sicken us, hospitalize us or kill us, because of the germs or parasites with which they're combined or packaged.

From the above Emerging Pathogens Institute data I've extracted information about the Top 50 pathogen-food combinations, ordered by pathogen. This info appears in the following table.

Top 50 pathogen-food combinations, ordered by pathogen

	Top 50 pathogen-food combinations, ordered by pathogen				
Pathogen	**QALY loss**	**Cost of illness ($ mil.)**	**Illnesses**	**Hospitalizations**	**Deaths**
Clostridium perfringens	731	259	806,193	366	21
Campylobacter	12,773	1,682	814,211	8,154	73
Cryptosporidium	203	28	34,286	125	2
E. coli O157	1,343	233	54,189	1,834	18
Listeria monocytogenes	9,652	2,656	1,590	1,454	257
Norovirus	4,884	1,946	5,310,280	14,256	144
Salmonella	16,781	3,309	1,027,560	19,337	378
Shigella	245	54	58,930	654	4
Toxoplasma	8,667	2,350	68,521	3,500	259
Vibrio vulnificus	541	282	93	90	35
Yersinia enterocolitica	1,186	211	81,806	446	25
	57,006	13,010	8,257,659	50,216	1,216

(The EPI's figures tally with the CDC figures cited earlier; figures which the CDC said represent only about 20% of reality.)

Just eleven pathogens are implicated in the top 50 food/pathogen combinations that cause acute poisoning when we eat them. Unsurprisingly, we covered all eleven in our discussion of the CDC's 31 worst pathogens.

Three pathogens – *Cryptosporidium*, which is listed as causing 2 deaths in produce-eaters; *Shigella*, 4 deaths in complex food eaters ("foods" that combine several categories, such as dairy, plants and meats); and *Vibrio vulnificus*, killing 35 people who ate "Seafood" – appear only once.

The remaining eight "food"-borne "disease" vectors appear in multiple un-foods and one food:

- *Clostridium perfringens* in Beef, Complex foods and Poultry
- *Campylobacter* in Beef, Eggs, Dairy, Pork, Poultry and Produce
- *E. coli O157* in Beef, Complex foods and Produce
- *Listeria monocytogenes* in Complex foods, Dairy, Deli Meats, Pork, Poultry, Produce and Seafood
- Norovirus in Beef, Breads and Bakery, Complex foods, Dairy, Deli/Other Meats, Pork, Poultry, Produce and Seafood

- *Salmonella* in Beef, Beverages, Breads and Bakery, Complex foods, Dairy, Deli/Other Meats, Eggs, Pork, Poultry, Produce and Seafood, [i.e. everywhere]
- *Toxoplasma* in Beef, Dairy, Deli/Other Meats, Pork, Poultry and Produce
- *Yersinia enterocolitica* in Dairy and Pork

(Produce is starting to look real dangerous. Maybe George Bush Sr. was on to something with his childish disparagement of broccoli. Actually, no. Produce may appear often but it's always a minor actor, present almost invariably because of contamination with animal shit.)

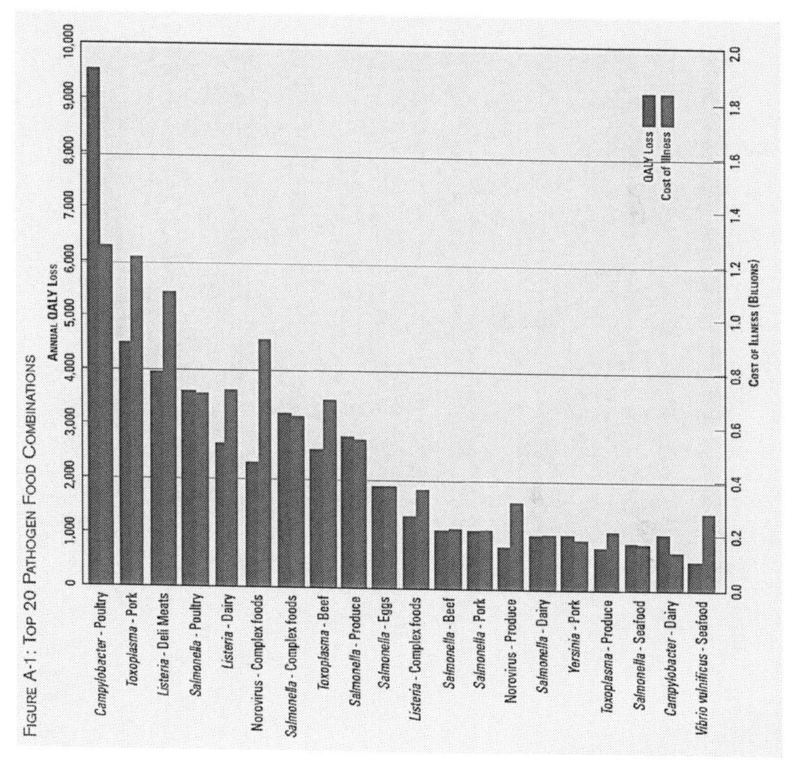

Batz et al: Figure A-1: Top 20 Pathogen-Food Combinations

On the previous page, there's a graphic representation of the top 20 edible/poison combos (Batz et al 2011, p. 65) showing how insignificant plants are in comparison to animals when it comes to "disease" Eatiology.

The top 5 Meater Eatiologies: *Campylobacter* in Poultry, *Toxoplasma* in Pork, *Listeria* in Deli Meats, *Salmonella* in Poultry and *Listeria* in Dairy cause more health and financial damage than all the rest combined.

Animals look even worse if we remove the top plant culprit combo, *Salmonella* in Produce, clearly a case of cross-contamination with animal feces.

We can easily remove it from our plates by eating shit-free organic, veganic or home-grown produce.

Norovirus and *Toxoplasma*, two other pathogens which also put produce in the top 20, can also be minimized by not infecting plants with animal shit.

On the following page, there's another table from the CDC (from www.cdc.gov/foodborneburden/) showing how just 5 pathogenic Meater Eatiologies contribute almost all the "disease" burden:

- 91% of illnesses
- 88% of hospitalizations
- 88% of deaths

"Eight known pathogens account for the vast majority of illnesses, hospitalizations, and deaths," according to the CDC.

The pathogens in the CDC's Tables 2-4 below account for between 88 and 91% of the "food"-borne illness burden: roughly 90% of illnesses, hospital stays and deaths.

Pathogens causing the most illnesses, hospitalizations, and deaths each year

Eight known pathogens account for the vast majority of illnesses, hospitalizations, and deaths. Tables 2–4 list the top five pathogens causing illness, hospitalization, and death.

Table 2. Top five pathogens causing domestically acquired foodborne illnesses

Pathogen	Estimated annual number of illnesses	90% Credible Interval	%
Norovirus	5,461,731	3,227,078–8,309,480	58
Salmonella, nontyphoidal	1,027,561	644,786–1,679,667	11
Clostridium perfringens	965,958	192,316–2,483,309	10
Campylobacter spp.	845,024	337,031–1,611,083	9
Staphylococcus aureus	241,148	72,341–529,417	3
Subtotal			91

Table 3. Top five pathogens causing domestically acquired foodborne illnesses resulting in hospitalization

Pathogen	Estimated annual number of hospitalizations	90% Credible Interval	%
Salmonella, nontyphoidal	19,336	8,545–37,490	35
Norovirus	14,663	8,097–23,323	26
Campylobacter spp.	8,463	4,300–15,227	15
Toxoplasma gondii	4,428	3,060–7,146	8
E. coli (STEC) O157	2,138	549–4,614	4
Subtotal			88

Table 4. Top five pathogens causing domestically acquired foodborne illnesses resulting in death

Pathogen	Estimated annual number of deaths	90% Credible Interval	%
Salmonella, nontyphoidal	378	0–1,011	28
Toxoplasma gondii	327	200–482	24
Listeria monocytogenes	255	0–733	19
Norovirus	149	84–237	11
Campylobacter spp.	76	0–332	6
Subtotal			88

February 2011 www.cdc.gov/foodborneburden

CDC Tables: Pathogens causing the most illnesses, hospitalizations & deaths each year

http://www.cdc.gov/foodborneburden/

Here's another table from the EPI, listing 14 Meater pathogens and their body count:

The EPI's Top 14 ~~Food~~borne Pathogens

TABLE ES-1: ANNUAL DISEASE BURDEN CAUSED BY 14 FOODBORNE PATHOGENS

PATHOGEN	COMBINED RANK*	QALY LOSS	COST OF ILLNESS ($ MIL.)	ILLNESSES#	HOSPITAL-IZATIONS#	DEATHS#
Salmonella spp.	1	16,782	3,309	1,027,561	19,336	378
Toxoplasma gondii	2	10,964	2,973	86,686	4,428	327
Campylobacter spp.	3	13,256	1,747	845,024	8,463	76
Listeria monocytogenes	3	9,651	2,655	1,591	1,455	255
Norovirus	5	5,023	2,002	5,461,731	14,663	149
E.coli O157:H7	6	1,565	272	63,153	2,138	20
Clostridium perfringens	6	875	309	965,958	438	26
Yersinia enterocolitica	8	1,415	252	97,656	533	29
Vibrio vulnificus	8	557	291	96	93	36
Shigella spp.	10	545	121	131,254	1,456	10
Vibrio other+	11	341	47	57,616	210	4
Cryptosporidium parvum	12	149	107	52,228	183	12
E.coli non-O157 STEC	13	327	26	112,752	271	0
Cyclospora cayetanensis	14	10	2	11,407	11	0
TOTAL		61,461	14,114	8,914,713	53,678	1,322

* Combined rank is the rank order when QALY rank and COI rank are averaged
# Incidence estimates are mean estimates reported in Scallan et al. (2011a).
+ includes *Vibrio parahaemolyticus* and other non-choleric *Vibrio* species

Batz et al. Ranking the Risks, p. 8.

The next two tables are a summary of our top 50 pathogen-food combos, by food or "food," followed by a breakdown of contaminated plants' contribution to eating-related illness.

Table: Top 50 pathogen-food combos, by food/non-food

	Top 50 pathogen-food combinations, by food				
Food	**QALY loss**	**Cost of illness ($ mil.)**	**Illnesses**	**Hospitalizations**	**Deaths**
Beef	5,512	1,304	693,221	4,504	128
Beverages	171	34	10,455	197	4
Breads and Bakery	977	271	461,803	1,819	25
Complex foods	7,494	2,075	2,991,896	11,653	188
Dairy	5,209	1,202	259,856	2,697	114
Deli/Other Meats	4,810	1,293	159,548	1,647	126
Eggs	2,219	415	136,752	2,382	44
Pork	7,748	1,866	364,614	4,291	198
Poultry	14,621	2,438	1,511,895	11,730	178
Produce	5,950	1,357	1,113,496	6,809	131
Seafood	2,295	755	554,123	2,487	80
Total	57,006	13,010	8,257,659	50,216	1,216
Plants only	**QALY loss**	**Cost of illness ($ mil.)**	**Illnesses**	**Hospitalizations**	**Deaths**
Beverages	171	34	10,455	197	4
Produce	5,950	1,357	1,113,496	6,809	131
Total	6,121	1,391	1,123,951	7,006	135

Table: Produce compared to the non-foods:

Comparison of Produce to the remaining top 50 pathogen-food combinations

Data from: Batz et al - Ranking the Risks: The 10 Pathogen-Food Combinations with the Greatest Burden on Public Health (Emerging Pathogens Institute, 2011)

Rank	Pathogen	Food	QALY loss	Cost of illness ($ mil.)	Illnesses	Hospitalizations	Deaths
8	*Salmonella*	Produce	2,781	548	170,264	3,204	63
14	*Norovirus*	Produce	779	311	847,184	2,274	23
17	*Toxoplasma*	Produce	772	209	6,104	312	23
26	*L. monocytogenes*	Produce	439	121	72	66	12
28	*Campylobacter*	Produce	693	91	44,178	442	4
41	*E. coli O157*	Produce	283	49	11,408	386	4
47	*Cryptosporidium*	Produce	203	28	34,286	125	2
	Totals (Produce only)		**5,950**	**1,357**	**1,113,496**	**6,809**	**131**
	Totals (All foods 1 - 50)		57,006	13,010	8,257,659	50,216	1,216
	Produce percentage of pathogen burden		10.44%	10.43%	13.48%	13.56%	10.77%

This last table, comparing produce to non-foods, shows that roughly 90% of our risk of getting ill, landing up in hospital or pushing up daisies in the shade of a cypress tree because of ingested pathogens, disappears when we eat nothing but whole plants.

We remove 90% of "food"-borne illnesses with a single dietary modification. Those who eat nothing but plants have about 10% of the risk of "food" poisoning as omnivores. Most of the remaining 10% of risk could be removed too, if animal farmers would desist from polluting the world and cross-contaminating whole plant foods with fecal-bacteria-containing animal feces.

50 million cases of zoönosis eradicated; thousands of hospital visits avoided; billions of dollars saved… when we become Planters.

Surely that should be worth a mention by the CDC?

Speaking of golden silence…

Why won't the largest environmental groups talk about the largest environmental villain?
SIERRA CLUB
GREENPEACE
RAINFOREST ACTION NETWORK
According to the United Nations, animal agriculture is one of the leading causes of every single form of environmental destruction everywhere in the world. It is also the easiest villain to defeat – we simply have to stop using animals. It's time for the people who are supposed to be protecting our planet to address these facts and promote a vegan diet.
Source: UN FAO report Livestock's Long Shadow
Learn more at cowspiracy.com
VeganStreet.com

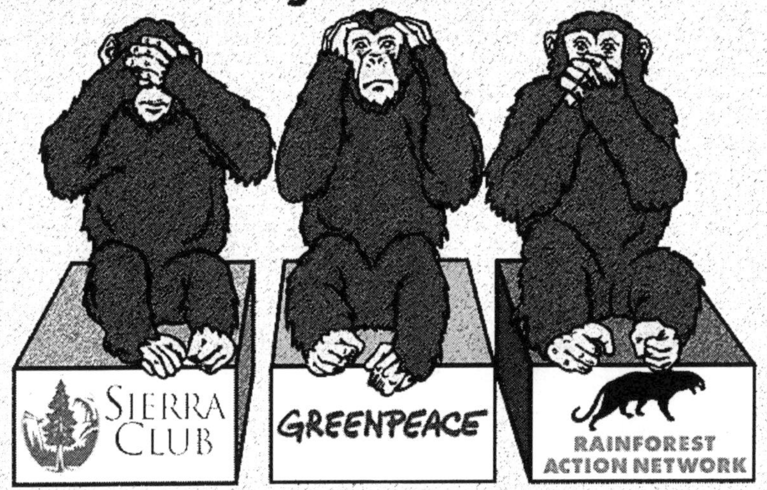

Refusing to face facts. Source: VeganStreet.com

Summary of ~~Food~~borne Pathogens – Eating accidents

In his poem "Casualty," Miroslav Holub writes "And while we are suturing inch after inch, night after night, nerve to nerve, muscle to muscle, eyes to sight, they bring in even longer daggers, even more dangerous bombs, even more glorious victories, idiots."

Just as driving badly can lead to car accidents, eating badly can cause eating casualties, as when we accidentally eat animals or when we eat animals on purpose, accidentally thinking they're food, idiots.

In Part 1A (Components) I showed that Planting removes 90% of our risk of chronic, degenerative symptoms of Meating and Junking such as heart "disease", diabetes and high blood pressure. And I've just shown that Planting removes 90% of our risk of infectious "food" poisoning and septicemia, caused almost entirely by Meating.

Planting has the power to keep us alive longer, and healthier and younger-looking and younger–feeling too during the extra years we live.

While I've said that Planting removes 90% of the risk of death via heart "disease" and un-food poisoning, Planting removes almost 100% of the *excess risk*, meaning Planting gives us the best survival odds.

We all die.

We all go into that good night, but there's no reason to accelerate towards the wall; there's no reason for us to stick our heads up above the nutritional parapet.

Meating and Junking cause 90% of degenerative and "food"-borne symptoms. And Meating and Junking cause 100% of the excess nutritional risk, as near as dammit.

In the third part of this section on Pathogens, I'm going to take a look at a few more Meater fellow travelers that mess with us and kill us when we eat animals.

~

Part 2C (~~Food~~borne Pathogens – Other)

In this section, we're going to look at another 35 ways that Meating can destroy our lives, via other animal/pathogen combinations that cause severe illness and death.

Other "food"-borne pathogens not in the CDC's top 31 list

Here are the new pathogens we're going to cover. Some are particular species, other are general classes of Meater pathogens:

Viruses

- Adenovirus 36
- Avian leukosis/sarcoma virus
- Bacteriophages
- Bovine leukemia virus
- Hepatitis E
- Human papilloma virus (HPV)
- Marek's disease virus
- Oncogenic (cancer-causing) viruses, in general
- Porcine endogenous retroviruses
- Poultry viruses, in general
- Rabies
- Reticuloendotheliosis virus
- Wart viruses, in general

Bacteria

- *C. diff* (*Clostridium difficile*)
- *Enterococcus*
- Fecal bacteria, in general
- *Proteus mirabilis*
- *Staphylococcus*
- MRSA (Methicillin or Multi-drug Resistant *Staphylococcus aureus*)

Parasites – helminths – nematodes (roundworms)

- *Anisakis* spp.
- Gnathostomiasis & Neurognathostomiasis
- *Linguatula serrata*
- *Toxocara*

Parasites – helminths – cestodes (tapeworms)

- Cysticercosis and Neurocysticercosis
- *Diphyllobothrium* spp.
- *Taenia* spp.

Pathogens – other – prions (infectious proteins)

- Prions & Transmissible Spongiform Encephalopathies (TSEs)
- Bovine spongiform encephalopathy (BSE/Mad cow disease)
- Kuru
- Creutzfeldt-Jakob disease (CJD)

Pathogens – other – miscellany

- BMAA
- Ciguatera
- Domoic acid
- Keriorrhea
- Scombroid poisoning
- Tetrodotoxin

Zoönoses

- Anthrax
- Swine flu

We're also going to look at 2 serious outcomes of Meater "food"-poisoning:

Resistance to drugs as a result of Meating, and

Chronic sequelae of animal-borne "diseases".

As John McDougall, Michael Greger and others have pointed out, there are no leaf molds, thrips, Dutch elm diseases or leaf blights that cause illness in humans. While zoönoses exist – diseases that escape the confines of their animal hosts to affect humans – there are no "phytoses" – diseases that mutate in plants to become deadly in humans.

We're animals, and we face a far reduced parasitic burden from plants. And when we eat plants only, and forgo animals altogether, autoimmune conditions between plants and humans other than celiac disease (a genetic condition affecting 0.67% of the US population) are unheard of.

Here we go then…

Other pathogens – viruses

Adenovirus 36 et al

In section 1, under the Eatiology of obesity, we came across the concept of Infectobesity: Obesity of Infectious Origin.

Nikhil V. Dhurandhar told us that Ad-36 is an oncogenic adenovirus that causes obesity. "In addition," he said: "the involvement of some pathogens in etiology of obesity suggests the possibility of a similar role for additional pathogens." Meaning, there's more where that came from.

The infectobesogens are in the chickens we eat. 20% of obese humans have been exposed to these viruses, and 15% of the population as a whole. These Meater viruses are part of the reason why only Planters have ideal body weight, as a group.

For more, see under: Obesity, in Part 1B (Mechanisms)

Avian leukosis/sarcoma virus

See under: Oncogenic viruses

Bacteriophages

Bacteriophages are 'bacteria-eaters.' They're viruses that Big Animal now legally sprays on dead animals to eat up the deadly shit-borne bacteria with which animals are contaminated: *E. coli*, *Campylobacter*, *Listeria*, *Proteus mirabilis*, *Salmonella*, etc.

Think about this for a moment… Does anyone really know the consequences of the microscopic DNA wars that the FDA has unleashed, by adding viruses to the bacterial load of animals? Who guards the guardians? Will any of the chopped-up DNA recombine in odd ways? I don't know; neither does anyone else.

To me, this is unbridled hubris, and I wouldn't be surprised if the Law of Unintended Consequences didn't show its ugly face. I've never been enamored of drone strikes, with their 'collateral damage.' Well, that's what may happen invisibly in our non-foods – mini-drones causing chaos, killing what they're not supposed to kill.

I've got to ask this question: If dead animals routinely carry such a potentially lethal load of pathogens that we add extra pathogens to eat the original pathogens in an attempt to make the animals safe to eat, should we really be thinking of animals as food? Wouldn't it be simpler and safer to eat bacteria-free food?

Bovine leukemia virus

Leukemia virus in cows is suspected as a cause of the blood cancer in humans known as Non-Hodgkin or Non-Hodgkin's lymphoma. 60,000 Americans get this "disease" each year and 20,000 die.

BLV is in most cattle and it gives them cancer. 75% of humans have antibodies to BLV, showing exposure, via Meating. Stockyard and slaughterhouse workers have greatly increased risk of lymphoma – actually, just about any cancer we can think of.

My heart bleeds for these poor people, many of whom are undocumented migrants, who have the worst working conditions in the country, are paid pitiful wages, and who're discarded when they're inevitably sickened or injured. Slaughterhouse work both attracts and extracts the worst of human behavior from people. And then they go home…

For more, see under: Oncogenic viruses

Butcher's warts

See under: Oncogenic viruses

Fish viruses

The oncogenic viruses that cause tumors in fish can cause stomach cancer in humans: E. S. Johnson, M. F. Faramawi, M. Sall, K.-M. Choi. Cancer and noncancer mortality among American seafood workers. *J Epidemiol* 2011 21(3):204 – 210.

As usual, Meater industry workers are the most exposed and, therefore, the most infected.

Hepatitis E

According to the CDC (http://www.cdc.gov/hepatitis/hev/), "Hepatitis E is a liver infection caused by the Hepatitis E virus (HEV). Hepatitis E is a self-limited disease that does not result in chronic infection. While rare in the United States, Hepatitis E is common in many parts of the world. It is **transmitted from ingestion of fecal matter**, even in microscopic amounts, and is usually associated with contaminated water supply in countries with poor sanitation."

Usually… but this infectious virus is now in the pigs we eat in the USA. The more pigs we eat, the better our chances of destroying our livers.

Elsewhere (http://wwwnc.cdc.gov/travel/yellowbook/2016/infectious-diseases-related-to-travel/hepatitis-e), the CDC says: "In Japan and Europe, sporadic disease can be **zoonotic** and **foodborne**, associated with **eating meat and offal (including liver) of deer, boars, and pigs**.

In France, disease can be acquired from eating **figatellu, a sausage delicacy prepared from raw pig liver**. [And to think the French are famous for their kissing!] Sporadic disease also is observed in the United States and other temperate countries, but **its cause is generally unknown**. **Shellfish** can transmit HEV."

What *is* generally known is that hepatitis E is now a zoönosis (animal-borne disease) in the US too, mainly via Meaters' predilection for pig flesh. It's also generally known that eating pigs correlates better to liver "disease" than alcohol consumption. (That's a stunner, by the way.)

Transmission of this form of hepatitis can also occur between infected humans, via the fecal-oral route, so Planters should be extra-careful around Meaters.

Human papilloma virus (HPV)

HPV is mostly a sexually transmitted disease, but eating pigs has been proven to cause cancerous warts of the anus and genitals. Low cervical cancer is reported in Jewish populations who forswear pig-eating. Islamic population should be similarly protected, as are Planters of all creeds. Butcher's warts cause cervical cancer, not in butchers but their sex partners. The same must apply to all Meaters, at a lower level of butchery.

For more, see under: Oncogenic viruses

Marek's disease virus

See under: Oncogenic viruses

Oncogenic, or cancer-causing, viruses

There are cancer-causing viruses in all the animals we eat. They're in cows (bovine viruses), sheeps (ovine), pigs (porcine), chickens (avian), fishes (unknown… pesky?) and goats (capricious?)

The viruses that cause warts and other nasty skin conditions in the workers whose hands come in contact with dead animals most often, also cause cancer. Workers on Meater disassembly lines or in animal dis-factories have far more cancer than any other occupational group. (I wouldn't deny that stress must be a huge contributory factor.)

To me, this is one of the most important papers of our generation, showing the dose-dependent relationship between the poison – Meating – and cancer:

Eric S. Johnson, Yi Zhou, C. Lillian Yau, Deepak Prabhakar, Harrison Ndetan, Karan Singh, Nykiconia Preacely. Mortality from malignant diseases—update of the Baltimore union poultry cohort. *Cancer Causes Control.* 2010 Feb;21(2):215-21. (DOI 10.1007/s10552-009-9452-6)

Johnson et al say: "Compared to the US general population, an **excess of cancers of the buccal** [mouth] **and nasal cavities and pharynx (base of the tongue, palate and other unspecified mouth, tonsil and oropharynx, nasal cavity/middle ear/accessory sinus), esophagus, recto-sigmoid/rectum/anus, liver and intrabiliary system, myelofibrosis** [bone marrow]**, lymphoid leukemia** [blood and marrow] **and multiple myeloma** [blood] was observed in particular subgroups or in the entire poultry cohort. We hypothesize that **oncogenic viruses** present in poultry, and exposure to **fumes**, are candidates for an etiologic role to explain the excess occurrence of at least some of these cancers in the poultry workers."

"Chronic exposure to animal proteins" giving rise to antigen production has been given as another Eatiology of cancer among animal 'processors,' who also have more **bladder, pancreatic and penis cancer**.

Here's more from Johnson: "Workers in poultry slaughtering and processing plants are exposed to **oncogenic viruses** that naturally infect and cause a variety of cancers in chickens and turkeys. These viruses include the **avian leukosis/sarcoma viruses (ALSV), reticuloendotheliosis viruses (REV)**, and **Marek's disease virus (MDV),** some members of which are **the most potent cancer-causing agent known in animals**. Other potentially carcinogenic occupational exposures include exposure to **fumes** emitted from the wrapping machine, **nitrosamines during the curing** of poultry, and to smoke or **aerosol** emitted during smoking or cooking of poultry products that contain **polycyclic aromatic hydrocarbons** and **heterocyclic amines**."

(Also: using compressed air hoses to remove brains and spinal cords from dead animals does a good job of spreading contagion in slaughterhouses, aerosolized brain matter contributing to neurodegenerative "diseases" among animal factory workers.)

In another paper (Johnson ES, Yau LC, Zhou Y, Singh KP, Ndetan H. Mortality in the Baltimore union poultry cohort: non-malignant diseases. *Int Arch Occup Environ Health.* 2010 Jun;83(5):543-52), Johnson's team found: "Poultry workers as a group had an overall **excess of deaths** from **diabetes**, anterior horn disease, and **hypertensive disease**, and a deficit of deaths from intracerebral hemorrhage. Deaths from zoonotic bacterial diseases, helminthiasis, **myasthenia gravis** [an autoimmune condition], **schizophrenia**, other diseases of the spinal cord, diseases of the esophagus and **peritonitis** were non-significantly elevated overall by all analyses…"

They conclude: "Poultry workers may have excess occurrence of disease affecting several organs and systems, probably originating from widespread infection with a variety of microorganisms." Is anyone surprised?

According to http://oshWikipedia.eu/Wikipedia/Work-related_skin_diseases, **occupational diseases** of butchers and other Meater workers include "**recurrent pyodermas** (folliculitis, furuncle, carbuncle, impetigo, ecthyma, paronychia, etc.), erysipelas," **milker's nodules** and **salami brusher's disease**. Got lots of animals, got lots of disease.

Toxicology is the study of poisons. The prime directive of toxicology is that "the dose makes the poison." So it makes sense that those who have the greatest exposure to animal poisons will be the most poisoned, whether by the viruses in the animals or the proteins of which animals are made or the incomplete combustion products of animals when they're smoked or cooked.

When we're amateur Meaters we poison ourselves less often than professional slaughterhouse workers, and with smaller cumulative doses.

Johnson et al provide the proof of animal toxicity: people like the Baltimore union poultry cohort, with the highest exposure to dead animals are among the most cancer- (and other disease-) packed people in the world. Virtually no one starts out life wanting to become a slaughterhouse worker. The consequences are horrific for these poor people, the Meatiest of all Meaters. (They're so sick, we should be asking them where they get their protein.)

When we're Meaters we kill not only the animals we eat, but the humans who prepare the dead animals for our eating pleasure.

Porcine endogenous retroviruses

There are cancer-causing viruses in pigs, some of which are common among other animals too, and some which are special to pigs. Hep E is one such oncogen. And, as with all poisons, those with the greatest exposure to these viruses are at the greatest risk of "disease" and death: hyper-Meaters such as meat packers and slaughterhouse disassembly line workers.

Pig consumption is also associated with increased dementia, such as Alzheimer's "disease". "Auto-immune attack triggered by the exposure to aerosolized brain" can cause "inflammatory neurological disease in workers" including "unrelenting seizures" and coma.

[See: http://nutritionfacts.org/video/eating-outside-the-kingdom/]

Poultry viruses

Three of the cancer-causing groups of viruses in chickens and turkeys, ducks and geese are avian leukosis/sarcoma viruses, reticuloendotheliosis viruses, and Marek's disease virus, and they're among the most powerful known oncogens. These bird viruses are also in the birds' eggs. Eggs should be boiled so hard they bounce, to make them virus-free (I almost said "safe to eat," but I caught myself in time – the virulence remains.)

Dear Meaters, you can forget sunny side up or over easy, forever. Just as bartenders should take car keys away from drunks, diner chefs should be legally bound to hard-boil eggs, if they serve them at all.

Eating chickens and their eggs is dangerous. For example, eating just a quarter of a chicken's breast a day doubles our risk of lymphoma and triples our risk of leukemia.

For more, see under: Oncogenic viruses

Rabies

Eating animals of different species is very much a cultural decision. Some people abhor eating pigs; others "dig on swine flesh." Some people eat primates as "bush meat"; others look upon sea life as the bush meat of the oceans. There was a big outcry in the UK recently about horses in the un-food supply, though Brits happily eat and drink cows. And we Westerners tend to frown on the eating of dogs and cats…

(Call me old-fashioned, but I *really* love animals, so I don't love eating any of them.)

Rabies is caused by a virus, and it's on the rise in parts of Asia. Eating rabies-laden cats and dogs can cause rabies in the people who eat the animals, particularly if the brains are under-done. One doesn't have to be bitten by a rabid dog to get rabies. Cat sushi is a no-no. I'd be suspicious of all street "food" and kebabs, if I were a Meater.

Reticuloendotheliosis virus

See under: Oncogenic viruses

Wart viruses

See under: Oncogenic viruses

Viruses – summary

Lies, lies, damned lies… and statistics.

Death statistics list the proximate cause of death, so if viruses cause diabetes or Alzheimer's or liver failure or cancer, and they do, the cause of death will probably be listed as diabetes or Alzheimer's or liver failure or cancer.

Under oncogenic viruses above, we saw that the more Meater we are, the more cancer we get, with slaughtered animals being a lethal occupational hazard for animal industry workers.

The viruses in animals are an under-recognized source of morbidity and mortality via both malignant and non-malignant "diseases" caused by Meating.

Viruses make Meating an occupational hazard for all humans.

~

Other pathogens – bacteria

Clostridium difficile

C. diff is a bacterium that *must* be in dead animals. Must? Yes. In Michael Greger's words:

> "*Clostridia* bacteria like *C. diff* comprise one of the main groups of bacteria involved in natural carcass degradation, and so by colonizing muscle tissue before death, *C. diff* can not only transmit to new hosts that eat the muscles, like us, but give them a head start on carcass break down."

[See: http://nutritionfacts.org/video/c-difficile-superbugs-in-meat/]

Just like the cadaverine and putrescine we met in Part 1A (Components), *C. diff* arises in response to an animal's death. It's also a fecal bacterium – it comes from the animal shit we eat.

The CDC lists *C. diff* as an Urgent Threat, one of only three organisms to achieve this highest threat level (higher than Serious and Concerning.) (CDC. *Antibiotic Resistance Threats in the United States*, 2013, p. 7.)

Here's the image and text on p. 51 of this CDC publication:

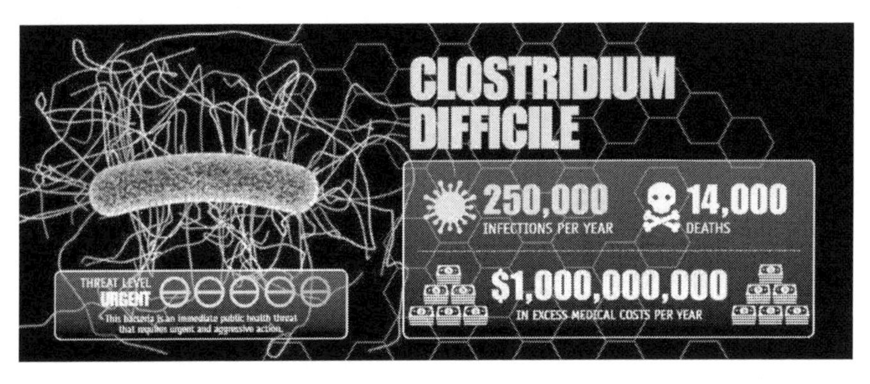

CDC. *Antibiotic Resistance Threats in the United States*, 2013.

"*Clostridium difficile* (*C. difficile*) causes life-threatening diarrhea. These infections mostly occur in **people who have had both recent medical care and antibiotics**. Often, *C. difficile* infections occur in hospitalized or recently hospitalized patients.

Resistance of Concern

- Although resistance to the antibiotics used to treat *C. difficile* infections is not yet a problem, **the bacteria spreads rapidly because it is naturally resistant to many drugs used to treat other infections.**
- In 2000, a stronger strain of the bacteria emerged. This strain is resistant to fluoroquinolone antibiotics, which are commonly used to treat other infections.
- This strain has spread throughout North America and Europe, infecting and killing more people wherever it spreads.

Public Health Threat

- **250,000 infections** per year requiring hospitalization or affecting already hospitalized patients.
- **14,000 deaths** per year.
- At least **$1 billion** in excess medical costs per year.
- Deaths related to C. difficile increased 400% between 2000 and 2007, in part because of a stronger bacteria strain that emerged.
- Almost half of infections occur in people younger than 65, but more than 90% of deaths occur in people 65 and older.
- About half of *C. difficile* infections first show symptoms in hospitalized or recently hospitalized patients, and half first show symptoms in nursing home patients or in people recently cared for in doctors' offices and clinics."

I'll dispute this last claim presently...

C. diff is one of a new tribe of bacteria known as "superbugs" that are becoming resistant to our most powerful antibiotics. Once found mainly in places where antibiotics are most-often used – animal industry and hospitals – drug-resistant strains of *C. diff* are now becoming widespread in the "food" supply, with ground-up turkeys, and chickens being the most contaminated.

C. diff usually has no effect on our intestines (which is good, considering their role as undertakers), but if our gut flora become deranged, most commonly by antibiotic use (see above) and by Meating, an infection called **pseudomembranous colitis** can arise, and, if unchecked, may morph into deadly **toxic megacolon**. Little can be done for those with toxic megacolon, infected with a drug-resistant strain of *C. diff*, except possible surgical removal of the infected colon.

(When it comes to destroying our beneficial gut bacteria, eating animals is the equivalent of taking antibiotics.

Anti- = against; bios = Greek for 'life.' Eating animals = anti-life.)

C. diff is highly resistant to both heat and chemicals, and its spores are easily transferred, which gives those of us who don't eat animals good reason not to want to touch those who do.

Under Fighting the Spread of Resistance, we find What CDC Is Doing. They say they're:

- "Tracking and reporting national progress toward preventing *C. difficile* infections.
- Promoting *C. difficile* prevention programs and providing gold-standard patient safety recommendations. [!!]
- Providing prevention expertise, as well as outbreak and laboratory assistance, to health departments and healthcare facilities."

I find that strange. Here's what I would have liked to have seen from a science-based CDC that's fighting the spread of resistance and providing "prevention expertise":

- Mounting education programs to teach animal agriculturalists to decrease antibiotic use.
- Lobbying Congress to pass stricter limits on antimicrobial drug use by Big Animal and Club Medical.
- Mounting grassroots Planter nutrition education programs to show the benefits of reduced *C. diff* intake.

My three recommendations would begin the "urgent and aggressive action" the CDC says is necessary to contain this top-level public health threat. Sadly, the CDC is too politicized an organization to make sound scientific recommendations, so we get wishy-washy bureaucratese instead...

Anyway, it appears that the CDC may be wrong about their half and half stats. Remember? They said earlier: "about half of *C. difficile* infections first show symptoms in hospitalized or recently hospitalized patients, and half first show symptoms in nursing home patients or in people recently cared for in doctors' offices and clinics."
They're saying: We're Meaters and we don't know why people come to health care facilities and then get sick. Yet Planters know why.

(D W Eyre, M L Cule, D J Wilson, D Griffiths, A Vaughan, L O'Connor, C L Ip, T Golubchik, E M Batty, J M Finney, D H Wyllie, X Didelot, K E Dingle, R M Harding, D W Crook, M H Wilcox, T E Peto, A S Walker. Diverse sources of *C. difficile* infection identified on whole-genome sequencing. *N Engl J Med.* 2013 Sep 26;369(13):1195-205.)

This 2013 paper says that therapeutic settings are involved only a third of the time: "In conclusion, we found that the transmission of *C. difficile* infection from symptomatic patients accounted for slightly more than a third of such cases in a region with a typical incidence of infection, which suggests that many cases arise from genetically diverse sources."

Eyre et al continue: "Over a 3-year period, 45% of *C. difficile* cases in Oxfordshire were genetically distinct from all previous cases [not from iatrogenic or healthcare causes]… Person-to-person transmission of *C. difficile* infection and surrounding contamination have been well documented. However, there are multiple other potential sources, including patients with asymptomatic colonization and sources in the wider environment, such as **water, farm animals or pets, and food**."

Finally… the Eatiology. It's not in the chickpeas and papayas; it's in the chickens and pigs. It's in more than 40% of the US animal supply.

Meating is what's causing the endemic spread of the drug resistance of *C. diff* and other microbes. Meating works on two fronts: first, Meater farmers stuff their animals full of antibiotics, allowing surviving generations to build up drug immunity, and then the animals spread the bacteria throughout the populace in their flesh.

And then Meater physicians cause more problems when they overprescribe the antibiotics that derange our beneficial gut flora, thus allowing *C. diff* to run amok. That's why the old belief persists that "half of *C. difficile* infections first show symptoms in" hospitals, and half in nursing homes, doctors' offices and clinics. It's not brain surgery.

Only by telling the public to (1) stop the prophylactic over-use of antibiotics in animals and (2) to stop eating animals (or at least to cut back radically), the CDC will never be able to provide the "gold-standard patient safety recommendations" they're deluded enough to think they're dispensing.

Enterococcus

Much of what I've said about *C. diff* applies to *Enterococcus* too, though the main dietary reservoir of *Enterococcus* is turkeys, rather than pigs. 90% of the turkeys we eat in the USA are contaminated with this potentially drug-of-last-resort-resistant bacterium.

VANCOMYCIN-RESISTANT
ENTEROCOCCUS (VRE)
20,000
DRUG-RESISTANT ENTEROCOCCUS INFECTIONS
1,300
DEATHS FROM DRUG-RESISTANT ENTEROCOCCUS INFECTIONS
66,000
ENTEROCOCCUS INFECTIONS PER YEAR
SOME ENTEROCOCCUS STRAINS ARE RESISTANT TO VANCOMYCIN
LEAVING FEW OR NO TREATMENT OPTIONS
THREAT LEVEL
SERIOUS

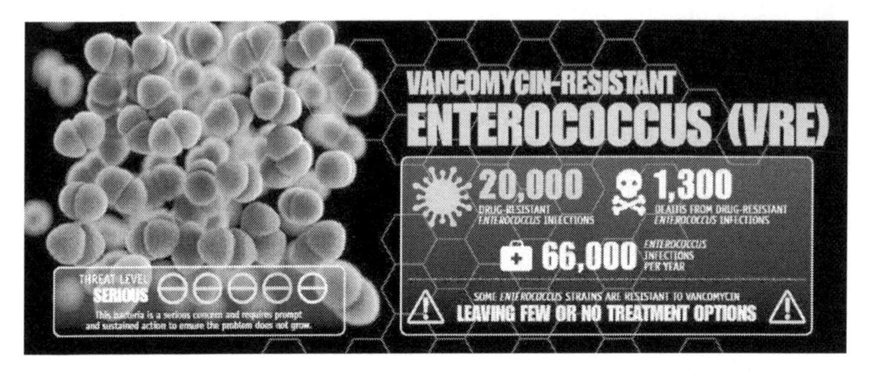

CDC. *Enterococcus*

This graphic is from p. 67 of the CDC's *Antibiotic Resistance Threats in the USA*, 2013.

The CDC says: "*Enterococci* cause a range of illnesses, mostly among patients receiving healthcare, but include bloodstream infections, surgical site infections, and urinary tract infections."

That bit about UTIs is interesting, and we'll come back to it. Remember: *E. coli* bacteria that cause UTIs may also be causing thousands of deaths extra-intestinally.

"Resistance of Concern

- *Enterococcus* often cause infections among very sick patients in hospitals and other healthcare-settings.
- Some *Enterococcus* strains are resistant to vancomycin, an antibiotic of last resort, leaving few or no treatment options.
- About 20,000 (or 30%) of *Enterococcus* healthcare-associated infections are vancomycin resistant.

Public Health Threat
An estimated 66,000 healthcare-associated Enterococcus infections occur in the United States each year. The proportion of infections that occur with a vancomycin resistant strain differs by the species of *Enterococcus*; overall 20,000 vancomycin-resistant infections occurred among hospitalized patients each year, with approximately 1,300 deaths attributed to these infections."

Here's what happens. Patients who're in hospitals are given antibiotics to combat a microbial threat. (And where did that microbe come from? 90% of the time, from Meating!) The antibiotics destroy our beneficial gut bacteria. Other less-friendly bacteria then take over, causing sepsis and other ill-effects. These other bacteria may be *C. diff* or *Enterococcus*, or any of the other usual "healthcare setting" suspects. They've been there all along, lying doggo, and it's the destruction of their friendly gut flora controllers that allows them to multiply unchecked.

The *Enterococci* aren't introduced into hospital patients – they were always there, just made to behave by a healthy gut flora. Now, what's a healthy gut flora? It's a gut flora fed on *tons* of fiber over the years, allowing the production of butyrate and propionate and other beneficial Planter substances. (See: Deranged Gut Flora)

So where did the *Enterococcus* and *C. diff* come from originally? They came from Meating. They're in the animals we eat; *Entero* particularly in **turkeys**, both *E. faecium* and *E. faecalis*, but also in other Meatertainments. They're fecal bacteria, for crying out loud – they're animal shit-borne bacteria.

The CDC said above: "*Enterococcus* often cause infections among very sick patients in hospitals and other healthcare-settings."

That's just plain wrong.

The *Enterococcus* infections in healthcare settings happen when patients swallow prescribed antibiotics (such as the vancomycin to which *Entero* is fast becoming accustomed) and they wipe out the bacteria that suppress *Enterococcus*. No antibiotics; no *Enterococcus* bloom; no resulting E-infection.

The more we use antibiotics, the less useful they become. The more we use antibiotics today, the less we'll be able to use them in the future. And, as we see with health-care related *Enterococcus* and *C. diff* infections, sometimes the more we use antibiotics to combat one microbe, the more deaths we cause via another.

The best way not to be among the 1,300 *Enterococcus* infection deaths each year is not to require antibiotics that will cause *Enterococcus* infection. We do this best by cutting our total bacterial load to a minimum by NOT EATING ANIMALS.

Am I shouting loud enough for you to hear me, dear CDC? Meating causes a whole host of fecal bacterial infections, and using antibiotics to combat them may cause other bacterial infections instead. It's like pressing down on a bad water bed: it rises somewhere else.

It's rare to eat plants that are contaminated with fecal bacteria such as *E. coli*, *Enterococcus* and *C. diff*; and then it only happens when animal feces have been added to the plants.

In contrast, it's rare to be able to eat animals that *aren't* covered in shit – not on the macroscopic level, but where it counts: on and in the flesh and liquids of the animals we eat, microscopically. Meaters eat these pathogens by the billion every day without seeing a single one. That doesn't mean they aren't there.

Planting → low intake of pathogenic bacteria → little need for antibiotics → little chance of gut flora disturbance → low chance of overgrowth with other pathogens → tiny chance of sepsis. Plus Planting promotes the optimal fiber-eating gut flora to begin with.

The CDC is limited in the good it can do by its Meater bias and its lack of Planter insight.

Postscript – not on the same page, or even in the same book?
Interestingly, on April 22, 2013, the FDA published the following: FDA Cautions in Interpretation of Antimicrobial Resistance Data (http://www.fda.gov/AnimalVeterinary/NewsEvents/CVMUpdates/ucm348794.htm)

They say: "Recently, the Environmental Working Group issued a report of its interpretation of the 2011 Retail Meat Annual Report of the National Antimicrobial Resistance Monitoring System (NARMS). **While FDA is always concerned when we see antimicrobial resistance** [actions would speak louder than words], we believe the EWG report oversimplifies the NARMS data and provides misleading conclusions. We do not believe that EWG fully considered important factors that put these results in context, including:

• whether the bacterium is a foodborne pathogen. The report highlights resistance to ***Enterococcus***, but this is **not considered a major foodborne pathogen**. Instead, we include it because its behavior is helpful in understanding how resistance occurs."

Yipes. While the CDC's telling us *Enterococcus* is killing thirteen hundred people a year, and others are telling us that 90% of retail turkeys are *Enterococcus*-positive, the FDA's singing 'Don't worry, be happy.'

What does FDA stand for again? Oh yeah, Food and Drug Administration. This troupe of clown is aces at pushing drugs, but they seem to know diddlysquat about food. It's time that these two mutually exclusive, even antagonistic, programs were separated.

We're all in dire need of a Food Administration, to keep us safe from the predations of Big "Food," Big Farmer, Big Pharma, Big Chemical and Big Pork Barrel government.

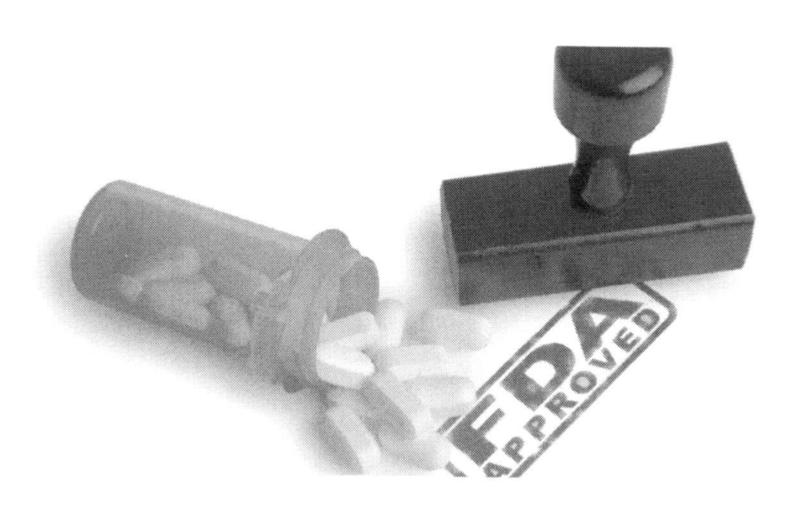

Image: Huffington Post
http://www.huffingtonpost.com/peterschwartz/what-if-we-had-no-fda_b_8732988.html

Fecal bacteria

Fecal bacteria is a general term for the bacteria which are in animal shit. Transmission of fecal bacteria usually happens via the 'fecal-oral' route – via what we eat and drink. It can be in the water we drink, but most often it's in the "food" we eat. *E. coli* is the bellwether for animal feces bacteria, and between about 70 and 90% of the animals we eat are contaminated with *E. coli.*

Proteus mirabilis

For those of us who've ever wondered why women are more prone to getting rheumatoid arthritis than men, here's one good explanation: higher chicken consumption and more frequent urinary tract infections.

It goes like this. As we saw earlier, several strains of *E. coli* bacteria that cause UTIs get into us via the animals we eat, particularly chickens. Another animal fecal bacterium we get by Meating is called *Proteus mirabilis.* It appears to provoke an auto immune response via molecular mimicry, fooling our bodies into attacking our own joints, causing inflammation, pain, stiffness: a crippling, disfiguring non-disease caused by the Meater eating disorder.

As previously mentioned, the mechanism is similar to the way strep throat infections can lead to damage of our kids' heart valves in rheumatic fever.

Staphylococcus aureus **and MRSA (Methicillin-resistant *Staphylococcus aureus*)**

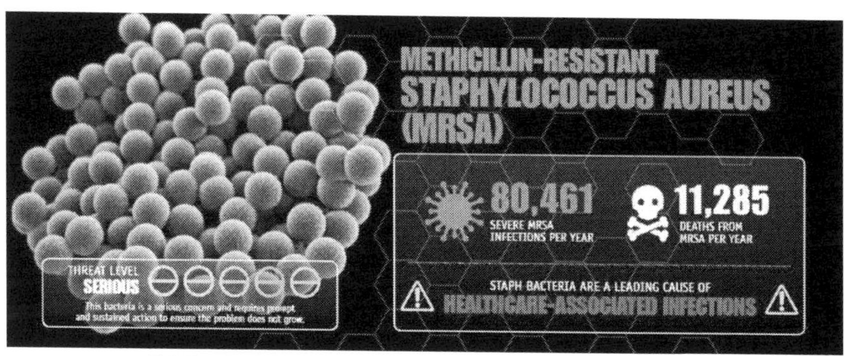

CDC: *Antibiotic Resistance Threats in the United States*, p. 77

There's staph… and then there's *staph*… the antibiotic-resistant kind.

Waters AE, Contente-Cuomo T, Buchhagen J, Liu CM, Watson L, Pearce K, Foster JT, Bowers J, Driebe EM, Engelthaler DM, Keim PS, Price LB. Multidrug-Resistant *Staphylococcus aureus* in US Meat and Poultry. *Clin Infect Dis*. 2011 May;52(10):1227-30.

"*Staphylococcus aureus* is **among the most prevalent causes of clinical infections globally** and has garnered substantial public attention due to **increasing mortality associated with multidrug resistance**. A **new multidrug-resistant *S. aureus* strain, ST398**, has emerged that **predominantly colonizes people working in food animal production**. First discovered in 2003, ST398 now makes up a **substantial proportion of the community-acquired methicillin-resistant *S. aureus* (MRSA) cases** in the Netherlands. Multiple studies have demonstrated the high prevalence of multidrug-resistant *S. aureus*, including ST398, among **intensively raised swine** in the European Union, Canada, and the **United States**, but few studies have been conducted to measure its prevalence in US food products.

In the current study, we evaluated the prevalence and antibiotic susceptibility profiles of *S. aureus* in retail meat and poultry samples from 5 US cities. We found that ***S. aureus* contamination was common among the samples** and that distinct *S. aureus* populations were associated with each meat and poultry type. We further demonstrated the **prevalence of multidrug resistance**, including resistance to clinically important antibiotics such as ciprofloxacin, quinupristin/dalfopristin, clindamycin, erythromycin, oxacillin, and daptomycin."

What more do we need to know? Potentially lethal *Staph aureus* is in the animals. We feed the animals antibiotics, which make the bacteria immune to the antibiotics. We eat the animals full of drug-resistant bacteria, which makes us need to take antibiotics. But the antibiotics no longer work well, because we've fed them to the animals, which we eat, and they're full of the bacteria that are now immune to our antibiotics, so we need to come up with more powerful antibiotics, which we feed to the animals, which we eat… Do we not see how crazy this is?

How lethal is *staph* infection? Methicillin- (or multidrug-) resistant *Staph aureus* strikes 11,285 times a year, according to the CDC:

As we've seen with other drug-resistant species of bacteria, according to CDC's *Antibiotic Resistance Threats in the United States*, 2013, pp. 77-8:

"Severe MRSA infections mostly occur during or soon after **inpatient medical care**." [This information appears three times on the same page, so they must believe it. Perhaps this belief is so strong, they can't see beyond it?]

"Methicillin-resistant *Staphylococcus aureus* (MRSA) causes a range of illnesses, from **skin and wound infections** to **pneumonia** and **bloodstream infections** that can cause **sepsis** and **death**. *Staph* bacteria, including MRSA, are one of the most common causes of healthcare-associated infections."

Commentary

Round and round the circle goes. Where it'll stop nobody knows.

Bacteria get into us from the external environment. At least 80% of our interaction with the environment comes from what we eat. At least 90% of all dietary bacterial infections come from eating animals; Planting supplying less than 10%, and even less when un-cross-contaminated with animal shit. Meating is therefore our greatest source of bacterial infection, by a country mile.

Meating is also our greatest source of antibacterial resistance – Big Animal uses antibiotics by the thousands of tons, while Club Medical uses them to a lesser extent. So, when we're Meaters who land up in hospital (which we do far more often than when we're Planters), we've already have tribes of potentially lethal bacteria living in our colons, such as *E. coli* (from animal shit, in general), *C. diff* (from pigs et al), *Enterococcus* (from turkeys et al) and *Staphylococcus* (from pigs et al), and these bacteria are barely being kept in check by our fiber-deprived, less-than-optimal gut flora.

Well-meaning physicians may then prescribe antibiotics to us to combat an entirely different microbe, let's say pneumococcal pneumonia, thereby also wiping out the friendly bacteria that are subduing our many sub-clinical bacterial infections. Like the right water temperature causing an algae bloom or red tide in the oceans, the conditions become iatrogenically (doctor-created) perfect for an often-resistant strain of bacteria to flourish.

The primary reservoir of infectious microbes isn't the healthcare setting (where even the most draconian hygiene measures can't eradicate them); they're in the patient, waiting for the healthcare genie to polish the infection lamp with antibiotics and let them out.

"Resistance of Concern
Resistance to methicillin and related antibiotics (e.g., nafcillin, oxacillin) and resistance to cephalosporins are of concern.

Public Health Threat
CDC estimates 80,461 invasive MRSA infections and **11,285 related deaths** occurred in 2011. An unknown but much higher number of less severe infections occurred in both the community and in healthcare settings."

[Infections in the community are directly Meater-related, while those in healthcare settings are indirectly Meater-related, as described above. That's a lot of "food" poisoning deaths that go uncounted; unattributed to Meater mal-nutrition.]

"Fighting the Spread of Resistance
Although still a common and severe threat to patients, invasive MRSA infections in healthcare settings appear to be declining. Between 2005 and 2011 overall rates of invasive MRSA dropped 31%; the largest declines (54%) were observed among infections occurring during hospitalization.

Success began with preventing central-line associated bloodstream infections with MRSA, where rates fell nearly 50% from 1997 to 2007. [Good news.] **During the past decade, rates of MRSA infections have**

increased rapidly among the general population (people who have not recently received care in a healthcare setting)."

"During the past decade, rates of MRSA infections have increased rapidly among the general population" because, as Waters et al demonstrated above, *Staph* is entrenched in the "food" supply now.

CAFOs (Concentrated Animal Feeding Operations) are so vile that MRSA is concentrated in the very air we breathe when we venture too close to some pig concentration/extermination camps. If it's in the air, it's definitely concentrated in the animals we eat. Strains that are resistant to our top-of-the-line antibiotics are in the chunks of pig, cow, chicken and turkey we put on our plates. MRSA is in at least 1 in 9 American pigs, with other species infected to a lesser extent. Maybe that's something we should concentrate on.

Animal agriculture makes the bacteria drug-resistant, and then serves up mega-doses of the bacteria for people to eat. MRSA is a zoönosis, able to move from non-human into human animals. It's not rocket science, people. Dr. Michael Greger says that MRSA is "now killing more Americans than AIDS every year in the United States."

[See: http://nutritionfacts.org/video/airborne-mrsa/]

According to www.cdc.gov/hiv/statistics/basics/ataglance.html, "An estimated **13,712 people with an AIDS diagnosis died in 2012**, and approximately 658,507 people in the United States with an AIDS diagnosis have died overall."

Dr. Greger may have access to better information than I do. Still, it's pretty darn close. AIDS and MRSA are two acronyms we don't want to die from. Both are preventable; MRSA largely by cutting animals out of our diet.

Antibiotic/Antimicrobial Resistance

According to the CDC (http://www.cdc.gov/drugresistance/index.html):

"Antibiotics and similar drugs, together called antimicrobial agents, have been used for the last 70 years to treat patients who have infectious diseases. Since the 1940s, these drugs have greatly reduced illness and death from infectious diseases. However, these drugs have been used so widely and for so long that **the infectious organisms the antibiotics are designed to kill have adapted to them, making the drugs less effective**."

"Each year in the United States, at least **2 million people become infected with bacteria that are resistant to antibiotics** and at least **23,000 people die each year** as a direct result of these infections."

It's my contention that most of these 23,000 deaths are caused by Meating.

Pretty much all that needs to be said about the danger of increased microbial resistance to antibiotics is this: Meating leads to drug resistance… Meater agriculture, Meater nutrition and Meater medicine.

According to the CDC, here's how it happens:

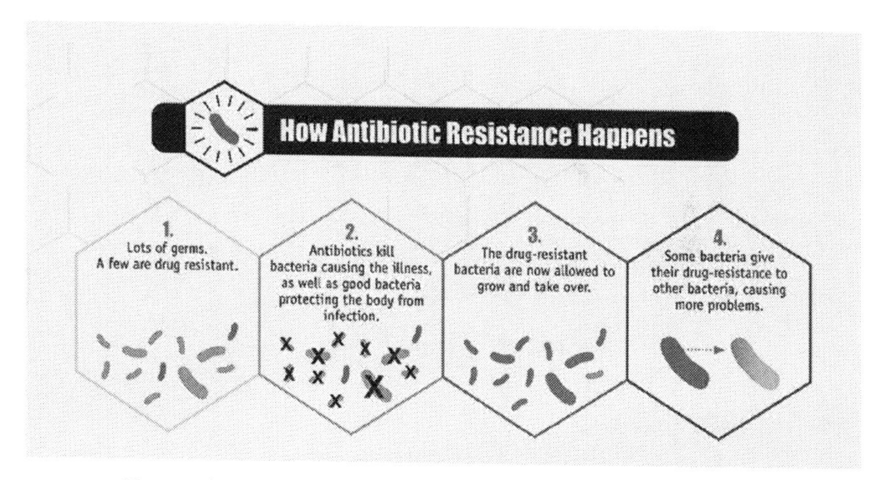

How antibiotic resistance happens. www.cdc.gov/drugresistance

Antibiotic resistance isn't quite that simple, so I'll amplify a little…

Our present societal-scale desire to eat animals can only be satisfied by industrial-scale animal dismemberment operations. Industrial Meating is only possible because of massive applications of antimicrobial drugs.

Continued massive applications of veterinary drugs will create industrial- and societal-scale medical drug resistance. Industrial-scale Meater drug resistance will lead inevitably to the loss of most, if not all antibiotics.

The loss of antibiotics will lead to increased morbidity and mortality in humans, reversing history's arrow and creating a post-antibiotic era of mega-death due to infection (just like the pre-antibiotic era, except without the hope of salvation). Many surgeries, now routine, will become impossible because of sepsis. Modern industrial medicine will cease to function, and human societies will decline… (unless we start Planting on a massive scale.)

All for the want of a horse shoe nail… Humanity, deluded into thinking animals are food, is Meating itself quickly and surely to death.

The good news is that if we accept Planting's innate healing, and couple Planting to our bodies' own enormous ability for self-healing, then rapid and beautiful blessings flow down on us automatically.

In her keynote address at the conference on "Combating antimicrobial resistance: time for action" in Copenhagen on 14 March 2012, Dr Margaret Chan, Director-General of the World Health Organization, spoke out about "Antimicrobial resistance in the European Union and the world."

Dr. Chan called drug-resistant pathogens "a serious, growing, and **global threat to health**."

She said: "The EU has its eyes wide open to the problem. This is readily seen in the number of recent policies, directives, technical reports, strategies, and regulatory decisions designed to **reduce antibiotic consumption, in humans and animals**, ensure the prudent use of these **fragile medicines**, and protect specific agents that are **critically important for human medicine**."

Please listen carefully: "fragile medicines… critically important for human medicine." The D-G of WHO isn't prone to exaggeration. Her measured tones are the equivalent of the rest of us running down the road like Chuck Heston shouting hysterically: "Soylent Green is people!" We have a small garret window of opportunity to avert a human catastrophe every bit as perilous as climate change, and one which climate change will only make worse, as pathogens extend both their virulence and their range (to greater latitudes and to higher altitudes).

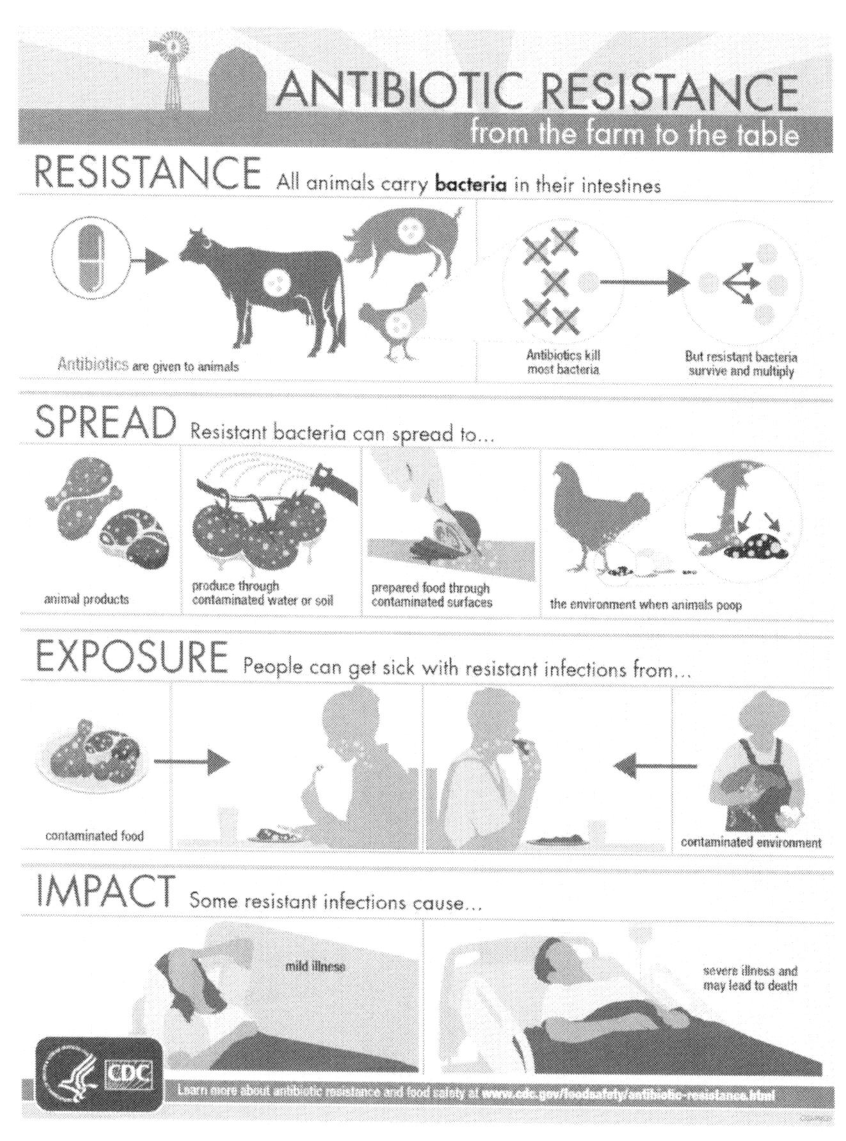

From the CDC: How antibiotics select for resistance http://www.cdc.gov/media/pdf/dpk/dpk-antibiotics-week/antibiotic-resistance-farm-to-table.pdf

Dr. Chan said: "Worldwide, the fact that **greater quantities of antibiotics are used in healthy animals than in unhealthy humans** is a cause for great concern." That's the nub of the issue: animals are dosed with antibiotics to promote the growth of healthy animals (and to prevent symptom-free animals succumbing to hideous CAFO conditions). Every present use of antibiotics in animals is contributing to future human deaths.

"In particular, Denmark has tackled the problem of antibiotic use in food-producing animals in a pioneering way. Recognizing the potential for a **health crisis**, this country progressively **ended the administration of antibiotics as growth-promoters** [still legal in the US] in the late 1990s, well before the EU-wide ban.

[On 8 September 2015 I read at http://organicveganearth.com/ that "The Danish government has announced that it will convert the entire country's agriculture into organic and sustainable farming, making it the first country in the world to become 100% organic." Russia subsequently announced that they're outlawing GM crops. May Monsanto rot in hell.]

An international review panel, set up by WHO at the request of the Danish government, concluded that **the ban reduced human health risks without significantly harming animal health or farmers' incomes**.

In fact, Danish government and industry data showed that **livestock and poultry production actually increased** following the ban, while antibiotic resistance on farms and in meat declined.

What began as the Danish "experiment" became the Danish "model"."

The Danish model = no antibiotics used prophylactically on animals (i.e. only as needed) → improved animal health and productivity + reduced human health risks **+ increased income to farmers.**

It shouldn't be what makes the difference, but the profit factor is absolutely vital. Animal farmers make more money when they stop dosing their herds, both because of reduced inputs and increased yields.

Clearly, as the world's greatest health authority shows, a win-win-win situation arises when we stop feeding antibiotics to animals – animals, humans and animal farmers all benefit. (Yes, of course, there'd be a winnest-winnest-winnest situation if animal slaughter stopped altogether.)

Dr. Chan said that "...pathogens are developing resistance to multiple drugs, some to nearly all. Hospitals have become hotbeds for highly-resistant pathogens, like MRSA, ESBL [Extended Spectrum B-lactamase producing *Enterobacteriaceae*], and CPE [Carbapenemase-producing *Enterobacteriaceae*], increasing **the risk that hospitalization kills instead of**

cures. These are **end-of-the-road pathogens** that are **resistant to last-line antimicrobials**.

If current trends continue unabated, the future is easy to predict. Some experts say we are moving back to the pre-antibiotic era. No. This will be a **post-antibiotic era**. In terms of **new replacement antibiotics, the pipeline is virtually dry**, especially for gram-negative bacteria. **The cupboard is nearly bare**."

You know, if I were an American public health official, my hair would stand up on end, all over my body, when I heard those words. I'd be electrified – galvanized – into action, driven to ban the use of antibiotics in symptom-free cattle in the USA.

As Dr. Esselstyn says: "Now is the time for heroic – legendary – work!"

The European Centre for Disease Prevention and Control, or ECDC, is on top of the situation. The CDC in the US? The FDA and the USDA? Not so much. Entrenched Meater special interest groups control the levers of power in the USA, and these corporates are too short-sightedly greedy and too set in their ways to realize that their present Meater practices are both less profitable and, ultimately, unsustainable, and, with a high degree of probability, humanicidal.

American Meaters, in particular, suffer from what Dr. Chan calls an "inability to combat the gross misuse of these medicines… A post-antibiotic era means, in effect, **an end to modern medicine** as we know it. **Things as common as strep throat or a child's scratched knee could once again kill**.

Some sophisticated interventions, like hip replacements, organ transplants, cancer chemotherapy, and **care of preterm infants** [!], would become far more difficult or even too dangerous to undertake. At a time of multiple calamities in the world, we cannot allow the loss of **essential antimicrobials, essential cures** for **many millions of people**, to become the next **global crisis**."

This is what Meating's doing to us all; the future that Meaterialism's mandating. We need to start behaving as if we give a shit about our children and our children's children, because they're the ones who'll be bearing the post-antibiotic and climate-changed brunt of our societal Meating disorder.

For the sake of our future loved ones, we need to stop eating animals. Now.

Bacteria – summary

We spent a long time looking at the CDC's numbers for pathogenic illnesses, hospitalizations and deaths. The CDC says that they've underestimated those numbers, by perhaps a factor of 5. Instead of ten thousand illnesses caused by "food" poisoning, they think perhaps 50,000.

Well, I think I've shown good evidence that the CDC is, like little Georgie Bush, mis-under-estimating its under-estimation. Considerably.

Using the CDC's own numbers just for *C. diff*, *Enterococcus* and *Staphylococcus* infections – all of which have a very strong dietary component – we get the following:

	Infections	Deaths
C. diff	250,000	14,000
Enterococcus	66,000	1,300
Staph (MRSA only)	80,461	11,285
Total:	396,461	26,585

It turns out that these 3 bacteria, not included in the CDC's top 31 "food" poisoners, may account for up to forty times more illnesses and up to 20 times more deaths than the top 31. Even in the highly unlikely event of Meating causing only 10% of the "disease" burden from *C. diff*, *Enterococcus* and MRSA, that's still four times and double what the CDC accounts for.

Eating animals is a fundamentally dis-understood cause of disease and death from non-food poisoning.

So why aren't *C. diff*, *enterococcus* and *staph* included among the 31 foodborne pathogens of concern? My guess is that Meaters just don't see what a dangerous, filthy habit Meating is. (Forgive them, Lord, for they know not what they do.) How can Meaters be self-critical of Meating? It's an unconscious addiction that breeds unconsciousness.

Of course, publicizing *34* pathogens that kill us when we eat them might mean admitting that eating the animals (which we mistakenly think of as food) kills tens of thousands of Americans each year with their inescapable xeno-pathogens. (As well as with their inescapable inherent endo-pathogens – animal proteins, animal fats, animal cholesterol etc. etc. etc. etc. etc… so exhaustively covered in Part 1A (Components).)

This reminds me of the >100,000 American deaths from ADRs (adverse drug reactions) that prescription drugs cause each year. We swallowed what we were told, but they killed us. Same with "food": we swallowed what we were told – animals – but they killed us. Swallowed… hook, line and sinker.

(Incidentally, "iatrogenic deaths," medical errors and ADRs are NOT listed as causes of death in the US's official mortality statistics… almost 200,000 of them a year, out of about 2.5 million deaths. That's a number substantial enough to make the rest of the statistics questionable.)

Because of their toxic bacterial load, animals aren't food.

Now let's take a look at some gruesome animal parasites.

Some general information about animal-borne parasites

Seeing as some of us are going to come into close contact with them after Meating them, let's start off with a little more background detail on parasites. Here's the CDC (www.cdc.gov/parasites/food.html) on Parasites, some of whom we've already met. I've highlighted the newcomers:

"Numerous parasites can be transmitted by food [read: animals] including many protozoa and helminths [parasitic worms and flukes]. In the United States, the most common foodborne parasites are protozoa such as *Cryptosporidium* spp., *Giardia intestinalis*, *Cyclospora cayetanensis*, and *Toxoplasma gondii*; **roundworms** such as ***Trichinella*** spp. and ***Anisakis*** spp.; and **tapeworms** such as ***Diphyllobothrium*** spp. and ***Taenia*** spp.

Many of these organisms **can also be transmitted by water, soil, or person-to-person** contact. Occasionally in the U.S., but **often in developing countries**, a wide variety of **helminthic roundworms, tapeworms, and flukes are transmitted in foods** such as

- undercooked **fish, crabs, and mollusks**;
- **undercooked meat**; **raw aquatic plants** such as watercress;
- raw vegetables that have been **contaminated by human or animal feces**;

Some foods are contaminated by food service workers who practice **poor hygiene** or who work in unsanitary facilities.

Helminthic infections can cause abdominal pain, diarrhea, muscle pain, cough, skin lesions, malnutrition, weight loss, neurological and many other symptoms depending on the particular organism and burden of infection."

Helminthic Parasites

According to http://parasite.org.au/para-site/contents/helminth-intoduction.html:

"The word 'helminth' is a general term meaning 'worm'… Many helminths are free-living organisms in aquatic and terrestrial environments whereas others occur as parasites in most animals and some plants. **Parasitic helminths are an almost universal feature of vertebrate animals**; most species have worms in them somewhere.

Biodiversity

Three major assemblages of parasitic helminths are recognized: the Nemathelminthes (nematodes, or round worms) and the Platyhelminthes (flatworms), the latter being subdivided into the Cestoda (tapeworms) and the Trematoda (flukes):

Nematodes (roundworms) have long thin unsegmented tube-like bodies with anterior mouths and longitudinal digestive tracts. Worms use longitudinal muscles to produce a sideways thrashing motion. Adult worms form separate sexes with well-developed reproductive systems.

Cestodes (tapeworms) have long flat ribbon-like bodies with a single anterior holdfast organ (scolex) and numerous segments. Segments exhibit slow body flexion produced by longitudinal and transverse muscles. All tapeworms are hermaphroditic and each segment contains both male and female organs.

Trematodes (flukes) have small flat leaf-like bodies with oral and ventral suckers and a blind sac-like gut… They exhibit elaborate gliding or creeping motion over substrates using compact 3-D arrays of muscles. Most species are hermaphroditic (individuals with male and female reproductive systems) although some blood flukes form separate male and female adults."

Worms and flukes are in the animals we eat, and then they take up residence within us. A disease caused by a particular parasite is usually indicated by adding the suffix –sis to the species name; the prefix neuro- lets us know the parasite is living in our brain, e.g. neurocysticercosis = tapeworm larvae in our brains, usually a result of eating pigs.

"Unlike other pathogens (viruses, bacteria, protozoa and fungi), helminths do not proliferate within their hosts. Worms grow, moult, mature and then produce offspring which are voided from the host to infect new hosts. Worm burdens in individual hosts (and often the severity of infection) are therefore dependent on intake (number of infective stages taken up).

Worms develop slowly compared to other infectious pathogens so any resultant diseases are slow in onset and chronic in nature. Although most helminth infections are well tolerated by their hosts and are often asymptomatic, subclinical infections have been associated with significant loss of condition in infected hosts.

Other helminths cause serious clinical diseases characterized by high morbidity and mortality. Clinical signs of infection vary considerably depending on the site and duration of infection. Larval and adult nematodes lodge, migrate or encyst within tissues resulting in obstruction, inflammation, oedema, anaemia, lesions and granuloma formation. Infections by adult cestodes are generally benign as they are not invasive, but the larval stages penetrate and encyst within tissues leading to inflammation, space-occupying lesions and organ malfunction.

Adult flukes usually cause obstruction, inflammation and fibrosis in tubular organs, but the eggs of blood flukes can lodge in tissues causing extensive granulomatous reactions and hypertension."

It's fascinating to know more about the micro-fauna who're eating us after we've eaten the macro-fauna that host them.

~

Other pathogens – parasites

Roundworms [nematodes]

Anisakis spp.

According to the CDC, "Anisakiasis is a parasitic disease caused by anisakid nematodes (worms) that can invade the stomach wall or intestine of humans. The transmission of this disease occurs when infective larvae are ingested from **fish or squid** that humans eat raw or undercooked. In some cases, this infection is treated by removal of the larvae via **endoscopy or surgery**." (http://www.cdc.gov/parasites/anisakiasis/) What they're not saying is that some susceptible people have an allergic reaction to cooked anisakis worms too. They're in 2/3 fishes in the US.

As Michael Greger says:

> "…we're finding some people that are "allergic" to fish really aren't; they're allergic to the dead worms in the fish. In fact, because we feed fishmeal to chickens, you can have an allergic reaction to a parasitic fish worm and not even eat fish at all!"

He continues:

> "Anisakis worms are found particularly in cod, anchovies, and squid, and can also cause **chronic hives** and **intractable chronic itching**. Because of these worms, researchers recommend people stop eating seafood sushi altogether because besides inducing allergenic reactions, the worms may cause a **leaky gut syndrome**, which often is unrecognized and it can predispose to other, more important pathologies than just being itchy all over."

[See: http://nutritionfacts.org/video/tick-bites-meat-allergies-and-chronic-urticaria/]

Gnathostomiasis & Neurognathostomiasis

Gnathostomiasis is another problem caused by eating raw or undercooked fishes: worms that tunnel around under our skin. They cause skin swellings and open sores which move as they move – disconcertingly, we can watch them at work. Neurognathostomiasis is when the worms wriggle into our brains, via our nerves. They sometimes also get into our eyes. Symptoms include agonizing pain, intracranial bleeding, paralysis and death. Treatment is by surgery.

Linguatula serrata* and *Armillifer arminilatus

Per www.fhi.no/dav/6a12e57215.pdf, *L. serrata* and *A. arminilatus* "belong to the *Pentastomida*, a group of **worm-like, bloodsucking parasites**… Dogs and other canines are the main definitive hosts while most herbivores, including ruminants, serve as intermediate hosts. The parasites inhabit the upper respiratory tract of terrestrial, carnivorous vertebrates, mostly reptiles and birds. All species of **tongue worms** infecting humans are currently classified as Porocephalida; the species *L. serrata* and *Armillifer arminilatus* are responsible for most human cases of infection."

After we're infected either through drinking water of eating animals containing the parasites' eggs, they can grow within us and then burrow through our gut walls and enter our blood, making their way to other parts of our bodies, including our tongues and our eyes. Fortunately, these tongue worm aren't very common.

Toxocara

According to Wikipedia: "Toxocariasis is an illness of humans caused by larvae (immature worms) of either the dog roundworm (*Toxocara canis*), the cat roundworm (*Toxocara cati*) or the fox (*Toxocara canis*)… This zoonotic, helminthic infection is a **major cause of blindness** and may provoke rheumatic, neurologic, or asthmatic symptoms. Humans normally become infected by ingestion of embryonated eggs… from contaminated sources (soil, fresh or unwashed vegetables, or improperly cooked paratenic hosts [any animal we eat that may be contaminated with but unaffected by the parasite]).

Foie gras may be made more dangerous than it already is because of amyloid, when the ducks' livers are undercooked, possibly playing host to *toxocara*.

Tapeworms
Cysticercosis, Neurocysticercosis and Taeniasis

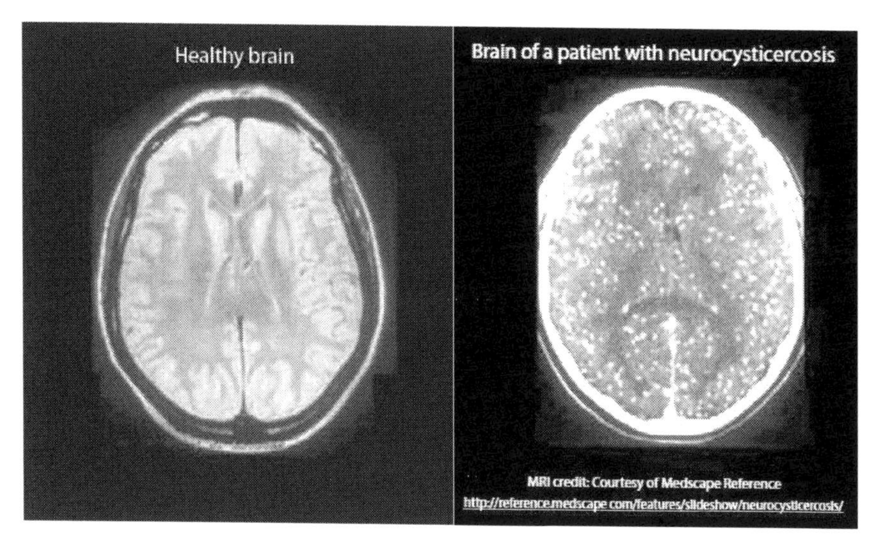

Image: Medscape Reference – http://reference.medscape.com

In the MRI scan on the right, each of the white dots represents a cyst containing tapeworm larvae, a result of eating pigs. There is no one on whom I'd wish this Meater condition.

Cysticercosis, Neurocysticercosis and Taeniasis are slightly complicated.

The CDC explains (http://www.cdc.gov/parasites/cysticercosis/):
"Cysticercosis is a parasitic tissue infection caused by **larval cysts of the tapeworm *Taenia solium***. These larval cysts infect brain, muscle, or other tissue, and are a major cause of **adult onset seizures** in most low-income countries [and, increasingly, in the United States]. A person gets cysticercosis by swallowing eggs found in the feces of a person who has an intestinal tapeworm. People living in the same household with someone who has a tapeworm have a much higher risk of getting cysticercosis than people who don't.

People do not get cysticercosis by eating undercooked pork. Eating undercooked pork can result in intestinal tapeworm if the pork contains larval cysts. Pigs become infected by eating tapeworm eggs in the feces of a human infected with a tapeworm."

[To say that people don't get cysticercosis by eating undercooked pork is true. However, if we eats pigs that contain larval cysts, we can get **taeniasis** (infection with intestinal tapeworms) and, when those tapeworms lay their eggs and we poop them out, if we aren't hygienic, we can self-infect ourselves and get cysticercosis that way.]

"Both the tapeworm infection, also known as taeniasis, and cysticercosis occur globally. The highest rates of infection are found in areas of Latin America, Asia, and Africa that have poor sanitation and free-ranging pigs that have access to human feces. Although uncommon, cysticercosis can occur in people who have never traveled outside of the United States. For example, a person infected with a tapeworm who does not wash his or her hands might accidentally contaminate food with tapeworm eggs while preparing it for others."

(Neuro)cysticercosis is infection with tapeworm larvae. Taeniasis is infection with *Taenia* tapeworms, of which there are many species, such as *T. solium* in pigs and *T. saginata* in cows.

On the following page, there's a depiction of the life cycle of taeniasis and cysticercosis, courtesy of the CDC.

In their publication, Neglected Parasitic Infections in the United States: Neurocysticercosis, the CDC writes:

"Neurocysticercosis is a **preventable parasitic infection** caused by larval cysts (enclosed sacs containing the immature stage of a parasite) of the **pork tapeworm** (*Taenia solium*). The larval cysts can infect various parts of the body causing a condition known as cysticercosis. Larval cysts in the brain cause a form of cysticercosis called neurocysticercosis which can lead to **seizures**.

Neurocysticercosis, which affects the brain and is the most severe form of the disease, can be **fatal**. Neurocysticercosis is considered a Neglected Parasitic Infection, one of a group of [five] diseases that results in significant illness among those who are infected and is often poorly understood by health care providers.

How people get neurocysticercosis:

A person gets neurocysticercosis by **swallowing microscopic eggs passed in the feces of a person who has an intestinal pork tapeworm.**

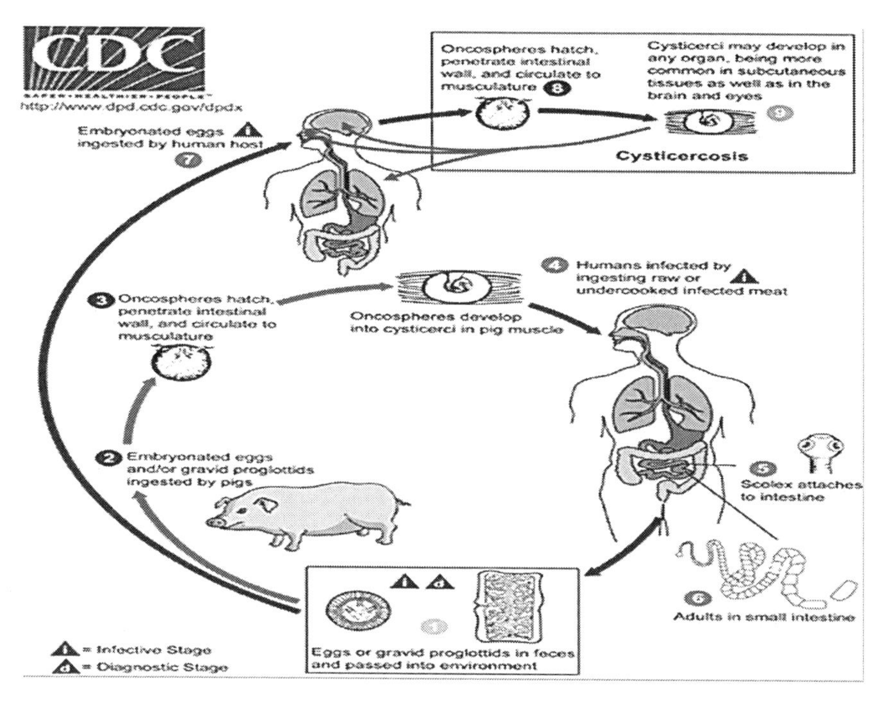

Taeniasis. http://www.cdc.gov/parasites/taeniasis/biology.html

For example, a person eats undercooked, infected pork and gets a tapeworm infection in the intestines. She passes tapeworm eggs in her feces. If she doesn't wash her hands properly after using the bathroom, she may contaminate food or surfaces with feces containing these eggs. These eggs may be swallowed by another person if they eat contaminated food. Once inside the body, the eggs hatch and become larvae that find their way to the brain. These larvae cause neurocysticercosis.

Why be concerned about neurocysticercosis in the United States?

Neurocysticercosis is a **leading cause of adult onset epilepsy worldwide**. It is costly to diagnose and treat but entirely preventable.

There are an estimated **1,000 new hospitalizations for neurocysticercosis in the United States each year**. [CDC: "Up to 1 out of 10 hospitalized patients will die. Symptoms include neurological disorders such as dizziness, headaches and seizures.]"

...neurocysticercosis creates a tremendous economic burden. In a recent study, the average charge of hospitalization due to neurocysticercosis was $37,600, with the most common form of payment being Medicaid (43.9%).

Currently, there is little being done to monitor, prevent, or identify and treat neurocysticercosis."

I'll say, especially about prevention, when our leading health body won't tell us that the best way to prevent infection with a pig parasite is to stop eating and farming the pigs. Really. The lady above who "passes tapeworm eggs in her feces" shouldn't bear the blame for the tapeworm infection (taeniasis) that she probably got from eating pigs (or cows).

Tapeworm larvae in the brain are the worldwide #1 cause of epilepsy in adults. As they burrow through our brains, they may also cause aneurysms, tumors and depression. (Who wouldn't be depressed, with parasites eating our brains?)

Tapeworms are found in pigs, cows, fishes and humans. None of them is food.

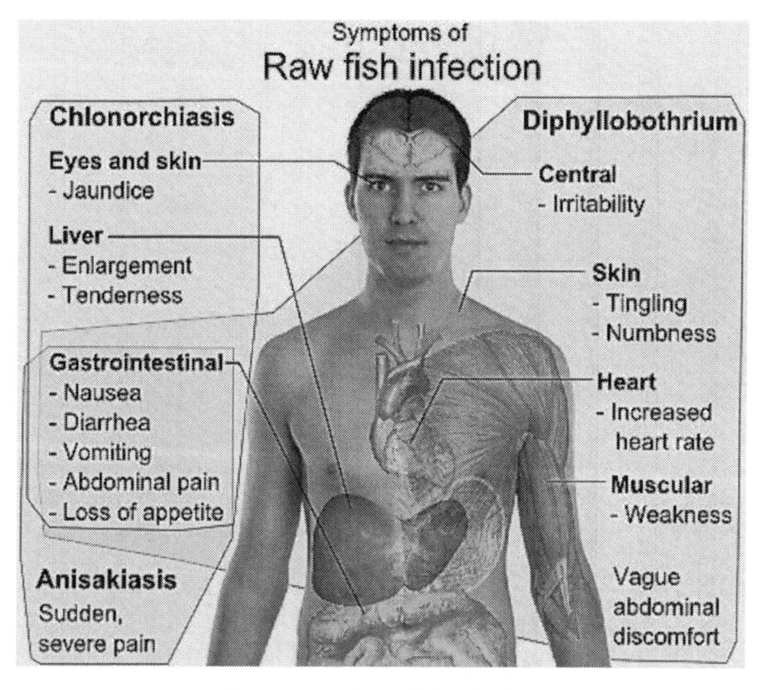

Symptoms of raw fish infection
https://en.wikipedia.org/wiki/Clonorchiasis:

Diphyllobothriasis & Clonorchiasis

Diphyllobothriasis is an infection with the fish tapeworm *Diphyllobothrium.*

Clonorchiasis is infection with the trematode *Clonorchis sinensis* (Chinese or oriental liver fluke), also from eating fishes.

According to Wikipedia, "Diphyllobothriasis occurs in areas where lakes and rivers coexist with human consumption of **raw or undercooked freshwater fish**. Such areas are found in Europe, newly independent states of the former Soviet Union, North America, Asia, Uganda, Peru (because of Ceviche), and Chile. It is particularly common in Japan, because of Sushi or Sashimi.

Around the middle of the 20th century in Japan, before advancements in refrigeration, many sushi/sashimi connoisseurs suffered great morbidity and mortality from *Diphyllobothrium* after eating unrefrigerated sashimi. Through research in parasitology, scientists came to realize that the primary cause was the **relatively favorable parasite-breeding conditions that raw fish offered**.

The disease is rare in the United States. It was, however, once more common and was referred to as "Jewish housewife's disease" because Jewish housewives preparing the traditional "gefilte fish" frequently tasted the fish before it was cooked."

Fishes aren't food, except for worms (and bigger fishes).

Other pathogens – prions

Prions – TSEs – Transmissible Spongiform Encephalopathies

Bovine spongiform encephalopathy (BSE)
"What fresh hell is this?" as Dorothy Parker used to say.

Mad cow "disease" was invented and created by Meater farmers. Despite related conditions such as kuru and scrapie and Creutzfeldt-Jakob "disease" being (fairly) common knowledge, some bright Meaters thought it would be a clever idea to feed leftover sheep's brains to cows, or vice versa, or to other sheep – waste not, want not – a penny saved is a penny earned – thereby transforming herbivores into carnivores or cannibals.

WTF? What the fudge were they thinking?

Prions are the "infectious proteins" responsible for Bovine Spongiform Encephalopathy. BSE can be loosely translated as "cow-borne disease which turns one's brain into a sponge." A sponge, not because it holds a lot of liquid; a sponge because it's full of holes.

These infectious proteins – they don't even have DNA, for Pete's sake! – are semi-alive, and they eat cows' brains away, driving them insane.

In the related conditions of kuru and CJD (see below), prions eat people's brains away. One slowly, inevitably loses one's mind, conscious all the while it's happening. It's a terrible death.

Mad cow "disease" is in the American flesh and milk supply. And so is mastitis, in 1 in 6 dairy animals, and the inflammation from the infection is thought to increase the risk of prion infection. Include me out.

Scrapie
Scrapie is the equivalent of 'ovine' spongiform encephalopathy – it occurs in sheeps instead of cows.

Kuru
Kuru is a rare spongiform encephalopathy that humans get from eating animal brains; the animals in questions being other humans, as used to happen in Papua New Guinea.

According to the NIH (https://www.nlm.nih.gov/medlineplus/ency/article/001379.htm):

"Kuru is a disease of the nervous system. Kuru is a very rare disease. It is caused by an infectious protein found in contaminated human brain tissue. Kuru is found among people from New Guinea who practiced a form of cannibalism in which they ate the brains of dead people as part of a funeral ritual. This practice stopped in 1960, but cases of kuru were reported for many years afterward because the disease has a long incubation period.

Kuru causes brain and nervous system changes **similar to Creutzfeldt-Jakob disease**. Similar diseases appear in cows as **bovine spongiform encephalopathy (BSE),** also called mad cow disease. The main risk factor for kuru is eating human brain tissue, which can contain the infectious particles [prions].

Symptoms of kuru include:

- Arm and leg pain
- Coordination problems that become severe
- Difficulty walking
- Headache
- Swallowing difficulty
- Tremors and muscle jerks
- [Death].

Difficulty swallowing and being unable to feed oneself can lead to malnutrition or starvation. The average incubation period is 10 to 13 years, but incubation periods of 50 years or even longer have been reported... There is no known treatment for kuru. Outlook (Prognosis) – Death usually occurs within 1 year after the first sign of symptoms."

Encephalopathies involving prions have been seen in cows (BSE), in sheep (scrapie), in fishes, and in humans (CJD and kuru.) Knowing that humans get infected with prions when eating some animals (humans) makes it seem far more likely to me that transmission also occurs when we eat other infected animals. Although the NIH says below that there's isn't a direct link proving that mad cow disease causes human cow disease, why risk it?

Creutzfeldt-Jakob "disease"

We have a one-in-a-million chance of getting CJD; low odds, but better than our chances of winning most lotteries.

According to Wikipedia: "Creutzfeldt–Jakob disease or CJD is a degenerative neurological disorder that is **incurable** and **invariably fatal**.

CJD is at times called **a human form of mad cow disease** (bovine or BSE)."

The NIH's Medline says: "Cattle can get a disease related to CJD called bovine spongiform encephalopathy (BSE) or "mad cow disease." **There is concern that people can get a variant of CJD from eating beef from an infected animal, but there is no direct proof to support this**."

Frankly, my dear, I don't give a damn whether there's direct proof or not. I invoke the precautionary principle – by eating whole plants I guard against a multitude of malefic possibilities.

I'm convinced that animals transmit this kind of TSE (transmissible spongiform encephalopathy) to humans. It's a prion disease; prions being "infectious proteins" invented by animal agriculturalists who fed "leftovers" of animals they'd killed to herbivores they were trying to fatten prior to killing.

Meating *may* not cause this brain-eating condition, but even the possibility should make a prudent being avoid eating animals. "You've got to be in it to win it," I remember Mayor Ed Koch saying of the New York lottery. We shouldn't buy a CJD ticket, my friend, we may win.

I don't want anything to do with prions. Planting holds no such terrors: there are no brain-devouring infectious proteins in spinach.

~

Other pathogens – miscellany

BMAA

β-methylamino-L-alanine is an amino acid that isn't among the 21 we build proteins out of (it's non-proteinogenic). It's a neurotoxin made by blue-green algae, sometimes found as a contaminant in spirulina, and it bio-accumulates in the flesh of fishes that eat algae (or other fishes). It's also been found in the brains of animals further up the "food" chain – human patients with Alzheimer's or Lou Gehrig's or Parkinson's "diseases". Interesting, no?

When we imprudently behave like peak predators, rather than the low-level Planters we're cut out to be, we often pay the price with neurodegenerative symptoms. In an appalling irony, our cognitively-impaired eating choices can lead to actual cognitive impairment.

Ciguatera

Ciguatera is an illness that starts out as a fish-borne Meating disorder that can morph into a very painful sexually transmitted "disease". Let that sink in for a moment…

Some of the tropical or subtropical fishes we eat contain biomagnified quantities of the neurotoxin-producing dinoflagellates they eat. (A dinoflagellate is "a single-celled organism with two flagella [like wings], occurring in large numbers in marine plankton and also found in fresh water. Some produce toxins that can accumulate in shellfish[es and fishes], resulting in poisoning when eaten."

(https://www.google.co.za/#q=dinoflagellate+definition)

The dinos – particularly *Gambierdiscus toxicus* – create several toxins besides ciguatoxin – gambieric acid, maitotoxin, palytoxin and scaritoxin. The small herbivores eat the dinoflagellates; the large carnivorous fishes eat the smaller ones; we eat the largest carnivores, getting the maximum dose of ciguatoxins et al. We can't smell or taste them, and cooking doesn't remove them, and their impact can last for decades.

Symptoms of ciguatera poisoning are mainly neurological, with people sometimes unable to distinguish between hot and cold. Sequelae include polymyositis (muscular aches and pains) and chronic fatigue syndrome – which sometimes is nothing more than "food" poisoning! And the STD part? Those with ciguatera poisoning can pass it on to their lovers, causing weeks of agonizing genital pain (and understandable suspicion). Planters make safer lovers.

Domoic acid

Retrograde amnesia is the kind in which we can't remember things that happened in the past. Anterograde amnesia is the rarer kind in which we can remember the past just fine; we just can't lay down any new memories after a certain point. Long-term memory's fine; short-term's shot. If we think about it for a moment, we'll realize how difficult it would be to function if we couldn't even remember meeting someone new, let alone their name, immediately after they've spoken.

Domoic acid is a rare but increasingly common fish-borne neurotoxin that can paralyze us, comatize us and kill us; it can also obliterate the hippocampal region of our brains responsible for creating new memories.

The diatoms that create domoic acid bioaccumulate up the "food" chain in anchovies, halibuts, mackerels, mussels, sardines, soles and tunas. They're odorless, tasteless and unaffected by cooking. For the love of our babies, domoic acid is yet another reason why the pregnant or would-be mothers among us should avoid eating fishes like the plague.

Keriorrhea

Diarrhea, we all know. Keriorrhea is when an oily, waxy orange goop comes out of our butts.

Where does this stuff come from? It comes from some of the fishes we eat who accumulate this wax in their flesh.

According to Wikipedia: "Keriorrhea (oily diarrhea, **oily orange diarrhea**, anal leakage, orange oily leakage) is the production of greasy, orange-colored stools which results from the consumption of indigestible wax esters found in oil fish and escolar" [a tropical and temperate deep-water fish].

"Escolar's wax ester content can cause keriorrhea (Greek: flow of wax), **gempylotoxism** or **gempylid fish poisoning**. Symptoms range from stomach cramps to **rapid loose bowel movements** [projectile diarrhea?], occurring 30 minutes to 36 hours following consumption. This condition may also be referred to as steatorrhea.

Two known ways to reduce the likelihood of escolar-induced keriorrhea are to limit portions to six ounces (170 g) or less and to consume portions close to the tail, which typically have a lower wax ester content."

Another known way to reduce the likelihood of keriorrhea is not to eat fishes. Animals can keep us alive, but on them we cannot thrive.

Scombroid poisoning

Earlier we met spermine, cadaverine and putrescine; the chemical breakdown products that bacteria release after animals die, to begin their decomposition. They give dead animals their distinctive smell of rotting flesh.

Scombroid poisoning comes from the tasteless, odorless, heat-stable toxins that form in the flesh of dead fishes before they've noticeably started to go "off." When we get an upset stomach after eating fishes or other sea creatures, it's often because of these flesh-rotting chemicals. We can get scombroid poisoning from "fresh" fishes or canned tunas.

Shellfish poisoning

According to Wikipedia: "There are four syndromes called shellfish poisoning, which share some common features and are primarily associated with bivalve molluscs (such as mussels, clams, oysters and scallops). These shellfish are filter feeders and, therefore, accumulate toxins produced by microscopic algae, such as dinoflagellates and diatoms, and cyanobacteria."

Shellfish poisoning comes about because of bio-accumulation; and we humans become the greatest bio-accumulators of all when we eat specialized filter feeders and peak predator fishes.

The four syndromes of shellfish poisoning are:

- Amnesic shellfish poisoning (ASP): See domoic acid, above
- Diarrheal shellfish poisoning (DSP): See keriorrhea, above
- Neurotoxic shellfish poisoning (NSP): See ciguatera, above
- Paralytic shellfish poisoning (PSP)

According to http://www.epi.alaska.gov/id/dod/psp/ParalyticShellfishPoisoningFactSheet.pdf, "Some of these toxins [in contaminated shellfishes] are **1,000 times more potent than cyanide**, and toxin levels contained in a single shellfish can be fatal to humans."

They continue: "What are **the symptoms of PSP**? Early symptoms of PSP include **tingling** of the lips and tongue, which may begin within minutes of eating toxic shellfish or may take an hour or two to develop. Symptoms may progress to tingling of fingers and toes and then the **loss of muscle control** in the arms and legs, followed by **difficulty in breathing**. Some people have experienced a sense of floating or nausea. Muscles of the chest and abdomen may become paralyzed. With high toxin exposures, **death** can occur in as little as 2 hours from paralysis of the breathing muscles."

They helpfully answer their own question: "Are there any other illnesses associated with shellfish? Yes, a person may have an allergic reaction to shellfish or become ill due to bacteria or viruses in shellfish."

I think I'll stick to pasta shells.

Eating blue-green algae in concentrated form can also cause these toxicities, as when spirulina supplements contain hepato- or neuro-toxins. Whole plants are best.

Tetrodotoxin

Fugu fugs up only a few people each year: the Japanese macho dish of specially prepared puffer- and related fishes in the *Tetraodontiformes* family that contain tetrodotoxin (TTX), a very powerful, bacterial neurotoxin. TTXs can paralyze us completely, blocking nerve impulses and preventing our muscles from working. When our diaphragms and intercostal muscles stop working, so do our lungs, and we die.

Or we could eat veggie California rolls.

~

Other pathogens – zoönotic diseases – zoönoses

A zoönosis or zoönotic disease is one that can cross over from one animal species to another. For example, there are human diseases which infect other animals, and vice versa. What can be inoffensive in the original host can become extremely virulent in the new target.

A partial list of zoönoses

Anthrax; Babesiosis; Balantidiasis; Barmah Forest virus; Bartonellosis; Bilharzia; Bolivian hemorrhagic fever; Brucellosis; Borrelia (Lyme disease and others); Borna virus infection; Bovine tuberculosis; Campylobacteriosis; Cat Scratch Disease; Chagas disease; Chlamydophila psittaci; Cholera; Cowpox; Creutzfeldt-Jakob disease (vCJD)*; Crimean-Congo hemorrhagic fever; Cryptosporidiosis; Cutaneous larva migrans; Dengue fever; Ebola; Echinococcosis; Escherichia coli O157:H7; Erysipelothrix rhusiopathiae; Eastern equine encephalitis virus; Western equine encephalitis virus; Venezuelan equine encephalitis virus; Giardia lamblia; H1N1 flu; Hantavirus; Helminths; Hendra virus; Henipavirus; Human Immunodeficiency Virus [HIV]; Korean hemorrhagic fever; Kyasanur forest disease; Lábrea fever; Lassa fever; Leishmaniasis; Leptospirosis; Listeriosis; Lymphocytic choriomeningitis virus; Marburg fever; Mediterranean spotted fever; Mycobacterium marinum; Monkey B; Nipah fever; Ocular larva migrans; Omsk hemorrhagic fever; Ornithosis (psittacosis); Oropouche fever; Pappataci fever; Pasteurellosis; Plague; Puumala virus; Q-Fever; Psittacosis, or "parrot fever"; Rabies; Rift Valley fever; Ringworms (Tinea canis); Salmonellosis; Sodoku; Sparganosis; Streptococcus suis; Toxocariasis; Toxoplasmosis; Trichinosis; Tularemia, or "rabbit fever"; Typhus of Rickettsiae; Venezuelan hemorrhagic fever; Visceral larva migrans; West Nile virus; Yellow fever; Yersiniosis.

* The unknown Wikipedia-author describes vCJD (variant Creutzfeldt-Jakob disease) as "a transmissible spongiform encephalopathy (TSE) from bovine spongiform encephalopathy (BSE) or "mad cow disease.""

Obviously not all of these animal-related diseases is related to diet. For example, we don't get parrot fever from eating parrots. (I hope.) While the link between HIV and "bush meat" is strong, we don't get HIV from eating hamburgers. The organism has changed its way of doing business and infection is now through blood. At one point, each of these diseases was confined to its original animal host, and then something happened to allow the micro-organism to broaden its horizons.

Zoönoses are beyond the scope of this book, so I thought I would just mention a couple. I thought of doing an A and a Z, but there's no Z, and we've already covered Yersinia, so here's anthrax and swine flu, as representative of dozens of animal-hosted pathogens that infect and sicken humans.

Anthrax

Of Anthrax, Wikipedia says: it's "an acute disease caused by the bacterium *Bacillus anthracis*. Most forms of the disease are lethal, and it **affects mostly animals**. It is contagious and can be **transmitted through contact or consumption of infected meat**."

The likelihood of anthrax infection is higher in the USA than other developed nations because Big Animal keeps "downers" in the "food" supply – animals that are too sick or damaged to walk are routinely dragged or bulldozed to their final end.

Anthrax spores can survive for decades, in the harshest of conditions. Anthrax is virulent and multiplies quickly, so it's easily weaponized.

"Diseased animals can spread anthrax to humans, either by direct contact (e.g., inoculation of infected blood to broken skin) or by consumption of a diseased animal's flesh… After the bacterium invades the bowel system, it spreads through the bloodstream throughout the body, while also continuing to make toxins. GI infections can be treated, but usually result in fatality rates of 25% to 60%, depending upon how soon treatment commences."

Anthrax infections are very, very rare. Still, we're more likely to be infected with anthrax by Meating than by other forms of terrorism.

Swine flu

Pigs are the reservoirs of influenza viruses that infect us when we breathe them in, so swine flu isn't a food poisoner. Yet the swine are there because some people mistakenly think of them as food, and they provide the reservoir for the virus. As with most transmissible pathogens, downer pigs are particularly infected… and we eat plenty of those in the US.

Of the 2009 flu pandemic in the United States, Wikipedia says:

It "was a pandemic experienced in the United States of a novel strain of the Influenza A/H1N1 virus, commonly referred to as 'swine flu', that began in the spring of 2009. As of mid-March 2010, the U.S. Centers for Disease Control and Prevention (CDC) estimated that about 59 million Americans contracted the H1N1 virus, 265,000 were hospitalized as a result, and **12,000 died**."

Meating killed these people. Hyper-concentrated animals in CAFOs and sick downers provide the perfect incubators for a multitude of pathogens, including novel strains of lethal viruses.

~

A Word on Meating and Antibiotic Resistance

According to the CDC's *Antibiotic Resistance Threats in the United States*, 2013, pp. 36-7:

"Improving Antibiotic Use

Antibiotics are widely used in food-producing animals, and according to data published by FDA, **there are more kilograms of antibiotics sold in the United States for food-producing animals than for people**…

[By the end of this book, hopefully many of us will be jarred by the oxymoron in the previous sentence: "food-producing animals." If we'd like to have any hope of saving the antibiotics for future human use, we need to stop thinking of animals as food.]

"This use contributes to the emergence of antibiotic-resistant bacteria in food-producing animals. **Resistant bacteria in food-producing animals are of particular concern because these animals serve as carriers.**

Resistant bacteria can contaminate the foods that come from those animals, and people who consume these foods can develop antibiotic-resistant infections. Antibiotics must be used judiciously in humans and [NOT AT ALL IN] animals because both uses contribute to not only the emergence, but also the persistence and spread of antibiotic-resistant bacteria.

Scientists around the world have provided **strong evidence that antibiotic use in food-producing animals can harm public health** through the following sequence of events:

▪Use of antibiotics in food-producing animals allows antibiotic-resistant bacteria to thrive while susceptible bacteria are suppressed or die. [Check]
▪Resistant bacteria can be transmitted from food-producing animals to humans through the food supply. [Check]
▪Resistant bacteria can cause infections in humans. [Check]
▪Infections caused by resistant bacteria can result in adverse health consequences for humans." [Check]

[The CDC gets it. They understand everything that's necessary to prevent antimicrobial resistance, except… they suffer Milan Kundera's "fundamental debacle… a debacle so fundamental that all others stem from it": they think animals are food or that they can produce food. Try rereading the CDC's four points again; this time with the certain knowledge that animals aren't food. We don't have to use antibiotics to suppress bacteria in food-producing plants! There are no prions in food.]

"Because of the link between antibiotic use in food-producing animals and the occurrence of antibiotic-resistant infections in humans, antibiotics should be used in food-producing animals only under veterinary oversight and only to manage and treat infectious diseases, not to promote growth."

[Yes, using antibiotics as a growth promoter in animals is insane, but so too is thinking that we can eat animals and still be healthy.]

"CDC encourages and supports efforts to minimize inappropriate use of antibiotics in humans and animals,"

[All uses of antibiotics in non-human "food" animals are inappropriate, because the animals are inappropriate as food.]

"…including FDA's strategy to promote the judicious use of antibiotics that are important in treating humans… [i.e., zero use] CDC supports FDA's plan to implement draft guidance in 2013 that will operationalize this strategy… CDC has also contributed to a training curriculum for veterinarians on prudent antibiotic use in animals."

How much training would it require for vets to use the truly prudent quantity of antibiotics in animals-as-food, which is zero? Giving antibiotics to animals we're not going to eat, who need them, is a very different matter.

The only prudent thing to do is not to breed, raise, kill and eat animals – that's the way to get antibiotics and drug-resistance out of the "food" chain: we simply redefine the food chain, et voila! Real food, no drugs, and no more increasing drug resistance.

Look, I know that most people aren't going to stop eating animals any time soon. One reason is that the four most important government departments, as related to food and health, the NIH, CDC, FDA and USDA, are all controlled by Meater interests, or are peopled by Meaters, so even if they have the scientific knowledge, they lack the political and public health will to act as the totality of the Planter nutrition science should require.

As long as Meater agriculture continues, drug resistance will continue. They can't be separated. Industrial Meating is impossible without the drugs. Big Meat and Big Pharma walk hand in hand. As with animal milk, we need to wean ourselves off an outmoded, unhealthy, lethal way of feeding ourselves. The Meater path leads to suicide, ecocide and Gaiacide.

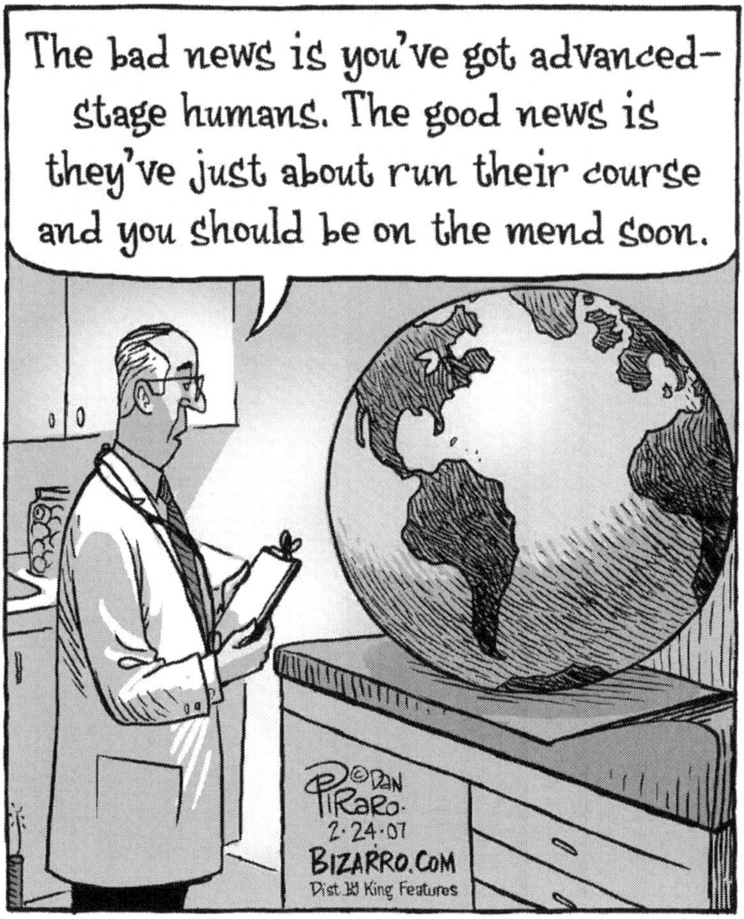

Cartoon courtesy of Dan Piraro, Bizarro.com

Current Antibiotic Resistance Threats in the United States, by Microorganism

(CDC. *Antibiotic Resistance Threats in the United States*, 2013.)

Microorganisms with a Threat Level of Urgent
Clostridium difficile
Carbapenem-resistant *Enterobacteriaceae*
Drug-resistant *Neisseria gonorrhoeae*

Microorganisms with a Threat Level of Serious
Multidrug-resistant *Acinetobacter*
Drug-resistant *Campylobacter*
Fluconazole-resistant Candida (a fungus)
Extended spectrum β-lactamase producing *Enterobacteriaceae* (ESBLs)
Vancomycin-resistant *Enterococcus* (VRE)
Multidrug-resistant *Pseudomonas aeruginosa*
Drug-resistant non-typhoidal *Salmonella*
Drug-resistant *Salmonella Typhi*
Drug-resistant *Shigella*
Methicillin-resistant *Staphylococcus aureus* (MRSA)
Drug-resistant *Streptococcus pneumoniae*
Drug-resistant tuberculosis

Microorganisms with a Threat Level of Concerning
Vancomycin-resistant *Staphylococcus aureus* (VRSA)
Erythromycin-resistant Group A *Streptococcus*
Clindamycin-resistant Group B *Streptococcus*

Let's close by taking a brief look at the microbes the CDC says are the biggest threats to antibiotic resistance right now. Other than two non-dietary pathogens that cause conditions like pneumonia and gonorrhea, they're mostly the Meater "food"-borne pathogens we've met before, while candida is a condition brought on by fiber and phytonutrient deficiency.

If we rounded up the usual suspects that cause drug-resistance, we'd find they're the Meater animal-borne pathogens that enter us when we eat animals: *C. diff*, *Enterococcus*, *Campylobacter*, *Salmonella*, *Shigella*, *Staph*, some *Strep*... They're mostly animal-borne, the very same animals that Big

Animal is dosing with antimicrobials and in which they're creating drug-resistant microbes. We need to break this silly cycle, once and for all.

We need to ask the CDC to stop manufacturing the public's consent to Meating.

~

Chronic Sequelae of "Food"-borne "Diseases"

James A. Lindsay. Chronic Sequelae of Foodborne Disease. *Emerging Infectious Diseases* Vol. 3, No. 4, 1997:443-452.

James A. Lindsay concludes his 1997 paper about the long-term repercussions of foodborne disease [!] with these words:

"Foodborne diseases are for the most part preventable; however, there is an inherent risk associated with the consumption of certain types of uncooked foods. Recognition by the public health community and the public that **many foodborne illnesses may have serious chronic sequelae** would help eliminate many illnesses and reduce health-care cost. Public health authorities could make a substantial impact by **reducing poor or unhygienic food production or food-handling practices** and by educating the public about **how harmful microorganisms enter the food chain and how they can be avoided**."

Lindsay's words take on a new meaning if we adopt a truly scientific definition of Food: nothing but whole plants; those known to be healthy and nutritious. (In other words, not belladonna and hemlock: whole isn't always healthy.)

I'm going to rewrite Lindsay's conclusion, amending it to reflect our current understanding of what is and what isn't food.

"Animal-caused symptoms are almost always preventable on a whole Planter diet. There is an inherent risk with the consumption of all animal un-foods, whether cooked or not (but especially when not). Recognition by the public health community and the public that many animal-borne illnesses may have serious chronic sequelae would help eliminate a great many illnesses and slash health-care cost. Public health authorities wouldn't have to make a substantial impact by reducing poor or unhygienic animal production or animal-handling practices, but they could make a substantial impact by educating the public about how harmful micro-organisms enter the food chain mainly from animals and how they can be avoided by avoiding eating animals."

My best estimate is that we avoid at least 90% of the pathogen burden associated with eating – and therefore at least 90% of the chronic sequelae associated with infection – when we stop considering animals to be food, and we eat nothing but whole plants, un-cross-contaminated with animal shit.

The prions, bacteria, viruses, parasites and biological toxins that invariably accompany dead animals are another reason why we're deluded when we think of animals as food.

~

Part 3 (~~Food~~borne Contaminants)

Contaminants – Pollutants and Additives

Chico Marx: "You can't fool me – there ain't no Sanity Clause."

Pollutants get into what we eat by accident; we put the additives in on purpose – and both harm us.

Part 1 of *Why Animals Aren't Food* summarized what animals are made of and showed that even the purest animals aren't food. Pure animals cause us too much harm for them to be considered food. The eating of animals and junk is responsible for about 90% of annual US morbidity and mortality. Most people who die in America each year are dying of "food" poisoning brought on by Meating and Junking.

Part 2 built on this knowledge, showing how animals play host to dozens of baleful biological life-forms such as worms, flukes, viruses, diarrheagenic and extraintestinal bacteria, and prions which sicken millions and kill hundreds of thousands of people worldwide. Plants are usually free of these pathogens, unless contaminated with animal wastes.

Part 3 will now show that animals are so contaminated with human industrial wastes that it's hard to find un-contaminated animals to eat. They're "unsafe at any feed," as Michael Greger jokes.

(Don't tell me you don't remember Ralph Nader's 1965 classic exposé, *Unsafe at Any Speed: The Designed-In Dangers of the American Automobile*? Well, our "foods" have designed-in dangers too.)

[See: http://nutritionfacts.org/video/unsafe-at-any-feed/]

Some basic principles apply.

Environmental toxins *do affect plants* but at orders of magnitude lower than animals. This is because animals eat plants, **bio-accumulating** and then **bio-magnifying** the pollution in plants and storing lipophilic (fat-loving) toxins in their **fat** cells. When we eat animals we eat the environment, at up to hundreds of thousands of times greater concentrations than if we merely ate the food. Therefore, Planters are at a great advantage when it comes to food contamination. For this reason alone, it's better to Plant than to Meat… way better.

There are basically four sources of industrial poisons in the things we eat (most of which we wrongly call food):

- Industry at large (Big Business; mainly Big Chemical)
- Animal Aggro-business (Big Farmer)
- The pharmaceutical and medical industries (Big Pharma and Club Medical)
- Big "Food"

Meating is made possible on an industrial scale today only by **hyper-concentrating animals** in CAFOs and battery operations. Grass-fed cows are for financiers and their cronies; we'd need several more planets to feed all Meaters grass-fed animals. As we saw with pathogens such as *E. coli*, *salmonella* and *campylobacter*, hyper-confining animals makes matters far worse than they already are. To take just one example: in the USA, thousands of tons of a Group 1 carcinogen (arsenic) are routinely added to chicken feed to combat parasite infestations in chicken "assault-and-batteries." Hyper-confinement concentrates toxic chemicals.

Almost invariably, aquatic creatures are the most contaminated animals. All rivers flow into the sea eventually. As badly contaminated as caged terrestrial animals are with persistent environmental pollutants, aquatic creatures – particularly farmed fishes – are the most contaminated animals we eat, just about every time. They live in our **oceans** of sewage.

Just about all fishes in the "food" chain contain some mercury. There's no safe lower limit for this neurotoxin. Besides, as we saw under "Fish Oil," the people with the highest blood levels of EPA and DHA (the long-chain omega acids found in fishes) have higher cancer rates, particularly of the prostate.

Almost invariably, hyper-confined animals, such as caged, warehoused chickens and CAFOed cows and pigs, are the second most contaminated. Farmed fishes get the worst of both worlds, enduring miserable CAFO conditions in the water.

Another thing we should keep in mind – mind-boggling as it is – is that many of the poisons we eat when we eat animals have been put there deliberately. They're additives as well as pollutants. Such is the modern-day disequilibrium of the combined corporate insanity practiced by Big Chem, Big "Food," Big Pharma and Big Farmer.

These are the five most common mal-effects industrial pollutants produce:

- Obesogenesis
- Insulin resistance
- Endocrine disruption → infertility, diabesity, cancer
- Neurotoxicity → neuropathy, sometimes → dementia
- Mutations → teratogenesis (birth defects) and cancer

In other words, because of the multiplied contaminants in animal flesh and secretions, Meating mutates us and gives us cancer (possibly causing birth defects), damages our nervous systems, messes with our hormones, makes us fat and gives us diabetes… conditions which set the stage for the full catastrophe of arterial "disease", heart and brain "disease", prolonged morbidity and early death.

As I'll show, though much pollution enters our food environment as a consequence of our heedless modes of production, a great deal enters because people have put it there deliberately. This is particularly true of animal aggroculture and the "food" industry, which quite legally inserts thousands of different environment-polluting chemotoxins into Junk (after they've supposedly self-tested them for safety and presented them to the FDA as GRAS, or 'generally regarded as safe').

As we've seen in the section on parasites, when we eat large animals, we eat all the smaller animals and animal-like creatures with which all animals are riddled. [A supersized bonus for animal lovers: buy one, get a few dozen million for free.] "Wee beasties and ghoulies" come along for the ride.

We also get the animals' considerable toxic burden of environmental contaminants, both from what the animals are exposed to during their short, sad lives and from what we've done to them pre- and post-mortem to prevent them from causing us too much harm in too noticeable a fashion. That's the subject of this section.

Much of the information in this section comes from four sources:

Firstly, the National Institute for Occupational Safety and Health's publication, *NIOSH Pocket Guide to Chemical Hazards*. It's available as a free download at http://www.cdc.gov/niosh. I'll refer to it simply as NIOSH.

Secondly, The Persistent Organic Pollutants Toolkit website at http://www.popstoolkit.com/, which I'll refer to as POPs Toolkit.

Thirdly, the US's Environmental Protection Agency (EPA) website at http://www.epa.gov/. The EPA refers to POPs as "persistent, bioaccumulative, and toxic (PBT) pollutants" or PBTs.

"A rose by any other name would smell as sweet." Or not.

Fourthly, Dr. Michael Greger's inimitable www.nutritionfacts.org, a reliable secondary source which points the way towards hundreds of primary sources.

Keeping in mind that human industries projectile-vomit tens of thousands of different chemicals into the environment each year, here follows an alphabetical listing of a few of the chemical treats we swallow when we're Meaters and Junkers, further annihilating animals' and junk's status as food...

An incomplete list of environmental contaminants and additives found in animals and junk

2,4,5-TP

2,4,5-TP is an endocrine-disrupting agricultural pesticide listed by The Breast Cancer Foundation as a cause of breast cancer. It's a persistent organic pollutant that concentrates in the animals we eat.

Acetaldehyde

Although acetaldehyde, a chemical intermediary product, does bioaccumulate in animals, it's more of a Junker issue than a Meater one. The beneficial, commensal bacteria that live under our tongues begin to metabolize alcohol as soon as we put it into our mouths. The first metabolite of alcohol is a carcinogen called acetaldehyde. All alcoholic drinks are carcinogenic, according to the World Health Organization. Our oral bacteria turn Dr. Jekyll Alcohol into Mr. Acetaldehyde.

NIOSH has this to say of acetaldehyde: "Incompatibilities and Reactivities: Strong oxidizers, acids, bases, alcohols, ammonia & amines, phenols, ketones, HCN, H_2S Note: Prolonged contact with air may cause formation of peroxides that may explode and burst containers; easily undergoes polymerization."

Does this stuff sound like it belongs in food?

Sidebar: the J-shaped curve for alcohol intake and mortality.

Why does one alcoholic drink a day make many of us live longer than those who drink either zero or two or more drinks a day? Because alcoholic drinks such as red wine provide some desperately needed phytonutrients to Meaters and Junkers who're pathetically starved of them.

The pitifully small increase in plant nutrients like resveratrol is enough to counter the carcinogenic effects of alcohol at low intake. Reality kicks in again when we have two or more drinks a day. The healthier, Planter way to get the benefits of the resveratrol from a glass of red wine is to eat the grapes from which the wine was made, or to drink the unfermented grape juice.

Additives

Real foods don't need additives. They simply… are. They're fresh apples and berries, beets and carrots, or sun-dried raisins, tomatoes or plums, without the sulfur dioxide. Frozen foods are next best, followed by canned or bottled… depending on how much salt or sugar's been added.

Food additives [oxymoron alert] include but aren't restricted to:

> Acidity regulators, Acids, Added fiber, Anticaking agents, Antifoaming agents, Antioxidants, Artificial flavors, Artificial sweeteners, Bulking agents, Color retention agents, Emulsifiers, Fat, Flavor enhancers, Flavorings, Flour treatment agents, Flow agents, Food dyes/colors, Glazing agents, Humectants, Nanoparticles, Other nutrient supplements, Preservatives, Rising agents, Salt, Stabilizers, Sugar, Sweeteners, Thickeners, Tracer gases, Vitamins and minerals, and Whiteners.

Wikipedia says: "Food additives are substances added to food to **preserve flavor** or **enhance its taste and appearance**. Some additives have been used for centuries; for example, **preserving** food by pickling (with vinegar), salting, as with bacon, preserving sweets or using sulfur dioxide as with wines. With the advent of processed foods [oxymoron alert] in the second half of the twentieth century, many more additives have been introduced, of both natural and artificial origin."

You'll note that none of the items they name is food. According to my criterion of phoods being substances that "first do no harm," bacon, sweets and wine don't qualify. They're wreck-creational eating materials.

A better definition of additives is: substances that are put into non-foods in an attempt to overcome their shortcomings (i.e. to fool us into thinking they're food) OR substances put into foods to improve their shelf life or their perceived palatability, for reasons of profit and convenience of the manufacturer rather than the health of consumers.

The presence of any of these substances is enough to convert a once-food into a UFO, an undigestible foodlike object, unfit for human consumption. (My single exception in the list above is vinegar's use in pickling.)

By the way, we'd expect The United States Food and Drug Administration (FDA) to have our backs when it comes to what goes into stuff we eat: they list all legal food additives as "generally recognized as safe" (GRAS). That's great. They must spend a lot of time, money and energy testing all those thousands of chemicals. Kudos.

Er, no.

Big "Food" tells the FDA which additives they've decided are safe, just as Big Chemical does with their poisons. (And, of course, there's never any testing done on cross-reactivities between all the shit they shovel in there.) As an illustrative example, Big "Food" told us for decades that Red Dyes 1 through 4 were good to go… until suddenly they were no good and they were gone, most of them, proven to be dangerous carcinogens. Oops, wait a mo'… Red 3 is still legal to use, even though the FDA recognized in 1990 that it's a thyroid carcinogen in animals.

The take-home message should be this: we shouldn't give up sovereignty over our own bodies. Especially not to the Meaters running government organizations like the FDA. The revolving doors between organizations like the FDA and EPA and the gigantic industries they're supposed to regulate means that conscience is absent from nutrition and health decision-making: corporations (at present, legal individuals (!) have only one moral obligation, and that's to maximize profits for their members.

There will always be a lag time of years or decades between the scientific consensus about the dangers of non-foods and policy implementation to ban their use. We need to defend ourselves during this time between the knowledge and the action – we need to "mind the gap!" – and trust our own knowledge and intuition about what is and what isn't food.

There's only one way to get around this governmental charade of "food" safety: it's to eat only food; no animals, no junk. Anything with a list of ingredients on a package probably isn't food. Fruits and vegetables come in often-nutritious peels and skins, not plastic wrappers.

I'll cover some food additives separately and in more detail.

For more, see under: Aluminum (in cheese); Arsenic (in chickens); Food coloring ~ Food dyes; Phosphates (in animal flesh)

Aldrin/dieldrin

A.k.a. 1,2,3,4,10,10-Hexachloro-1,4,4a,5,8,8a-hexahydro-endo-1,4-exo-5,8-dimethanonaphthalene, "aldrin is readily metabolized to dieldrin by both plants and animals," per the EPA.

As we'll see under dieldrin, Meaters are exposed to this carcinogenic pesticide mainly by eating fishes and shellfishes, and eating and drinking cows. Meater mothers pass it on to their breastfed infants.

Alkylphenols ~ Endocrine Disruptors
Alkylphenols are endocrine disrupting chemical toxins that persist in the environment and bioaccumulate in animals, including us humans.

They're particularly implicated in causing and exacerbating allergic conditions such as eczema and hay fever. They're used in cleaners and other household products, and they're biomagnified by the animals we eat.

We saw in Part 1A (Components) that estrogen is a double-edged sword. In appropriate concentrations estrogen is just part of being alive; one of our hormones, entirely appropriate and necessary. However, human animal estrogen and animal animal estrogen are identical. More isn't better; so eating animals leads to estrogen overload – also longer life-time exposure, thanks to Meating-induced earlier menses in girls and later menopause in women – factors which combine to cause cancer.

The animals we eat disrupt our endocrine system… our hormonal balance. So-called xeno-estrogens (strange or foreign estrogens) are human-made chemicals that do the same. They're called endocrine disruptors – chemicals that behave like excess estrogen, particularly causative of breast cancer.

As we'll see many, many times, seafood [oxymoron alert] is the most common source of these industrial chemicals.

It's worth mentioning again that benign or protective phytoestrogens bind to estrogen receptor sites, lowering the effects of estrogen and xenoestrogens.

For more, see under: Endocrine disruptors; Xenoestrogens

Aluminum
We're right to worry about aluminum exposure: it's strongly implicated in neurodegenerative conditions such as Alzheimer's. After atherosclerotic damage to our blood-brain barrier and cranial blood vessels, secondary damage occurs via deposits of toxic metals such as aluminum and copper; while amyloid plaques are forming.
How do we avoid becoming contaminated with aluminum? Several ways. We can:

- Avoid aluminum-containing vaccines in childhood
- Avoid baking powders that contain aluminum
- Avoid antiperspirants ditto
- Avoid antacids ditto

- Avoid junk like candy with aluminum dye-binders
- Avoid junk in general
- Avoid using cookware made of aluminum
- Never eat shellfishes and other aquatic species that bioaccumulate aluminum
- Never eat cheese.

I've listed these top sources of aluminum contamination in increasing order of severity. By far the most aluminum enters our bodies when we eat cheese. Why? Because cheese makers put it in there on purpose.

According to Michael Greger:

> "The aluminum salts produce a "smooth, uniform film around each fat droplet" to prevent something called fat bleeding and to give the cheese a softer texture and "desirable slicing properties.""

[See: http://nutritionfacts.org/video/aluminum-in-vaccines-vs-food/]

So if we're parents worrying about the aluminum in vaccines, every grilled cheese sandwich we give our kids is like injecting them with a dozen aluminum-containing vaccines." (I'd still be worried about mercury.)

Just one grilled cheese sandwich provides more than 5 days' worth of the World Health Organization's tolerable daily intake limit for aluminum. If we're eating more than one a week, consistently, even without considering the animal fats, proteins, hormones and cholesterol, we're setting ourselves up for a future health crisis.

Dairy products help cause Parkinson's, that "food"-borne condition born out of Meating. Considering its connection to Alzheimer's, adding aluminum to dairy probably doesn't help. Got milk? Got dis-ease. This muck isn't food.

By the way, there's plenty of aluminum in tea, but its bioavailability and absorption are extremely low. It's not what we drink that counts; it's how much we absorb. So let's drink our phytonutrient-packed green tea every day. Without milk. White tea with lemon has the most antioxidants of the non-herbal teas.

Ammonia

While our urinary tracts need to be slightly alkaline (high pH), our bowels operate best at a slightly acidic or low pH level. When we eat lots of nitrogen-containing substances (and, by definition, proteins are nitrogen-containers par excellence), when we eat animal proteins, in particular, our gut flora (which thrive by fermenting indigestible-to-us-humans plant fibers) start a process called putrefaction in our colons.

Animal proteins literally rot, giving rise to metabolites such as ammonia (NH_3) which is alkaline. Ammonia disturbs the acid environment of our gastro-intestinal tract, setting the stage for a cascade of ill-effects.

So, hands up anyone who thinks that eating ammonia would be a good idea? Apparently Big Burger thinks so. For years, they've been adding thousands of tons of the stuff to fast "food" burgers (1) to kill off all the pathogens in the dead animals, and (2) to cheaply bulk out their low- to-almost-no-meat product. In the industry, it's come to be known as "Pink Slime."

These aren't good people. This isn't food.

For more, see under: Pink slime

AMPA

AMPA (α-amino-3-hydroxy-5-methyl-4-isoxazolepropionic acid) is a toxic metabolite of Monsanto's toxic roundup herbicide. It's a good reason not to eat contaminated, genetically modified crops. Fortunately for Planters – less so for the animals and the Meaters who eat *them* – most GM crops in the USA are fed to animals.

According to the International Service for the Acquisition of Agri-Biotech Applications' Pocket K No. 11: Contribution of GM Technology to the Livestock Sector, found at http://www.isaaa.org/resources/publications/pocketk/11/default.asp:

"Current Use of GM Feed Ingredients in Livestock Diets

Feed grain usage as a percentage of total crop production ranges from 18% for wheat, 52% for sorghum, 70% for corn, 75% for oats, to more than 90% of oil seed meals…

About 90 million metric tons of GM corn grains are produced worldwide. Given that 70% of total corn grain production are used for livestock feed, then at least 65 million metric tons of GM corn grains are used in livestock diets annually. In the case of soybean, about 70 million metric tons of soybean meal derived from GM soybean are fed to livestock per annum."

Rather them than me.

Antibiotics

The looming, tragic end of the antibiotic era because of their overuse, which is often guesstimated at 80% by animal agriculture and 20% by the medical industry (but no one knows really, because Big Medicine doesn't keep tabs very well), should be sufficient reason for a rational species to stop eating animals, even if vets and doctors use different drugs.

What possible good can it do humans to swallow residues of veterinary or human-bound antibiotics in animal flesh?

According to a Meater apologist website called meatmythcrushers.com, in Myth: 80 Percent of Antibiotics are Used in Animals: "It is true that more antibiotics are used in animals than humans, but there are far more animals in the U.S. than people. There are more than 90 million cattle, 5.3 million sheep and lambs, 66 million hogs, 200 million turkeys and eight billion chickens on U.S. farms. The combined weight of livestock and poultry in the U.S. is roughly 3.5 times that of the combined weight of American men and women. A 1,200 pound steer is equal to roughly six men. If a steer needs treatment for pneumonia, it is logical will tell you that it will require a larger dose than a person. Similarly, it is logical that our combined U.S. livestock and poultry herds and flocks will require more antibiotics by volume than our combined human population."

Oh, that's alright then.

Actually, that's the problem. Because they're not food, there's not any good reason for us to breed so many animals into existence, simply to kill them quickly… and then have them kill us slowly or, after enough time has gone by and enough plaque builds up, very suddenly indeed. (Not to mention the greenhouse gases.)

Eight billion chickens… 25 per American man, woman and child…

Are we insane?

Antibiotic Resistance

For almost a century, antibiotic drugs have been able to prevent millions of people dying from infection or sepsis. Thanks to Big Animal Farmer, antibiotics are losing their effectiveness, and may even be useless within a decade or two.

Hyper-confined animals live in such squalid conditions that preventative use of antibiotics is absolutely necessary. Bacteria, which live for hours or days, multiply quickly, especially in foul, under-aired, over-manured conditions, and only those individual bacteria that survive the antibiotics pass on their genes, so the species quickly become drug-resistant.

Parents in the future whose children die of tetanus– acquired from a rusty nail in the foot, for example – may well look back and blame us oxy morons who're busy eating ourselves, our animal neighbors, our children and our grandchildren and our planet to death.

There are residues of antibiotics in most conventionally reared animals in the USA.

For more, see under: Drug residues

Antidepressants

If we're eating animals, we're more depressed to begin with. Vegans have the best global mood scores, the least depression and the lowest suicide rates. Already with compromised brain health as a result of Meating, we also take in a cocktail of drug residues when we eat animals. There can be prozac and zoloft and a concoction of other psychoactive drug residues biomagnified in the flesh of the animals we eat, especially the fishes.

Antihistamines

Conditions are so foul in "assault-and-battery" poultry operations, with so many thousands of birds packed ruthlessly on top of each other, that respiratory problems are a major killer. So, with the milk of human unkindness, instead of unprofitably providing more space for the beleaguered birds, chicken farmers profitably add antihistamines to chicken feed to help the poor birds breathe. Some even add prozac to calm them down.

Antihistamines are some of the drug residues that accumulate in chicken fats, which we later eat.

Arsenic

Here's where things get plain weird. Arsenic is a carcinogenic and neurotoxic heavy metal that berserker chicken and egg farmers add to chicken feed by the millions of pounds in the USA to prevent parasitic infestations and thus boost growth rates within their animal concentration camps. (In the words of Isaac Bashevis Singer: "In relation to them, all people are Nazis; for the animals it is an eternal Treblinka.") These farmers are killing us, not with Zyklon B, but with arsenic, and it's quite legal for their toxic waste to end up in the soil, in our water, and in us.

And it's not just fed to chickens, although they're the largest 'beneficiaries' of Big Farmer arsenic largesse. Of the more than 75% of arsenic we get from animal products, it's mostly in chickens, but also in their eggs, in cows and their milk, and in pigs. As we'd expect, hot dogs are quite contaminated: hot dogs are the end of the line when it comes to waste products masquerading as food.

These are cases of deliberate arsenic additives. Fishes get contaminated mainly by agricultural runoff and other industrial pollution.

To reiterate: there's so much arsenic in fishes that blood levels of arsenic are the best biomarker we have for total fish intake. Same with mercury. Arsenic levels are better predictors of how much fish we eat than our levels of omega-3 fatty acids, supposedly the reason why fishes are considered "brain food." (Why do vegan kids have the highest IQs then? Just asking…) After chickens, tuna fishes are the largest contributor of arsenic to the "food" supply.

Arsenic helps cause cancer, diabetes, heart "disease", neuropathy and "neurocognitive deficits in children."

Because there's some of this Group 1 carcinogen in Chinese rice, as a result mainly of contamination with chicken shit, it's probably better to eat local; organic is best. A kind of sea plant called hijiki or hiziki may also contain excess arsenic; best to avoid. Even with these veggie issues, far and away the worst source of arsenic is Meating, particularly of chickens and fishes.

Artificial flavors

Artificial flavors are a concoction of chemicals in non-foods that are, at best, inert, and, at worst, incredibly poisonous. There's never anything positive about them, and they're everywhere in Junkland. We shouldn't eat any of them.

Diacetyl is one of them. It's the chemical in the butter flavor pollutant we put on popcorn. It causes something called 'popcorn lung,' for which the medical term is 'bronchiolitis obliterans.' The name says it all: diacetyl obliterates the bronchioles (air passages) of our lungs.

We should let diacetyl be our poster child for all things artificial in the "food" chain. Popcorn is fabulous food, but diacetyl converts it into toxic waste. Artificial stuff isn't food and we shouldn't eat it.

Artificial sweeteners

I've already made my pitch for shunning all things artificial that masquerade as food, but artificial sweeteners are such widespread and widely accepted poisons I thought I'd say something about them.

We all have sweet tooths. We're human; we're powered by glucose. Our bodies have been programmed over millions of years to seek out sources of sugar for energy. Here are the opening lines of Chapter 1 ("Exploiting the Biology of the Child") from Michael Moss's 2013 *Salt Sugar Fat*:

"The first thing to know about sugar is this: Our bodies are hard-wired for sweets. Forget what we learned in school from that old diagram called the tongue map, the one that says our five main tastes are detected by five distinct parts of the tongue. That the back has a big zone for blasts of bitter, the sides grab the sour and the salty, and the tip of the tongue has that one single spot for sweet. The tongue map is wrong. As researchers would discover in the 1970s, its creators misinterpreted the work of a German graduate student that was published in 1901; his experiments showed only that we might taste a little more sweetness on the tip of the tongue. In truth, **the entire mouth goes crazy for sugar, including the upper reaches known as the palate. There are special receptors for sweetness in every one of the mouth's ten thousand taste buds, and they are all hooked up, one way or another, to the parts of the brain known as the pleasure zones**, where we get rewarded for stoking our bodies with energy. But our zeal doesn't stop there. Scientists are now finding **taste receptors that light up for sugar all the way down our esophagus to our stomach and pancreas**, and they appear to be intricately tied to our appetites." [emphases added]

Moss, Michael. *Salt Sugar Fat: How the Food Giants Hooked Us* (Kindle Locations 373-382). Random House Publishing Group. Kindle Edition.

Sugar-containing plants are anything but "evolutionarily novel."

We're sugar-powered beings – and we should all be eating sugar-containing whole foods all the time. Sugar isn't a problem, as long as it stays in the food and comes packaged with everything else that's in food, like…

nutrients, especially fiber. (Yes, "we" *can* digest fiber; it is a nutrient – see later.)

Isolated, refined sugar is a problem. Sugar on its own is "empty calories" – energy without nutrition – and as Planters we're looking for energy with maximum nutrition.

And sugar substitutes are also a problem – few calories, but extra chemicals to go.

Anything that contains stuff like acesulfame K, aspartame, cyclamate, high fructose corn syrup (HFCS), nutrasweet or sucrose isn't food and we should love ourselves well enough not to defile our body temples with them. This stuff is pure garbage.

Isolated sugar and sugar substitutes can both make us fat, which of course is ironic considering that sugar substitutes exist to help with weight loss.

The good news is that our taste buds are all new after about 3 weeks, so if we can switch to Planting and maintain it for just 3 weeks, we should be rid of our sugar addiction. After learning to love the taste of sweet peaches and grapes, sugar will taste too sweet and substitutes will taste like what they are: noxious chemicals.

At first we'll feel real shitty as we go through chemical and psychological withdrawal… we just need to make it through the first week or so. It gets easier after that. And then, after three weeks on a pure Planter diet, no non-foods, we'll have lost so much weight, reversed our insulin resistance and dropped our cholesterol by so much our Meater doctors will do a double take and order a re-test. But we'll be feeling so darn good that the detox, the change, and our loved ones' pitying or sarcastic comments, will all be worthwhile. We'll need some new jeans and belts to fit our new skinnier frames, and we'll have learned a whole bunch of stuff… about food, about ourselves, about animals, about the world.

That's why I call Planting the Enlightenment Diet.

Back to the here and now…

Three sweeteners that qualify as food, because they're "full calories," are blackstrap molasses (not my favorite taste), erythritol and date sugar (actually just powdered whole dates).

Asbestos

This category 1 carcinogen isn't a nutritional issue. I mention it here because the same legal, PR and advertising companies that fought asbestosis claims for decades, even though the industry knew of the lethality of its product, are the same legal, PR and advertising companies that fought on behalf of Big Smoke, even though the industry knew of the lethality of its tobacco products, and, guess what?

The same legal, PR and ad firms, using the same "white coat" strategy of co-opting scientists and publishing spurious 'ghost-written' studies, are now representing Big Meat and Big Egg and Big Cheese, even though they know of the lethality of their products.

To quote the late great Bill Hicks: "By the way, if anyone here is in marketing or advertising...kill yourself. Thank you. Just planting seeds, planting seeds is all I'm doing. No joke here, really. Seriously, kill yourself, you have no rationalization for what you do, you are Satan's little helpers. Kill yourself, kill yourself, kill yourself now. Now, back to the show. Seriously, I know the marketing people: 'There's gonna be a joke comin' up.' There's no f**kin' joke. Suck a tail pipe, hang yourself...borrow a pistol from an NRA buddy, do something...rid the world of your evil f**kin' presence."

Benzene

Sodium benzoate, a preservative widely used in sodas, breaks down to form carcinogenic benzene in the presence of ascorbic acid, a vitamin C analog, also routinely added to sodas or present in real food.

Here's what NIOSH has to say about benzene on p. 56: They call it a "Class IB flammable liquid." Yum. Under 1st Aid it says: "Breathe: Resp support; Swallow: Medical attention immed." If we inhale it, we should receive respiratory support. If we swallow it, we should receive immediate medical attention.

But I guess it's okay to put stuff in sodas that turns into benzene inside our kids. We wouldn't want our cola drinks to turn black, would we? *That* would be terrible. They may be killing our kids, but at least our sodas are a nice brown color. What a relief.

Benzene can also be found in cigarette and car exhaust fumes, and in canned tunas. In industrial wastes, junk and animals.

For more, see under: Hexachlorobenzene; Sodium benzoate

Benzo(a)pyrene [B(a)P]
According to the EPA [http://www.epa.gov/pbt/pubs/benzo.htm]:

"Benzo(a)pyrene (B(a)P) is a member of a class of compounds known as **polycyclic aromatic hydrocarbons (PAHs)** which generally occur as complex mixtures and not as single compounds. PAHs are primarily **by-products of incomplete combustion**. These combustion sources are numerous, including natural sources such as wildfires, industrial processes, transportation, energy production and use, **food preparation, smoking tobacco**, and disposal activities such a as open trash burning.

Why Are We Concerned About B(a)P?

B(a)P along with other PAHs are suspected of causing cancer in humans. It is **bioaccumulative, does not break down easily in our environment**, and is subject to long range air transport.

What Harmful Effects Can B(a)P Have On Us?

Likely **causes cancer** in humans

Causes **skin disorders** in humans and animals

Causes **harmful developmental and reproductive effects**

How Are We Exposed To B(a)P?

- In the home by breathing air contaminated by smoke from **fireplaces**, wood stoves, furnaces burning coal or oil and from **food preparation**.
- **Eating meats and fish that have been smoked or charbroiled**
- **Smoking tobacco products**
- Inhaling vehicle exhaust
- Inhaling fumes from working with coal tar and asphalt, working near **charbroiling** and **high temperature frying equipment**, working in coal coking operations and other industrial operations such as asphalt and aluminum production.

Where Can B(a)P Be Found?
B(a)P has no specific uses. It is generated by various combustion sources and is also a component or contaminant of such materials as tar and asphalt."

B(a)P and the other PAHs come from industrial sources. However, our most common exposure to these carcinogens is through cooking animal muscles at high temperature, smoking cigarettes and eating smoked animals.

B(a)P exposure is strongly linked to the Meater dietstyle – at least those who're exposed to industrial PAHs are usually required to wear safety equipment such as respirators. Kids at BBQs or in kitchens where bacon's cooking don't usually have that option.

Beta-carboline alkaloids

These are neurotoxic chemicals such as harmane, found particularly in chickens, which are responsible for our most common neurological movement disorder, essential tremor. Harmane is often also found in the brains of Parkinson's sufferers.

Need I say it? Chickens aren't food.

For more, see under: Harmane

BHA

Butylated hydroxyanisole is an antioxidant "food" preservative that turns out, unfortunately, to be carcinogenic. We're better off sticking to food.

Bio-identical hormones

Bio-identical hormones are something the medical industry thought might be a good idea. Well, let's take all of ten seconds to think this through. If excess hormones such as estrogen and testosterone are known to be carcinogenic (and they are), what might be the effect of ingesting excess hormones that are identical to the harmful ones? Might they be bio-identically harmful? Yes, they are.

Phyto-hormones such as the estrogens from plants, on the other hand, are protective against cancer. They bind to estrogen receptors, preventing estrogen from misbehaving there. This is why long-term isoflavone-packed soy eaters such as Asian women (until their recent nutrition transition to more animals and junk) have historically had little or no breast cancer.

Bisphosphonates

This is a trifle unfair, picking on one particular family of chemicals, and one particular drug, but I want to point out that medicinal drugs or pharmaceuticals don't have side-effects: they only have effects. For example, viagra came out of tests for something else, chest pain I think. Penile engorgement was a side-effect which complicated those trials. So the corporates switched their drug's use to erectile dysfunction, and now the once-side-effect is the desired effect, and the so-called side-effects are things like temporary blindness or everything looking blue (from blue balls perhaps?) (Is the name viagra supposed to conjure up a subliminal image of Niagara, whispering to us that we'll ejaculate with the same liberal liquid bounty as the famous waterfalls?)

Fosamax is one of the bisphosphonate-based anti-osteoporosis drugs which occasionally causes the side-effect/effect of osteonecrosis or "bone death," particularly in the jaw. I'm not sure that osteo-sufferers will appreciate the irony.

Pharmaceuticals are environmental contaminants which we willingly put into ourselves. In the future, people will look back with bemused bewilderment on this benighted, mesmerized medical era of "better living through chemistry," radiation and surgery and shake their heads, much as we do now when we think of bleeding, cupping and leaching as first-line medical treatments.

If I'd tried to be a completist about medical environmental toxins, this book would never end. All pharmaceutical drugs are liver-toxic at the very least; often mutagenic; sometimes teratogenic. We need to treat drugs as the serious environmental pollutants they are.

Of course, pharmaceuticals and their residues are problems for Meaters, not Planters. Planters don't eat the contaminated animals, for one, and also don't need to pop as many pills. Anyone get the connection?

(Anyone who'd rather take a drug to get or maintain an erection rather than be a Planter should go to this web page and check out the side effects of viagra: http://www.drugs.com/sfx/viagra-side-effects.html. I had to click my scroll bar seven times to see them all. I did a double take when I saw this effect: "• sexual problems in men (continuing), including failure to experience a sexual orgasm." What? All that money for a shag, and failure to launch can still be an issue? What they're really saying, of course, is: no money back if our drug doesn't work and you don't get wood.)

Viagra is an industrial product, not a food like watermelon, whose citrulline boosts arginine levels in us, which in turn boosts our nitric oxide levels, which in their turn improve our vasodilation and male sexual function.

Bovine growth hormone (rBGH/rBST)

Now, we know that excess human growth hormone (IGF-1), provoked by eating animal protein, causes human cancers. And we know that the natural growth hormones in animals cause human cancers. What are the infinitesimally low chances that artificial growth hormones shot into cows to boost their growth won't also cause cancer cells to grow rapidly in us when we eat them? Zero.

If I'm wrong, please let me know.

BPA (Bisphenol A)

Bisphenol A is a chemical found in epoxy resins and polycarbonate plastics used for lining some food cans and plastic bottles.

It's banned in many countries but not the USA. (What's their problem, those wimpy foreigners? Do they want to live forever?) So, as well as what's listed on the already abysmally inadequate food label, we might also be getting some free plastic along with our over-salted, -fatted and –sugared baked beans.

The Mayo Clinic says: "Exposure to BPA is a concern because of possible health effects of BPA on the brain, behavior and prostate gland of fetuses, infants and children. However, the Food and Drug Administration (FDA) has said that BPA is safe at the very low levels that occur in some foods."

Phew, that's ok then… Not.

As with most government agencies at this sorry juncture of early 21st Century America, the constituency of the corrupt FDA is the industries they're meant to regulate – in this case, the "food" and drug industries, and ne'er the twain should meet – and not the general populace they're supposed to represent.

(Incidentally, having one group to regulate these two 'commodities' – Food and Drugs – is ridiculous. Except that we're dealing with Meater and Junker non-foods that make drugs essential. Real foods *are* drugs and make most exogenous drugs superfluous.)

JAMA (*The Journal of the American Medical Association*) links BPA to diabetes, and liver and heart conditions. I think I'll go with what they say, not the FDA. Other sources link BPA – found also in turkeys – to erectile dysfunction, decreased libido, decreased "ejaculation strength" – now there's something we don't measure in a gym! Is it measured by distance? –

and decreased overall sexual satisfaction. Combined with lower testosterone levels and sperm counts in Meaters, I've got to ask: what price 'first class protein' now, Mr. Meater Macho Man?

Cadmium

NORD, The National Organization for Rare Disorders, says: "The heavy metals most commonly associated with poisoning of humans are lead, mercury, arsenic and cadmium. **Heavy metal poisoning** may occur as a result of industrial exposure, air or water pollution, foods, medicines, improperly coated food containers, or the ingestion of lead-based paints."

[See: https://rarediseases.org/rare-diseases/heavy-metal-poisoning/]

Cadmium, arsenic, lead and mercury are four toxic industrial 'heavy metals' that bioaccumulate in animals, particularly fishes; and especially in the case of cadmium, tunas. And the older and larger (and thus the more sought-after) the fish (or cow), the more contaminated it is with toxins.

Our bodies can't detoxify cadmium, so it may persist in us for many years. The riskiest behaviors we indulge in, when it comes to cadmium, are: eating animals – particularly sea creatures and the organs of land creatures – and smoking cigarettes.

Increased tuna intake/smoking → increased cadmium → decreased fertility (longer time to conception).

At tiny concentrations, cadmium also contributes to cancer (particularly 'hormonal' cancers such as breast and prostate), cognitive impairment, diabetes and heart "disease". We really want to maintain the lowest possible levels of this toxic heavy meatal.

Planting, by removing animals from one's diet, drops one's heavy metal levels precipitously. While there is cadmium in grains and other plants, 'animal cadmium' is much more absorbable than 'plant cadmium.'

(Note: high absorbability isn't necessarily a good thing. We see this same difference between plant and animal absorption rates with heme (animal) iron and 'animal' phosphorus. In every case, the lower absorbability of the plant mineral proves beneficial.)

Plant cadmium isn't associated with the negative health outcomes that animal cadmium is, partly because of its (plants-only) phytate- and fiber-induced lower bioavailability, partly because of the thousands of beneficial phytonutrients which accompany plant cadmium.

"Food is a package deal."

Higher fish consumption = more cadmium = more breast or prostate cancer.

Higher grain and veggie intake = more cadmium = less breast or prostate cancer.

We may always retain some cadmium in us but the less the better: vegans (again) are at an enormous advantage over those who eat even a few animals. Organically grown plants contain about half as much cadmium as plants doused with industrial fertilizers: another good reason to be as pure a Planter as we can.

Carbon monoxide

CO gas is deadly because it binds to hemoglobin hundreds of times more tenaciously than CO does$_2$ and then it doesn't relinquish its grip. It's the bull terrier of gases. CO levels build up in us and we die. This deadly gas is used by Big Animal to keep red animal flesh looking red, instead of the normal postmortem grey. Flesh is red because of the iron in hemoglobin.

When flesh breaks down, carbon monoxide is released. It's linked to inflammatory bowel "diseases" such as Crohn's and ulcerative colitis.

Canthaxanthin

Not everything natural is good for us. Dragon's blood, or sangre de grado, for example, taken from an Amazonian tree, is so high in phyto-antioxidants that it can mutate our DNA. I think I'll pass.

Canthaxanthin is a plant pigment added to the flesh of dead salmons to keep them looking artificially pink. The real color of dead animal muscles is a flat grey/brown.

Canthaxanthin is also used as a 'skin bronzing' potion.

Overconsumption can cause a malady known as gold dust or canthaxanthin retinopathy, in which this phytonutrient forms blobby deposits in the retinas of our eyes, displacing the pigments that are in healthy eyes: zeaxanthin+lutein, which are best obtained anywhere besides eggs.

Carcinogens

As a rule of thumb, animal 'ingredients' such as animal proteins, animal fats, cholesterol, heme iron, and growth and steroid hormones are carcinogenic, while plants contain anti-carcinogens such as phytoestrogens and chlorophyll. When it comes to environmental contamination, Meating concentrates carcinogens at levels which can be 4 or 5 orders of magnitude higher than Planting. The disparity is so great that Planting becomes almost irrelevant in comparison.

Because of their benign constituent parts and their comparatively much lower level of contamination with environmental pollutants, Pure Plants are the best prevention and the best possible cure for cancer.

The Breast Cancer Foundation lists some industrial mutagens they find relevant:

1. 1,3 butadiene
2. Aromatic amines
3. Benzene
4. Cadmium and other metals
5. Chlordane
6. DDT
7. Diethylstilbestrol (DES)
8. Ethylene oxide
9. Hormone replacement therapy (HRT) Estrogen; Progesterone
10. Oral contraceptives
11. Polybrominated diphenyl ethers (PBDEs)
12. Polychlorinated biphenyls
13. Polycyclic aromatic hydrocarbons (PAHs)
14. Tobacco smoke
15. Vinyl chloride (PVC)

#s 1 and 15 are the only two for which I have no evidence that they're bioaccumulated within animal flesh.

While the animals we eat are innately carcinogenic, animals also play host to many carcinogenic pollutants which they biomagnify massively, sometimes $>10^5$ x the environmental level.

We shouldn't be eating carcinogens. Animals aren't food.

Cesium

Cesium is a radioactive element that concentrates in the bodies of large fishes… yet another reason to avoid eating them, particularly in the Pacific Rim countries, as Fukushima continues to spew out radioactive isotopes.

Chlordane

The EPA says [http://www.epa.gov/pbt/pubs/chlordane.htm]: "Chlordane was used in the United States from 1948 to 1978 as a **pesticide** on agricultural crops, lawns, and gardens and as a fumigating agent. In 1978, EPA canceled the use of chlordane on food crops and phased out other above-ground uses for the next 5 years. From 1983 to 1988, chlordane's only approved use was to control termites in homes. The pesticide was applied underground around the foundation of homes. In **1988**, all approved uses of chlordane in the United States were terminated; however, **manufacture for export still continues.** [!? As if we don't all live in one world.] Chlordane is a **persistent, bioaccumulative, and toxic (PBT) pollutant** targeted by EPA.

Why Are We Concerned About Chlordane?

Everyone in the United States has been exposed to low levels of chlordane due to its wide spread use. Because chlordane is **bioaccumulative**, it builds up in our food chain and becomes more concentrated as it moves up our food chain to humans and other wildlife. **Fish consumption** advisories for some species are in effect for chlordane in the Great Lakes ecosystem. Chlordane remains in our food supply because it was commonly used on crops in the 1960's and 1970's.

What harmful effects can Chlordane have on us?

- Likely causes **cancer** and may cause liver cancer
- Can cause **behavioral disorders** in children if they were exposed before birth or while nursing
- **Harms the endocrine system, nervous system, digestive system, and liver**

How are we exposed to Chlordane?

- Infants may be exposed through **breast milk**
- By **eating contaminated fish and shellfish**
- **Unborn children exposed through the mother's blood stream**
- Highest exposure from living in homes that were treated with chlordane for termites"

Although the EPA claims that the highest exposure comes "from living in homes that were treated with chlordane for termites," "EPA no longer updates this information" and I suspect it's somewhat out of date. Homes have gradually become less contaminated, while our lakes and rivers and oceans have become progressively more so. Eating fishes is probably the most relevant source of chlordane toxicity today; fish eating and being in the womb of (or being breastfed by) a Meater mother. I may be wrong about home exposure, so it might be a good idea to have your place checked…

Cholesterol

The reason why many dairy farmers force their cows to become cannibals is that the cholesterol in the dead animals they feed back to their cows increases their cows' milk production. It's a purely financial decision. (By the way: f**k you.)

Copper

Alzheimer's appears to be a multi-factorial condition, due in part to metal toxicity, including iron, aluminum and copper. Almost non-existent a century ago, Alzheimer's now affects tens of millions of people. What's changed about our copper intake? Well, for one thing, we're living longer. For another, we've introduced copper plumbing – remember what happened to Rome after their hydraulic engineers, the aqualegi, introduced lead plumbing? – and copper-containing supplements (a no-no), and… we're eating far more animals.

Here's the thing about 'animal copper': it's far more easily absorbed than 'plant copper.' As with aluminum, cesium and iron, the differential absorbability of plant vs. animal minerals always seems to favor the beneficial plant mineral. Better absorption isn't always better for us, especially not of an oxidant like copper. There's a lot of copper in the animals we Americans eat, and we absorb too much of it, setting us up for copper toxicity and its neurological consequences.

The USA hasn't set upper safety limits for copper in "food". Excess copper is yet another reason not to eat animals.

DDD and DDE

DDD (Dichlorodiphenyldichloroethane) and DDE (Dichlorodiphenyldichloroethylene) are metabolites of DDT (see below) and pesticides in their own right, and they're more persistent than their baleful parent. They occur in plants and soil, but bioaccumulate in far greater amounts in animals, with consequently greater ill-effects on Meaters than Planters.

DDT

The pesticide DDT (dichlorodiphenyltrichloroethane) was banned in the USA in 1972, a decade after 'flaky,' alarmist environmental activist Rachel Carson pointed out in *Silent Spring* that its continued use might lead to springtimes silent of birdsong… all the birds being dead. (Will springs soon lose their buzz as the bees die off?)

According to the EPA, who Carson dragged kicking and screaming to ban DDT [http://www.epa.gov/pbt/pubs/ddt.htm]:

"Prior to 1972 when its use was banned, DDT was a commonly used **pesticide**. Although it is no longer used or produced in the United States, we continue to find DDT in our environment. Other parts of the world continue to use DDT in agricultural practices and in disease-control programs.

Therefore, atmospheric deposition is the current source of new DDT contamination in our Great Lakes. DDT, and its **break-down products DDE and DDD**, are **persistent, bioaccumulative, and toxic (PBT) pollutants** targeted by EPA.

Why Are We Concerned About DDT?

Even though DDT has been banned since 1972, it can take more than 15 years to break down in our environment. Fish consumption advisories are in effect for DDT in many waterways including the Great Lakes ecosystem.

What harmful effects can DDT have on us?

Probable human **carcinogen**
Damages the **liver**
Temporarily damages the **nervous system**
Reduces reproductive success
Can cause liver cancer
Damages reproductive system

How are we exposed to DDT?

By eating **contaminated fish and shellfish**
Infants may be exposed through **breast milk**
By eating **imported food** directly exposed to DDT
By eating **crops grown in contaminated soil.**"

We're exposed to DDT, DDD and DDE via what we eat (or what our Meater breastfeeding mothers feed us as infants). Overwhelmingly, this means through Meating, particularly through eating aquatic animals, in whom bioaccumulation is always the greatest.

DES (Diethylstilbestrol)

I'm going to quote Michael Greger at length here because he puts matters so succinctly [the highlights are mine]:

> "…DES was fed to chickens for years after it was shown to cause human vagina cancer.
>
> Between 1940 and 1971, the synthetic estrogen DES was prescribed to several million pregnant women with the promise that it would help prevent miscarriages. **Problems were first highlighted in 1953** when it was clear that not only was DES ineffective, but might actually be harmful. However, **a powerful and emotive advertising campaign ensured that its use continued until 1971**, when it was found to cause **cancer of the vagina in the daughters of the mothers who took it.** DES was also used to stunt the growth of girls who were predicted to grow "abnormally tall"…
>
> But most people don't know that **the greatest usage of DES was by the livestock industry**, improving feed conversion in cattle and chickens. Within a year of approval it was fed to millions of farm animals, and **although it was shown to be a human carcinogen in 1971, it was not until 1979 that all use of DES in the meat industry production was banned**. Not. They just use different synthetic estrogen implants, but even now decades after DES was banned, we're still seeing the effects, an **elevation in birth defects even down to the third generation**."

[See: http://nutritionfacts.org/video/illegal-drugs-in-chicken-feathers/]

This is the appalling way things work at the pharmaceutical/medical/animal agriculture/regulatory agency nexus. Problems with DES first seen in 1953… ad campaign, i.e. disinformation campaign, for close on twenty years until… 1971, shown to cause vaginal cancer in the 2nd generation of women… switched to livestock for eight years until 1979… now causing birth defects in the 3rd generation. Scum. They knew exactly what harm they were causing and still they did everything they could to keep the money rolling in, millions of women be damned.

This mutagenic, carcinogenic, teratogenic, synthetic growth-promoting hormone and others like it persist today within the animals we eat.

(Absolute scum.)

Diacetyl

This is the fake butter that's put on movie house popcorn. It obliterates our lungs. It's not food. (Neither is real butter.)

For more, see under: Artificial flavors

Dieldrin

Dieldrin is a carcinogenic insecticide commonly found in the animals we eat.

According to the EPA webpage on Aldrin/Dieldrin [http://www.epa.gov/pbt/pubs/aldrin.htm]:

"Dieldrin is an insecticide and a by-product of the pesticide Aldrin. From 1950 to 1974, dieldrin was widely used to control insects on cotton, corn and citrus crops. Also, dieldrin was used to control locusts and mosquitoes, as a wood preserve, and for termite control. Usually seen as a white or tan powder, most uses of dieldrin were banned in 1987, however, dieldrin is **no longer produced in the United States due to its harmful effects on humans**, fish, and wildlife. Dieldrin is a **persistent, bioaccumulative, and toxic (PBT) pollutant** targeted by EPA.

Why Are We Concerned About Dieldrin?

Because dieldrin is **bioaccumulative**, it **does not break down easily** in our environment and **becomes more concentrated as it moves up the food chain to humans** and other wildlife.

What Harmful Effects can Dieldrin Have On Us?

- Decreases the effectiveness of our **immune system**
- May increase **infant mortality**
- Reduces **reproductive** success
- May cause **cancer**
- May cause **birth defects**
- Damages the **kidneys**.

All uses of dieldrin were **banned in the United State in 1985** except for subsurface termite control, dipping of nonfood roots and tops, and moth-proofing in a closed manufacturing process. **Dieldrin is still found in our environment from past uses**.

"Potential Sources from our Environment" include:

- Contaminated **fish and shellfish**
- Contaminated **dairy products and meat**
- **Breast milk.**

While the US no longer allows the use of Dieldrin, it persists in the environment three decades after its last legal use. According to the POPs Toolkit: "Dieldrin binds strongly to soil particles and hence is very resistant to leaching into groundwater." Swings and roundabouts, I guess… ["http://www.popstoolkit.com/about/chemical/dieldrin.aspx]

The US milk supply is particularly contaminated with POPs, making dairy products even more lethal than they already are – there's a very strong link between swallowing dairy products and getting Parkinson's. Also, the US imports much of its food from 3rd World countries, where the use of dieldrin may or may not be allowed.

Planting reduces our risks of contamination significantly, especially if we grow our own fruits and veg veganically.

Dioxins and furans

According to the EPA [http://www.epa.gov/pbt/pubs/dioxins.htm]:

"What is Dioxin (2,3,7,8-TCDD)?

The term Dioxin is commonly used to refer to a family of toxic chemicals that all share a similar chemical structure and a common mechanism of toxic action. This family includes seven of the polychlorinated dibenzo dioxins (PCDDs), ten of the polychlorinated dibenzo furans (PCDFs) and twelve of the polychlorinated biphenyls (PCBs). PCDDs and PCDFs are not commercial chemical products but are **trace level unintentional byproducts of most forms of combustion** and several industrial chemical processes. PCBs were produced commercially in large quantities until production was **stopped in 1977**. Dioxin levels in the environment have been declining since the early seventies and have been the subject of a number of federal and state regulations and clean-up actions; however, **current exposures levels still remain a concern.**

Why Are We Concerned?

Because dioxins are **widely distributed throughout the environment in low concentrations**, are **persistent and bioaccumulated**, **most people have detectable levels of dioxins in their tissues**. These levels, in the low parts per trillion, have accumulated over a lifetime and will persist for years, even if no additional exposure were to occur. This background exposure is likely to result in an increased risk of cancer and is uncomfortably close to levels that can cause subtle adverse non-cancer effects in animals and humans.

What Harmful Effects Can Dioxin Produce?

Dioxins have been characterized by EPA as likely to be human **carcinogens** and are anticipated to increase the risk of cancer at background levels of exposure.

In 1997 the International Agency for Research on Cancer classified 2,3,7,8, TCDD, the best studied member of the dioxin family, a known human **carcinogen**. 2,3,7,8 TCDD accounts for about 10% of our background dioxin risk.

At body burden levels 10 times or less above those attributed to average background exposure, adverse non-cancer health effects have been observed both in animals and, to a more limited extent, in humans. In animals these effects include changes in hormone systems, alterations in fetal development, reduced reproductive capacity, and immunosuppression. Effects specifically observed in humans include changes in markers of early development and hormone levels. At much higher doses, dioxins can cause a serious skin disease in humans called **chloracne**...

How Are We Exposed to Dioxins?

Most of us receive almost all of our dioxin exposure from the food we eat: specifically from the animal fats associated with eating beef, pork, poultry, fish, milk, dairy products. Most of us get these foods through the commercial food supply. Since most of the meats and dairy products we consume are not produced locally but have been transported hundreds or thousands of miles, the majority of our dioxin exposure does not come from dioxin sources within our own community. Additionally, because we are all being exposed from the same national food supply, we are all receiving a similar exposure with **the main difference between individuals being individual food preferences.** [True: Planters approach zero.]

Important exceptions to this pattern of general population exposure are individuals who, over an extended period of time, eat primarily locally grown meat, fish or dairy products that have significantly

greater dioxin levels than those found in the commercial food supply. Individuals in this situation receive greater exposure and are at greater risk than the general population. These elevated dioxin food levels can be the result of nearby local sources or from past contamination of soil or sediments. Another example of elevated exposure is **nursing infants**; however, health experts generally agree the overall benefits to infants of nursing far outweigh potential risks."

Dioxins and furans are environmental carcinogens that find their maximum concentrations in the animals we eat, making them even more carcinogenic than they already are naturally via animal protein stimulation of IGF-1, heme iron and estrogenic effects. D+F are present in Plants, but in microscopic amounts, comparatively.

Drugs ~ Pharmaceuticals

If we're Meaters and Junkers, we're taking far more drugs than Planters. Fact. Planters take far fewer drugs of just about every category – laxatives, antidiarrhetics, analgesics, tranquilizers, antihistamines, you name it, we need fewer of them when we Plant. (Except vitamin B_{12} supplements!) Certainly fewer cholesterol- and blood sugar- and blood pressure-lowering drugs, that's for sure.

As a result, Meaters and Junkers are far more likely to fall prey to drug side-effects than Planters. As more than 100,000 Americans die each year as a result of ADRs – adverse drug reactions – caused not by prescription or physician error, but by correctly taking one's prescribed drugs – that's a not inconsiderable factor to consider when choosing what or who to eat.

Drug residues

Drug residues of all description bioaccumulate in the flesh of animals, especially lake and river dwellers. Although they're present at low concentrations, these substances may first accumulate in animal fat and then in our own fat, particularly our brains, which are very fatty organs. For the best health, we should be eating plants, which should all be free of drug residues, unless contaminated with animal manure.

Antibiotic residues

Just one of the terrible things about eating organic cows [oxymoron alert – 'organic' cannot apply to animals] is that sick beasts aren't allowed to be treated with antibiotics when they're ill. Even if beeves are organically reared – "grass-fed, poetry-read, tucked-in-bed," as Colleen Patrick-

Goudreau says – and then "humanely slaughtered" [vile oxymoron alert], they're killed just as dead as their CAFO-grown brothers and sisters; probably sliced and diced in the same slaughterhouses. (Unless do-it-yourselfer Joel Salatin happened by your house over the weekend, and Daisy went missing, perhaps?)

The vast majority of cows we eat are dosed regularly, and prophylactically, with antibiotics. Few warehoused chickens would survive without regular antibiotics (and arsenic!) in their feed. Animal agriculture dwarfs the medical industry when it comes to profligate use of antibiotics.

Discovered by bacteriologist Alexander Fleming in 1928, penicillin has saved millions of lives in the intervening years. Less than a century later, we're faced with the situation that Fleming himself warned of: the overuse of antibiotics has allowed bacteria to adapt to them to such an extent that antibiotics may soon disappear from the pharmacopeia. Despite warnings from the UK's chief medical officer and the Director General of the World Health Organization, animal agriculture continues to shove millions of pounds of antibiotics down animals each year.

Climate change, zoönoses (with the strong possibility of future pandemics) and antibiotic resistance are the three most serious legacies of animal farming for which future generations won't thank us.

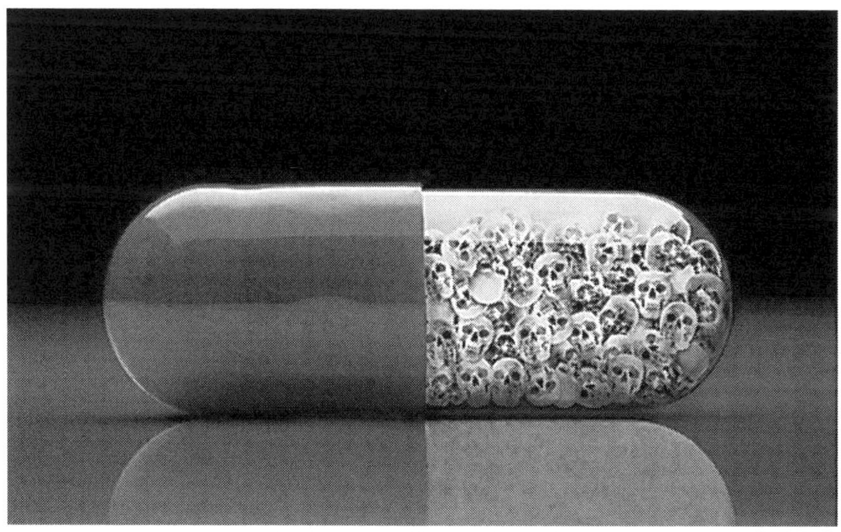

Reid Jenner @TrueDiagnosis
https://twitter.com/TrueDiagnosis/status/650437755953127424/photo/1

Drugs other than antibiotics

Streams and lakes near highly populated areas have high concentrations of all the medications that people take, mainly to combat the effects of the animals they've eaten. Fishes, who live full-time in these waterways, bio-magnify the drug residues, which people then recycle unintentionally when they eat the fishes.

Extra prozac, anyone?

Endocrine disruptors

According to the NIH (at http://www.niehs.nih.gov/health/topics/agents/endocrine/), "Endocrine disruptors are chemicals that may interfere with the body's endocrine system and produce adverse developmental, reproductive, neurological, and immune effects…

A wide range of substances, both natural and man-made, are thought to cause endocrine disruption, including **pharmaceuticals**, **dioxin and dioxin-like compounds**, **polychlorinated biphenyls** [PCBs], **DDT** and **other pesticides**, and plasticizers such as **bisphenol A**.

Endocrine disruptors may be found in many everyday products – including plastic bottles, metal food cans, detergents, flame retardants, food, toys, cosmetics, and pesticides. The NIEHS supports studies to determine whether exposure to endocrine disruptors may result in human health effects including lowered fertility and an increased incidence of endometriosis and some cancers.

Research shows that endocrine disruptors may pose the **greatest risk during prenatal and early postnatal development** when organ and neural systems are forming."

Plants contain phytoestrogens which mitigate the effects of xeno- [foreign] estrogens. Isoflavones from soy and lignans from flax seeds combat and even reverse estrogenic cancers such as breast and prostate. Plants don't cause negative endocrine disruption or harbor many endocrine disruptors.

Animals, on the other hand, are crammed full of endogenous steroid hormones, plus they bioaccumulate to crazy levels all the endocrine disruptors such as dioxins, PCBs, DDT, BPA and PBDE flame retardants, making Meating the prime cause of endocrine disruption within the general population.

Foods don't disrupt our hormones. Animals aren't food.

Feather meal

The use of feather meal [euphemism alert] is another disgusting practice of animal aggroculture. After killing bajillions of chickens on their disassembly lines, there's tons of leftovers, like feathers and heads and entrails and feet and stuff. What to do with it all? I know, why don't we mix it all together with some manure, throw in some additives and drugs, and feed it to the next batch of chickens, or maybe some other animals? What could possibly go wrong with that idea?

One consequence of this foul practice is the biomagnification of the carcinogenic toxins such as arsenic they fed to the previous generation. It was exactly this kind of forced carnivorism and cannibalism which created TSEs (transmissible spongiform encephalopathies), the prion infections such as mad cow "disease". Greek investigators have created "mad fish disease" by duplicating fish farming conditions. Can "mad chicken disease" be far behind? Maybe they just don't live long enough to display symptoms?

Sometimes when we're Meaters we behave so callously and carelessly I wonder if we're not already brain-diseased.

Feed additives

A better question to ask than "What do we industrial animal farmers add to our feeds?" would be "What don't we add when we're Meaters?"

We add all the leftover parts of dead animals, turning herbivores into carnivorous cannibals without blinking an eye. The cholesterol in animal parts boosts milk production in cows. Sick. We make feather meal out of dead chickens to feed back to live chickens. We add sawdust. We add cement. We add caffeine. We add growth hormones. We add antibiotics and antihistamines and antidepressants. We add Ractopamine, a drug like adrenaline, which keeps pigs constantly jittery, with pounding hearts. We add every drug you ever heard of, including many that were banned years ago; anything to fatten up an animal while trying to keep it alive under appalling conditions. It's a tightrope walk between losing animals and spending pence on their rearing.

Of course, I'm not saying that all farmers do all these things. These are some of the things that many farmers do. Cattle are best adapted to eating grass, and nothing but. Farmers persist in feeding them corn and other grains and soy, most of which are genetically modified, and which cows can't properly digest anyway. But, hey, the government subsidizes it, so we may as well feed it to the animals. And there isn't enough grass for a tenth of the animals, so CAFOs ('concentration camp' animal feeding operations) are here to stay if everyone's to get *their* meat.

It's a hideous mess.

Fertilizers

N-P-K fertilizers contain nitrogen, phosphorus and potassium in mega-doses. American farmers use 4.7 million tons of the stuff annually.

The nitrogen in fertilizers is often in the form of ammonium nitrate. We've already seen the ill-effects of ammonia, and later on we'll see the ill-effects of carcinogenic nitrosamines.

Earlier, under Cadmium, we saw that crops grown with N-P-K fertilizers contain twice as much of this toxic heavy metal as organic crops… which is all the reason we should need to avoid conventionally fertilized "foods". As Maria Rodale asks in her *Organic Manifesto*, why is poisoning us with chemical fertilizers called conventional? [I have a question for Ms. Rodale: because animals aren't food, how can their dead bodies be called organic?]

Eutrophication is the oxygen death of water bodies caused by fertilizer run-off into streams and resultant algal growth. This is happening everywhere 'modern' agricultural methods are used. Dead zones are areas of our oceans where there isn't enough oxygen to support life, the result of fertilizer runoff. The mouth of the Mississippi River in the Gulf of Mexico is the most obvious of these animal agriculture-deadened swathes of sea, extending over thousands of square miles.

(Most grain crops are fed to the animals we eat, and they can't digest them.)

The bad news about chemical fertilizers is their very existence. (By 'fixing' nitrogen, Haber and Bosch broke our planet.) The good news is that we won't be able to carry on much longer, wantonly destroying The One Planet, artificially fertilizing the hell out of it so we can grow crops to feed to animals so we can eat the animals. My guess (hope!) is that that custom is going to end within the next generation, perhaps within the next decade.

I pray for the day. Every one of us will benefit, even the Meaters who'll be deprived of the animals we protest to love while loving to eat.

Fish oil

Well, it's made from dead fishes so you can guess it's not on my list of beneficial items to swallow. Why do I bother to mention it at all? Because so many people have bought into the I'll-die-if-I-don't-get-my-omegas-like-the-Inuit myth.

The latest science shows that people with the highest long-chain omega levels, gotten from fishes, live shorter lives.

Fishes don't make omega fatty acids. If you want a marine source, go for the phytoplankton that the fish themselves eat. I wouldn't though, because of the consequences for the oceans. Even the best fish oils are often contaminated with heavy metals and other pollutants. I'd also be concerned about excess vitamin A.

Ground-up flaxseeds or whole walnuts are the best sources of omegas, even if they are of the short-chain variety. Flax oil is also 100% fat and it goes rancid in a hurry. Imagine how quickly the oil of dead fishes rots.

Flame retardant chemicals

PBDEs (polybrominated diphenylethers) are a class of fire retardant chemicals whose use has sky-rocketed in the last half century, while other persistent pollutants have gradually been dissipating.

PBDEs do what it says on the box: they slow down fires. And that's a worthy goal in our consumer society, full of stuff, much of it liable to combustion, like curtains and carpets and mattresses and fluffy toys. The problem is that these chemicals are carcinogenic, they disrupt our endocrine and thyroid function, and they're developmental neurotoxins. This last means they cause nerve and brain damage to fetuses and infants while they're growing.

How do we get contaminated with PBDEs? By eating the animals that have most bioaccumulated them in their fats – cows, pigs, dairy, eggs, chickens and... drum roll... fishes, by far the most riddled with these poisons. American women have up to 100 times more PBDEs in their bloodstreams than Europeans.

This is of major concern in pregnant women, especially Meaters. Though Planters may also be contaminated, Meater mothers are far more so, literally carrying their unborn babies swimming in an amniotic fluid soup of PBDEs and other pollutants, just as the fishes who contaminated them once swam in our polluted oceans. Almost 100% of American women have some chemicals in their blood. Shockingly, the average number of pollutants in each prospective mother is 35! Imagine how toxic that is to a fetus who's relying on us for nutrition.

All our mothers want the best for our kids. Surely if we knew the dangers we're creating for our womb-dwellers, we'd do our best to prevent causing them brain damage? We do that by becoming Planters; by completely cutting out the animals, the overwhelming source of all environmental toxins, and thus removing them from our blood and our breast milk.

Fluoroquinolones

A family of antibiotics that show up in animal feeds such as feather meal and, therefore, in the animals we eat. According to the NIH, "The fluoroquinolones currently available in the United States include ciprofloxacin, gemifloxacin, levofloxacin, moxifloxacin, norfloxacin, and ofloxacin. These agents are well absorbed orally and well tolerated with a low rate of adverse effects.

The currently available fluoroquinolones appear to cause idiosyncratic liver injury rarely, at an estimated rate of 1:100,000 persons-exposed.

Several quinolones and fluoroquinolones were introduced, but were subsequently withdrawn after spontaneous reports of severe adverse events including **hepatotoxicity**: temafloxacin (1992), gatifloxacin (2006), and trovafloxacin (1999)."

http://livertox.nih.gov/Fluoroquinolones.htm

Liver damage from accumulated residues of discontinued drugs may be one consequence of eating chickens.

"Food" additives

If it's got additives in it, it ain't food.

See under: Additives

"Food" coloring ~ "Food" dyes

Natural isn't necessarily good. A most glaring example is mercury. What could be more natural than a physical element? It's a deadly poison. And it used to be legal in the US to add it to food. During the early Atomic Age, just after WWII, adding radioactive ingredients to consumer items was all the rage. So adding natural dyes to foods isn't always safe.

Who are we going to trust about what's safe and what's not? The FDA, with its abysmal track record of approving lethal chemicals for use (some of which have contaminated the entire planet), followed by decades of foot-dragging, causing tens of thousands of extra deaths while they dithered and pandered to their corporate owners? Not me.

I trust the Center for Science in the Public Interest. No one owns them. Here's a free publication from them called "Food Dyes: A Rainbow of Risk." It's downloadable at https://cspinet.org/new/pdf/food-dyes-rainbow-of-risks.pdf.

Here's some of what they have to say, with some emphasis added:

"**Blue 1 may not cause cancer**, but confirmatory studies should be conducted. The dye can cause hypersensitivity reactions." Phew, that's a relief… it *may not* cause cancer. Food doesn't cause hypersensitivity reactions.

"**Blue 2** cannot be considered safe given the statistically significant incidence of **tumors**, particularly brain gliomas, in male rats. **It should not be used in foods**."

Citrus Red 2: "The dye poses minimal human risk, because it is only used at minuscule levels and only on orange peels, but it still has **no place in the food supply**."

"**Green 3** caused significant increases in bladder and testes **tumors** in male rats. Though the Food and Drug Administration **(FDA) considers it safe**, this little-used **dye must remain suspect** until further testing is conducted."

"**Red 3** was **recognized in 1990 by the FDA as a thyroid carcinogen** in animals and is banned in cosmetics and externally applied drugs. All uses of Red 3 lakes (combinations of dyes and salts that are insoluble and used in low-moisture foods) are also banned. However, the **FDA still permits Red 3 in ingested drugs and foods**, with about **200,000 pounds of the dye being used annually**. The **FDA needs to revoke that approval.**"

But what would we use to make our popsicles red if we didn't have Red 3? That would be a national calamity! So what if a few kids die ghastly deaths… The FDA's stubborn refusal to outlaw Red 3 is mind-boggling. Especially after Red 1, Red 2 and Red 4 finally bit the dust, after killing thousands. How do these scum sleep at night?

"**Red 40**, the most-widely used dye, may accelerate the appearance of immune-system tumors in mice. [Fortunately or unfortunately, depending on our point of view, researchers are increasingly finding mouse studies to be useless for extrapolating to the human condition – RM.] The dye causes **hypersensitivity** (allergy-like) reactions in a small number of consumers and might trigger **hyperactivity** in children. Considering the safety questions and its non-essentiality, Red 40 **should be excluded from foods** unless and until new tests clearly demonstrate its safety."

Exactly. The burden of proof should be on industrialists to prove safety before use, not to deny harm retroactively. We avoid all danger by eating whole apples, beets, chickpeas, dates, kumquats and rutabagas…

"**Yellow 5** was not carcinogenic in rats, but was not adequately tested in mice. It may be contaminated with several cancer-causing chemicals. In addition, Yellow 5 causes sometimes-severe **hypersensitivity** reactions in a small number of people and might trigger **hyperactivity** and other behavioral effects in children. Posing some risks, while serving **no nutritional or safety purpose**, Yellow 5 **should not be allowed in foods**."

"**Yellow 6** caused **adrenal tumors** in animals, though that is **disputed by industry and the FDA**. It may be **contaminated with cancer-causing chemicals** and occasionally causes severe hypersensitivity reactions. Yellow 6 adds an **unnecessary risk to the food supply**."

This last paragraph says a mouthful: "disputed by industry and the[ir wholly-owned subsidiary, the] FDA." Listen up, dear hearts, the Food and Drug Administration does not have our best interests at heart. There has been a coup d'état at the heart of government, and the industry rats are in charge. Nowhere is this clearer than at the EPA, the FDA and the USDA's Meater- and Junker-controlled nutrition guidelines committees.

CSPI has this to say about the FDA's flawed food dye tests: "Almost all the toxicological studies on dyes were commissioned, conducted, and analyzed by the chemical industry and academic consultants. Ideally, dyes (and other regulated chemicals) would be tested by independent researchers."

Do you hear what the CSPI is saying? In much more polite language than I'll use, they're saying: "You crooks are biased. You're paying shills to give you the result you want." Should we even have to bring up the concept of fairness and independent tests when the lives of every single eater in the world is in the balance? I don't think so.

Remember Upton Sinclair? He was the author of *The Jungle*, the blockbuster book which first revealed the depravity of the Chicago stockyards more than a hundred years ago. He said: "It is difficult to get a man to understand something, when his salary depends on his not understanding it." He could have been speaking about the FDA.

It would be great if the goons running the FDA or the USDA were to follow the science, not the money. Until that day, we need to protect ourselves from them by eating nothing but pure food.

Formaldehyde

Formaldehyde is the single word answer to why we shouldn't eat junk containing aspartame: it's a carcinogenic, neurotoxic metabolite of the methanol that forms when aspartame breaks down. Formaldehyde can cause neurological damage to a fetus and also result in premature births. 'Nough said, I think.

Fungicides

Fungicides – like herbicides and insecticides – may persist for decades in the environment. As with the other persistent pollutants, they congregate in animal fats, making animals far more dangerous to eat than plants.

Some of the organotin compounds can also behave as obesogens – chemicals that promote obesity in their consumers. They do this by converting fat stem cells into adipocytes, meaning that we end up with more fat cells than normal. (Usually we have the same number of fat cells throughout our leaves, and they just become fuller or emptier. Obesity may result when we have more fat bags to fill.) As usual, these obesogens are found mainly in fishes, the most pollution-filled species of all.

For more, see under: Obesogens; Persistent Organic Pollutants (POPs)

Gaiacides

My word for anything we make that harms our planet. I'm thinking artificial fungicides, herbicides, insecticides, pesticides, genetically modified organisms and crops, and terminator seed technology, stuff like that. Surely it's a coincidence that a Monsanto product is next up…

Glyphosate

Three cheers for California!

Finally, a US state with the cojones to take on Monsanto. Glyphosate is now listed by our most public health-conscious state as a human carcinogen. Halle-frigging-lujah. All roundup-ready crops can now truthfully be labeled cancer-spready crops.

And yet, as Monsanto scientists have pointed out, glyphosate on its own is indeed not as dangerous as it's made out to be. Testing has shown repeatedly that glyphosate on its own doesn't cause much tissue damage or hormonal disruption in humans. But… who cares? Glyphosate is added to crops with a bunch of other chemicals in the roundup formulation.

To single out glyphosate from roundup and calling roundup harmless is like singling out vitamin B_{12} (the only beneficial contaminant in animals) and saying, look: vitamin B_{12} is wonderful, so eating animals must be wonderful too.

Here's what's been found when we test roundup, not just glyphosate. While glyphosate may be almost harmless as the active ingredient in roundup, when all the other chemicals that are sprayed on roundup-ready GM crops are added and tested together mal-synergistically, roundup is a hundred times more damaging to human tissues than glyphosate on its own. In fact, roundup is worse than most other pesticides that have been tested.

So… let's all join Billie Burke and Judy Garland and the Munchkins in singing "Ding-Dong! The Witch Is Dead" while I propose a toast to the State of California.

Sticking with Monsanto and their putrid ilk…

GMOs

Genetically modified organisms are different to animals or plants bred and selected for desired heritable traits. GM shoots gene fragments into DNA and sees what sticks. GM takes DNA from one species (or class or phylum or kingdom) and transplants it into another.

I'm no Luddite. I love science. But I don't see what good can come out of tinkering in areas that are way, way beyond our understanding. (We don't even know what food is.) We can't even understand the simplest of ecosystem equations. We kill all the raptors like coyotes and wolves, usually to benefit cattle farmers, then act surprised when the ecosystem doesn't prosper. We remove the nautilus shells from coral reefs, then act surprised when crown-of-thorn nasties destroy the coral.

Humans are past masters of the unintended consequence.

So I'm not going to even bother to get technical about GM. Just seeing who's involved is enough to make me throw up in my own mouth.

GMs are pushed by giant chemical corporations to create larger markets for their poisonous chemicals. They're not making new strains of drought-resistant crops or other such gifts to humanity, which is the big lie of GM; they're making patented, terminator seeds that are modified to be resistant to their expensive pesticides which kill everything else. And then they have the temerity to bully and sue non-GM neighbors whose crops become wind-contaminated with their unsought, un-paid for product!

I'm sorry to say this: there isn't much good science showing that GM crops are harmful. (I didn't think you'd like hearing that. I didn't like saying it.) I still don't want to eat them. I'm happy eating food. And I want to know where they are. Along with about 90% of Americans, I'd like there to be labels showing clearly where this international nutrition experiment is being conducted upon our bodies. But, as our bought-and-sold government no longer cares about the wishes of American citizens, this isn't likely to happen in the face of corporate spending.

The authorizing bureaucrats at the FDA and USDA have a consistent record of claiming things are safe, finding out they're not, sitting on the information for decades while more people die, then finally recalling the product. (I'm thinking in particular of the 1962 publication date of *Silent Spring* and the 1972 banning of DDT.) I don't want to have to be nervously whiling away the decades, waiting for the GM shoe to drop on my head. Besides, organic plants suit me fine, thank you. They're the outcome of billions of years of evolution and millennia of human breeding, and they provide optimum health… with no fears of frankenfoods… and no corporate owners to loathe.

The psychic benefits of that last is considerable. (You know who you are, you dreary drones.)

If GM promoters really wanted the best for humanity, they'd be recommending that we all become Planters – the single best piece of public and private health advice it's possible to give. In the end, that's my largest issue with GM: even when it creates GM plant crops, it's all about Meating… finding a cheap way to pack pounds onto animals so that we can kill them and eat them and, by so doing, kill ourselves.

No, thank you.

Synthetic growth hormones

Look, an excess of our own natural growth hormone, IGF-1, produced by eating animal proteins, is so cancer-causing, who in their right minds would consider adding more growth hormones to the animals we eat, just so they can make more money?

"Ah," as Phil Larkin wrote in his poem Days, "solving that question brings the priest and the doctor in their long coats running over the fields." By that I mean that it's a moral and medical question: who would do these crazy things? The pure animals already cause us harm; why would anyone make them worse?

Meaterialists, is the answer. Meater industrialists who're so dead to mercy or constraint that some may even think they're acting in our best interests as their profiteering kills us.

Time is money. Growth hormones speed the growth of animals. Less time to slaughter weight, lower feed expenses, greater profits. Don't talk to me about free-range. We've reached peak range, as well as peak oil and peak water. Garagiste animal production is for the super-entitled only; it's not a possible way to feed a world population that's been infected with our omnivoraciousness.

HAs or HCAs

See under: Heterocyclic amines

Harmane (Harman)

Meating is tremorogenic… it induces permanent tremors in people.

Harmane, harmine and harmaline belong to a family of neurotoxic β-carboline alkaloids that cause **essential tremor (ET)**, "a widespread, predominantly late-life neurological disease that affects 4% of individuals aged 40 years and older, and an estimated 20% or more of individuals in their 90s and older… As such, it is one of the **most common neurological diseases**… In addition to action tremor, which may range from mild to severe, ET patients may exhibit other neuropsychiatric signs, including gait ataxia and incoordination… and various levels of **cognitive impairment**… Both genetic and non-genetic (environmental) factors… are likely to play a role in disease etiology."

Elan D. Louis, MD MSc, Wendy Jiang, MD PhD, Marina Gerbin, MPH, Amanda S. Viner, BA, Pam Factor-Litvak, PhD, and Wei Zheng, PhD. Blood Harmane (1-methyl-9h-pyrido[3,4-b]indole) Concentrations in

Essential Tremor: Repeat Observation in Cases and Controls in New York. *J Toxicol Environ Health* A. 2012 June 15; 75(12): 673–683. –

While I respect the good scientists' findings, I find it highly unlikely that genetic abnormalities are going to be the prime cause of a condition that affects 4% of those over 40. How many tens of millions is that? If genetics played the major role, there'd be a whole lot more shakin' goin' on, not just here but rockin' all over the world, and there isn't. Why not?

We need to understand the Eatiology, not the etiology, when looking for the cause of ET. Essential tremor is mostly caused by eating animals, particularly chickens, the most concentrated source of harmane and the other β-carbolines. Also cows, pigs and fishes. **Meating causes our most common movement disorder.** It's an elective non-disease. It's a dietary choice. If we like to eat animals, we should accept that other consequences of Meating, besides heart "disease", stroke and diabetes, are essential tremor (and a worse animal-induced movement disorder called Parkinson's).

The more animals we eat, the greater our risk of getting ET: up to 21 times higher. Not 21% higher; 2100% higher. That's much worse than our odds of getting lung cancer from smoking cigarettes. Harmane is the smoking gun of essential tremor. Unsurprisingly, elevated harmane levels have also been found in the brains of some Parkinson's sufferers. Harmane's high fat solubility makes our fatty brains an ideal spot for this neurotoxin to take up residence.

Long-term vegans and the residents of the world's Blue Zones don't choose to get essential tremor (or Parkinson's or Alzheimer's). We too can elect not to get these elective conditions by electing to eat no animals.

For more, see under: Heterocyclic amines

Heavy metals

Under heavy metal poisoning, NORD, the National Organization for Rare Diseases, at https://rarediseases.org/rare-diseases/heavy-metal-poisoning/, lists Poisonings by:

Aluminum, Antimony, Arsenic, Barium, Bismuth, Cadmium, Chromium, Cobalt, Copper, Gold, Iron, Lead, Lithium, Manganese, Mercury, Nickel, Phosphorous, Platinum, Selenium, Silver, Thallium, Tin and Zinc.

Most of these conditions are caused by industrial contamination. For example, lithium poisoning happens most often in battery factories. (And gold poisoning, in James Bond movies, no doubt.)

NORD says: "Heavy metal poisoning is the accumulation of heavy metals, in toxic amounts, in the soft tissues of the body. Symptoms and physical findings associated with heavy metal poisoning vary according to the metal accumulated. Many of the heavy metals, such as zinc, copper, chromium, iron and manganese, are **essential to body function in very small amounts.**

But, if these metals accumulate in the body in concentrations sufficient to cause poisoning, then serious damage may occur. The **heavy metals most commonly associated with poisoning of humans** are **lead, mercury, arsenic and cadmium**. More isn't better. Heavy metal poisoning may occur as a result of industrial exposure, air or water pollution, foods, medicines, improperly coated food containers, or the ingestion of lead-based paints."

Hopefully most of us will avoid industrial exposure (and swallowing paint), so excellence in nutrition becomes vital. Nutrition is highly relevant in all four of the most common heavy metal poisonings (arsenic, cadmium, lead and methyl-mercury poisoning), with Meaters consuming far more of each than Planters. Remember: bioaccumulation.

For more, see under: Arsenic; Cadmium; Copper; Iron; Lead; Mercury; Phosphorus

Herbicides

Organic produce is better than 'conventional' produce is better than GM produce: no chemical contamination is better than some contamination is better than a lot of contamination.

Herbicides are chemicals; chemical aren't food; we should only eat food.

For more, see under: Persistent Organic Pollutants (POPs)

Heterocyclic amines (HAs or HCAs)

For very good health reasons, humans tend to cook animal flesh before eating it, but it's a case of damned if we do, damned if we don't. Assuming that we're not paleotarded enough to eat our animals raw, thus increasing our risk of potentially deadly parasitic or bacterial infections, we run the risk of cancer from estrogenic carcinogens called heterocyclic amines that form when we cook animals at high temperatures, such as when we fry, grill or barbecue them.

There are at least 20 different heterocyclic amine carcinogens which arise as a reaction between creatine or creatinine and the glycogen, or stored sugar in muscle tissues.

For more on creatine and creatine, see the list of animal baddies in Part 1 (Animals, Themselves).

Heterocyclic amines also form in cigarette smoke. Remember, as Dr. Neal Barnard says, "Meat is the new smoking." So if we'd still like to get our daily dose of mutagenic heterocyclic amines and we don't smoke cigarettes, we're in luck because they're easy to get from smoking-hot cows, pigs, chickens and fishes. Don't forget eggs and cheese; they're good sources too.

As we saw with AGEs – the Meater gerontotoxins that age us – some cooking methods are healthier than others; boiling being much safer than higher temperature methods such as deep-frying, broiling or barbecuing.

Unlike many other carcinogens which are cancer initiators or promoters, HAs often do it all: they can cause the original DNA mutation, stimulate growth and angiogenesis, and then fuel invasiveness and metastasis too.

For example:

PhIP

Kathy Freston, well-known and gorgeous plant nutrition writer, calls 2-Amino-1-methyl-6-phenylimidazo(4,5-b)pyridine, better known as **PhIP**, "The Three Strikes Breast Carcinogen" because it initiates breast cancer, it promotes cancer cell growth and it causes the cancer to spread, or metastasize.

In his "Estrogenic Cooked Meat Carcinogens" video, Michael Greger says:

> "DNA-damaging chemicals formed when meat is cooked stimulate breast cancer cells almost as much as pure estrogen and can infiltrate the ducts where most breast cancers arise."

PhIP is a major cancer culprit, because it's almost as powerful a carcinogen as estrogen itself.

For more information on estrogen, see under: Hormones.

Harmane

Meating causes essential tremor, our most common neurological movement disorder. When we see someone with shaky hands or shaky head, they may have this animal-borne condition. Harmane, which we met earlier, is an HA neurotoxin found mainly in cooked chickens and pigs. Neurotoxins poison nerves, and harmane is lipophilic, meaning fat-loving, so it concentrates in the fatty brain. It's almost 100% certain that it's the harmane, but it may be something else in animals, in which case harmane serves as a good bio-indicator not to eat flesh.

Harmane is also linked to cancer – those unlucky enough to have both ET and cancer have the highest harmane levels.

We'll never, ever, ever hear about these animal health hazards from Low-Carb Bullshit Artists with tawdry books to sell.

The top things to avoid if we want to keep a healthy brain are cigarette smoke and cooked animals (especially chickens, fishes, pigs and cows).

Grain Brain? Bollocks. Sheer unadulterated low-carb bullshit artistry of a type Dr. John McDougall calls "*Eat More Animals to Lose Weight.*"

Is Junking bad for us? Of course it is. Meating? Obviously. Planting? Hardly ever - only a tiny minority of people have issues with grains. They should avoid them. It's worth asking how *Grain Brain* author Dr. David Perlmutter can write in his *Brain Maker* that "the two key mechanisms that lead to brain degeneration are chronic inflammation and the action of free radicals" without warning us against Meating, the main cause of inflammation and oxidation. Planting is our best remedy for oxidation and -inflammation.

For more, see under the individual Harmane entry above.

IQ4,5b

This potent cooked animal carcinogen is also found in cheese and eggs. IQ production is stimulated by eating creatine-containing items – animals.

MeIQx

Michael Greger calls this heterocyclic amine "one the most potent mutagens ever tested." Fortunately, animal eaters can quickly drop their blood concentrations of this carcinogen by stopping eating cooked animals, even for a day. Of course, levels rise rapidly upon resumption of Meating.

[See: http://nutritionfacts.org/video/heterocyclic-amines-in-eggs-cheese-and-creatine/]

Hexachlorobenzene

According to the EPA [http://www.epa.gov/pbt/pubs/hexa.htm]:

"HCB is a white crystalline solid which was commonly used as a **pesticide** until **1965**. In the past, HCB was also used as a **fungicide** to protect seeds of wheat and for a variety of industrial purposes. HCB is a **persistent, bioaccumulative, and toxic (PBT) pollutants targeted by EPA**.

Why Are We Concerned About HCB?

Because HCB is persistent and bioaccumulative, it stays in our environment for a long time and **contaminates our food chain**. HCB can cause **severe health problems for humans and other wildlife.**

[I like that: humans and *other* wildlife.]

What harmful effects can HCB have on us?

Damages bones, kidneys, and blood cells
Can harm the immune system
Lowers the survival rates of young children [!?]
Can cause **abnormal fetal development**
Harms the liver, endocrine, and nervous system
May cause **cancer**

How are we exposed to HCB?

Infants exposed through **breast milk**
During pregnancy, unborn children can be exposed through the **mother's blood stream**
By eating foods such as **meat and poultry** if those animals are exposed from **contaminated feed**
By drinking **dairy products** where the cattle have been exposed through their feed
By eating **contaminated fish and shellfish**
Breathed in in urban air"

HCB "lowers the survival rates of young children." To me, that sounds like a euphemism for "HCB kills kids."

Besides air pollution, all the exposures to carcinogenic, teratogenic HCB come from Meating, either via our mothers or on our own: animal flesh, poultry, dairy, fishes. Not watermelons; not grapes; not corn; not bread: animals.

HFCS – High fructose corn syrup

Yipes! Sugar on steroids. A way of slipping empty calories into us by the dozens of pounds each year. Sodas aren't food. Neither is anything else that contains HFCS. We should dare to eat a peach instead.

For more, see under: Gout; Insulin resistance; Obesity

Hydrogen sulfide (H_2S)

When we put any high-sulfur substances into our bodies, we favor the wrong gut flora (such as *Bilophila wadsworthia*) which form 'rotten egg' hydrogen sulfide gas in our colons and create unhealthy alkaline conditions, making it difficult for our healthy plant-fed flora to break down fiber into cancer-preventative and immune system-modulating substances like butyrate and propionate, and generally setting the stage for inflammatory bowel "diseases" such as ulcerative colitis, and colorectal cancer.

What substances are high in sulfur? Culprit #1 is **animal proteins**, high in the sulfur-containing amino acids we met earlier. Every time we eat animals, a small amount of leftover animal protein putrefies or rots in our colons, releasing the sulfur from the 'animal amino acids.'

Culprits #2 & 3 are the preservatives **sulfites** and **sulfur dioxide**, used in a wide variety of foods and un-foods, not just the most commonly known applications: sulfites in wines and sulfur dioxide in dried fruit.

H_2S is just another reason to stop Junking and Meating.

Industrial pollutants

'Industrial pollutants' is a general term for harmful pollution created by human industry. We tend to think of these substances being in the air we breathe and the water we drink. However, by far the greatest exposure we have to industrial pollutants is through the animals we eat and drink. As we'll see later, compounds like PCBs can concentrate in animal fats at many tens of thousands of times the ambient concentration.

For more, see under: Persistent organic pollutants (POPs)

Industrial toxins

Poisons made by humans, present in the environment, most concentrated in the milk and flesh of the animals we consume.

For more, see under: Persistent organic pollutants (POPs)

Iron

The best way we get the iron we need, particularly for building blood hemoglobin, is by Planting. As mentioned earlier, we humans lack a mechanism for regulating the intake of animal, or heme iron. Heme iron just blows straight through our intestinal walls, whether we have enough or not. A pro-oxidant, iron is something we really should not have in excess.

The last thing we should consider doing if we think we may be anemic, unless advised to do so by a lifestyle medical practitioner – not an MD untrained in plant nutrition – is to take iron supplements. The best way of getting optimal iron levels is to eat lots of beans and greens, while also maximizing vitamin C intake; vitamin C boosts iron absorption. And, if we're tea or coffee drinkers, it's best to drink those bevvies between meals, not during them, because they may hinder iron absorption.

Iron supplements are toxic pollutants – we needn't choose to put them in us. They aren't food.

Insecticides

Insecticides are poisons that target insects but can then persist for decades in the environment. Insecticides tend not to discriminate between so-called pests and beneficial pollinators such as bees. These POPs threaten the very basis of the planet's food web. As with all POPs they're present in animal bodies at far greater concentrations than in plant bodies.

I'd like to ask Meater mothers a question: Would we be doing right if we sprayed our kids with Doom or some such poison, every day? If the answer's No, and it should be, shouldn't we also give our kids clean, insecticide-free amniotic fluid and blood and milk, to bathe in and feed on before and after they're born? To be a Meater mother is to boost fetus and infant exposure to insecticides. Developmental and cognitive impairment often result; childhood leukemia too.

Not smart, not cool.

If we eat peak predators like tunas, or if we supplement with even the purest fish or shark oil available, we're inviting DDT and other half-century-old insecticidal maniacs (and their heavy metal, PCB and dioxin sidekicks) to take up residence in our body-homes.

Pregnant and even would-be mothers should never, ever eat fishes again.

Nor should our children.

Or our adults.

Carbamates, organophosphates and the more recent, controversial neonicotinoids are three families of insecticide. None of them should be eaten.

For more, see under: Persistent Organic Pollutants (POPs), below

Lead

The National Organization for Rare Diseases, NORD says:

"In adults, overexposure to lead may cause **high blood pressure** and damage to the **reproductive organs**. Additional symptoms may include fever, headaches, fatigue, sluggishness (lethargy), vomiting, loss of appetite (anorexia), abdominal pain, constipation, joint pain, loss of recently acquired skills, incoordination, listlessness, difficulty sleeping (insomnia), irritability, **altered consciousness**, hallucinations, and/or **seizures**. In addition, affected individuals may experience low levels of iron in the red blood cells (**anemia**), **peripheral neuropathy**, and, in some cases, **brain damage** (encephalopathy). Some affected individuals experience decreased muscle strength and endurance; kidney disease; wrist drop; and **behavioral changes** such as **hostility, depression, and/or anxiety**. In some cases, symptoms may be **life-threatening**."

https://rarediseases.org/rare-diseases/heavy-metal-poisoning/

Lead poisoning is pretty darn serious. Scallops and shrimps are the animals most contaminated with neurotoxic lead; aquatic animals in general being more toxic than their terrestrial sisters and brothers.

For optimum health we need to get the lead out. We do that by avoiding both industrial exposure and Meating. Pure Planter diets are lead-free.

Lindane

Lindane is a banned endocrine disrupting, neurotoxic insecticide that persists in the environment and – you guessed it – bio-accumulates in the flesh of animals that people love… to eat.

According to the EPA: "Lindane is used as an insecticide on fruit and vegetable crops, for seed treatment, in forestry, and for livestock and pet treatment. Lindane is no longer produced in the United States (however, it is still formulated in this country)… [For the benefit of lucky foreigners, no doubt.] Lindane is also used topically for the treatment of head and body lice and scabies."

http://www3.epa.gov/airtoxics/hlthef/lindane.html

This toxin should only be used as a treatment for lice as a last resort.

There's a coconut-based treatment that's far safer than Lindane and many times more effective than permethrin, a common treatment.

See: M. Connolly, K. A. Stafford, G. C. Coles, C. T. C. Kennedy, and A. M. R. Downs. Control of head lice with a coconut-derived emulsion shampoo. *Journal of the European Academy of Dermatology and Venereology*, 23(1):67-69, 2009.

Sadly, I don't know of a commercial version of this "coconut-derived emulsion (CDE) shampoo" that contains what Connolly et al call "Paramide plus." [Business opportunity alert.]

Lindane's yet another once-approved, now-discontinued carcinogen that persists in the environment, bioaccumulating in the animals we eat. "EPA has classified lindane as a Group B2/C, possible human carcinogen." If even the EPA admits it's probably bad, then we know it must be reaaaaallllly bad.

Lindane affects Meaters; Planters, not so much.

Meat glue

Times are tough, I know, but are things so bad for Big Meat that they have to resort to fraud, using an enzyme called **transglutaminase** to stitch together animal offcuts, even tendons, probably from several different animals (or species!), into something that resembles a single large hack of animal?

Well, that's what they do. They make more money out of us that way, and they endanger our health at the same time. Search in vain on our packaged gobbets of flesh for the words: "This product is made up of surgically reattached lambs." Par… no… bogie for the course in Meaterland.

How common is this glue? It's used in about 4,000 tons of animals each year in the US. It's found particularly in salmons and turkeys. Yeah, but it's approved by the EPA and FDA and USDA and NRA and NASA, so it must be harmless, right?… hell, even beneficial? Not so much.

Firstly, the gumming together process often introduces fecal bacteria such as *E. coli* O157:H7, and we saw in the Pathogens section earlier what those little sweethearts can do.

Then, weirdly, transglutaminase may act as an antigen, provoking an antibody allergic reaction in those with gluten sensitivity. Eating animals may be life-threatening for the 0.67% of the population with celiac disease, who never venture within a country mile of eating a breakfast roll!

Here's a promise I feel quite comfortable making: I will stop eating all fruits and vegetables the day I discover that unscrupulous people have secretly been gluing my papayas together with an epoxy resin they've "harvested" from guinea pig livers.

Mercury

The EPA says [at http://www.epa.gov/mercury/about.htm]:
"In a nutshell: What's mercury and why is it a concern?

Mercury is a naturally occurring element (Hg on the periodic table) that is found in air, water and soil. It exists in several forms: elemental or metallic mercury, inorganic mercury compounds, and organic mercury compounds. Elemental or metallic mercury is a shiny, silver-white metal and is liquid at room temperature. If heated, it is a colorless, odorless gas.

Exposures to mercury can affect the **human nervous system** and harm the **brain, heart, kidneys, lungs, and immune system**...

The most common way we are exposed to mercury is by eating fish or shellfish that are contaminated with mercury."

We don't get mercury poisoning from eating kale chips. Or potato chips. We get poisoned with mercury when we eat animals, especially aquatic animals. Mercury seriously damages our brains and often leads to brain damage in children born to Meater mothers with high blood mercury levels. If for no other reason, all prospective mothers should avoid eating animals during (and possibly two years prior to) their pregnancy, to avoid causing '**fetal mercury syndrome**.'

With Mercury, less is always more. As Michael Greger jokes, Planters shouldn't eat thermometers. Otherwise, we're good to go, mercury-wise.

Mirex (Dechlorane)

According to the EPA website [at http://www.epa.gov/pbt/pubs/mirex.htm]:

"The insecticide mirex was used for 16 years (1962-1978) in the Southeastern United States to control the imported fire ant. Eight of the infested states border on the Atlantic Ocean or the Gulf of Mexico or both, making fire ant control programs an issue in the use and management of estuaries. Mirex as a control chemical for fire ants became controversial when it was found to be highly **toxic to a variety of marine crustaceans**, including commercially important species of shrimps and crabs. Extensive public hearings were held during the period 1973-1976. All uses of mirex were cancelled in 1978. This chemical is usually seen as a snow-white crystalline solid, is odorless, and does not burn easily. When mirex does break down, it turns into **photomirex**, which also can have harmful health effects. Mirex has been listed as **a persistent, bioaccumulative, and toxic (PBT) pollutants target by EPA.**

Why Are We Concerned About Mirex?

Because mirex is **bioaccumulative**, it **does not break down easily** in our environment. This is why mirex is still found in our environment after being banned. **Mirex becomes more concentrated as it moves up the food chain to humans and other animals. Mirex is not broken down in the body and is stored in our fat.**

What harmful effects can Mirex (Dechlorane) have on us?

Classified by the EPA as probably causing **cancer** in humans
Harmful effects on **stomach** and **intestines**
Damages the **liver and kidneys**
Harms the **eyes** and **thyroid** gland
Causes damage to the **nervous system** and the **reproductive system**
May be the cause of increased **miscarriages**

How are we exposed to Mirex (Dechlorane)?

Infants may exposed through **breast milk**
Eating **contaminated fish and shellfish**
To some extent it may be in drinking water
Inhalation"

What I'd like to know is: What on earth was the EPA doing all those years ago when they happily legalized all the lethal toxins they're now working so hard to eliminate? Were they just as in thrall to corporate interests then as they are today? It appears so.

Mirex is another doozy, isn't it? Besides breathing and drinking it in low concentrations, we get it in high concentrations from animals: either from our own mothers or from the mothers and fathers of other species. As ever, with environmental pollutants, sea creatures are the most in-toxin-ated.

I know that sea creatures were never healthy items to eat, being as they are chock-full of harmful animal proteins, animal fats and cholesterol. But today I'm more certain of it: water-dwelling animals the world over are now so contaminated with industrial toxins that none of them are safe to eat. Would-be and pregnant mothers and their unborn or young offspring should all avoid eating sea animals at any cost.

Mutagens

Mutagens are substances that cause mutations in our DNA, leading to cancer formation and accelerated aging.

Wikipedia says: "In genetics, a mutagen is a physical or chemical agent that changes the genetic material, usually DNA, of an organism and thus increases the frequency of mutations above the natural background level. As many mutations can cause cancer, mutagens are therefore also likely to be carcinogens."

Many environmental toxins are mutagens; almost all of them are lipophilic (fat-soluble) and therefore bioaccumulative; therefore Meating causes far more mutations than Planting, there being up to hundreds of thousands more mutagens in animals than the ambient level. This is particularly true of aquatic animals and the water they inhabit, while most aquatic plants remain near the same concentration as the surrounding water.

Nanoparticles ~ Microparticles

These are tiny particles of substances like titanium dioxide which are used in industry by the millions of tons to whiten or brighten paints. It's known as Pigment White 6, titanium white, or CI 77891 when it's used as a pigment. Does that sound like food? Some bright spark thought it would be a good idea to use them to add some glow to our foods too, so Junkers may now be eating trillions of these littlies every day without even knowing they're there or even having heard of them.

Supposedly inert, micro- and nanoparticles have been found to be just as destructive to our colons as animal proteins… and that's saying a lot. They're key causes of inflammatory bowel "disease" and colorectal cancer.

At least with stuff like saturated fat and cholesterol, most of us know it's bad for us, so we can make our own decision about whether to eat animals or not. With TiO_2 most of us don't even know it's there let alone that it may be trashing our guts and killing us. Junk isn't food.

Neonicotinoids

Neos are the latest family of FDA-approved insecticides that may or may not be ridding our planet of those pesky bees. With names like acetamiprid, clothianidin, dinotefuran, imidacloprid, nitenpyram, thiacloprid, and thiamethoxam, I'm certain that humans shouldn't be eating them, even in the unlikely event of their being proven innocent of causing Colony Collapse Disorder (CCD).

I don't know of any clear science proving dire toxicity to humans. (We'll need to wait decades while the chemical companies perform their global-scale human trials on us, the general populace; then, at some time in the future, they'll probably be found to be hepatotoxic and carcinogenic and teratogenic and be withdrawn, to be replaced by a new, more powerful class of gaiacidal chemical maniacs, averred to be benign by an ever-accommodative EPA.)

However, is it likely that a nicotine-containing chemical is going to add years to our lives? Will Californians line up to buy neonicotinoid-supplemented smoothies? Will neonicotinoid patches become the rage at Smokenders? No, no, no, Nanette.

As ever, the best way of avoiding neonicotinoids is to avoid eating animals.

Neurotoxins

Neurotoxins – substances that poison our nerves or brain – are of two main kinds: biological toxins such as BMAA, from blue-green algae, or industrial pollutants such as flame retardant PBDEs.

Whether biological or chemical, we become contaminated with neurotoxins most often by Meating. They're in the animals we eat, particularly the mercury-laden fishes… which makes them un-foods… which is why we should stop eating them.

Nitrites

Plants, especially the leafy green veggies like rocket (arugula), kale and beet greens (and beets, too), are packed full of nitrates. NitrAtes, with an A. Animals are a pathetically bad source of nitrates.

Why are they important? Nitrates are amazing.

Here's something I bet 99 out of 100 people don't know about digestion. When we eat plants, the nitrates in the plants get absorbed by our stomachs, then pumped back up into our mouths. They enter our mouths via our salivary glands, where our commensal sublingual bacteria (mutually beneficial bacteria that live under our tongues) turn the nitrates into nitrites. NitrItes, with an I.

We re-swallow and re-absorb the nitrites, which don't cause us harm because "food is a package deal" and the nitrites are accompanied by antioxidant vitamin C, another plant-only nutrient. The nitrites enter our blood and make their way to every single cell. There, in the presence of arginine, nitrites get turned into a gas called nitric oxide (NO).

There's plenty more amazing stuff that NO does, such as maximizing our proton pump efficiency etc., but NO is the signaling molecule our endothelial cells use to tell our arteries when and how much to dilate. It's this arginine/NO pathway that erectile dysfunction-combatting drugs like viagra target so that Meaters with compromised arterial function can achieve an erection. By the way, watermelons and other fruits contain a phytochemical called citrulline which boosts arginine production, relieving ED without the druggy side-effects.

I find nitrates fascinating. We should all be eating leafy greens every day, every meal.

Back to nitrites…

Nitrites, as I intimated above, are damaging. However, 'plant nitrites' are different to 'animal nitrites.' Plant nitrites are temporary intermediary metabolites between nitrates and nitric oxide; plus they come packaged with antioxidant phytonutrients that prevent damage by free radicals (oxidation or oxidative stress).

The nitrites we get from Meating, whether the nitrites that are naturally in all animals or the more harmful nitrite additives that are added to animal parts to stop them rotting too quickly, are dangerous. In our bodies, they get converted into toxins called nitrosamines; amines being other nitrogenous compounds found more in animals than in plants.

To be continued…

Nitrosamines

Nitrosamines are carcinogenic, DNA-altering toxins that can form out of the nitrites we eat. Not the nitrates/nitrites from plants; the nitrites from Meating. Nitrosamines are one of the chemicals that cigarette manufacturers use to cause lung cancer.

Not many parents actively encourage kids to smoke. It's sad then that many of us feed kids hot dogs, each with the equivalent death-dealing ability of five cigarettes, particularly from brain cancer and blood cancer (childhood leukemia). A kid who eats four wieners may as well smoke a pack of cigarettes. At what point does nutritional ignorance become criminal neglect?

Nitrosamines are yet another piece of the evidence showing that animals aren't food.

Obesogens

In the Pathogens section, we encountered a poultry virus that causes obesity in other chickens and also in humans. These viruses are called obesogenic viruses; they cause obesity. We also came across the concept of 'infectobesity,' the infectious transmission of obesity from one animal to another. How weird is that? An online search for the word 'infectobesogen' came up empty, (please can I have dibs?), but there's no reason why the word shouldn't exist: it's an agent that causes infectious obesity, infectobesity.

There are also endocrine-disrupting environmental pollutants that have an obesogenic effect. They're called obesogens.

Any guess which is more likely to be contaminated with obesogens, beefsteak or beefsteak tomatoes? Animals win, hands down. As always, when it comes to any environmental pollution, the lower down the food chain we eat – preferably at grassroots level, or even below – the less polluted we become. Not by a little; by tens, even hundreds of thousands of times.

Organotin compounds have many industrial applications; they're used as biocides – bactericides and fungicides, often in boat antifouling. The tri-n-alkyltins are so phytotoxic (planticidal!) they can't be used in agriculture. Organotins are thought to be especially obesogenic and, as usual, the poor fishes bear the heaviest loads of these poisons.

We eat Godzillions less pollution on a Pure Planter diet.

Octachlorostyrene

"Octachlorostyrene is a persistent, bioaccumulative, and toxic (PBT) pollutant targeted by EPA.

Current uses:

Formed when graphite anodes are used during electrolytic production of magnesium from magnesium chloride.

Past uses:

By-product of wastes from the electrolytic production of chlorine prior to 1970 when graphite anodes and coal tar pitch binder were used."

http://www.epa.gov/pbt/pubs/octa.htm

I feel justified in assuming that Octa, because it's bioaccumulative, is present in animals more than plants, and that if "OCS is one of the 12 Level 1 priority PBT pollutants identified for the initial focus of action in the PBT Strategy," as a toxin it must be harmful to humans.

Confirmation comes from this EPA report [at http://www.epa.gov/pbt/pubs/octaaction.htm]:

"Potential human exposure pathways for OCS are through ingestion (especially of contaminated **fish**), inhalation, and absorption through the skin… OCS may act as a "promoter" of **mutagenicity**, and thus also as a promoter of **carcinogenicity** (Holme and Dybing, 1982)… **Pregnant women** (i.e., the **developing embryo and fetus**) and subsistence and sport fishermen [oxymoron alert] may be suspected as **sensitive subpopulations**."

[Sensitive isn't a word that trips lightly off the tongue when used about fisherfolk.]

OCS concentrates, as usual, in aquatic animals. And, as usual, Planting produces better health outcomes than Meating.

Organochlorines

The 1st generation carbon- and chlorine-containing insecticides such as chlordane, DDT, dieldrin and toxaphene are particularly persistent and bioaccumulative organic pollutants that are literally everywhere. There is no place on Earth that is unbesmirched by these chemicals; they're in the ice at both Poles. Take the "second star to the right, and straight on till morning" and we'll find them there too.

Because of their extremely low water-solubility/extremely high fat-solubility, these poisons accumulate in the fats of the animals we eat at thousands of times the concentration in air, water or soil. Meating is by far our most profound source of organochlorine intake.

For more, see under: POPs (persistent organic pollutants)

Organophosphates

If we did away with all organophosphate compounds, we'd be in for a big surprise: DNA and RNA are Ops. The ones that affect us most nutritionally and health-wise are the organophosphate chemical herbicides, insecticides and nerve agents.

Wikipedia says: "Organophosphates are widely used as solvents, plasticizers, and EP additives… The United States Environmental Protection Agency lists organophosphates as very highly acutely toxic to bees, wildlife, and humans. Recent studies suggest a possible link to adverse effects in the neurobehavioral development of fetuses and children, even at very low levels of exposure."

You must be getting used to this by now: Organophosphates are neurotoxic, and they cause birth defects. They bioaccumulate in animals in astronomically higher concentrations. Fishes are the most contaminated. We shouldn't eat them. They're not food.

(Should I just write the words Boilerplate or Ditto from now on, to indicate: Neurotoxic, carcinogenic, mutagenic, endocrine disruptive… Hyper-concentrated… Meating-related… Aquatic life the most toxic… Contamination of children via blood- and breast milk-stream… Planting the only logical behavior?)

Organotins

Organotin compounds are a highly toxic family of chemicals, often used as biocides, which have obesogenic effects. Yes, they bioaccumulate in animals such as ourselves when we behave like predators.

Meating is the ultimate Predator Diet. (No, that's not a good thing.)

For more, see under: Obesogens

PAHs ~ polycyclic aromatic hydrocarbons

More cooked animal carcinogens, mostly from fried animals.

For more, see under: Benzo(a)pyrene [B(a)P]; Polycyclic aromatic hydrocarbons

PBDEs (polybrominated diphenylethers)
PBDEs are a class of fire retardant chemicals that bioaccumulate in animals, causing endocrine disruption, cancers and impaired neurological and brain development in fetuses and infants.

For more, see under: Flame retardant chemicals

PCBs (Polychlorinated Biphenyls)
Another generous gift to humanity from the fine people at Monsanto…

According to the EPA [http://www.epa.gov/pbt/pubs/pcbs.htm]:
"There are no known natural sources of PCBs in our environment. PCBs are either oily liquids or solids, are colorless to light yellow, and have no smell or taste. Because they do not easily burn and are good insulators, PCBs have been used widely as coolants and lubricants. PCBs are **persistent, bioaccumulative and toxic (PBT) pollutants** that have been targeted by EPA.

Why Are We Concerned About PCBs?
PCBs do not break down in our environment and can have severe health effects on humans. PCBs in the air eventually return to our land and water by settling or from runoff in snow and rain. In our water, **PCBs build up in fish** and **can reach levels hundreds of thousands of times higher than the levels in water. Fish consumption advisories** are in effect for PCBs in all five of the Great Lakes. **PCBs are the leading chemical risk from fish consumption.**

What harmful effects can PCBs have on us?
Probable human **carcinogen**
Damages the **stomach**
Skin irritation
Liver and **Kidney** damage
Thyroid gland injuries

How are we exposed to PCBs?
By eating contaminated **fish and shellfish**
Infants may be exposed through **breast milk**
Unborn children may exposed while in the womb
May be in **milk, meat, and their by-products**
Breathing indoor air in buildings where electrical equipment contains PCBs

Where can PCBs be found?
Manufacturing of PCBs stopping in the Unites States in **1977** because they were found to build up in our environment and cause harmful effects. However, we can still find them in our environment, **especially in our lakes, rivers, and streams.**"

When the EPA says "Fish consumption advisories are in effect for PCBs in all five of the Great Lakes," they're saying that everything that lives in the Great Lakes is too poisonous to eat. Forgetting about all the other contaminants found in sea, lake and river animals, PCBs should be a good enough reason for everyone to stop eating these poor poisoned creatures. Eating them brings us nothing but harm. PCBs poison us when we eat animals, and then they poison our fetuses and neonates via our blood and our breast milk.

Fishes aren't food. Unhealthy in their own right, they're trebly so because of all the contaminants they harbor [aquatic pun alert].

Perfluorochemicals
At http://www.cdc.gov/biomonitoring/pdf/PFCs_FactSheet.pdf, there's a pretty inadequate CDC download on PFCs. They say:

"Perfluorochemicals (PFCs) are a group of chemicals used to make fluoropolymer coatings and products that resist heat, oil, stains, grease, and water. Fluoropolymer coatings can be used in such varied products as clothing, furniture, adhesives, food packaging, heat-resistant non-stick cooking surfaces, and the insulation of electrical wire. Many chemicals in this group, including perfluorooctane sulfonic acid (PFOS) and perfluorooctanoic acid (PFOA), have been a concern because they **do not break down in the environment**, and they **build up in wildlife**. PFCs have been found in rivers and lakes and **in many types of animals on land and in the water**.

How People Are Exposed to PFCs
How people can be exposed to PFCs is **as yet unclear**. Some PFCs persist in the environment, and **people are mostly likely exposed by consuming PFC-contaminated water or food**. Exposure may also occur by using products that contain PFCs."
Okay, why do I call this (obviously Meater-written) factsheet inadequate? It's got some pretty good info in it. I think it's inadequate because it misses the point completely, the one I've been making over and over and over in

this Pollutants section. It's not at all "unclear" how people are exposed to PFCs.

Here's what we know: PFCs don't break down in the environment; they build up in wildlife. They're POPs, persistent organic pollutants. As such they behave like all the other POPs out there. They're biomagnified in animals, who store them in their fats. Yes, we may get some from the air we breathe and the water we drink, but the overwhelming majority of our PFC intake comes from Meating.

WE are the environment in which PFCs don't break down. WE are the wildlife in which PFCs build up, causing thyroid disorders in us, causing birth and brain defects in our kids via Meater mother's blood and breast milk.

Our best and only protection from PFC intoxification is Planting, without the added chemical cocktails.

Persistent, bioaccumulative, and toxic (PBT) pollutants
PBTs are the Environmental Protection Agency's version of POPs, or persistent organic pollutants, below. They're poisonous chemicals that were once used by industry (in agriculture, mainly), that have been outlawed for decades, but which persist in the environment, wreaking health havoc. Especially in the way they build up in concentration the higher one moves up the "food" ladder, until we peak predator humans eat them at their greatest concentrations when we eat the animals on the next rung down the ladder. (A very good reason not to be a cannibal.)

The "EPA's First 12 Priority PBT Pollutants From the Canada-US Binational Toxics Strategy" – their worst of the worst – are:

- Aldrin/dieldrin
- Alkyl-lead
- Benzo(a)pyrene
- Chlordane
- DDT, DDP, DDE
- Dioxins and furans
- Hexachlorobenzene
- Mercury
- Mirex (Dechlorane)
- Octachlorostyrene

- PCBs
- Toxaphene

Most PBTs are known carcinogens (cancer causers) and teratogens (causers of birth defects).

Each of these PBTs/POPs is covered individually in this section. In every single case, bioaccumulation or biomagnification causes Meaters to be between hundreds to hundreds of thousands of times more contaminated than Planters. Consequently, Meaters can never approach the health status of Planters who're eating organically or veganically grown food (and taking their B_{12} supplement regularly).

Persistent organic pollutants (POPs)

According to L. Ritter et al, in their paper entitled Persistent Organic Pollutants, "Persistent organic pollutants (POPs) are organic compounds that, to a varying degree, resist photolytic, biological and chemical degradation. POPs are often halogenated and characterized by low water solubility and **high lipid solubility**, leading to their **bioaccumulation in fatty tissues**. They are also semi-volatile, enabling them to move long distances in the atmosphere before deposition occurs."

In other words, they're carbon-containing compounds that resist sunlight, digestion and chemical breakdown; they often contain chlorine or fluoride; and they're very soluble in fats, which is central to why Meaters become far more contaminated with environmental toxins than Planters do.

Ritter et al continue: "Although many different forms of POPs may exist, both natural and anthropogenic, POPs which are noted for their persistence and bioaccumulative characteristics include many of the **first generation organochlorine insecticides** such as **dieldrin**, **DDT**, **toxaphene** and **chlordane** and several industrial chemical products or byproducts including polychlorinated biphenyls (**PCBs**), dibenzo-p-dioxins (**dioxins**) and dibenzo-p-furans (**furans**). Many of these compounds have been or continue to be used in large quantities and, due to their environmental persistence, have the ability to bioaccumulate and biomagnify. Some of these compounds such as **PCBs**, may persist in the environment for periods of years and may **bioconcentrate by factors of up to 70,000 fold**."

Besides eating roughly three times as much fat as Planters, it's animal fats that massively concentrate POPs. Chicken fats, not chickpea fats.

"Humans can be exposed to POPs through diet, occupational accidents and the environment (including indoor). Exposure to POPs, either acute or chronic, can be associated with a wide range of adverse health effects, including illness and death."

Perhaps we should avoid them? The best way to do that is to stop Meating.

Pesticides

To avoid just one of the myriad Meater-caused degenerative conditions, Parkinson's, we should avoid getting hit in the head, one, and two: we should stop drinking cows' milk or eating stuff made out of it.

For two reasons: all of the stuff that comes in pure cows' milk, like animal fats and hormones and cholesterol, which lead to atherosclerosis in the brain, setting us up for various forms of dementia, one, and two: all the pesticides and other pollutants which come along for free in animal milk. Pesticides and Parkinson's go together like Bogie and Bacall.

For more, see under: Persistent Organic Pollutants, above

Phosphate additives

As we saw earlier, 'animal phosphorus' is different to 'plant phosphorus.' Animal phosphorus bioavailability and absorption are about 50% higher than plant phosphorus. As is true with other metals like cadmium, copper and iron, Meaters are also in danger of getting too much phosphorus (and too little magnesium).

The higher our phosphate levels, the shorter our lifespans. More isn't better. More can damage our arteries, kidneys and hearts, and contributes to osteoporosis.

Does it make any sense then to eat phosphate additives? Well, that's what we do when we're Meaters and Junkers.

Junkers get it mostly in sodas, in which phosphates are used as preservatives, and Meaters get it from injected additives which (1) give (along with carbon monoxide!) dead animals a more pleasing pink color than their natural grey and (2) slow down "purge." As we'll see, purge is the fecal stew that chicken body parts, for example, are swimming in behind their plastic wrappers in the supermarket. It's the stuff that oozes out of the plastic-wrapped packages of dead animals as they rot. 90% of retail chickens are plumped up with phosphates.

Unlike plant phosphorus (>50%) and animal phosphorus (~75%), phosphate additives are almost 100% absorbable. So, not only are we getting excess phosphorus when we Junk and Meat, we're getting phosphorus on steroids.

Animals, already high in phosphorus, thus gain an extra dose of phosphorus. Excess phosphorus damages our arteries and our kidneys, can lead to metastatic calcification, and shortens our lives.

Well, maybe we can just check out the nutrition label to see how much phosphorus we're getting. Good luck with that, dear Meaters and Junkers… even though excess may be killing many of us, phosphorus isn't listed. Why not? Probably because we'd all see how unhealthy Junker and Meater products truly are. Chickens are probably the worst, by the way.

Phthalates

As above, so below… Chickens are also the worst source of phthalates; dairy and eggs are often contaminated too. What in phthunder's name are phthalates? The NIH says "Phthalates are a family of chemicals used in plastics and many other products. Phthalates are a group of chemicals used to soften and increase the flexibility of plastic and vinyl. Polyvinyl chloride is made softer and more flexible by the addition of phthalates. Phthalates are used in hundreds of consumer products."

[http://toxtown.nlm.nih.gov/text_version/chemicals.php?id=24]

Why should we care? Because pregnant Meater mothers who eat the most chickens are ten times more likely to give birth to "undervirilized" sons with, in Michael Greger's words: "one or both testicles incompletely descended, their scrotum categorized as small and/or "not distinct from surrounding tissue," and a significantly smaller penis volume, a measure of penis size taking into account both length and girth."

[See: http://nutritionfacts.org/video/chicken-consumption-and-the-feminization-of-male-genitalia/]

MEHP (mono 2-ethylhexyl phthalate) is particularly associated with undervirilization.

It's dreadfully unfair that the nutrition sins of one generation should be visited on the next, but that's exactly what can happen when Meater mothers don't eat nothing-but-food during pregnancy.

How much does the NIH page cited above say about nutrition and phthalates? Precisely zero. To them, bad medical tubing and kids chewing on toy ducks are more relevant than the #1 cause of phthalate exposure: Meating.

Some phthalates are confirmed carcinogens; some are thought to be endocrine disruptors; some are teratogenic. We should avoid them all. The best way to do that is by eating nothing but food. The good news is that phthalates disappear from our systems rapidly when we quit Meating, within days or weeks.

Pink slime

WE IN THE INDUSTRY DON'T LIKE THE TERM PINK SLIME! WE PREFER THE MORE ACCURATE NAME -
- SOYLENT PINK!
WHERE'S THE BEEF?
BEEF

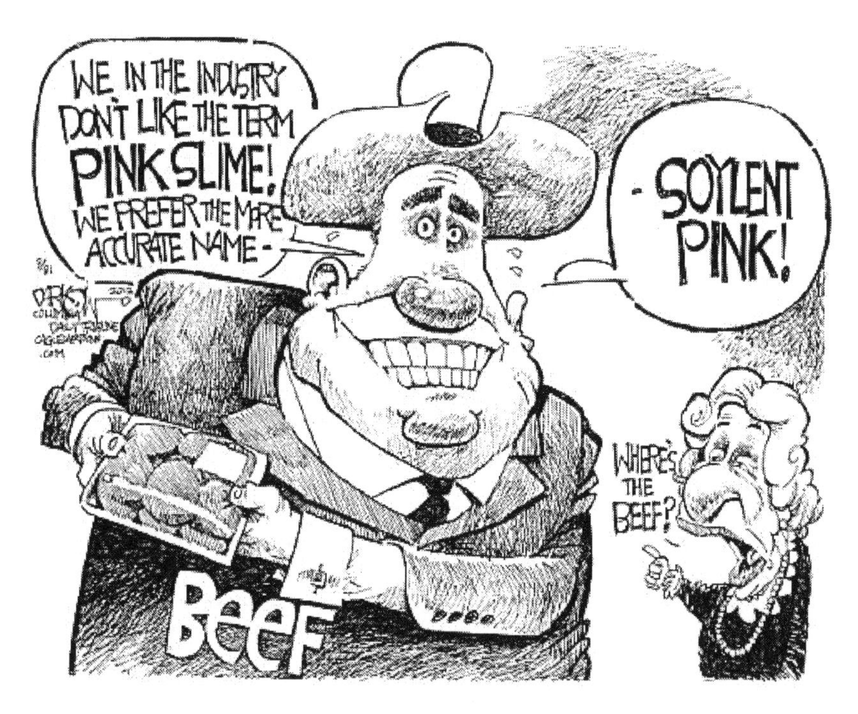

Cartoon by John Darkow, with thanks

When some pathologists – let that word sink in for a moment – took a look under the hood of fast "food" burgers, made by, yes, all the giant corporations that you just thought of, they found between 2.1% and 14.8%

animal muscles. The *best* burger they tested was about one part animal muscle and 6 parts…what? And what is meat if it's not muscle? Well, I don't think you'd like to know. Let this 'meat' remain a mystery.

Except for pink slime, which is what happens when corporate entities decide it's good for their bottom line to add ammonia to their products. Besides killing the rampant bacteria, ammonia has the benefit of cheaply bulking out burger goop and making it more easily extrudable. Except it stinks… and it's caused a riot in at least one prison whose inmates told the warden they were mad as hell and they weren't going to take it any more.

When we purée strawberries, they don't turn into pink slime.

For some of the many ways ammonia damages our health, see under: Ammonia

Polonium

Radioactive polonium forms as uranium breaks down. It occurs naturally in the oceans and then bioaccumulates in sea creatures, especially in crustaceans such as shrimps. So eating shrimps may cause mutations of our DNA and cancer as a result of radiation.

Two other polonium exposures may be worse: I bet you didn't know there was polonium in cigarette smoke. It's what gets the blame for infertility in smokers. The worst exposure appears to be pediatric CAT scans, which causes a few hundred cases of cancer in kids each year in the US.

For non-smokers not undergoing radioactive scanning procedures, Meating remains the prime source of exposure to this radioactive mutagen.

Polycarbonate plastic

Polycarbonate plastics are the kind that contain BPA (bisphenol A), which is involved in causing diabetes, liver conditions and heart conditions.

For more, see under: BPA (Bisphenol A)

Polychlorinated Biphenyls (PCBs)

"PCBs are persistent, bioaccumulative and toxic (PBT) pollutants that have been targeted by EPA."

For more, see under: PCBs

Polychlorinated naphthalenes (PCNs)

Per Wikipedia: "Polychlorinated naphthalene (PCN) products are made by chemically reacting chlorine with naphthalene, a soft, pungent solid made from coal or petroleum and often used for mothproofing.

PCNs started to be produced for high-volume uses around 1910 in both Europe and the United States… After about twenty years of commercial production, health hazards began to be reported in workers exposed to PCNs: severe skin rashes and liver disease that led to deaths of workers… There was a lag of about forty years between disclosure of PCN hazards and government regulation.

[Forty years!]

While some PCNs can be broken down by sunlight and, at slow rates, by certain microorganisms, many PCNs persist in the environment. After more than 80 years of use and total production of several hundred million kilograms, PCN residues are widespread. Acute exposure causes chloracne. Chronic exposure increases risk of liver disease."

PCNs are chlorinated polycyclic aromatic hydrocarbons, or PAHs (see below) that can behave like dioxins, i.e. dangerously.

The things we eat that are most contaminated with PCNs are farmed fishes like salmons, then wild fishes, chickens, turkeys and eggs, lambs, pigs and cows, cow's milk, cheese and butter, with the lowest levels in fruits and veggies, a.k.a. food. Food has a hundred times lower PCN concentration than fishes. Not two or three; one hundred times safer.

Polycyclic aromatic hydrocarbons (PAHs)

Whereas we get our largest intake of carcinogenic HAAs (heterocyclic aromatic amines) from eating the flesh of animals cooked over high heat, we get our largest dose of carcinogenic PAHs (polycyclic aromatic hydrocarbons) from the gases emitted while the HAAs form in grilled, fried or BBQed animal muscles.

PAHs are carcinogenic and teratogenic. Respiratory tract cancers abound among Meater BBQ chefs, and birth deformities abound among the children of Meater women who inhale too many PAH fumes.

"Meating is the new smoking." As by-products of incomplete combustion, PAHs occur as much in cigarette smoke as in animal smoke and smoked animals. We'd also do best not to live near trash-burning incinerators or to be a wildfire firefighter with a substandard respirator.

This is a seriously dangerous family of Meater substances.

For more, see under: Benzo(a)pyrene (B(a)P)

Potassium sorbate

Potassium sorbate is "the preservative used to prevent mold growth in foods such as cheese, yogurt, wine, dried meat, pickles, apple cider, and many herbal dietary supplements," according to Michael Greger.

[See: http://nutritionfacts.org/video/is-potassium-sorbate-bad-for-you/]

He cites a paper which concludes:

> "Based on our results, consumers should be made aware that PS [potassium sorbate] should be considered a genotoxic and mutagenic compound."

[See: Mamur S, Yüzbasioglu D, Unal F, Yilmaz S. Does potassium sorbate induce genotoxic or mutagenic effects in lymphocytes? *Toxicol In Vitro.* 2010 Apr;24(3):790-4.]

What's the difference, genotoxic vs. mutagenic, you ask?

Here's John Tainer answering that question over at ResearchGate: [http://www.researchgate.net/post/What_is_the_difference_between_mutagenicity_and_genotoxicity]

"Mutagens cause direct or indirect damage to DNA that results in mutations, which are changes in the DNA sequence that are retained in somatic cell divisions and passed onto progeny in germ cells. Mutagenicity refers to a chemical or physical agent's capacity to cause mutations (genetic alterations). Agents that damage DNA causing lesions that result in cell death or mutations are genotoxins. All mutagens are genotoxic, but not all genotoxins are mutagens as they may not cause retained alterations in DNA sequence."

Got that?

Anyway, pure plants are best. If we like pickles, they're easy to make at home; the vinegar's easy to make too. When we make our own we aren't exposed to mutation-causing preservatives, which turn potential foods into non-foods.

Preservatives

When we eat whole, fresh, seasonal, ripe, raw, organic, local/home-grown plants as the mainstay of our diet, what use do we have for preservatives? Dry legumes and grains last almost indefinitely so they don't need chemical preservatives either.

Essentially preservatives are for the convenience of "food" manufacturers [oxymoron alert - "Only God can make a tree"], not for the benefit of consumers. They're certainly not a boon to consumer health or safety. Anything that contains potassium sorbate, sodium benzoate, sulfites or sulfur dioxide shouldn't be thought of as food. Dried fruit, for example, preserved with sulfur dioxide, might not be the worst thing in the world, but I think we deserve the best, so we should hold out for sun-dried, and hold the chemicals.

Each of these four near-ubiquitous preservatives causes serious health issues, so we should put as few of them in our bodies as we can. Remember Caldwell Esselstyn's dictum: "Moderation kills." Moderation means mediocrity; let's eat most excellently.

For those signed up for the crewed flight to Mars, preservatives in the food may be a good idea, though I did see a short video recently of astronauts in the permanent space station proudly sprouting some lentils. That might be the way to go. I can't think of one good reason to use preservatives, except if it's non-foods we're trying to keep from rotting.

I'm a fan of pickled and fermented foods. Prebiotics, if you will, rather than the probiotics those with gut flora deranged by eating animals or antibiotics often have to take. Dill pickles, pickled onions, sauerkraut, low-salt olives, pickled beets, just love them all, even if they're not the best form of plants to eat. They've been well preserved; just without chemical preservatives like sodium benzoate which can break down into carcinogenic benzene, mutagenic potassium sorbate, or the nitrite preservatives in processed meats that form carcinogenic nitrosamines.

Don't get me started on salt as a preservative. Salt and sugar are almost as deadly as the animals we eat.

See also: Potassium sorbate; Sodium benzoate; Sulfites; Sulfur dioxide

Psyllium husks

Sometimes sold as Metamucil, psyllium husks are a lousy fiber supplement for the constipated Meater. A far better solution for constipation is to stop the Meating and Junking which cause constipation, and to eat the fiber that's naturally contained in plants. The plants don't even have to be prunes, though they work great. Sorry, dried plums, as prune producers have rebranded them.

Food trumps supplements, every time out to infinity… except for B_{12}.

Ractopamine

Ractopamine is a growth-promoting drug used mainly to bulk up pigs and turkeys, residues of which have been found in about 1 in 5 samples in the US. If we feel our hearts pounding like crazy after a meal of pig or turkey, maybe that's because Ractopamine acts like adrenaline, our "fight or flight hormone," usually secreted by our adrenal glands in response to stressful situations. Other symptoms include raised blood sugar levels, twitching muscles and high anxiety levels.

God alone knows how stressed out the already stressed-out animals must get, constantly on this stuff. Do animal farmers really not feel any empathy for animals? Or is the bottom line all that ever counts? Bastards.

Roundup®

Monsanto's Gaiacidal pesticide, whose active ingredient, glyphosate, is now deemed carcinogenic by the State of California.

My heroes. Roundup-contaminated crops aren't food.

For more, see under: Glyphosate

Salt

Added salt is another way, besides added fats and industrial sugar, that "food" synthesizers enslave us through our taste buds. Food technologists [oxymoron alert] know exactly how much sugar and salt to add to their addictive concoctions to reach the 'bliss point,' that Goldilocks amount of dopamine-spiking sugar and salt that's just right, not too much, not too little… so that we'll buy their product [oxymoron alert] and not their competitor's. Bliss point and mouth feel have nothing to do with food; blissifying mangoes already feel perfect in my mouth.

Reducing our salt intake by about a teaspoon a day would save tens of thousands of lives each year, mainly via decreased blood pressure, but also through reduced arterial damage, independent of blood pressure. As a Planter, I've become accustomed to what food tastes like without added salt. As a Meater, my taste buds were so clogged up with fats that I couldn't taste much of anything, so I added lots of salt. Now, tastes are like shafts of the rainbow, vibrant and colorful… no additives required… and dishes with added salt taste… well, unhealthy to me now.

Sodium benzoate

As mentioned under benzene above, sodium benzoate breaks down in the presence of ascorbic acid to produce benzene, a powerful poison. The most common place sodium benzoate and ascorbic acid get together is in sodas. Benzene is a known carcinogen, which also causes hyperactivity. So, besides killing us with sugar, Coke and Pepsi and their ilk are poisoning our kids and us with benzene.

Tell me, what do these people think is going to happen when they put a preservative into a non-food, a preservative made of sodium (salt) + benzene (a carcinogen)? Do they think: Gee, I hope they stick together? Or, what would happen if they don't stick together? Or, I don't care if they stick together or not, it wasn't us that split them apart? Or, I hope that salt isn't bad for them? How on earth can putting benzene+salt into a digestive tract be sane? What a digestive tract does is split things apart: we have enzymes that do nothing but split chemical bonds.

Bottom line: we have three choices. Like the Low-Carb Bullshit Artists, these people are either stupid, insane or evil. You choose.

Benzene has been found in 60% of soda brands tested and, as with most other environmental pollutants, fishes are the most contaminated: yet another reason not to eat canned tunas.

Statins

In their paper 'Statins for the primary prevention of cardiovascular disease,' one of the most respected sources, The Cochrane Collaboration, says this of cholesterol-lowering statin drugs:

"Reductions in all-cause mortality, major vascular events and revascularisations were found with no excess of adverse events among people without evidence of CVD treated with statins."

[http://www.cochrane.org/CD004816/VASC_statins-for-the-primary-prevention-of-cardiovascular-disease]

Cochrane approves of using statins to prevent cardiovascular "disease" – angina, heart attacks and strokes – from happening in lower-risk populations before clinical symptoms appear. The risk of side-effects is low.

As far as drugs go, statins aren't the worst. They work, sort of, and they're not very dangerous.

But statins have a "number needed to treat" of 1,000… that is, with a thousand people taking the drug, we'll expect to save one life a year.

Compare this with, say, Dr Caldwell Esselstyn's experience with putting 28 banana peelers on a Planter diet and keeping all of those who stuck to Planting (27) alive for decades, and we'll see how much more potent Planting is than Drugging. (Banana peelers are desperately sick people who're so close to death's door that they have one foot permanently on a figurative banana peel.)

"Number needed to treat" isn't a metric we should apply to nutrition, and yet… Esselstyn's (and Ornish's and Barnard's and… and… and…'s) number to treat approaches 1. Almost everyone who Plants gets better. Of course, Planters do die… but not often from cardiovascular "disease". Planters have no use for statins, and no need to be embroiled in the statin controversy. Planters are the CVD no-risk population.

Statins are a Meater and Junker issue.

And, for all their much-vaunted safety, here's the Mayo Clinic's discussion of statin side-effects (at http://www.mayoclinic.org/diseases-conditions/high-blood-cholesterol/in-depth/statin-side-effects/art-20046013):

They say "Statin side effects can be uncomfortable, making it seem like the risks outweigh the benefits of these powerful cholesterol-lowering medications."

Admittedly rare statin effects include:

- "Muscle pain and damage… Rhabdomyolysis can cause severe muscle pain, liver damage, kidney failure and death.
- Liver damage… unusual fatigue or weakness, loss of appetite, pain in your upper abdomen, dark-colored urine, or yellowing of your skin or eyes.
- Digestive problems… nausea, gas, diarrhea or constipation
- Rash or flushing
- Increased blood sugar or type 2 diabetes
- Neurological side effects… memory loss or confusion"

"Uncomfortable." Ya reckon? Oh, and we have to take our statins every day for the rest of our lives. Well, here's another thing we could do every day for the rest of our lives without rolling the dice on rhabdomyolysis and dementia: we could just eat food and give up our Meating-induced heart "disease". That way we won't need any statins, ever.

Pfizer would be out $8.4 billion a year for their lipitor and Merck would be out $4.4 billion a year for their zocor. In the US alone. All taken electively by Meaters who elect to have a malnutrition-caused elective "disease", and who elect to have the unpleasant side effects brought on by swallowing the environmental pollutants packaged as cholesterol-lowering drugs.

Heart "disease" and strokes aren't statin-deficiency diseases; they're simple cases of junk- and animal-caused indigestion. Mal-nutrition. Heart burn.

Sugar

Refined white sugar is pure rubbish, the original junk "food" that fueled the trans-Atlantic and Caribbean slave trade. ~~Food~~ corporations profit from it as much today as plantation owners did in the 18th and 19th Centuries. We, the general populace, are Big "Food"'s sugar slaves.

As I've said in other parts of this book, glucose is our primary fuel. Sugar in whole plants is what we're adapted to eating. Whole sugars in foods are solidified sun energy. However, industrial sugars such as high fructose corn syrup are toxic, leading us down the high glycemic highway that leads from insulin resistance to obesity, diabetes, artery and heart "disease", kidney failure, blindness, dementia and amputations through gangrene.

The sugars in whole plants are food; the sugars in junk are slow-acting, but certain poison.

But, please remember: just because isolated sugar is bad, that doesn't mean that whole plants are bad. Just because industrial sugar is sickening, that doesn't make animals food.

Sugar and cancer; Sugar and atherosclerosis

Cholesterol denialists and other medical and nutrition science fringe-dwellers need a credible-sounding alibi for how Meating can be thought of as healthy. As I've said, there are only three things we eat: animals, junk and whole plants. I've made a strong case for how harmful both animals and junk are, explaining the Eatiology of most degenerative and auto-immune conditions as responses to Meating and Junking, in hundreds of ways.

So, because Low-Carb Bullshit Artists, paleofantasists and other quackpots want to sell us on doing even more Meating, they need to come up with alternative "plausible biological mechanisms" for degenerative conditions; cancer and heart "disease", in particular. They blame the kitchen sink on sugar.

Here's Joseph Mercola, D.O., speaking in episode 8 of a 9-part, 14-hour series called *The Truth About Cancer*, which aired online from 14-22 October 2015, in which a lovely, caring man by the name of Ty Bollinger interviewed more than a hundred physicians, healers, scientists and cancer survivors, and yet managed not to mention a single Meater mechanism of cancer. That must be an all-time record for obscurantism.

Here's what Dr. Mercola has to say [*The Truth About Cancer*, episode 8, from 1:05:27 on]:

"Well, I believe it [the ketogenic diet in the treatment of cancer] has great value and, in my view, should be seriously considered as an adjunctive therapy in the treatment of most malignancies. You might say why? Because of the basic understanding we have of the physiology of cancer cells.

Otto Warburg was awarded the Nobel Prize, I believe in the 30,s for the understanding that the primary fuel for cancer cells is glucose, or sugar. And our non-cancerous cells have the ability to use glucose or fat: those are the two primary fuels. And cancer cells seem to have lost this ability."

Firstly, glucose is our primary fuel. Fat is our secondary, back-up fuel, used when we run low on glucose. Glucose is so crucial that, in an emergency, via a process known as gluconeogenesis, our bodies can turn just about anything into glucose: fats, proteins, nucleic acids...

Then, in *The Prime Cause and Prevention of Cancer* (1966), Otto Warburg wrote this:

"Cancer, above all other diseases, has countless secondary causes. But, even for cancer, there is only one prime cause. Summarized in a few words, **the prime cause of cancer is the replacement of the respiration of oxygen in normal body cells by a fermentation of sugar**. All normal body cells meet their energy needs by respiration of oxygen, whereas cancer cells meet their energy needs in great part by fermentation. All normal body cells are thus obligate aerobes, whereas **all cancer cells are partial anaerobes**... Oxygen gas, the donor of energy in plants and animals is dethroned in the cancer cells and replaced by an energy yielding reaction of the lowest living forms, namely, a fermentation of glucose."

People like Mercola and Noakes who misuse Warburg to make their case for glucose being the main cause of cancer, while exonerating animals, have thus got things 180° wrong. Warburg, a real scientist, would be appalled by such cynical misapplication of his work. Sugar doesn't cause cancer cells to become anaerobic, i.e. cancerous; anaerobic conditions in the cells force them to ferment sugar.

Oxygen starvation causes the cancer, and sugar fermentation is a symptom of the cancer. Sugar fermentation is our cells' desperate attempt to stay alive in low oxygen conditions.

Here's how the energy pathways diverge, for normal and cancer cells, according to Warburg, who was *not* a cholesterol denialist:

"...Biochemistry can explain already today why **fermentation arises, when respiration decreases**."

These five words sum up Mercola's foolishness: "fermentation arises when respiration decreases." The logical healing solution is therefore to increase respiration, isn't it?"

Mercola's witness, Warburg continues:

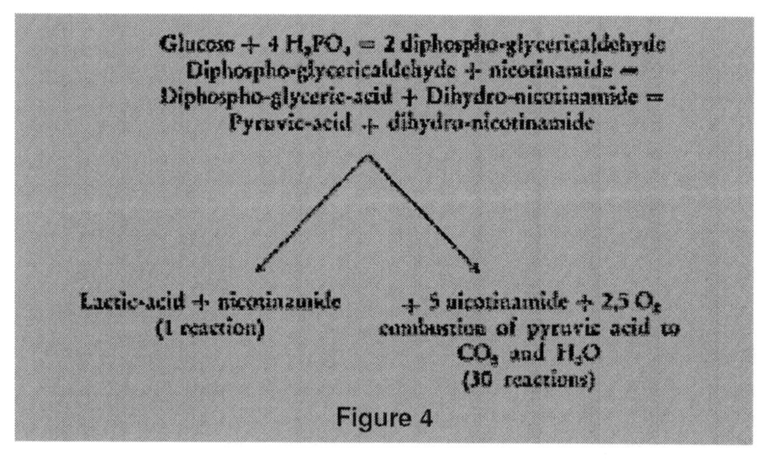

Figure 4

How sugar does *not* cause cancer, according to Otto Warburg.
Figure 4 from Otto Warburg. *The Prime Cause and Prevention of Cancer* (1966)

"Figure 4 shows that the pathways of respiration and fermentation are common as far as pyruvic acid. Then the pathways diverge. The end-products of fermentation [are] reached by one single reaction, the reduction of pyruvic acid by dihydro-nicotinamide to lactic acid. On the other hand, the end-products of the oxidation of pyruvic acid, H_2O and CO_2, are only reached after many additional reactions. Therefore, **when cells are harmed, it is probable that first respiration is harmed."**

(I've found it's always good to scrutinize the references that Meaters and cholesterol denialists and sugar meshuganahs give. (Especially retired journalists like Gary Taubes, Nina Teicholz and Bryan Walsh.) Often, as here, the sources they cite say the very opposite of what they claim. Why do they do this? They have no option because there's zero science that shows eating animals can be beneficial to cancer or cardiac patients.)

Warburg says, in effect, that a condition of low oxygen causes cancer, not that a condition of high sugar causes cancer. High sugar usage by cancer cells is the symptom; low oxygen is the cause. Yet Mercola wants us to starve the left-hand reaction, fermentation caused by hypoxia, while ignoring restoring the right-hand reaction, oxygen respiration, by increasing oxygen supply.

There's no reason to contort our physiology by putting it into a life-shortening, carb-deprived, fat-burning ketogenic state, just to stop burning our primary fuel, glucose. What we need to do is stop causing the anaerobic (low oxygen) state which causes cells to become cancerous and sugar-fermenting in the first place.

How do we do that?

Easy. Planter healers have done it millions of times. Whole-plant eaters do it every day.

We stop eating all animals and all junked-up, funked-up plants.

One of the hallmarks of Meating and Junking is atherosclerosis (hardened, damaged arteries), brought about mainly by eating the trans or hydrogenated fats in junk AND the saturated and trans fats in animals, both of which cause hypercholesterolemia, or elevated cholesterol levels, which in turn result (sequentially) in foam cells full of cholesterol in our arterial walls, then fatty streaks, then atherosclerotic plaques and narrowed arteries, leading to ischemia (reduced blood flow) and resultant hypoxic (lowered oxygen) states in tissues, which is what Warburg (but not Mercola) tells us causes cancer. Alzheimer' "disease" and other dementias, too.

It really is that simple. Apply Occam's Razor: the simplest, most apparent cause is usually the true cause. We don't need to bring in sugar to explain how the cholesterol gets into the arteries. Sugar can't build atheromas in the absence of cholesterol. There's no sugar in our artery walls.

Meating and Junking can cause cancer; pure Planting can prevent, stop and heal it.

Those heroes in *The Truth About Cancer* who managed to reverse their cancer did so to the extent that they stopped eating the two non-foods, animals and junk.

Those heroines who reversed their cancer while still eating animals (in reduced quantities), did so *despite the animals they ate*, not because of them. Their bodies' innate healing mechanisms, fortified by phytonutrients working in beautiful collaboration, overcame both the cancer and the animals.

So let's consider two approaches to reversing cancer: a Planter method and the ketogenic diet Dr. Mercola advocates.

Planting gradually improves vascular health. The arteries dilate better, delivering more blood and oxygen to all our cells, including the cancerous cells. This allows cellular respiration of oxygen to be favored over aerobic fermentation, and the cancer cells may even be returned to normal, without killing them. The root cause is removed. This is essentially a very high sugar diet. BUT this is a whole plant, high fiber diet, and we've known for decades now that it's the best anti-atheroma diet available (Ornish 1990).

The best that the ketogenic diet can do is to treat a symptom – the glucose fermentation that's caused by oxygen starvation – and then, instead of returning cells to health, we're trying to starve billions of cancer cells to death, by restricting glucose, while also depriving the body's tens of trillions of healthy cells. No wonder people on ketogenic diets live shorter lives. Why doesn't Dr. Mercola mention that little fact?

Sadly, the truth about *The Truth About Cancer* is that, while hours were devoted to the spectacular benefits of Planting and the demerits of Junking, not a single second was devoted to the hideous consequences of Meating. I don't know why. Sponsorships? Popularity? Personal Meating habit?

To heal from cancer, we do indeed need to stop eating processed sugars – Junk – but we also need to stop Meating.

We need to learn how to count to two, dear people. It's not just the sugar, and it's not just the animals; it's both. It's the animals AND the sugar. They're both non-foods. 'Meat + sweet' will be the death of most of us.

Sulfites

The preservative saga continues, unabated… The problem with putting one FDA-approved, GRAS (generally regarded as safe) chemical into our bodies is that our bodies like to get rid of the stuff we put in them, so they change the (supposedly okay) stuff into other stuff, and the other stuff may be poisonous. That's what happens to sulfur-containing sulfites. They get broken down and the sulfur is incorporated into hydrogen sulfide (see above), with potentially lethal consequences via inflammatory bowel "disease" and colon cancer.

As we can see in the table on the following page called "FDA Guide to Foods and Drugs with Sulfites," there are items that we should quite legitimately be able to label as food. Unfortunately, the addition of sulfur is enough to turn them into non-foods. We should try to avoid them.

If we eat items that have lists of ingredients and nutrients on labels on packets, then we need to read the labels carefully for a whole range of possible villains and take evasive action when necessary. A safer, more nutritious way to eat is simply to eat whole grains, nuts and seeds, fruits and vegetables: whole food, mostly label- and ingredient-list-free.

"The following foods and drugs MAY contain sulfites, according to the Food and Drug Administration. Not all manufacturers use sulfites in these products, and the amounts may vary. Remember to check the product label."

A word of caution: according to the list below, some asthma drugs may contain sulfites. This is ironic because somewhere between one in a hundred and one in two thousand people is allergic or sulfite-sensitive, so some asthmatics may be being put in danger by their medications.

(There's oceans more to be said about the dangers of medications, but now's not the time, nor this the place.)

Food Category	Type of Food
Alcoholic Beverages	Beer, cocktail mixes, wine, wine coolers.
Baked Goods	Cookies, crackers, mixes with dried fruits or vegetables, pie crust, pizza crust, quiche crust, flour tortillas.
Beverage Bases	Dried citrus fruit beverage mixes.
Condiments and Relishes	Horseradish, onion and pickle relishes, pickles, olives, salad dressing mixes, wine vinegar.
Confections and Frostings	Brown, raw, powdered or white sugar derived from sugar beets.
Modified Dairy Products	Filled milk (a specially prepared skim milk in which vegetable oils, rather than animal fats, are added to increase its fat content).
Drugs	Antiemetics (taken to prevent nausea), cardiovascular drugs, antibiotics, tranquilizers, intravenous muscle relaxants, analgesics (painkillers), anesthetics, steroids and nebulized bronchodilator solutions (used for treatment of asthma).
Fish and Shellfish	Canned clams; fresh, frozen, canned or dried shrimp; frozen lobster; scallops; dried cod.
Fresh Fruit and Vegetables	Sulfite use banned (except for fresh potatoes).
Gelatins, Puddings, and Fillings	Fruit fillings, flavored and unflavored gelatin, pectin jelling agents.
Grain Products and Pastas	Cornstarch, modified food starch, spinach pasta, gravies, hominy, breadings, batters, noodle/rice mixes.
Jams and Jellies	Jams and jellies.
Nuts and Nut Products	Shredded coconut.
Plant Protein Products	Canned, bottled or frozen fruit juices (including lemon, lime, grape and apple); dried fruit; canned, bottled or frozen dietetic fruit or fruit juices; maraschino cherries and glazed fruit.
Processed Vegetables	Vegetable juice, canned vegetables (including potatoes), pickled vegetables (including sauerkraut), dried vegetables, instant mashed potatoes, frozen potatoes and potato salad.
Snack Foods	Dried fruit snacks, trail mixes, filled crackers.
Soups and Soup Mixes	Canned seafood soups, dried soup mixes.
Sweet Sauces, Toppings	Corn syrup, maple syrup, fruit toppings, and Syrups high-fructose corn syrup, pancake syrup.
Tea	Instant tea, liquid tea concentrates.
The [above] foods and drugs MAY contain sulfites, according to the Food and Drug Administration.	Not all manufacturers use sulfites in these products, and the amounts may vary. Remember to check the product label.

FDA Guide to Foods and Drugs with Sulfites
Source: http://extoxnet.orst.edu/faqs/additive/sulf_tbl.htm.

(I lean towards the 1-in-2000 figure for sulfite-sensitivity: there's so much else that's life-threatening in non-foods besides sulfites that there's lots of room for confounding non-nutrients, especially when most researchers mistakenly think animals are food. I may be wrong.)

Sulfur dioxide (SO_2)

SO_2 continues our string of preservatives that are routinely added to foods and routinely mangle our health. SO_2 works in the same way as sulfites: by being metabolized into hydrogen sulfide, setting us up for bowel inflammation and cancer.

Its main use is in dried fruits. Fresh are better than dried, but sun-dried are better than sulfur-preserved; they just won't last as long. But, hey, we need to ask: why do we want to stop food from rotting? Rotting is what's supposed to happen over time. Food should rot. Only non-foods don't rot. Not rotting is a quality desired by the seller, not the buyer.

Supplements

Why do we take supplements? Because we're not getting enough of certain nutrients in our "food".

Which nutrients are we deficient in? Protein? Hardly – our protein problems are caused by eating too many, and of the wrong sort – animal rather than vegetable.

Different eaters may lack different nutrients.

Vegans often lack calcium, iodine, vitamin B_{12} and, sometimes, vitamin D, if we're not spending enough time out of doors.

Planters – people who eat nothing but whole plants, as opposed to vegans, who may be Junkers – get sufficient calcium and iodine; calcium from plants such as leafy greens like arugula and kale, or crucifers like broccoli, and iodine from sea vegetables. Plant calcium is absorbed twice as well as milk calcium. Most Planters need to supplement B_{12} forever. Either that, or eat enough fortified foods, which hopefully aren't unfoods such as sugary commercial breakfast cereals.

Vitamin D is the hormone made from cholesterol by the action of sunlight on our skins, so, if we live in boreal climes, where the sun never gets high enough in the sky for us to be getting the right sunrays to make D, or if we don't spend enough time outdoors, then we should take a vegan D supplement. That's it. Planters should take B_{12} for sure, and maybe D. We should be careful with D. Too much can be harmful. With B_{12}, we could swallow a kilo of the stuff and just pee out the excess. That's not a challenge.

Meaters are often deficient in eight nutrients; understandably because many of these are found only in plants: vitamins C and E, fiber, folate (all plants-only) and magnesium, potassium, calcium and iodine.

Calcium and iodine we touched upon under what Planters eat. It's ironic that Meaters are often calcium-deficient, considering the main supposed benefit of drinking cow's milk is its calcium content. C, E, fiber and folate are found only in plants, so Meaters should be eating more whole plants, not just the parsley garnish. Magnesium deficiency is a big reason why so many Meaters drop dead from heart attacks every year. Just getting the recommended amount of this single nutrient from food, not supplements, could save tens of thousands of lives. A daily small handful of nuts or seeds would do the trick. Potassium deficiency and stroke, ditto, sourced from beans and leafy greens.

Magnesium (Mg) is fascinating. It's the metallic ion at the heart of the heme portion of the chlorophyll molecule, the wondrous miracle that converts sunshine into sugar, our prime fuel. I'll go into more detail about magnesium in the Animal MIAs section. When we were discussing heme iron on page 53 we saw a picture that compares the structures of chlorophyll and the heme portion of hemoglobin, our blood's oxygen transport molecule, which has an iron (Fe) ion at its core.

The power particles in our blood (oxygen is fuel) and the sugar-making molecules in plants (glucose is fuel) are, with the easiest of substitutions, essentially identical. We are sun- and sugar- and oxygen-powered beings! I find that absolutely gobsmackingly miraculous. I'd love to know where your thinking takes you on that one. Till later…

Back to supplements.

All Planters need to do to achieve optimum nutrient intake is to get enough B_{12}, i.e. take a harmless supplement, and go out in the sun, with as much skin exposed as possible. Don't overdo it, and not with the sun overhead at high noon.

All Meaters need to do to achieve optimum nutrient intake is to become Planters, and take their B_{12}.

I used the word 'harmless' with B_{12} above on purpose, because many other supplements are harmful. Taking supplements such as multivitamins has been shown, at best, to make no difference in life expectancy, or, at worst, shorten our lives. Especially multis that contain copper or iron, both of which are associated with increased risk of dementia.

These supplements all cause damage or shorten our lives… In other words, taking these as supplements rather than getting them from plants damages us and kills us before our time:

- Vitamin A

- Beta carotene
- Vitamin E
- Lutein
- Folic acid (not the same as plant folate)
- Calcium!

The latest science tells us that the risks of supplementing with calcium outweigh the benefits. For healthy bones, be a Planter and exercise.

And, though I'm fond of the memory of twice-Nobel laureate Linus Pauling, vitamin C is very healthy for its manufacturers but does pretty much zilch for us on its own as an extracted, isolated, out-of-context micronutrient. It certainly doesn't do nearly as much for us as dietary vitamin C – we should dare to eat an orange or a grapefruit, every day, to prevent the need for C supplements, or for the need of megadoses of C as a cancer treatment. C supplements remind me of one definition of a sailboat: a hole in the water, surrounded by wood, into which we pour money. Supplements make expensive pee.

Here's the landmark study that laid bare the dangers of many nutrients taken as supplements:

G. Bjelakovic, D. Nikolova, L.L. Gluud, R.G. Simonetti, & C. Gluud. Mortality in randomized trials of antioxidant supplements for primary and secondary prevention: systematic review and meta-analysis. *JAMA*, 297(8):842-857, 2007.

If there's anything we eat that's "evolutionarily novel," it's nutritional supplements. Which is why it's hilarious to see how many paleo bro-scientists are supplement and/or fiber hucksters on the side.

"Food," as Dr Greger and I love to repeat, "is a package deal." There are a hundred thousand naturally occurring phytonutrients in nature. There are more than 500 different carotenes alone. They all come packaged together and work synergistically to create effects and inter-reactions that we will never be able to unravel, not with all the computing power in a googolplex (10^{100}) of universes. Different phytonutrients potentiate each other, so having one without the other is a waste of time and resources. An example is vitamin C's boosting of iron absorption.

To think that we can replicate what food does with nutrients by isolating one little nutrient at a time and then ingesting it in massive quantities is to fundamentally misunderstand food. This puerile scientific reductionism is costing many people their lives every day, killed by trying to be healthy… and taking deadly supplements. Their manufacture – that word should give us a clue about whether they're food or not – is idiocy, hubris, lunacy. I'm not against science; I'm against flawed science for profit.

Other than vitamin B_{12} (and D, taken with care, if necessary), all non-botanical supplements should be labeled with skulls and crossed bones. They're not food. We shouldn't swallow their makers' snake oil sales pitches, and we shouldn't swallow them.

(I really should learn to express my feelings. This reticence of mine isn't healthy.)

Supplements, the corporate way

Though supplements aren't food, and supplements aren't medicine, they can be powerful drugs. Many supplements are downright dangerous, taking years off our lives. Of course, if I were an educated Meater, I wouldn't worry about what the supplements are doing to me – I'd know that eating animals is far more dangerous to my health, so I'd supplement away… But maybe we should ask, Qui bono? Who benefits? Many supplements are sold by the very same drug companies health-conscious supplementers are seeking to avoid.

Caveat: If you're on an Atkins diet and you can't see your way clear to eating some fibrous plants, you'd be advised to stock up on all the fiber supplements they're itching to sell you. A diet that sells fiber supplements can't be taken very seriously by anyone with the first inkling of a nutrition education.

Teratogens

MedicineNet.com defines a teratogen as "Any agent that can disturb the development of an embryo or fetus. Teratogens may cause a **birth defect** in the child. Or a teratogen may halt the pregnancy outright. The classes of teratogens include radiation, maternal infections, chemicals, and drugs."

PBTs or POPs are very often teratogenic and, as mentioned above, **abortifacients**: they can cause miscarriages. Consequently, with POPs biomagnified by animals, Meaters are far more prone to giving birth to deformed children than Planters. As ever, fishes and other sea life are the worst of the worst when it comes to contamination.

Tetrahydroisoquinoline

Parkinson's is complicated. There are many neurotoxins associated with it, including BMAA and environmental pollutants such as aluminum and pesticide residues and metabolites.

Tetrahydroisoquinolines are a family of alkaloids also associated with Parkinson's, and, guess what? Just like aluminum – which cheese makers actively, consciously, deliberately put into their deadly wares – Tetra is found mainly in cheeses.

Though present in low concentrations, Tetra may bioaccumulate in animal fats; in our case, the fatty organ involved is our human brain.

So, while it may matter to researchers whether it's the dairy products that are causing neurodegenerative conditions such as Parkinson's or whether it's the neurotoxins which come in the dairy products, we consumers shouldn't give a hoot. We should simply not eat the wretched stuff, that is, not if we'd like to keep all our marbles.

Titanium dioxide

TiO_2, also known as paint Pigment White 6 or titanium white, is what some bright spark put into Junk to make some un-foods look whiter. Sadly, it's a major cause of inflammatory bowel conditions and colorectal cancer.

For more, see under: Nanoparticles ~ Microparticles

Tobacco smoke

Oscar Wilde said: "You must have a cigarette. A cigarette is the perfect type of a perfect pleasure. It is exquisite, and it leaves one unsatisfied. What more can one want?" In *The Importance of Being Earnest*, Algernon says: "When I am in trouble, eating is the only thing that consoles me. Indeed, as anyone who knows me intimately will tell you, I refuse everything except food and drink."

Perhaps Wilde would have appreciated the PCRM awareness campaign we saw earlier, called "Meat is the new smoking." Eating one hot dog has a carcinogenic effect equivalent to smoking five cigarettes. What price pleasure now, when faced with this 'competing risks analysis?'

And one of the agents is the same: the carcinogenic nitrosamines in cigarette smoke are the same nitrosamines our bodies make out of the nitrites we eat when we eat animals, either naturally present or when added as preservatives.

Actually, cigarette smoke can be called a persistent organic pollutant. Smoking indoors causes a deposition of residues (of hundreds of different toxins) that builds up over time on surfaces, causing harm via what's now known as 3rd hand smoking. The gift that keeps on giving…

Cigarettes, alcohol and HFCS are the ultimate in Junking, rivaled only in their ill-effects by Meating. Animals and cigarettes are so packed with carcinogens that, if they were new products just being introduced to the market, even our present corrupt bureaucracy would be forced to deny them a license to kill.

Toxaphene

The EPA website [at http://www.epa.gov/pbt/pubs/toxaphene.htm] says:

"Toxaphene is an **insecticide** which is usually found as a solid or gas. From 1947 to **1980** toxaphene was primarily used in the southern United States on cotton crops. Widespread use of toxaphene has been **banned** in the United States due to its **harmful effects** on us. Toxaphene is a **persistent, bioaccumulative, and toxic (PBT) pollutant targeted by EPA**.

Why Are We Concerned About Toxaphene?

Because toxaphene is **bioaccumulative**, it **does not easily break down** in our environment and **becomes more concentrated as it moves up the food chain** to humans and other animals. Levels may be high in some **predatory fish and mammals** because toxaphene **accumulates** in the bodies of those exposed to it. Toxaphene-like substances have been found in the **Great Lakes** ecosystem.

What harmful effects can Toxaphene have on us?

Injures the **kidneys** and **liver**; Damages the **immune system**; Harms the **adrenal gland**; Causes changes in the **development** of unborn children; May cause **cancer**; Damages the **lungs**; Damages the **nervous system**

How are we exposed to Toxaphene?
By eating **contaminated fish and shellfish**
By eating foods exposed to toxaphene
Infants may be exposed through **breast milk**
Unborn children can be exposed through the **mother's blood stream** if she is exposed

Where can Toxaphene be found?

Current uses:
Cattle dip for scabies control
Pineapples in Puerto Rico
Emergency treatment of cotton, **corn, and small grains**
Bananas in the Virgin Islands"
I hope for everyone's sake that this EPA information is out of date – are Dole pineapples and Chiquita bananas inundated with toxaphene? That's gross, if they are.

As with every one of the **PBTs**, as their name defines: they're **persistent**, lasting decades in the environment; they're **bioaccumulative**, becoming more deadly the further up the food chain we eat… until we reach us at the top; and they're **toxic**.

They're in the animals we eat, particularly fishes and shellfishes, and Meater mothers may contaminate their fetuses or neonates via their blood or breast milk.

Unlike other PBTs it appears that some outposts of Empire – Virgin Islands and Puerto Rico – may still be using toxaphene, and using it to bugger up otherwise healthy plant crops. So, as well as advising people to steer away from Meating, I'd have to counsel eating only organic fruits and veg from a reliable source, to avoid damage from this mutagen and teratogen.

Trans Fats

Trans fatty acids occur nowhere in nature except in animals. However, food scientists [oxymoron alert] have found them useful to give otherwise perishable items a long shelf-life [oxymoron alert: if it lasts a long time without rotting, it probably isn't alive.]

Trans fats are implicated in raising the cholesterol of those who believe in the cholesterol myth (but not the cholesterol levels of unbelievers, who are nutrition marvels, immune to atherosclerosis, as proven by no scientific study, nowhere, nowhen.)

The USDA's list of the top sources of trannies appears below.

Junk fats – hydrogenated vegetable oils and spreads – rule the roost. Vegetable oils chemically modified to behave like animal oils. But we don't eat a whole lot of those. Besides junk, animal muscles and dairy products account for most of the trans fats we eat.

USDA National Nutrient Database for Standard ReferenceRelease 27

Nutrients: Fatty acids, total trans (g)

Food Subset: All Foods
Ordered by: Nutrient Content
Measured by: 100 g
Report Run at: December 24, 2014 02:35 EST

NDB_No	Description
04667	Shortening, industrial, soy (partially hydrogenated) for baking and confections
04652	Oil, industrial, soy (partially hydrogenated), all purpose
04664	Oil, industrial, soy (partially hydrogenated), palm, principal uses icings and fillings
04654	Oil, industrial, soy (partially hydrogenated) and cottonseed, principal use as a tortilla shortening
04645	Oil, industrial, canola (partially hydrogenated) oil for deep fat frying
04665	Margarine, industrial, non-dairy, cottonseed, soy oil (partially hydrogenated), for flaky pastries
04668	Margarine, industrial, soy and partially hydrogenated soy oil, use for baking, sauces and candy
04655	Margarine-like shortening, industrial, soy (partially hydrogenated), cottonseed, and soy, principal use flaky pastries
04585	Margarine-like, margarine-butter blend, soybean oil and butter
04610	Margarine, regular, 80% fat, composite, stick, with salt
04617	Margarine, regular, 80% fat, composite, stick, without salt
04628	Margarine, 80% fat, stick, includes regular and hydrogenated corn and soybean oils
04691	Margarine, regular, 80% fat, composite, stick, with salt, with added vitamin D
04629	Margarine, margarine-type vegetable oil spread, 70% fat, soybean and partially hydrogenated soybean, stick
04666	Shortening, industrial, soy (partially hydrogenated) and corn for frying
04648	Oil, industrial, soy (partially hydrogenated), principal uses popcorn and flavoring vegetables
04615	Shortening, vegetable, household, composite
04651	Oil, industrial, soy (partially hydrogenated), multiuse for non-dairy butter flavor
04612	Margarine-like, vegetable oil spread, 60% fat, stick, with salt
04693	Margarine-like, vegetable oil spread, 60% fat, stick, with salt, with added vitamin D
04649	Shortening, industrial, soy (partially hydrogenated), pourable liquid fry shortening
04653	Oil, industrial, soy (partially hydrogenated) and soy (winterized), pourable clear fry
25014	Snacks, popcorn, microwave, regular (butter) flavor, made with partially hydrogenated oil
28111	KEEBLER, READY CRUST, Chocolate Pie Crust
28266	KEEBLER, READY CRUST, Graham Pie Crust (10"), Reduced Fat
04614	Margarine-like, vegetable oil spread, 60% fat, stick/tub/bottle, with salt
04695	Margarine-like vegetable-oil spread, stick/tub/bottle, 60% fat, with added vitamin D
21324	McDONALD'S, Baked Apple Pie

USDA National Nutrient Database for Standard Reference Release 27: Trans fats

Trans fats are lethal, worse than saturated fats even, and they raise blood cholesterol levels far more than dietary cholesterol itself. Eating animal fats – trans and saturated – is the dietary factor that best predicts Alzheimer's "disease". (So which is the disease, the Meater cause or the Alzheimer's effect?)

Any well-informed government free of corporate suasion would ban the production of trans-fat-like hydrogenated vegetable oils or the inclusion of trans fats in food. In a heartbeat. We shouldn't eat anything that has Meater or Junker trans fats in them – they're not food.

Transglutaminase

Transglutaminase is the enzyme used in meat glue, once taken from guinea pig livers, now of synthetic origin. It's used to gum together offcuts and waste products like tendons to make a solid-seeming, more commercially rewarding cut of animal flesh.

Wikipedia has this to say: "A transglutaminase is an enzyme that catalyzes the formation of an isopeptide bond between a free amine group (e.g., protein- or peptide-bound lysine) and the acyl group at the end of the side chain of protein- or peptide-bound glutamine. The reaction also produces a molecule of ammonia... [Ammonia; that doesn't sound good.]

Transglutaminases were first described in 1959. The exact biochemical activity of transglutaminases was discovered in blood coagulation protein factor XIII in 1968."

Let's unpack that a bit. Transglutaminases actually join the proteins of two different pieces of flesh together chemically, at the molecular level. That's why meat glue can't be detected with the bare eye. I picture a zipper pulling two pieces of fabric together... where the analogy breaks down is that the meat glue zipper spews out toxic ammonia in its wake.

Transglutaminase enzymes quite naturally knit together blood proteins when our blood clots. I would stick with that natural process and forego any extra glue enzymes from Meating.

For more, see under: Meat glue

Triclosan and Triclocarban

T&T are antibacterial compounds used in soaps and household products, reliably considered to be carcinogenic. If they're in our dishwashing liquid, I'd make certain I rinsed my plates thoroughly after using so I didn't accidentally eat any.

By the by: as a pure Planter, I haven't needed to use dishwashing soap in many years. I don't even use hot water to wash up. There's no need. I also don't have a fat trap in my sink drain: there's no need. I also don't need oven cleaner. These are all Meater products for which I have no use. Fat isn't a feminist issue; it's a Meater issue.

Vegetable oils

All veggie oils, even the supposedly heart-healthy ones, are 100% fat (meaning that all the energy they provide comes from fat). Olive oil is

~13% saturated fat, the same fat that makes animals so unhealthy to eat. We should keep these to a minimum in what we eat, especially if we're suffering from heart "disease", i.e. if we're Meating or Junking. Anyone facing a health challenge like atherosclerosis or cancer should cut out the oils altogether, at least until they're well again. (Anyone eating animals *is* health-challenged.)

Dr. John McDougall, of whose *Starch Solution* course I'm a graduate, thinks that vegetable oils potentiate carcinogens and are more relevant to cancer than animals, even. I don't think he's right, but that doesn't matter. He's got decades of practical experience and I haven't, so I' more likely to be wrong. We're both Planters and I agree that vegetable oils are junk. So does Caldwell Esselstyn who, along with Dean Ornish, is the most accomplished heart "disease" reverser alive today, and both of them use plant-based diets. Famously, one of Ess's mantras is: "No oil!"

"Why?" he asks. "Because of the data."

There's a fun YouTube clip from VegSource, called "No Oil – Not Even Olive Oil! – Caldwell Esselstyn MD" at https://www.youtube.com/watch?v=b_o4YBQPKtQ.

Salads make for famously nutrient-dense, low-calorie Planter meals. I eat mine with balsamic or flavored vinegars, or lemon juice, or plain. The addition of just a single tablespoon of oil undoes most of the low-calorie goodness of the food; with more calories coming from the oil than all the veggies, unless we've loaded up with avos, nuts or olives – all excellent high-fiber fat sources.

Vegetable oils are the liquid 'empty calorie' equivalent of white bread.

So, no – or at least very low – veggie oils.

Veterinary drug residues

About 320 million or so humans share the USA with about 100 million head of cattle, each, except for those unlucky enough to be organically reared, consuming pounds of veterinary drugs each year. Well, those thousands of tons of vet's drugs end up someplace… either in the animals we eat or in the water we often drink. This isn't ideal, shall we say?

Vinclozolin

Vinclozolin is a fungicide used by conventional farmers to control plant diseases, such as blights, molds and rots. Sadly it acts as an endocrine disruptor in humans and has anti-androgenic effects, meaning it messes with male hormonal development. It's known to cause hypospadias, "a congenital condition in males in which the opening of the urethra is on the underside of the penis."

The only way to be optimally healthy is to eat organically grown plants, free from teratogenic substances like vinclozolin.

Vitamins

Vitamin, a portmanteau word for 'vital amine,' is a misnomer, because they're not amines. They're vital in that our bodies don't make them, so we get them from food. Putting it the other way around explains the situation: because vitamins were everywhere around us as we humans developed over millions of years, we didn't bother to set up Darwinianly expensive metabolic pathways to make them when we ate them every day.

In my earlier sidebar rant about the word "essential" I showed how the word's meaning has become twisted. Vitamins are essential nutrients. It's essential that we eat them. They're ubiquitous (if we eat food) so it's entirely inessential for us to make them. Why set up a factory to make wild flowers, for example, when they're lolling around the countryside, brightening up the hedgerows?

Our bodies do make B_{12}, but in our colons, too far down our alimentary canals for it to be absorbed. Until very late in our history, we'd get our bacteria-made B_{12} from the dirty things we ate (just the way Meaters get it now). Today, in our antiseptic world, we need to supplement it.

Vitamin supplements are a no-no. They're a "brainer," not a no-brainer. We have to think about and understand holistic nutrition to grok that vitamins only come from plants (yes, B_{12} from bacteria and D from the sun/skin collaboration) and that vitamins from health food stores [oxymoron alert, when it comes to supplements] aren't food. No matter how earnest and persuasive the sandal-wearers may be, we should skip the life-shortening vitamin supplements and just eat food. They're environmental contaminants we can choose not to put into ourselves.

Vitamin B_{12} – a beneficial Meater contaminant

Now, at the risk of making you fall out of your chair in surprised disbelief, I've got to admit that this is the one nutrient that modern Planting doesn't supply as well as Meating.

That said, I'm now going to resume normal service by saying: Meating isn't a better source of B_{12} than Planting. That's because "food is a package deal" and when we're Meaters we can't get the cyanobacteria-produced B_{12} with which animals are contaminated without also getting the full catastrophe of animal proteins and fats, cholesterol, hormones and heme iron, and on and on… and the parasites and other pathogens… and the bioaccumulated environmental toxins.

Eating animals because it provides B_{12} – or not being a Planter because it doesn't supply B_{12} – is like refusing to go to the beach because we've taken umbrage at one particular grain of sand. In the larger scheme, it's irrelevant.

Animals don't make B_{12}; the bacteria that coat the entire planet make it, and animals get it by having their faces in the planet all day long, as they graze on plants. In olden times, when our plants weren't so sterilized, we used to get all the B_{12} we needed from contaminated plants. Now… now we eat fortified whole foods or we take supplements.

B_{12} is the single limiting factor of Planting. We accept it. It's the single mis-tied knot in our carpet, because only God – may his name be praised! – can make a perfect thing. It's the crack through which Leonard Cohen says the light gets in.

If the lack of B_{12} is what limits Planting, it's a minute drawback, compared to the advantages of being heart attack-proof and living years longer.

If getting B_{12} from dead animals is a Meater advantage, it's a miniscule one, especially when compared to all the major drawbacks of Meating… oh, like more of all the degenerative "diseases", more of the animal-borne infectious diseases, decreased intelligence, diminished sexual vigor and shorter lifespan.

When weighed against each other, Meating and Planting, B_{12} is seen for the non-issue it is.

Warfarin

Now, call me old-fashioned but… rat poison? Really? Having been told that veganism is "a little extreme" by people who think nothing of prescribing or imbibing a chemical that kills rats by thinning their blood, I wonder, along with Tina Turner, 'who's zoomin' who?' Why is it extreme to eat plants that naturally contain salicylic acid, aspirin's active ingredient, giving us all the blood-thinning benefit without the potentially lethal ulcerations?

NIOSH calls warfarin a 'rodenticide.' Why would we put it in our bodies? And why would we want to harm the gorgeous wittle wattywoos?

Xenoestrogens

Xenoestrogens (a sub-group of xeno-hormones) are foreign substances, either natural or human-made, that cause unhealthy effects similar to human estrogen, which is known to be carcinogenic when produced in excess. They're endocrine disruptors: they disrupt our hormonal balance.

The Breast Cancer Fund, at http://www.breastcancerfund.org/clear-science/radiation-chemicals-and-breast-cancer/, has a list of…

Chemicals and Radiation Linked to Breast Cancer

They say: "In our daily lives we are exposed to toxic chemicals and radiation from a wide range of sources, and a large and growing body of scientific evidence tells us that some of these exposures can increase breast cancer risk.

Exposures to breast carcinogens—chemicals that directly cause breast cancer—are an obvious concern.

But we also must pay attention to exposures to chemicals that disrupt the body's hormones—chemicals known as endocrine-disrupting compounds [EDCs]—as well as to physical agents such as ionizing radiation. Below is a catalogue of chemicals and physical agents that have been linked to breast cancer."

I've extracted the EDCs from their list of breast carcinogens. (Of course, many of these toxins cause mutations as well as disrupting our hormone signaling.)

Here's **the Breast Cancer Fund's list of endocrine disruptors**:

2,4,5-TP (Agricultural pesticide)
Alkylphenols (Used in many household products and cleaners)
Aromatic amines (Byproduct from manufacturing foams, dyes and more)
Atrazine (Triazine herbicide, used to control weeds)
Bioidentical hormones (Hormones used to treat the symptoms of menopause)
Bisphenol A (BPA) (Synthetic estrogen used in food can linings and everyday products)
Bovine growth hormone (rBGH/rBST) (Hormone injected into cows to increase milk production)
Cadmium and other metals (Naturally occurring heavy metals)

Chlordane, Malathion & 2,4-D (Pesticides used on termites)
DDT (Widely banned pesticide)
Dieldrin and Aldrin (Pesticides used from the 1950s-1970s)
Diethylstilbestrol (DES) (Drug found to cause vaginal cancer and breast cancer)
Dioxins (Group of chemicals formed when chlorinated compounds are burned)
Heptachlor (Pesticide banned in 1993; still persists in the environment)
Hormone replacement therapy (HRT) Progesterone (Pharmaceuticals used in post-menopausal hormone therapy)
Hormones in personal care products (Placental extracts containing high hormone levels)
Mycoestrogens (Fungal estrogens) (Estrogens produced by fungi; can contaminate grains)
Oral contraceptives (Birth control pills, which are most often a mixture of synthetic estrogen and progestin)
Parabens (Preservatives used in food, pharmaceuticals and cosmetics)
Perfluorooactinoic acid (PFOA) (Synthetic chemical used in non-stick cookware & stain resistant coatings)
Phthalates (Class of plastics found in plastics, personal care products, and fragrance)
Phytoestrogens [No explanation given in the main heading. Author]
Polybrominated diphenyl ethers (PBDEs) (Fire retardants used in consumer and industrial products)
Polychlorinated biphenyls [PCBs] (Class of banned chemicals still found in the environment and in products produced before the ban)
Polycyclic aromatic hydrocarbons (PAHs) (Class of chemicals that are products of combustion)
Sunscreens (UV filters) (Some chemicals used as UV filters are also endocrine disruptors)
Tobacco smoke (Contains hundreds of chemicals, including known carcinogens)
Triclosan and Triclocarban (Antibacterial compounds used in soaps and household products)
Zeranol (Synthetic growth factor used in cattle)

The majority of the BCF's endocrine disruptors show up as individual listings in this Contaminants section of *Why Animals Aren't Food.* What they all have in common is that they're not foods, and yet they're all consumed in vastly higher concentrations by Meaters and Junkers than by Planters.

This is because EDs are POPs, organic pollutants that persist in the environment. Animals eat them and biomagnify them in their fat, and we're the animals that eat the animals with their hyper-concentrated toxins.

Meater mothers bathe unborn babies in these toxins in the womb, then feed them more via breast milk. As I mentioned earlier, a cynic once said that the best way for a Meater woman to detox is to have a child and pass her poisons on. That sounds cruel and insensitive, but that's what happens all the time out here in Meaterland: mothers passing on teratogens and carcinogens to the next generation, raising Cain without knowing it.

After we've gotten rid of all our toxic household, cookware and personal care products, and stopped taking HRT and oral contraceptives, the best way to avoid endocrine disrupting chemicals is Planting.

Oops... Phytoestrogens are in the list of endocrine disruptors above... Plant hormones... How can that be? Let's take a look. It turns out that they're *beneficial* endocrine disruptors. Here's what the BCF says: "...current epidemiologic evidence from studies in humans suggests that eating soy products and other phytoestrogens during the adolescent period has a protective effect against subsequent breast cancer risk." Everyday, uncommon sense tells us this: until recently, Oriental women have been almost immune to breast cancer. One of the reasons cancer has skyrocketed in the East is because they're now eating *less* soy, not more; and more animals and junk.

But here's a news flash for those who remain unconvinced: we don't automatically have to eat soybeans just because we're vegans. "The prevailing evidence against synthetic estrogens must be understood alongside evidence about the effects of plant estrogens (phytoestrogens). Foods such as whole grains, dried beans, peas, fruits, broccoli, cauliflower and especially soy products are rich in phytoestrogens."

Getting back in character... turning away from the merits of Planter endocrine disruptors and back to the demerits of Meater endocrine disruptors...

It should be obvious why Meaters and Junkers have way, way more breast (and prostate and ... and... and...) cancer than Planters: when we Meat and Junk, we fill ourselves up with all the carcinogens and endocrine-disrupting pollutants that contaminate and magnify in and are inseparable from the animal package.

Except through accidental exposure to radiation, 9 times out of 10, we don't get cancer: we eat ourselves cancerous. Truer than compassionate eater Mahatma Gandhi knew: "The most violent weapon on earth is the table fork." After the insensate, pointless violence we do to animals, and to Gaia and God, the greatest violence we do with our cutlery is to ourselves.

PS Sadly, the banner of the Breast Cancer Fund's website reads: "Help us expose and eliminate the environmental causes of breast cancer. Together we can stop this disease before it starts." We stop the "disease" by not using our Meater knives and forks to put the environment inside ourselves.

Zeranol

Zeranol is a synthetic growth factor used on cows. Under the category Endocrine Disruptor, the Breast Cancer Fund describes zeranol like so:

"Zeranol is one of the most widely used chemicals in the U.S. beef industry. It is of special concern for breast cancer because it mimics the hormone estradiol. Cancer cells exposed to zeranol show significant increases in cancer growth."

http://www.breastcancerfund.org/clear-science/radiation-chemicals-and-breast-cancer/zeranol.html

That's fairly pithy. I think we should keep zeranol away from our food. That isn't difficult – it's used in animals:

"The synthetic compound zeranol is a potent non-steroidal growth promoter that mimics many of the effects of estradiol. Zeranol is used extensively in the United States and Canada to promote rapid and more efficient growth rates in animals used as sources of meat (Al-Dobaib, 2009)."

Planters don't eat this endocrine-disrupting, breast cancer-causing animal growth promoter.

Zinc

Multivitamin pills that contain metals such as copper, iron and zinc are problematic. I'm mentioning zinc here because the best science says that zinc in multivitamin supplements doubles our risk of prostate cancer.

Which is ironic, considering that men need to top up with zinc after sex, zinc being a component of semen. Our best source isn't oysters; it's beans, greens, whole grains, nuts and seeds, especially when accompanied by mineral absorption enhancers such as garlic or onions.

The take-home message about multivitamins and other non-whole-food supplements is that they're junk and that we take our lives in our hands when we eat anything that's not food.

Stick a fork in me… I'm done (with this animal contaminants section).

~

Part 4 (Missing in Action)

Animal MIAs – Animal Deficiencies

Daniel 5:27: "Thou art weighed in the balances, and art found wanting."

In Part 1 (Animals, Themselves), we saw that *all* the natural 'ingredients' of animals are naturally inimical to our health when we eat them.

In Part 2 (~~Food~~borne Pathogens), we saw that, besides inflicting zoönotic diseases on us, animals play host to dozens of species of micro-organisms and parasites that harm our health (except the bacteria that make B_{12}!)

In Part 3 (~~Food~~borne Contaminants), we saw that – through no fault of their own – animals bio-accumulate and bio-magnify thousands of environmental toxins to thousands of times the ambient concentrations, and harm our health when we eat them.

Not only do animals cause an endless litany of ill-effects, they crucially lack the following vital components and effects provided only by plants. These are the animal Missing in Action, which re-re-confirm that we are Planters:

50 Animal Deficiencies That Rule Them Out as Food

1. Water

Without knowing it, Meaters are often chronically dehydrated. First, the fluids – blood and lymph et al – are systematically drained from animals' bodies at slaughter. *All* slaughtered animals die the same way, by bleeding to death, while they're still conscious. Blood makes animal flesh soggy and unpalatable, and it's anathema to humans, except for outliers such as the Maa-speaking Maasai and Samburu pastoralists of East Africa.

Also, Meaters tend to cook animal flesh over high, dry heat until most of the moisture is gone – there's not much water, even in the juiciest of steaks. For this and other reasons such as avoiding the carcinogens and gerontotoxins produced by cooking flesh, animals are most healthily prepared over low, moist heat in stews and soups.

To be a Meater is to be dehydrated (and constipated).

2. Chlorophyll

Chlorophyll is incredible stuff. My mind boggles when I consider chlorophyll.

In the process known as photosynthesis, or 'making from light,' plants, algae and cyanobacteria use pigments to convert the sun's energy into chemical energy. They're called photoautotrophs, which means 'light-self-feeders.' Chlorophylls of various kinds are the pigments involved.

The plants take in carbon dioxide and water from the air and soil (nitrogen too), and, using solar energy to power the reaction, they create sugar and oxygen. Energy is stored in the sugar structures and later converted into molecules of ATP (adenosine triphosphate), our cells' energy currency.

The initial chemical reaction looks like this:

$$6CO_2 + 6H_2O \rightarrow C_6H_{12}O_6 + 6O_2$$

Carbon dioxide + water → sugar + oxygen

Plants are like solar arrays, with their chlorophyll-green leaves like phyto-solar panels pointed at the sun. They absorb the sun's rays and create sugar from carbon dioxide and water, and they exhale oxygen.

And then we come along, and we eat the sugar and breathe the oxygen – the two substances that fuel humans – and we breathe out carbon dioxide and pee out water – the two substances that fuel plants. And around and around the cycle goes, humans and plants in perfect synergy.

We humans are essentially solar-powered beings. Plants are the primary solar beings, the phyto-photo-auto-trophs. We're the secondary solar beings, powered by plants.

It's so beautiful, it makes me tear up sometimes when I think about it: us and nature in perfect, peaceful harmony… going around and around, them feeding us, us feeding them in an indefinitely sustainable partnership. (Understanding our nature as solar beings makes one understand a little clearer why Meating is such an abomination – a rending asunder of our perfect human-plant relationship.)

I mentioned nitrogen above. Plants absorb nitrogen from root bacteria which 'fix' the nitrogen for them, and plants then create the amino acids that make up the proteins that make up their leaves and stems and tubers. Plants also make fats and carbohydrates. Hydrated carbon = carbon + water, essentially – a convenient storage form of glucose, our universal power molecule.

Earlier I showed a diagram comparing the structures of chlorophyll and heme, the metalloprotein in hemoglobin which carts oxygen around in our blood. Isn't this miraculous? Plants use this molecule to create oxygen out of sunlight and carbon dioxide, and then we humans adapt the same molecule to ferry our oxygen fuel (and our carbon dioxide wastes) around inside ourselves. If we get this – really get it; understand to our core that we humans developed after billions of years in inseparable association with plants – then we know with absolute certainty that we're obviously and exclusively adapted to eating nothing but plants… who, in turn, developed inseparably from cyanobacteria and algae, yet other solar-powered beings.

In this direction lies our angel nature, in Pure Planting. Eating animals is our "fundamental debacle," upsetting the perfection of the energy cycle between humans and plants and bacteria and the sun: it's inefficient, cruel, selfish and spectacularly unnecessary. Meating is beyond pointless. For solar-powered beings to power ourselves by eating the bodies of other solar-powered beings is demonic.

Besides creating the human macronutrients – carbs, fats and proteins – plants also give us the micronutrients. Plants make all the vitamins, except for B_{12} – I told you we were partners with the bacteria! – and vitamin D – I told you we were solar powered beings! Plants serve up our minerals for us too, absorbing them from the soil and making them bioavailable to us in Goldilocks amounts. Organic minerals are different to inorganic rocks (which is what table salt is – pulverized rocks which we over-consume in deadly quantities).

As we'll see in the next entry (Phytonutrients) plant pigments, usually found in plant skins and peels, are the healthiest, most antioxidant parts of plants. They're the plants' chemical sunblock and raincoat, all in one.

Besides making our food, giving us life, the phytonutrient known as chlorophyll has one other spectacular property: it's a **carcinogen interceptor**. Chlorophyll binds to carcinogens, changing their shape and preventing them from slipping into our DNA and mutating it. That's just one of the many reasons why people who eat the most plants have the lowest cancer rates. Chlorophyll prevents what Meating causes. Isn't that amazing?

There's zero chlorophyll in animals. There's nothing amazing about Meating. Meating is a chlorophyll deficiency disease.

In the first two Meater deficiencies we've covered so far, we've met the three real macronutrients: water, air and sunlight. That's what we're made out of: water, air and sunlight. Without these three, life as we know it is impossible. Meating is deficient in water, in air and in sun power.

3. Synergistic phytonutrients

OK, saying that animals lack phytonutrients isn't saying much. As we know, the 'phyto' in phytonutrients or phytochemicals or phytoestrogens merely means 'plant,' so it shouldn't gobsmack us that there aren't many in animals – less than 1/64th on average. Here's the big hairy but, though, and it's enormous: there are estimated to be more than 100,000 phytochemicals all acting in synergy to bring us myriad health benefits. Only in plants.

Michael Greger says:

> "The leading candidate class of compounds responsible for the protection against Alzheimer's are the phenolics, like flavones, and flavonones, and flavonols, which in many cases can rapidly cross the blood-brain barrier. There are more than 5,000 different types of flavonoids in the plants we eat. Research suggests that within minutes of biting into an apple, for example, these phytonutrients are already starting to light up our brain."

[See: http://nutritionfacts.org/video/phytochemicals-the-nutrition-facts-missing-from-the-label/]

There are a few phytos in the animals we eat – cows and sheeps and chooks are, after all, plantivores, not raptors. That said, there are pathetically few. On average, there're more than 60 times as many phytonutes in plants than in the animals that eat plants. Plants *are* phytonutrients. (In fact, 'phytonutrient' is a tautology: because only plants are food, all nutrients are phytonutrients.) Every mouthful of nutrient-free animal displaces more than 60 mouthfuls of nutrient-packed plants.

Anyone interested in learning more about the healing powers of plants should read Dr. Michael Greger's *How Not to Die: Discover the Foods Scientifically Proven to Prevent and Reverse Disease.*

Meating is a phytonutrient deficiency disease.

4. Nutrient density

When we come down to it, animals and junk are the exact opposite of food. They're overly endowed with bad stuff – especially fat-stored energy – and underendowed with nutrients. Animals and Junk are calorie-dense but nutrient-poor. Food, on the other hand, is calorie-lean and nutrient-hyper-dense. Animals and Junk lack appropriate nutrient density. Insulin resistance is just one of the ways junky, processed plants affect us in the same bad way as processed animals.

In the words of T. Colin Campbell: "There is no nutrient in animals that's not better supplied by plants."

Meating and Junking are nutrient-to-energy ratio imbalance diseases.

5. Plant proteins

Plant proteins differ from animal proteins in most beneficial ways. For example, plant proteins have lower amounts of the acidifying sulfur-containing amino acids, and lower amounts of leucine and methionine, the limitation of which has been shown to be life-extending. Plant proteins also don't cause the cross-reactivity problems that lead to auto-immune responses.

Meating isn't only a plant protein deficiency disease; it's an animal protein overdose disease.

5a. Glutamic acid

Glutamic acid is an amino acid found in many plants, and it has a strong independent blood pressure-lowering effect; independent meaning that plants in general lower BP, but glutamine can do it on its own. Animals have much lower glutamic acid levels; Meaters have higher BP.

6. Plant fats

Plant fats are different to animal fats both in their relative amounts in food and in their constitution. While Meaters get >30%, Planters get about 10% of their calories from fats, an ideal amount both for weight maintenance and peak performance. Same paleo diets are way more than 50% fat. The fats in whole plants tend to be unsaturated and anti-atherogenic, while those in processed animals and processed plants tend to be saturated, pro-inflammatory and pro-atherogenic.

Meating is a dose-dependent animal fat disease; a plant fat deficiency syndrome.

7. Carbohydrates

Other than the lactose in mothers' breast milk, and a tiny amount of stored glycogen in muscles, animals make no sugars at all. Glucose is the simple sugar that makes up both digestible starches and 'indigestible' fiber.

Glucose is our most efficient fuel, though, in its absence, fats and proteins – even nucleic acids! – can be burned in an emergency situation.

As solar powered beings, we're adapted to eat liquid sunshine: sugar. Not table sugar. Not high fructose corn syrup. Sugar, as made by plants out of sunshine, water and our exhalations, then packaged with fiber and countless nutrients into… food.

Eating animals is a sugar-deficiency disease. The only healthy part of low-carb diets is the Planting.

8. Fiber

Fiber is fascinating stuff. I've been following the fiber story ever since 1974, when one of my heroes, Dr Dennis Burkitt gave a lecture in Cape Town titled "On Human Ordure." (As an English surgeon, I'm not sure he used the title 'Doctor.' In inverse snobbery, I suspect, surgeons in England tend to be called 'Mister.')

Burkitt and other physicians working in East Africa, like Hugh Trowell, noticed that constipation, diverticulosis and colorectal cancer weren't just rare among the predominantly plant-eating local population: they were absent. So too were the heart attacks, hypertension and strokes common in the West.

They put this down to the huge amounts of fiber in the traditional sub-Saharan African diet. Well, they were wrong… and they were right. Fiber itself may not be doing all the heavy lifting, so, when reductionists do experiments with fiber and nothing but the fiber, they sometimes fail to get good results. (This is why fiber substitutes like psyllium husks are a waste of time.) But…

When we use foods that are full of fiber then we get the results that Burkitt, Trowell et al got: a massive reduction in degenerative "diseases" across the board, particularly inflammatory bowel conditions.

Almost all Americans fail to meet the recommended daily fiber intake, including most vegans, who eat too much processed junk. 96% fail to eat adequate amounts of beans or greens. 99% don't eat enough grains.

There's zero fiber in animals, and precious little in junk. While Meating is a fiber-deficiency disease that causes a host of symptoms, from constipation to breast cancer, there are fiber-associated phytonutrients that are just as important as the fiber itself. One of them is:

9. Phytate ~ phytic acid

Discovered in 1903, phytates are a class of phosphorus-containing, saturated cyclic acid antioxidants found in all plant seeds: whole grains, beans, peas and lentils, nuts and seeds. They're what sprouting seeds feed on when they germinate, so you can imagine what wonderful nutrients they are – phyto-breast milk! Sprouts and micro-greens are intensely healthy.

Phytates have long been thought to be anti-nutrients because they were thought to lower our absorption of some minerals… but maybe we're looking at things the wrong way. Who says that lots of absorption is always a good thing? Unregulated heme iron absorption isn't good. Supplements are megadoses of micronutrients, and many of those shorten our lives. More isn't always better.

There are **mineral absorption enhancers** in plants, particularly in the allium family, that boost absorption, so if we're worried about our whole grain pasta inhibiting zinc or iron absorption, we can just add some onions or garlic, leeks or scallions to the tomato sauce. Oh, you do already? Great. Calamity averted.

(Someone once asked Winston Churchill to define the difference between a calamity and a catastrophe. He said: "If Clement Attlee fell into the Thames it would be a calamity. If someone fished him out again, that would be a catastrophe." He also said of Attlee that he was a modest man, who had much to be modest about, and that he was "a sheep in sheep's clothing." Some ill-feeling there, I think.)

But there wasn't a calamity anyway. The fear turned out to be fear of fear itself. The old anti-nutrient story about phytates was a canard based on ancient animal studies, now superseded by human data. Women who eat the most phytates have the best bone density – with higher calcium and phosphorus levels – so Planter phytate-eaters have the least osteoporosis.

To *not* eat phytonutrient-packed nuts and seeds, beans and grains every day is to eat our bones fragile. Late-life bone fractures are a consequence of lack of load-bearing exercise plus the eating disorder I've called Meating.

Besides lowering our risk of osteoporosis, phytates are powerful anti-cancer agents.

Do you remember how I said earlier (under Fiber) that there are phyto-nutrients that are bound to fiber that may be doing the heavy lifting on behalf of fiber (playing bellhop to fiber's concierge)? It's the phytate.

In Michael Greger's pithy words:

> "Dietary phytate, rather than fiber per se, might be **the most important variable governing the frequency of colon cancer,** as we know phytate is a **powerful inhibitor of the iron-mediated production of hydroxyl radicals**, a particularly dangerous type of free radical. So the standard American diet [Meating + Junking] may be a double whammy, the heme iron [a pro-oxidant or free radical producer] in muscle meat plus the lack of phytate in refined plant foods to extinguish the iron radicals."

[See: http://nutritionfacts.org/video/phytates-for-the-treatment-of-cancer/]

So, Burkitt and his colleagues were right to promote high fiber consumption, but maybe not for the fiber alone – we didn't know about phytate's marvelous anti-cancer properties back then. Diverticulosis and colorectal cancer are, indeed, fiber-deficiency conditions brought on by eating fiber-free animals and junk. Changing the magnification, we can say that Western "diseases" such as diverticulitis and colon cancer are also phytate-deficiency diseases.

Phytates are bound to fiber – no fiber, no phytates. Conversely, adding fiber to our diet doesn't add phytates. That's why Meater broscientists love to perform this following sleight of hand: fiber supplements don't prevent colon cancer (agreed, they don't, for the reason we now know – phytate deficiency); therefore eating plants doesn't prevent colon cancer. Gnur? No Planter has ever advocated eating isolated fiber as a proxy for Planting. Using it as one is a cheap shot. Planting drops our risk of inflammatory bowel symptoms like a put-ed shot.

The more animals we eat, the more cancer we get – not just bowel cancer. Cows double our risk. Chickens triple it. Beans and grains – all phytate-filled seeds – slice our risk like a knife through hot potatoes. (That's why the animal industry adds phytates to its dead products…)

Besides combatting cancer via antioxidation, phytates have multiple other anti-cancer mechanisms, beyond the scope of this discussion. Please just take it from me that these are powerful phytochemicals, and that we should eat whole plants every day to pack ourselves full of them (to phyte the good health phyte, daily).

(For more, see Dr. Greger's outstanding coverage in his book, *How Not to Die*, and in his online video "Phytates for Rehabilitating Cancer Cells.")

Also, high phytate intake → less diabetes + less heart "disease" + fewer kidney stones.

Plus phytates put their mineral-grabbing powers to use on heavy metals such as lead and cadmium, so that Planters could eat more mercury [it doesn't happen], and still have lower mercury blood levels than Meaters. Grain- and bean-eating lowers our risk of heavy metal toxicity! Double!!

I did an online search for a definition of 'vitamin' and I got "any of a group of organic compounds which are essential for normal growth and nutrition and are required in small quantities in the diet because they cannot be synthesized by the body."

Well, we need it and we can't make it, so phytic acid qualifies as a vitamin or essential-to-eat, unnecessary-to-make-because-ubiquitous-in-food nutrient, and may eventually make its way into the accepted canon, which presently numbers a last-supper-ish 13. (Were there waiters? No need, I guess, with such a simple meal.)

Historically, vitamins have come and gone, reflecting our current knowledge of physiology. For a while, laetrile – isolated from apricot pips – was called vitamin B_{17}. It's since been demoted. Sad, really; tasting glory, then blithely discarded. (As I'll mention later, there are two other phyto-candidates for vitaminhood (vitamancy would be too confusing.))

Meating and Junking are potentially lethal phytate vitamin-deficiency diseases.

10. Gut flora

The old view of 'indigestible' fiber or 'roughage' is that it's supposed to be the cellulose part of plants that we can't digest, and it's beneficial because it bulks out our stools, aids peristalsis, binds up cholesterol/bile acids and estrogens and flushes them out, while it itself remains undigested… a kind of poop catalyst.

As we now know, "we" *can* digest fiber. By "we" I mean, we humans working in tandem with the trillions of gut bacteria who live within us, particularly in our bowels, and who greatly outnumber our human cells.

Our gut flora digests fiber. They thrive on fiber. They ferment it and produce wonderful products, of use to them and to us. We feed them and they feed us.

I find our gut flora (and our enteric (gut) nervous system) fascinating. We can change our gut flora, depending on what we feed them. This is absolutely essential to understand:

We should think of our gut flora as making up a separate anatomical organ. That's how important they are to digestion and metabolism.

Different populations of bacteria take up residence in our guts depending on what we feed them.

Planters and Meaters have different gut flora: you won't see this on an anatomical chart or in a textbook, but **Planters and Meaters have different digestive tracts**. Different bodies! Meating changes our bodies by deranging our gut flora. Feeding our gut flora decomposing animals actively selects for gut flora that decompose dead animals. We live in harmony with our gut flora when we're Planters.

Within our gut flora, some species are definitely healthier than others. Phytonutrients such as the polyphenols found in green tea, in fruits like apples and grapes, and in the vinegars made from them encourage *Prevotella* species such as *Faecalibacterium prausnitzii* to flourish, while discouraging *Bacteroides* species (which is good, because the latter are associated with increased immune response and more inflammation.) Animals do the exact opposite.

If instead of feeding our intestinal bacteria with fiber to ferment, we feed them animal proteins to rot, we shouldn't be surprised when we get different, sulfur-emitting results. Fermentation is beneficial; putrefaction by baleful species such as *Bilophila wadsworthia* is decidedly not.

Meating is a gut flora-deranging disease.

For more, see The Eatiology of Obesity #15: Enterotypes, in Part 1C (Eatiology)

11. Propionate

When we feed our friendly gut bacteria on the fiber they love, they digest it for us and make a substance called propionate, which we absorb through our gut walls into our bloodstream. It turns out that fiber is digestible by humans – we just have to change our definition of human. We need to rewrite the human anatomy texts to include a virtual digestive organ known as our gut flora. It doesn't matter if it doesn't appear in *Grey's Anatomy*; it appears in us and has always done so. We're slowly getting wise to its/their existence.

Propionate slows the synthesis of cholesterol. (Here's another double whammy for Meaters, who get the negative of too much cholesterol to begin with, plus the lack of the positive propionate effect from plants.) Propionate also slows down our stomach emptying and creates a feeling of satiety, which combines in a **hypophagic effect**. Hypo = less, and phagic = eating. The propionate from bacteria-digested fiber makes us eat less.

The hypophagic effect of propionate, the effects of healthy *Bacteroides* gut flora species, the lower energy density (and higher nutrient density) of plants, the avoidance of animal-borne obesogenic viruses and chemical obesogens, the bulkiness of fiber that triggers pressure sensors in our intestinal walls signaling fullness, and the thermogenic effect (see later) and increased brown fat deposition (later), both of which speed up Planters' metabolisms, leading to more calories being expended as heat, are multiple mechanisms which combine to make Planters the only group of eaters to have ideal body weight (BMI < 25).

As a group, Planters are the slenderest people in the world. This isn't wishful thinking; it's demonstrated scientific fact. (We've seen some of the great Adventist studies, comparing different dietstyles' effects on obesity, diabetes, hypertension and heart "disease". Each of these conditions gets worse, dose-dependently, with increased animal consumption.)

While Meaters and Junkers feel the need to take probiotics to promote a healthy gut flora, Planters don't. Planters use prebiotics. In other words, Planters just eat food. Planting feeds our gut flora their meal of choice – fiber – and that encourages the healthiest possible gut flora to thrive. Eating fiber encourages fiber-eating bacteria, who in turn feed us propionate, with its amazing anti-obesity qualities. Eat plants… they will come.

Fiber-depleted Meating and Junking are propionate deficiency diseases.

12. Lignans

Lignans are a class of anti-carcinogenic phytonutrients found in seeds and nuts, particularly flax seeds and walnuts. Actually, there are zero lignans in flax: our gut flora makes them for us out of their lignan precursors in nuts and seeds.

Lignans are phytoestrogens that help prevent breast and prostate cancer in particular. Meaters' gut flora isn't purpose-built for making lignans. Meaters' gut flora, lacking in fiber and disturbed by sulfur, have adapted to eating dead animals. That's why Meaters become so farty when eating beans – the wrong bacteria for digesting beans, or nuts and seeds. So, it's a double whammy for Meaters – more carcinogens in what we eat when we Meat, and fewer of the cancer-fighters served up on Planters' plates.

Meating is a lignan-deficiency disease.

13. Butyrate

Butyrate is yet another substance that our gut bacteria make for us, also out of fiber, like propionate. Butyrate is a short chain fatty acid with anti-inflammatory and anti-cancer properties.

Butyrate is what fuels the cells that make up our colon walls. We and our bacteria are partners in dining: we feed each other… as long as we don't eat animals. Eating animals encourages the wrong species of bacteria to take over. There's no possible way for bacteria to make butyrate both out of carbohydrate and out of animals – there's zero carbohydrate in animals. We're sugar-powered sweeties, not ghouls.

The more fiber we eat, the more butyrate-producing bacteria there are in our colons. We don't change our genes by eating fiber, but epigenetic changes take place so that the more bacteria there are, the more butyrate-producing genes get switched on. Fiber eating upregulates the genes for butyrate production.

Butyrate is a large part of the reason why Planters get so much less colon cancer and ulcerative colitis than Meaters; the presence of butyrate, and the absence of the cytotoxic gas, hydrogen sulfide, that our gut bacteria produce from animal proteins.

(If something we eat induces our gut flora to make an oxidative, DNA-damaging cell poison out of it, should we call it food?)

Propionate, lignans and butyrate are three very large gifts our good bacteria give us; gifts that Meaters spurn, their bacteria not having been given the gift of fiber. Or, if Meaters do eat fiber, the animals they've eaten have encouraged animal-eating gut bacteria, who're less able to produce propionate or butyrate. Meating not only introduces obesogenic, inflammatory, and carcinogenic agents, but Meaters lose out on the wondrous anti-obesity, anti-inflammatory and anti-cancer agents produced by plant-fed bacteria.

Meating is a (sulfur overdose and) butyrate deficiency disease.

14. Minerals

Minerals are powdered rocks. They're the inorganic part of soil, from where they're incorporated into plants as they grow. Minerals need to be taken up by plants to become bioavailable at appropriate concentrations. Taking a rock and using a grater to sprinkle some stone particles into our food, as if we're cows at a salt lick, may work too well. Plants are the kitchen workers who prepare minerals for the dining pleasure of animals… like us humans. We don't need to pass minerals through animals before ingesting them. Other animals get their minerals from plants. So should we.

In some cases, Meating is a mineral deficiency disease. In others, Meating is a mineral overdose disease. Planters absorb minerals in Goldilocks amounts: not too many, not too few, right in the middle in the sweet spot, with phytonutrients that limit or boost absorption, depending on how much we need.

More isn't better. As we saw above, plant copper, plant iron and plant phosphorus are all better regulated than their animal counterparts, which are prone to overload, setting us up for kidney failure and dementia. On the other hand, plant calcium is far better absorbed than animal.

Junking and Meating are mineral-inefficiency diseases.

15. Magnesium

Unsurprisingly, animal eaters are often deficient in magnesium, the ion at the heart of the chlorin ring in chlorophyll. (Not chlorine; chlorin.) The majority of Americans don't meet the recommended minimum intake.

The following list shows the first of 311 online pages of magnesium-containing foods and non-foods adapted from the USDA's National Nutrient Database for Standard Reference Release 27. You'll notice that no non-foods make it onto the page. There's nothing but nuts, seeds, beans and grains… and molasses, though I think non-bears would find a cup of molasses hard to swallow.

Food is where we find magnesium. The only two animal sources to crack the top 100 are conch at #76 and (enhanced!) turkey at #80. So, one rare sea animal, and one animal + supplement.

NDB_No	Description	Weight(g)	Measure	Magnesium, Mg (mg) Per Measure
20060	Rice bran, crude	118	1.0 cup	922
19304	Molasses	337	1.0 cup	816
12014	Seeds, pumpkin and squash seed kernels, dried	129	1.0 cup	764
16078	Mothbeans, mature seeds, raw	196	1.0 cup	747
12007	Seeds, cottonseed flour, partially defatted (glandless)	94	1.0 cup	678
12160	Seeds, cottonseed kernels, roasted (glandless)	149	1.0 cup	656
12016	Seeds, pumpkin and squash seed kernels, roasted, without salt	118	1.0 cup	649
12516	Seeds, pumpkin and squash seed kernels, roasted, with salt added	118	1.0 cup	649
16067	Hyacinth beans, mature seeds, raw	210	1.0 cup	594
16133	Yardlong beans, mature seeds, raw	167	1.0 cup	564
12174	Seeds, watermelon seed kernels, dried	108	1.0 cup	556
16060	Cowpeas, catjang, mature seeds, raw	167	1.0 cup	556
16083	Mungo beans, mature seeds, raw	207	1.0 cup	553
16108	Soybeans, mature seeds, raw	186	1.0 cup	521
12201	Seeds, sesame seed kernels, dried (decorticated)	150	1.0 cup	518
43299	Soybean, curd cheese	225	1.0 cup	513
12023	Seeds, sesame seeds, whole, dried	144	1.0 cup	505
12078	Nuts, brazilnuts, dried, unblanched	133	1.0 cup	500
20001	Amaranth grain, uncooked	193	1.0 cup	479
12529	Seeds, sesame seed kernels, toasted, with salt added (decorticated)	128	1.0 cup	443
12029	Seeds, sesame seed kernels, toasted, without salt added (decorticated)	128	1.0 cup	443
16047	Beans, yellow, mature seeds, raw	196	1.0 cup	435
12065	Nuts, almonds, oil roasted, without salt added	157	1.0 cup	430
12565	Nuts, almonds, oil roasted, with salt added	157	1.0 cup	430
12665	Nuts, almonds, oil roasted, lightly salted	157	1.0 cup	430

National Nutrient Database for Standard Reference Release 27: Magnesium

Why's magnesium important? Magnesium is one of the minerals that maintain our bodies' electrical systems. Our heartbeats are controlled by electrical impulses, and magnesium is our drummer (Hi, Debs. Hi, Gary.) It's the positive ion that keeps the rhythm going. Arrhythmias result from magnesium deficiency (and bass players).

Being low in magnesium sets us up for Sudden Cardiac Death, which accounts for more than half of all deaths from our #1 killer, heart "disease".

Death via SCD is the first symptom, or warning, the majority of heart attack victims get of their heart "disease". 'Healthy' one moment; dead the next. Only about 2% of Americans meet their daily requirement of magnesium. Seeing as the top sources of magnesium are seeds, nuts and grains, I'll leave it to you to work out who makes up the bulk of the 2% of adequate mag-eaters. (I believe that vegans now make up about 2% of the population, but there may be many Junkers within the vegan ranks.)

Just an ounce (28g) of seeds or nuts a day, added to the crappy SAD diet could extend many tens of thousands of American lives each year.

Meating and Junking are magnesium deficiency diseases. Sudden Cardiac Death is often a first symptom of Meating with the unfortunate character flaw of being a 'last word freak.'

16. Calcium

For all that the dairy industries of the world tell us otherwise, their products aren't a particularly good source of calcium. (They're a pretty good source of pus though, in case we think we're running low?)

Countries that have the highest dairy consumption suffer from the highest rates of osteoporosis. (Yes, we'll correlate away, my friends – we know the difference between correlation and causation, and there's plenty of other evidence to back the epidemiology.) The Asians who have the good fortune to be lactose intolerant and who consume no dairy products at all have no osteoporosis. (Those who do, do.) Osteoporosis can be as much or more a consequence of lack of load-bearing exercise than lack of calcium or magnesium or phosphorus or boron. It's the result of a sedentary lifestyle coupled with the eating of animals. Having enough vitamin D is also important, so we should all bear our loads outdoors when we can.

Phyto-calcium is absorbed half again as well as animal milk and cheese calcium, without the side order of Parkinson's.

Meating is a calcium-deficient diet; but junk "food" veganism can be too – we need to eat our whole greens and beans, dear peeps, every day!

17. Potassium

Potassium is another mineral Meaters struggle to get enough of. Showing why, below, is the first page of the National Nutrient Database for Standard Reference Release 27, for potassium per 100g.

It looks like the word 'herb' isn't in the USDA's lexicon. I tend to use 'herb' for plant leaves and 'spice' for all the other parts. I wouldn't call tarragon a spice. But, hey, it took a court case to change tomatoes from fruits into vegetables, so I may have missed the Supreme Court's spice ruling.

Upping one's potassium levels seriously reduces one's risk of stroke, much the same way increased magnesium intake seriously cuts one's risk of arrhythmia and heart attack. 98% of Americans are deficient in potassium; meaning, basically, that all Meaters are potassium-deficient and at risk of stroke. Well, we knew that anyway, because stroke is the #4 cause of death, after heart "disease", cancer and lung "disease".

The best way to avoid stroke is to stop Meating and go on a high-potassium Planter diet, with plenty of beans and leafy green veggies. Sun-dried tomatoes and sweet peppers are great sources.

NDB_No	Description	Potassium, K (mg) Value Per 100g
18373	Leavening agents, cream of tartar	16,500.00
18371	Leavening agents, baking powder, low-sodium	10,100.00
11625	Parsley, freeze-dried	6,300.00
14353	Tea, instant, unsweetened, powder, decaffeinated	6,040.00
14366	Tea, instant, unsweetened, powder	6,040.00
2008	Spices, chervil, dried	4,740.00
2012	Spices, coriander leaf, dried	4,466.00
14203	Coffee, instant, regular, powder, half the caffeine	3,535.00
14214	Coffee, instant, regular, powder	3,535.00
14218	Coffee, instant, decaffeinated, powder	3,501.00
11432	Radishes, oriental, dried	3,494.00
14368	Tea, instant, unsweetened, lemon-flavored, powder	3,453.00
11955	Tomatoes, sun-dried	3,427.00
14222	Coffee, instant, with chicory, powder	3,395.00
2017	Spices, dill weed, dried	3,308.00
11634	Peppers, sweet, green, freeze-dried	3,170.00
11931	Peppers, sweet, red, freeze-dried	3,170.00
14409	Beverages, Orange-flavor drink, breakfast type, low calorie, powder	3,132.00
16425	Soy sauce, reduced sodium, made from hydrolyzed vegetable protein	3,098.00
2041	Spices, tarragon, dried	3,020.00
11615	Chives, freeze-dried	2,960.00
31019	Seaweed, Canadian Cultivated EMI-TSUNOMATA, dry	2,944.00
14196	Cocoa mix, no sugar added, powder	2,702.00
14538	Beverages, Cocoa mix, low calorie, powder, with added calcium, phosp	2,702.00
2029	Spices, parsley, dried	2,683.00

National Nutrient Database for Standard Reference Release 27: Potassium

Meating is a potassium deficiency disease.

18. Iodine

Getting enough iodine can be a problem for all of us, Meaters and Planters alike. For optimal health, we need to get adequate iodine, which is a component of thyroid hormones, otherwise we may get a thyroid growth called a goiter. Not pretty.

According to the NIH, under Food Sources, at https://ods.od.nih.gov/factsheets/Iodine-HealthProfessional/: "Seaweed (such as kelp, nori, kombu, and wakame) is one of the best food sources of iodine, but it is highly variable in its content... Other good sources include seafood, dairy products (partly due to the use of iodine feed supplements and iodophor sanitizing agents in the dairy industry, grain products, and eggs. Dairy products, especially milk, and grain products are the major contributors of iodine to the American diet."

The iodine in commercial dairy products is partly from supplements; also partly from iodine contamination with disinfectants used in milk tanks and on often-swollen, mastitic cow udders. (More than 15% of cows in the US have mastitis, a staph infection, so the odds of staph in milk tanks is 100%.) I think I'll pass. And I think I'll skip the seafood [oxymoron alert], because of the bonus heavy metals; and the eggs because of the free cholesterol (a single yolk putting us over our 'safe' daily upper limit). (Wouldn't it be nice if Kevin Bacon, egg tout for the American Egg Board, actually knew something about nutrition?) "Food is a package deal," so iodine is best found in sea vegetables (but not hijiki/hiziki because of arsenic contamination, and not kelp, because it contains too much iodine.)

Curiously, the USDA's National Nutrient Database for Standard Reference Release 27 doesn't list iodine as a nutrient. Which puzzles me, because the list is fairly comprehensive. For example, they do list alcohol, caffeine and theobromine, so boozehounds, Java junkies and chocoholics can all do a quick search to get the biggest bangs for their bucks. But no iodine…

And my other go-to source for nutrient numbers, SELFNutritionData at http://nutritiondata.self.com, is similarly reticent. Type in 'kelp' (a single gram of which, according to the NIH, provides between 11% and 1,989% (!!) of one's DV (daily value)), and we get the news that kelp is high in sodium, but not a single word about iodine. Using their 'nutrient search' tool also comes up empty. It looks like they get their info from the USDA database.

(There may be a quite logical explanation for this iodine coyness, one that's known to non-amateur nutrition enthusiasts such as myself: a kind of shibboleth, which allows outsiders to be slaughtered for mispronouncing the word. I'd love to know… Perhaps iodine is too dangerous to make recommendations about? The variation in kelp above is certainly concerning: 11 to 1,989 is an astonishing range of almost three orders of magnitude. My guess is that iodine is too variable in its sources to make concrete dietary intake recommendations.)

Iodine is tricky, so Planters, Junkers and Meaters – all of us, except the prana-sustained breatharians – are all at risk of iodine-deficiency, so we need to give it some thought.

Sidebar: A quick rant about the National Nutrient Database
The USDA's nutrition database is horribly flawed. It lists nutrients in two searchable ways – either by hundred gram portions or by household, in which they choose measures which they think are suitable, such as cups of

grains or kilo slabs of cow's ribs. This is absolute craziness. None of us has a daily intake requirement for weights and measures of food – we don't need to eat 2 cups of this or a thousand grams of that.

What we do each have is an energy requirement of (very) roughly 2000 - 2500 calories per day; an energy requirement that should be divided up among all the nutrients we need to eat each day. We need to get at least 100% of all our nutrients every day, or on average over a period of time, while staying within our calorie budget. What point is there in getting 100% of our nutrients, if it takes 150% of our energy requirement to get there? Listing nutrients by weight or household doesn't help with this.

All nutrients should be listed by multiples of calories, not by weight! This is an absolute fundamental principle of studying food, Nutrition 101, and the USDA gets it wrong.

Why?

Because the USDA caters to animal agriculture. Listing nutrients by weight instead of calories makes animals look better and plants look worse. Why? Because animals are energy-dense and nutrient-poor, while plants are nutrient-dense and energy-sparse. Meating and Junking provide at least three times as much fat as Planting, and fat itself provides 2.25 times as much energy per gram as the other macronutrients. (Fat, 9 calories per gram; alcohol, 7; protein and carbs, 4.)

Planters get more of all nutrients while eating fewer calories. This is the concept of nutrient density, popularized by Dr. Joel Fuhrman and others.

All that data… and the USDA hasn't presented it in a way that makes meaningful comparisons between plants, junk and animals possible. It's not quite useless, but it should be a lot better. The USDA should be ashamed of themselves for their incompetence or deviousness, whichever it is.

The Meater USDA as a whole, and their Meater dietary guidelines committees in particular, are probably the single major reason why the USA became the fattest population ever to exist. Them, and the inventors of HFCS. (Note: I believe we've recently lost this dubious #1 distinction… to populations who eat just like us, only more so.)

Kudos to SELFNutritionData for allowing us to search their nutrient database the right way: by 200 calorie servings.

19. Nitrates

When dealing with nitrites earlier, I went into the importance of nitrates for vascular health. While nitrites abound naturally in animals and also in preservatives used in animals, animals are spectacularly poor sources of nitrates. Leafy green vegetables are nitrate bonanzas.

When we're Meaters, the closest some of us come to this beneficial form of nitrogen may be from fertilizer residues or from the nitroglycerine tablet we suck on desperately, to counteract the crushing cardiac pain known as angina (a symptom of Meating).

Meating is a nitrate deficiency disease.

20. Phytoestrogens

This one's dead easy. Phytoestrogens are beneficial endocrine disruptors in plants that block out the effect of animal estrogens and environmental estrogen disruptors that bioaccumulate in animals, lowering our risk of estrogenic cancers. There aren't any in animals.

Meating is a phytoestrogen deficiency disease.

21. Vitamins

As I mentioned when discussing the miracle of chlorophyll, all the vitamins are made by plants, except for two, one of which is made by bacteria (B_{12}), and one (D) by the action of sunlight on animal skin, us being the animals in question.

This being the case, Meating is a vitamin deficiency disease, unless accompanied by liberal doses of Planting.

22. Vitamin A

Vitamin A supplements and beta-carotene supplements shorten our lives. Planters have higher levels of A than Meaters. Meaters who try to address their deficiency shouldn't do it by Junking – taking supplements – but by Planting.

Meaters should also not get their A from cod liver oil, even if it is the top-ranked source in the USDA database, below.

Supplements are dangerous non-foods and we shouldn't eat them… except for cobalamin (B_{12}).

USDA National Nutrient Database for Standard ReferenceRelease 27

Nutrients: Vitamin A, IU (IU)

Food Subset: All Foods
Ordered by: Nutrient Content
Measured by: 100 g
Report Run at: February 01, 2015 12:21 EST

NDB_No	Description
04589	Fish oil, cod liver
23425	Beef, New Zealand, imported, liver, raw
11931	Peppers, sweet, red, freeze-dried
17203	Veal, variety meats and by-products, liver, cooked, braised
23424	Beef, New Zealand, imported, liver, cooked, boiled
11683	Carrot, dehydrated
11615	Chives, freeze-dried

National Nutrient Database for Standard Reference Release 27: Vitamin A

23. Folate (Vitamin B_9)

Folate is another of the phytonutrients in which Meaters tend to be deficient. They're best obtained from beans and green foliage.

While plant folate is beneficial, folic acid in supplements is harmful. Folate is cancer-protective; synthetic folic acid, carcinogenic.

Meating is a folate deficiency disease.

24. B vitamins (thiamin, riboflavin, niacin, pyridoxine, folate et al)

In general, Planters have higher levels of the B vitamins than Meaters, always supposing we take our B_{12}.

As mentioned in section 1, homocysteine is an intermediary metabolite between two other sulfur-containing amino acids, methionine and cysteine. I went to some length describing how much more of these amino acids there is in animals, and also how damaging they can be to our health. For example, methionine restriction is an acknowledge method of slowing down the aging process.

Elevated levels of homocysteine are associated with blood clots, heart attacks and strokes; also with cognitive decline and Alzheimer's.

Three of the B vitamins are crucial for maintaining brain health by detoxifying homocysteine. It looks like this:

$B_6 + B_9 + B_{12} \rightarrow$ lower concentration of homocysteine $\rightarrow$ less cognitive decline or Alzheimer's.

A shortage of any of these three B vitamins can cause hyperhomocysteinemia (a fancy way of saying elevated homocysteine levels), so it's important to keep all three high. As borne out by population studies, Planters who keep topped up with B_{12} have better levels of the other two Bs and consequently better brain health than Meaters, but Planters who neglect B_{12} can end up with stiffened, enflamed arteries just like Meaters, and cognitive decline.

Most people get enough pyridoxine (B_6), so for Meaters, the limiting B vitamin for detoxing homocysteine is folate (B_9), found mainly in green leafies and beans.

(Only 4% of Americans meet the pathetically low suggested daily intake levels for either leafy greens or beans, which puts 96% of the population at risk for brain damage via homocysteine. I guess that makes dementia-by-malnutrition 'normal.')

Other Meater factors that worsen our risk for Alzheimer's include inflammation via arachidonic acid, amyloidosis via animal proteins, heme iron, increased copper and aluminum toxicity, and cardiogenic dementia, via cholesterol-induced atherosclerosis.

25. Beta- and the carotenes

No, not a 60s-era pop band from Liverpool. Beta-carotene is just the best-known of more than 500 carotene phytonutrients. All of them play a role, not just one, and they work synergistically... the total being immeasurably greater than the sum of the parts.

Beta-carotene supplements are life-shortening. They're not food and we shouldn't eat them.

26. Vitamin C

While vitamin C is a fabulous general-purpose antioxidant, it plays a special role in boosting iron absorption from plants. (We've already seen that we can't regulate intake of heme iron from animal blood.) Our bodies aren't dumb. Iron creates lots of free radicals, so how better to manage iron intake than to have the antioxidant responsible for defusing the iron be the one who's working the door for crowd control, deciding who and how many get in?

In plants, the bomb and the bomb disposal expert come packaged together in one food. With animals, we keep chucking bombs into the crowd, without a bomb techy anywhere in sight.

Take a look below at page 1 of old standby, the USDA's nutrient database page for vitamin C. There's not much there in the way of real food, but I think you get the drift. Animals need not apply.

Besides being a disease of heme iron toxicity, Meating is a vitamin C deficiency disease.

USDA National Nutrient Database for Standard ReferenceRelease 27

Nutrients: Vitamin C, total ascorbic acid (mg)

Food Subset: All Foods
Ordered by: Nutrient Content
Measured by: 100 g
Report Run at: February 01, 2015 12:05 EST

NDB_No	Description
14409	Beverages, Orange-flavor drink, breakfast type, low calorie, powder
43345	Fruit-flavored drink, powder, with high vitamin C with other added vitamins, low calorie
11634	Peppers, sweet, green, freeze-dried
11931	Peppers, sweet, red, freeze-dried
09001	Acerola, (west indian cherry), raw
09002	Acerola juice, raw
11615	Chives, freeze-dried
02012	Spices, coriander leaf, dried
42055	Fruit-flavored drink, dry powdered mix, low calorie, with aspartame
19703	Gelatin desserts, dry mix, reduced calorie, with aspartame, added phosphorus, potassium, sodium, vitamin C
25016	Formulated bar, MARS SNACKFOOD US, SNICKERS MARATHON Energy Bar, all flavors
35203	Rose Hips, wild (Northern Plains Indians)
25003	Snacks, candy rolls, yogurt-covered, fruit flavored with high vitamin C
43544	Babyfood, cereal, rice with pears and apple, dry, instant
14424	Orange-flavor drink, breakfast type, with pulp, frozen concentrate
11670	Peppers, hot chili, green, raw
08504	Cereals ready-to-eat, RALSTON Enriched Wheat Bran flakes
14407	Orange-flavor drink, breakfast type, powder
09139	Guavas, common, raw
08028	Cereals ready-to-eat, KELLOGG, KELLOGG'S ALL-BRAN COMPLETE Wheat Flakes
08058	Cereals ready-to-eat, KELLOGG, KELLOGG'S PRODUCT 19
08077	Cereals ready-to-eat, GENERAL MILLS, Whole Grain TOTAL
16262	SILK Hazelnut Creamer
14426	Orange drink, breakfast type, with juice and pulp, frozen concentrate
11951	Peppers, sweet, yellow, raw
09165	Litchis, dried
09083	Currants, european black, raw
25043	Snacks, candy bits, yogurt covered with vitamin C

National Nutrient Database for Standard Reference Release 27: Vitamin C

27. Vitamin E

On the next page is the USDA on antioxidant vitamin E. Junk tops the list in the form of processed vegetable oils and cereals, but the point is: Plants only. Sunflower seeds are the best whole-food source. Nuts like almonds, hazelnuts or filberts are also excellent. Other good sources are green leafies and whole grains.

Nuts and seeds, because of their high vitamin E content, are protective against asthma, slashing risk in half.

Meating is a vitamin E deficiency disease.

NDB_No	Description
04038	Oil, wheat germ
08504	Cereals ready-to-eat, RALSTON Enriched Wheat Bran flakes
08590	Cereals ready-to-eat, KASHI HEART TO HEART, Warm Cinnamon
08387	Cereals ready-to-eat, KASHI HEART TO HEART, Honey Toasted Oat
14047	Beverages, UNILEVER, SLIMFAST Shake Mix, powder, 3-2-1 Plan
14055	Beverages, UNILEVER, SLIMFAST Shake Mix, high protein, powder, 3-2-1 Plan
04532	Oil, hazelnut
08028	Cereals ready-to-eat, KELLOGG, KELLOGG'S ALL-BRAN COMPLETE Wheat Flakes
08058	Cereals ready-to-eat, KELLOGG, KELLOGG'S PRODUCT 19
08077	Cereals ready-to-eat, GENERAL MILLS, Whole Grain TOTAL
08610	Cereals ready-to-eat, KASHI Honey Sunshine
16155	Peanut butter, smooth, vitamin and mineral fortified
16156	Peanut butter, chunky, vitamin and mineral fortified
08611	Cereals ready-to-eat, KELLOGG's FIBERPLUS Cinnamon Oat Crunch
04060	Oil, sunflower, linoleic (less than 60%)
04506	Oil, sunflower, linoleic, (approx. 65%)
04545	Oil, sunflower, linoleic, (partially hydrogenated)
04584	Oil, sunflower, high oleic (70% and over)
04642	Oil, industrial, mid-oleic, sunflower
04529	Oil, almond
02009	Spices, chili powder
04687	Margarine-like spread, BENECOL Light Spread
12038	Seeds, sunflower seed kernels, oil roasted, without salt
12538	Seeds, sunflower seed kernels, oil roasted, with salt added
35232	Wocas, dried seeds, Oregon, yellow pond lily (Klamath)
04502	Oil, cottonseed, salad or cooking
04702	Oil, industrial, cottonseed, fully hydrogenated
12036	Seeds, sunflower seed kernels, dried

National Nutrient Database for Standard Reference Release 27: Vitamin E

28. Vitamin K

Herbs (and other, larger) green leafy vegetables are where K is found.

In "Plant vs. Cow Calcium ," Michael Greger calls vitamin K a "bone health superstar." Higher vitamin K levels are yet another reason besides superior calcium absorption from plants, decreased acidosis from plants, decreased phosphorus levels from Planting and increased levels of potassium and magnesium that Planters have better bone health than Meaters: reduced risk of bone fracture and osteoporosis.

Meating is a vitamin K deficiency disease.

NDB_No	Description
02003	Spices, basil, dried
02038	Spices, sage, ground
02042	Spices, thyme, dried
11297	Parsley, fresh
02012	Spices, coriander leaf, dried
02029	Spices, parsley, dried
11003	Amaranth leaves, raw
11236	Kale, frozen, cooked, boiled, drained, without salt
11791	Kale, frozen, cooked, boiled, drained, with salt
11147	Chard, swiss, raw
11234	Kale, cooked, boiled, drained, without salt
02034	Spices, poultry seasoning
11207	Dandelion greens, raw
11233	Kale, raw
11164	Collards, frozen, chopped, cooked, boiled, drained, without salt
11769	Collards, frozen, chopped, cooked, boiled, drained, with salt
02023	Spices, marjoram, dried
02027	Spices, oregano, dried
11271	Mustard greens, cooked, boiled, drained, without salt
11799	Mustard greens, cooked, boiled, drained, with salt
11208	Dandelion greens, cooked, boiled, drained, without salt
11203	Cress, garden, raw
11464	Spinach, frozen, chopped or leaf, cooked, boiled, drained, without salt
11856	Spinach, frozen, chopped or leaf, cooked, boiled, drained, with salt
11575	Turnip greens, frozen, cooked, boiled, drained, without salt
11892	Turnip greens, frozen, cooked, boiled, drained, with salt
35205	Stinging Nettles, blanched (Northern Plains Indians)
11245	Lambsquarters, cooked, boiled, drained, without salt

National Nutrient Database for Standard Reference Release 27: Vitamin K

29. Ergothioneine

Ergothioneine is the first of the two phytochemicals I mentioned earlier that could qualify as a new vitamin. I bent the rules slightly though. Ergothioneine isn't a phytonutrient; it's a myconutrient, found in fungi like white button mushrooms, and it's also made by bacteria in the soil, just like B_{12}. There's definitely none in animals.

We need ergothioneine in small amounts and we can't make it: that makes it a nutrient essential for us to eat. A mushroom a week probably does the trick.

What does it do for us? It's an amino acid that's a potent antioxidant and cytoprotectant – it protects our cells from DNA damage, even inside our cell nuclei and mitochondria, which are particularly full of free radicals because they're our little cellular nuclear reactors.

According to Michael Greger:

> "Ergothioneine concentrates in parts of our body where there's lots of oxidative stress—the lens of our eye and the liver, as well as sensitive areas such as bone marrow and seminal fluid."

[See: http://nutritionfacts.org/video/ergothioneine-a-new-vitamin/]

Although most people haven't heard of this amazing quasi-vitamin, Meating is an ergothioneine deficiency disease.

30. Salicylic acid

Well, I didn't keep the suspense going for long: salicylic acid, the active ingredient in aspirin, is another phytonutrient that should probably also be classed as a vitamin. We need it in tiny quantities and we can't make it: ergo, vitamin. Originally isolated from willow tree bark, salicylic acid is present in small amounts virtually throughout the plant kingdom.

Considering that cardiologists often prescribe a baby aspirin a day to patients with heart "disease" to prevent blood clots and heart attacks, wouldn't it be easier to stop the Meating that causes the heart attacks and start Planting, which contains the doctor's remedy already? Can the salicylic acid (that's naturally in plants) be another reason why Planters have so much less heart "disease" than Meaters?

Yes, it can.

Meating is an aspirin-deficiency disease, not a statin-deficiency disease.

31. Neurotransmitters, part 1: serotonin

Neurotransmitters are the chemicals that make nerves work. When nerves transmit information as electrical impulses, neurotransmitters are chemicals which are released into synaptic clefts between nerve cells, or neurons, and they activate other nerve cells, or muscles or glands.

Serotonin, dopamine, melatonin and adrenaline (epinephrine) are all neurotransmitters… and they're made by plants! Of course, plants, not having nervous systems, use these chemicals for other purposes. It's a bit speciesist of us to call them neurotransmitters when their creators have been using them for billions of years for protection and flowering etc. They only become neurotransmitters when they're in Johnny-come-lately animals such as ourselves.

Serotonin is known as the "happiness hormone." A shortage of serotonin in our brains causes depression. There's a class of anti-depression drugs known as SSRIs (selective serotonin reuptake inhibitors), a very lucrative class of drugs which don't work very well and have serious (side-) effects. They supposedly work by preventing serotonin's reabsorption after release, making it persist longer, but placebos have been shown to work just as well, and placebos do squat to serotonin absorption.

Another way of boosting brain serotonin (besides preventing reabsorption) is to put more of it into our brains. But serotonin doesn't cross the blood-brain barrier, so eating plants for their serotonin doesn't work. Happily, a precursor of serotonin, the amino acid tryptophan, does get into the brain, allowing us to make more serotonin.

Plant tryptophan is particularly beneficial. Michael Greger lists "plantains, pineapples, bananas, kiwis, plums, and tomatoes" as excellent sources. There's also some tryptophan in animals, but there are so many other more aggressive amino acids in animals that animal tryptophan loses out in the competition for receptor sites.

[See: http://nutritionfacts.org/video/human-neurotransmitters-in-plants/]

Planting is the best frontline remedy for depression. Meating is a depressing serotonin-deficiency disease. Prozac and zoloft and tryptophan supplements aren't food, and we shouldn't eat them.

And absolutely no one should have brain stimulants like Ritalin inflicted upon them. We should just make our kids food, dear hearts. And exercise.

32. Neurotransmitters, part 2: dopamine

If serotonin is the "happiness hormone," dopamine is the "pleasure hormone." It's released, for example, during orgasm, lighting up the 'pleasure center' of our brains.

Here's what Michael Greger has to say about dopamine and Parkinson's:

> "At its root, Parkinson's is a dopamine deficiency disease, because of a die-off of dopamine-generating cells in the brain. These cells make dopamine from L-DOPA derived from an amino acid in our diet [L-tyrosine], but just like we saw with the serotonin story, the

consumption of animal products blocks the transport of L-DOPA into the brain, crowding it out."

[See: http://nutritionfacts.org/video/treating-parkinsons-disease-with-diet]

Planting helps prevent Parkinson's, with coffee being a star performer. Not only is plants-only vitamin C a strong antioxidant, it's vital as a co-factor in dopamine production, so less Parkinson's for Planters and more well-being.

Exercise boosts dopamine and norepinephrine levels too, almost instantaneously. Perhaps we should all walk to the coffee shop and back every day?

The exercise would benefit obese people who've not only developed insulin resistance, requiring more pancreatic release of insulin, but also resistance to dopamine's effect on the brain pleasure center, requiring more and more fat or sugar for a diminishing return of happiness. Fat and sugar are now known to be addictive, and fat 'n' sugar highs are just like other highs – junkies always need to up the dose.

Anhedonia – the inability to experience pleasure – is part of an eating disorder that is a vicious circle of eating non-foods and becoming fatter and becoming unhappier and eating more to dull the unhappiness. Dietary anhedonia via dopamine resistance can spill over into our sex lives too, already compromised in Meaters by insufficient genital blood supply. Erectile dysfunction and decreased dopamine sensitivity are a powerful recipe for Meater unhappiness.

Planting breaks the dopamine deficiency cycle. Unlike people who practice omnivorism, Planters have no spurious dilemma. Planters eat only food.

Meating and Junking are dopamine-deficiency diseases.

33. Neurotransmitters, part 3: adrenaline (epinephrine)

Please note that my opinion on adrenaline is entirely speculative. I have zero information to back this up.

Webster's College Dictionary describes epinephrine as:

"1. a hormone secreted by the adrenal medulla upon stimulation by the central nervous system in response to stress, as anger or fear, and acting to increase heart rate, blood pressure, cardiac output, and carbohydrate metabolism.

2. a commercial preparation of this substance, used chiefly as a heart stimulant and antiasthmatic.

Also called adrenaline."

Adrenaline is animals' "fight or flight hormone."

Without any proof, and absolutely open to being proven wrong, I'm as certain as I can be that terrified animals in slaughterhouses, all of whom are conscious, after being 'stunned' by a captive bolt gun, while they're being dismembered – a truly awful word – release copious quantities of adrenaline, a goodly portion of which we eat when we're Meaters. I can't imagine that the outcome is beneficial. If dietary adrenaline is responsible for Meater aggression, I wouldn't be surprised.

By the way, using adrenaline from animals (or a facsimile thereof) to treat asthma caused by eating animals is bizarre form of homeopathy – using like to treat like. I guess it doesn't occur to Meaters that to stop Meating is the cure, any more than fish find water problematic.

Strictly speaking, adrenaline doesn't belong in this section of animal deficiencies. I'll admit, yet again, that adrenaline may or may not be a physical health issue. If it is, it's an overload issue, not a deficiency.

The deficiency is a deficiency of heart, a metaphysical ignore-ance of others' needs. Not ignorance. Everyone knows how animals suffer. At this late stage of the Holocaust of the Animals, "But I didn't know…" doesn't cut it any more, if it ever did.

I hope you've finally realized this, René Descartes, wherever you are.

A keen vivisectionist, Descartes thought the howls of the living dogs he carved up the mere reflexes of insensate mechanisms. "Cogito, ergo sum," and they don't cogitate. Has Descartes' "I think, therefore I am" been the most disastrous mantra we humans ever adopted? (Or was it our willful transformation of a benevolent Biblical "Dominion" into our birthright to dominate all others?) Fortunately for our non-human sisters and brothers, saner, kinder dicta are arising: I feel, therefore I am. I love, I play, I grieve, I know fear and joy; therefore I am worthy of consideration and respect.

Meating is an empathy-deficiency disease.

Now let's look at some of the Eatiological mechanisms of Meating …

Planter mechanisms of optimal health in which Meating is deficient

That's it for substances in which Meating and Junking are deficient. I'm sure there are others, but "that'll do, Pig, that'll do," as Farmer Arthur H. Hoggett said to Babe.

In section 2 we learned about many mechanisms by which Meating causes ill-health. Now I'm going to list some nutrition mechanisms of good health which are available when we're Planters but which are unavailable to Meaters.

Think of yin and yang; joined opposites; a dialectic between the positives of Planting and the mirrored negatives of Meating. For example, animals are pro-oxidative. Eating them promotes free radical formation, or oxidation. Plants are antioxidants – they counter the effects of Meating and Junking by dousing free radicals. Animals and Junk are seriously deficient in antioxidants.

Among the following few listings are qualities that plants have and animals don't. In effect, I'm just listing the opposite effects of what Meating causes. Meating causes problems like oxidative stress, ischemia, inflammation, so animals are deficient in their opposites, antioxidants, anti-ischemics and anti-inflammatories.

For whatever Meating causes, Planting has a remedy.

34. Antioxidants

Plants are antioxidants. Put another way, antioxidants are plants. If they occur in animals, they're there because the animals ate them (except for uric acid – an endogenous antioxidant so potent that we need to minimize our levels.) To eat animals to get at the antioxidants they got from eating plants is a perversion of nutrition sense. (Cough, cough… the same can be said of animal proteins.)

35. Anti-inflammatories

By and large, plants which counter oxidation also counter inflammation. Oxidation causes inflammation. When we eat them, animals cause inflammation, either through the direct action of animal proteins on arthritic joints, for example, or via Neu5Gc, "the inflammatory meat molecule," or by disrupting our colon's gut flora. (When the Meater wrecking ball swings into action, there are usually multiple pathways it takes.)

Animals are lovely, but they're not food. I love them, so I don't love eating them. I don't love "my meat" – it's not mine, it's theirs. It's their muscles. Meat is an artificial construct in human nutrition. Meat as food only exists for omnivores and carnivores, which it has been the aim of this entire book to prove that we are not.

36. Anticarcinogens

Anticarcinogens are mostly plants, just like the antioxidants. Just as most antioxidants are also anti-inflammatory, there's also wide overlap with anticarcinogens. One Bing cherry or one cling peach to rule them all.

The merest stub of a Wikipedia entry says: "An anticarcinogen (also known as a **carcinopreventive agent**) is a substance that **counteracts the effects of a carcinogen or inhibits the development of cancer.** Anticarcinogens are different from anticarcinoma agents (also known as anticancer or anti-neoplastic agents) in that anticarcinoma agents are used to selectively destroy or inhibit cancer cells after cancer has developed. Interest in anticarcinogens is motivated primarily by the principle that it is preferable to prevent disease (**preventive medicine**) than to have to treat it (**rescue medicine**).

When consumed as part of a low fat diet, fiber-containing **grain products, fruits, and vegetables** may reduce the risk of some types of cancer."

Exactly. Well said. Preventive medicine via Planting. Eggs, animal flesh, fishes and dairy will never, ever, ever be categorized as anticarcinogens.

And what is a true low-fat diet? It's a no-animal diet.

Whole grains are a great source of phytates, powerful anticarcinogens. As Michael Greger says:

> "Unlike most other anti-cancer agents, the phytates naturally found in whole plant foods may trigger **cancer cell differentiation**, causing them to revert back to behaving more like normal cells."

[See: http://nutritionfacts.org/video/phytates-for-rehabilitating-cancer-cells/]

(Planting, by removing the cause of cancer, can restore normal function in cancerous cells, while starving carcinomas of sugar is to kill them while targeting a cancer symptom, as we saw with Dr. Joseph Mercola earlier.)

Another antioxidant anticarcinogen is the curcumin in cooked turmeric, which boosts the activity of an enzyme called catalase, which can destroy millions of oxidative molecules per second. High turmeric consumption in curries is probably why Indian cancer rates have historically been so low. Low animal consumption doesn't hurt.

As well as being carcinogenic, Meating is an anticarcinogen-deficiency disease. So is Junking.

37. Anti-angiogenesis agents

Continuing with cancer… There are phytonutrients such as **apigenin**, **fisitin** and **luteolin** that prevent tumors from growing blood vessels to supply themselves with nutrients. These phytonutrients starve cancers, prevent them from growing, and kill them.

Fisitin may be why strawberries are protective against esophageal cancer; the other two are found in most plants, particularly citrus fruits and peppers.

Meating promotes inflammation; inflammation promotes angiogenesis. PhIP, Kathy Freston's "three strikes breast carcinogen" is particularly involved in Meating's carcinogenesis.

Meating is both an angiogenic and an anti-angiogenic-deficiency disease.

38. Aromatase inhibitors

Most breast cancer cells thrive on estrogen. Many of them are able to make their own estrogen out of testosterone, via aromatase, an enzyme. Mushrooms act as aromatase inhibitors, blocking estrogen formation, blocking breast tumor growth.

Animals supply the hormones that cause the cancer; plants (fungi, in this case) inhibit the hormones.

Meating is an aromatase inhibitor deficiency disease.

39. DNA repair enzymes

Continuing the Planter anti-cancer theme (or the Meater cancer theme)… Earlier we saw that amazing, plants-only chlorophyll is a "carcinogen interceptor," blocking mutagens from mutating our DNA and causing cancer. And plant antioxidant fire jumpers prevent DNA damage too by putting out free radical forest fires.

But what happens if carcinogenesis does begin? Can we repair our DNA?

Yes. There are phytonutrients that upregulate our genes to create more DNA repair enzymes – epigenetics in action, beneficially promoted by

Planting, via a home-made protein called P53 which binds to our DNA and mobilizes the DNA repair enzymes.

Planting (especially of berries) is what gets our repair enzymes cracking. Meating is a DNA repair enzyme deficiency disease.

40. Epigenetic up- and down-regulators

Populations of people who've long lived in association with grains have more copies of genes for digesting grains. They've evolved over eons to be efficient "starchivores." These are genetic adaptations.

Epigenetic changes are changes in gene expression without changing the physical genes themselves. We arrive in this world with our genes in place, but it's up to us whether we switch them on or leave them off. Genes get switched on and off through environmental interactions, and by now we should know that our most powerful environmental interactions occur thrice daily (if we're privileged Westerners) at breakfast, lunch and supper.

Foods and non-foods are the environment, up close and in our faces.

Eating food causes beneficial epigenetic changes all around. Meating and Junking cause epigenetic havoc. For example, after Dr. Dean Ornish proved that Planting can reverse prostate cancer in 2005, he showed in 2008 how Planting flipped the switches of hundreds of genes to new, beneficial settings to reverse cancer.

Ornish D, Magbanua MJ, Weidner G, Weinberg V, Kemp C, Green C, Mattie MD, Marlin R, Simko J, Shinohara K, Haqq CM, Carroll PR. Changes in prostate gene expression in men undergoing an intensive nutrition and lifestyle intervention. *Proc Natl Acad Sci U S A.* 17;105(24):8369-74, 2008.

(*The Proceedings of the National Academy of Sciences* (*PNAS*) is one serious scientific journal – the likes of ex-journalists Gary Taubes, Bryan Walsh and Nina Teicholz don't get published there.)

On the other hand, POPs like pesticides can cause cancer directly through DNA damage or through detrimental epigenetic changes in gene expression. It's as if a drunken singer mangles a song either by changing the words altogether or by slurring them so badly they can't be understood.

Genetics isn't destiny. What we eat is far more important. Planting trumps genes, 9 times out of 10. Genetics is passé; epigenetics rules.

Low-Carb Bullshit Artists hate epigenetics, just like they hate epidemiology, because neither branch of science tells them what they want to hear. In fact, epidemiology shows the exact opposite of what Meaters want to hear: that Planting prevents degenerative "diseases" and obesity, and creates ideal conditions for longevity; and then epigenetics provides one of the mechanisms whereby Planting causes positive outcomes and Meating, negative.

At each meal we can make a choice between eating ourselves epigenetically healthy with Plants. Or we can eat ourselves sick, as Meaters and Junkers.

Meating is an epigenetic sinkhole.

41. IGF-1 Binding Proteins

Still on carcinogenesis…

When we eat animals, animal proteins stimulate our livers to release IGF-1, our growth hormone, and our body is told to build, build, build. This is only supposed to happen in human neonates when our mothers feed us breast milk. Mother's milk proteins are the only animal proteins we're supposed to receive during our entire lifetimes. Okay, faced with this aberration – animals stampeding through our blood – our livers churn out IGF-1.

Another thing happens too: our levels of IGF-1-BP go down. BP stands for binding proteins, and their role is to remove carcinogenic growth hormones and steroid sex hormones like estrogen and testosterone from circulation. But, faced with animal amino acid building blocks to get rid of, the levels of IGF-1- BP plummet, further worsening IGF-1's carcinogenic effect.

Planters naturally have the healthy reverse condition: low IGF-1 levels and high liver and blood levels of IGF-1- BP. The higher our binding protein levels are, the more we're protected against cancer.

Meating is an IGF-binding protein deficiency disease.

42. Brown fat and the thermogenic effect

Meaters lack 'plant calories.' Of course, there's no such thing. What happens is this: Planting raises our metabolic rate slightly, shifting more calories to be burned as heat rather than stored as fat. This is known as the thermogenic effect, and it accounts for roughly a difference of 0.4 – 0.5kg (~1 pound) in body weight per year between Planters and Meaters on an isocaloric (equal energy) diet.

Meaters create more abdominal white fat, implicated in meatabolic syndrome. Planters create more brown fat, which is sparsely laid down over the neck and shoulder area, and which is burned to create heat.

Meating is a brown fat deficiency disease; a thermogenic inefficiency disease.

43. Adiponectin

Continuing with obesity… Adiponectin is a hormone which is protective against "gynoid lipodystrophy," aka cellulite. High adiponectin levels = low butt fat. (High butter fat = high butt fat.)

Meating drops our adiponectin levels by almost 20%. Planting raises them by almost 20%.

Meating is an adiponectin-deficiency disease.

Cellulite isn't a feminist issue; it's a Meater issue.

44. Leptin and ghrelin

According to Wikipedia: "Leptin (from Greek λεπτός leptos, "thin"), the "satiety hormone," is a hormone made by adipose cells that helps to regulate energy balance by inhibiting hunger. Leptin is opposed by the actions of the hormone ghrelin, the "hunger hormone." Both hormones… regulate appetite... In obesity, a decreased sensitivity to leptin occurs, resulting in an inability to detect satiety despite high energy stores." When we're overweight, our bodies can't tell we're full even when we're stuffed.

I find it fascinating that it's the fat cells themselves that release these two hormones that tell us whether *they're* hungry or not! Talk about minds of their own.

So, these two hormone antagonists duke it out constantly, satiety (fullness) vs. hunger. When we're obese, our bodies become resistant to leptin, the satiety hormone, (in much the same way that we become resistant to another hormone, insulin), and ghrelin – Mr. Hunger – wins, so we eat more and we gain weight.

What boosts leptin levels? Planting. What drops leptin levels? Meating. Planting leads to skinny people; Meating leads to fat. Leptin/ghrelin is one of the Eatiology mechanisms that explains the epidemiology of skinny Planters and overweight Meaters.

Meating is a leptin deficiency disease.

45. Mineral absorption enhancers & 'dis-enhancers'

We've seen that several minerals are absorbed differently depending on whether they come packaged in animals or plants. Animal iron and animal phosphorus are notable rebels, refusing to obey limits. Plant mineral absorption, on the other hand, is much easier for our bodies to regulate, sometimes with better absorption (e.g. calcium); some plant nutrients like phytates may slightly decrease iron and zinc absorption, while vitamin C boosts iron absorption from plants. Meating lacks this finesse – Meater iron blows through our gut walls regardless of whether we have enough or not.

There are phytonutrients that behave as mineral absorption enhancers – the entire allium family, which includes garlic, onions, leeks, scallions, spring onions and shallots.

Unregulated heme iron absorption causes oxidative stress; phosphorus overload can lead to kidney damage; and systemic acidosis leads to muscle wasting as calcium is stripped from our muscles (not our bones) to buffer acid. There are no Meater mechanisms which advance or retard mineral absorption the way that the onion family, phytates and vitamin C do.

Meating is a mineral absorption regulator deficiency disease.

46. Detoxification enzymes

There's something about broccoli and it's cruciferous cousins, cabbage, kale, Brussels sprouts and others, that upregulates our livers' production of detoxification enzymes. It's probably the cancer-busting sulforaphane. Berries do the same thing, causing our livers to clean house (that is, more than they already do, all the time.)

Animals supply the toxins; plants supply the detox enzymes.

47. Xenohormesis

When plants are stressed they produce antioxidants and anti-inflammatories. This process of producing beneficial substances to cope with bad situations is known as hormesis. We take advantage of plant hormesis by eating the plants and getting *their* anti-stress phytonutrients. We're the xeno- foreigners practicing xenohormesis.

When animals are stressed they produce adrenaline and stress hormones and, probably, metabolites of metaphysical compounds known as "anguish" when their calves are stolen from them and "bewilderment and terror" as they go to slaughter.

Meating is a xenohormesis (and compassion) deficiency disease.

48. Apoptosis

Apoptosis is "programmed cell death." Our immune systems clear cancer cells from our systems, alerting them when it's time to die. On a constant diet of animals, cancer cells become immortal, dividing and metastasizing. Planting boosts apoptosis.

Meating is an apoptosis-deficiency condition.

49. Natural killer cells

Berries are outstanding at increasing the numbers of our immune system's natural killer cells, vital for defense against cancer. Other immune components need to meet up with an antigen before our bodies start manufacturing clones of the antibodies needed to combat the intruder. NK cells are our standing army; the rest are reserves and new recruits, enlisted on demand.

We have billions of NK cells constantly circulating through us, on the lookout for intruders. Some phytonutrients in berries (and the spice cardamom) can double the number of NK cells we have, thus boosting our immunity.

Planting confers high levels of immune function. Meating confers an immunocompromised condition.

50a. Small intestine immune system activators: Aryl receptors

This book is about why animals aren't food, and, if there are 50 Ways to Leave Your Lover, then there are 50 Ways to Retrieve Your Liver in this Animal Deficiency section.

> "Just snip out the back bacon, Jack
> Make an eggless diet plan, Stan
> You don't eat the koi, Roy
> Just set the chickens free
> Stay off the pus, Gus
> You won't feel disgust much
> Just drop off the turkey, Lee
> And get yourself free."

With apologies to Paul Simon.

Pigs, chicken's eggs, fishes, cow's milk, turkeys… none of them is food.

For the last two entries in this Meater deficiency section, I'd like us to put on our evolutionary biologist hats (or our creationist hats, if we'd prefer). It doesn't matter which.

We've established that the time the environment impinges on us the most is when things we've eaten are a single enterocyte cell's width away from our real innards. To facilitate absorption of nutrients, these gut cells must let the environment in, and wastes out, all the time.

Eating is when we're at maximum danger of environmental poisoning, so it's natural that our immune systems should be at DefCon1 while we're eating. Right? We need our immune system to be on high alert, looking out for would-be assassins and saboteurs. Between meals our immuneteers can relax and stand down.

What activates our small intestine immune system when we eat? That should be obvious. Animals. They're the most endotoxin-, pollutant-, parasite- and pathogen-encrusted things we eat. Our bodies have to know straight away when crut-filled animals hit town.

Except… plants are our immune system activators, not animals.

Now, while some Meaters might crow, saying: See, plants are so bad for us, they cause our immune systems to be flashing red, that's not right. As I've shown over and over, whole plants bring nothing but benefits, unless contaminated by animals.

We're either the culmination of billions of years of incremental evolution or God's sudden creation. Either way, activation of our intestinal tract's immune system only by plants shows that we are adapted to eating plants only. Would either God or evolution have enabled us to eat animals without activating our gut's immune systems? Does that make any sense?

Animals are far and away the dirtiest things we put in our mouths. Or do Meaters think early hominins always ate an hors d'oeuvre of grass to activate gut immunity before chowing down on a stegosaurus steak?

We know that Planters have superior immune function and that Meaters have compromised immune function, by comparison. And Planting primes the small intestine's immune pump.

This is how it works:

Intraepithelial lymphocytes (IELs) are small, round white blood cells, immune system components that live between the epithelial cells that make up the mucosal lining of our gastrointestinal (GI) tracts. (Our reproductive tracts too.) Their surfaces are covered with receptors known as aryl hydrocarbon (Ah) receptors. They're the ignition switch for starting up our immune system motors, and the key is plants, particularly cruciferous vegetables such as broccoli, cabbage, cauliflower and kale.

What this means, in evolutionary biology terms, is that we humans (and the species before us) grew up over millions of years in tight association with the plant kingdom, with not enough animal input to change our basic frugivore, herbivore, starchivore, plantivore, phytophage genetic makeup. We lack the genetic code, even now, after geological ages of eating animals, for Meating to activate our intraepithelial response the way that Planting does. Our ancestors ate plants for so long before we started to eat animals that we'd already established how to alert our immune system to incoming food… with plants.

We saw confirmatory evidence with chlorophyll, how our blood and plant blood are almost identical; heme and chlorophyll. Further evidence of our non-Meater nature is that atherosclerosis is an immune response to Meating. If anyone can name me one omnivore or carnivore that forms atherosclerotic plaques in response to animal cholesterol, I'll give them a small house. There aren't any. The notion of human nutritional exceptionalism is a costly one, with millions of us ignorantly succumbing to Meating each year.

The overwhelming tower of evidence for our Planter nature, listed throughout the pages of this book, is capped by this semi-final piece of the puzzle; plants activate our small intestine's immune function when we eat them; not animals. Plants and humans go together like two peas in a pod.

It's clear that we're Planters.

Meating is an immune system activator deficiency disease.

50b. Immune system deactivators in the colon: T_{regs}

In Part 1B (Mechanisms), under Deranged gut flora, I described how beneficial bacteria colonize our colons when we feed them on a high-fiber, whole-plant diet. We feed our bacterial digestive-and-immune 'organ' on fiber and phytates and other phytonutrients, and in return they make nutrients for us and they regulate the colon's immune function and prevent cancer.

One Meater deficiency may lead to another. Continuing with the thread I started earlier in this Animal MIAs section, discussing Planter deficiencies in fiber, phytates, gut flora, propionate, lignans and butyrate, out greatest Meater deficiency may come as a result of suppressing *Faecalibacterium prausnitzii*, and other beneficial colon bacteria like the 'clostridial clusters' who've been living as part of the human intestines for millions of years.

One of the many reasons why Meaters have worse immune function (and more inflammation) in the colon – and are thus more susceptible to inflammatory bowel and leaky gut conditions such as ulcerative colitis, Crohn's "disease" and colorectal cancer – is because Meaters create conditions which are inhospitable to our fiber-eating bacteria.

The final deficiency in my list of 50 comes at the end of this chain:

Low fiber diets (Meating and Junking) → ↓ *F. prausnitzii* et al → ↓ butyrate and other fatty-acid production → ↓ Regulatory T cell, or T_{reg} production.

Meating and Junking combine to cause a T_{reg} deficiency disease.

Aryl receptors in our small intestine *activate* our immune system when they perceive a threat. In our colons, T_{regs} actively *suppress* our immune system. They keep the immune system from attacking our intestinal flora.

Remember, our intestinal flora are us. They're a vital part of us, tantamount to a bodily organ. Therefore, when we eat low-fiber (low-whole-carb, high-animal) diets we're causing an auto-immune response in our colons. We make our immune systems attack other parts of ourselves; in this case, our intestinal bacteria. Animals and junk aren't food… not for us, and not for our bacterial fellow travelers.

Meating is a form of unintentional slow-motion self-murder, as opposed to suicide, which stems from a conscious desire to do away with one's self. If somnambulists are sleepwalkers, Meaters and Junkers are "somnophages" – sleep-eaters. We don't know how to eat. We eat ourselves to death, in part because we eat our multi-part bacterial gut organs to death. And we're oblivious to the fact that we're doing it.

Animals and junked plants aren't food.

Sidebar: On PREbiotics, PRObiotics and 'RETRObiotics'

Vegetarians and other non-vegans make much of the probiotics they get from eating the refrigerated, fruit-flavored goop otherwise known as yogurt.

WebMD says "Probiotics are live bacteria and yeasts that are good for your health, especially your digestive system. We usually think of bacteria as something that causes diseases. But your body is full of bacteria, both good and bad. Probiotics are often called "good" or "helpful" bacteria because they help keep your gut healthy."

Probiotics are supplements that Meaters and Junkers have to take to artificially create a healthy microbiome, because their diets are devoid of the fiber upon which a healthy gut bacteria population thrives.

Yogurt is bacterially fermented milk. Being fermented, it's got less lactose in it, so it's not as terrible for us as regular milk. But it's still milk. It's just as laden with animal hormones, animal fats and animal proteins, and just as contaminated with environmental pollutants. It's not food for humans, or for cows. No cow has ever wittingly fed a fermented milk culture to her calf, and no adult cow drinks any kind of milk.

Probiotics are, in effect, retrobiotics. We add them to our diet to retrofit our bacteria, while we wipe out the same bacteria with other parts of our diet: animals and junk.

(It's like Low-Carb Bullshit Artists with diabetes having to take metformin to control their Meater-induced diabetes.) If we quit Meating and Junking, we can quit taking probiotics (and metformin and statins and… and… and…)

Prebiotics, on the other hand, are just whole plants, packed full of fiber and fiber-associated nutrients. They're food for humans and food for bacteria. They feed us all. Prebiotics aren't supplements; they're merely whole food.

That said, Meaters and Junkers would be well-advised to carry on swallowing their probiotics and their drugs to make up for the ill-effects of their immune- and otherwise deficient diets.

Those of us who'd prefer to live long healthy lives should ditch the yogurt, and just eat the fruit.

Stop Press Bonus Meater Deficiencies

51. Natural Products That Target Cancer Stem Cells

Here's an exciting paper, out in November 2015, just in time to make it into the first edition of this book early in 2016:

Moselhy J, Srinivasan S, Ankem MK, Damodaran C. Natural Products That Target Cancer Stem Cells. *Anticancer Res.* 2015 Nov;35(11):5773-88.

"The cancer stem cell model suggests that tumor initiation is governed by a small subset of distinct cells with stem-like character termed cancer stem cells (CSCs). CSCs possess properties of self-renewal and intrinsic survival mechanisms that contribute to resistance of tumors to most chemotherapeutic drugs. The failure to eradicate CSCs during the course of therapy is postulated to be the driving force for tumor recurrence and metastasis."

Cancer stem cells are resistant to chemotherapy. Not only does chemo not kill CSCs – it can make them more virulent.

This is really important: "Recent studies evaluating NPs against CSC support the **epidemiological evidence linking plant-based diets with reduced malignancy rates**."

Epidemiology shows Planters get less cancer. Here's just one of the many reasons why… **Planters get less cancer because Planting wipes out Cancer Stem Cells.**

Moselhy et al list 25 Natural Products (NPs) that selectively target cancer stem cells, without harming normal cells:

1. Baicalein – Chinese skullcap [Chinese herb of the mint family]
2. β-Carotene – Carrots, leafy greens
3. Curcumin – Turmeric
4. Cyclopamine – Corn lily [not to be eaten – a lethal teratogen]
5. Delphinidin – Blueberry, raspberry
6. Epigallocatechin-3-gallate (EGCG) – Green tea
7. Flavonoids (Genistein) – Soy, red clover, coffee
8. 6-Gingerol – Ginger
9. Gossypol – Cottonseed [not to be eaten – may cause paralysis; sometimes used in China as a male contraceptive]
10. Guggulsterone – Commiphora (myrrh tree)
11. Isothiocyanates – Cruciferous vegetables
12. Linalool – Mint
13. Lycopene – Grapefruit, tomato
14. Parthenolide – Feverfew
15. Perylill alcohol – Mint, cherry, lavender
16. Piperine – Black pepper
17. Placycodon saponin – Playycodon grandifloruim [Chinese bellflower]
18. Psoralidin [a coumarin] – Psoralea corylilyfolia [Babchi, in Ayurveda]
19. Quercetin – Capers, onions
20. Resveratrol – Grapes, plums, berries [not red wine – carcinogenic]
21. Salinomycin – Streptomyces albus [a bacterium which generates mycelia]
22. Silibinin – Milk thistle
23. Ursolic acid – Thyme, basil, oregano
24. Vitamin D3 – [Sunlight on skin] Fish, egg yolk, beef, cod liver oil
25. Withaferin A – Withania somnifera (ashwagandha) [Indian ginseng, a nightshade, also used in Ayurveda.]

What do we notice about all these anti-cancer stem cell agents? With the exception of #24, which is best obtained by the action of sunlight on human skin, they're all plants; not necessarily edible plants, but plants all the same. All the animal products suggested in #24 as sources of vitamin D3 are themselves carcinogenic, so we'd be better off getting D3 from fortified non-junk-foods or a supplement, in the case of us not getting enough sunshine. We should stock up with this vital hormone whenever we can – on holiday, or during non-wintry months.

The reason why chemotherapy is a poor treatment of cancer, and why regression is so common after traditional therapies, is that they tend to kill the cancer daughter cells and so reduce tumor size, but they leave the stem cells untouched, leading to the false hope that the tumor is going, as it shrinks, while the cancer 'seeds' are left to germinate again later.

Using these Natural Products goes right to the root of the cancer, wiping out the stem cells. Plus... they boost our immune systems, which conventional "treatments" such as chemo and radiation are notorious for eradicating. We know that whole plants and their phytonutrients can synergize powerfully. Knowing this, we should eat a wide variety of plants that contain these (and other yet-to-be-discovered) NP substances such as gingerols, isothiocyanates, flavonoids and carotenes, all washed down with a nice cup of EGCG, for spectacularly, synergistically beneficial results. I'd pick them over chemo or radiation every time. [I'm not giving medical advice; merely pointing out the power of the new medicine: lifestyle medicine. Please consult a physician, preferably one versed in nutrition.]

Because we're sweet solar-powered beings (via sunlight and plants), Meating is a sunlight-deficiency condition, lacking in the natural, healing plant products that combat cancer stem cells.

Meating is not only carcinogenic; it's a Natural Product-deficiency disease.

52. Primordial prevention

If "The purpose of primary prevention is to limit the incidence of disease by controlling causes and risk factors," as says Sorin Ursoniu, MD, PhD, then primordial prevention begins even earlier: "Primordial prevention deals with underlying conditions leading to exposure to causative factors."

Planting is automatically primordially preventative of degenerative "diseases".

Why? Because Meating and Junking *are the risk factors* for most chronic ailments.

Meating and Junking are primordial prevention disaster zones.

Summary of MIAs

To aid my summary of missing-in-action animal nutrients [oxymoron alert] and MIA beneficial health mechanisms, I'm going to refer to a 2014 paper by Jennifer Di Noia PhD:

Defining Powerhouse Fruits and Vegetables: A Nutrient Density Approach. *Preventing Chronic Disease* 2014:11:130390 [downloadable at http://www.cdc.gov/pcd/issues/2014/pdf/13_0390.pdf],

In her paper, Dr Di Noia writes: "This article describes a classification scheme defining PFV [**powerhouse fruits and vegetables**] on the basis of **17 nutrients of public health importance** per the Food and Agriculture Organization of the United Nations and Institute of Medicine (i.e., potassium, fiber, protein, calcium, iron, thiamin, riboflavin, niacin, folate, zinc, and vitamins A, B_6, B_{12}, C, D, E, and K)" (3).

Her reference (3) is to Drewnonwski A. Concept of a nutritious food: toward a nutrient density score. *Am J Clin Nutr* 2005;82(4):721-32.

Let's take a look at Dr Di Noia's 17 nutrients "of public health importance":

calcium
fiber
iron
potassium
protein
vit. A (retinol, retinal, and 4 carotenoids incl. beta carotene)
vitamin B_1 (thiamine)
vit. B_2 (riboflavin)
vit. B_3 (niacin)
vit. B_6 (pyridoxine)
vit. B_9 (folate)
vit. B_{12} (cyano-, hydroxy- or methylcobalamin)
vit. C (ascorbic acid)
vit. D (cholecalciferol (D_3), ergocalciferol (D_2))
vit. E (tocopherols, tocotrienols)
vit. K (phylloquinone, menaquinones)
zinc

Magnesium doesn't make the list. That surprises me. Just upping our magnesium levels with a few nuts and seeds a day could prevent tens of thousands of fatal heart attacks in the US annually. I guess the FAO had to draw the line somewhere. I think they stopped one nutrient too soon.

This list contains two nutrients we should never, ever get from animals: **iron** and **protein**. As I've shown repeatedly, heme iron and animal protein are extremely toxic carcinogens, via nitrosamines and IGF-1 respectively.

To their detriment, there is no **fiber** in processed animals or plants.

Calcium and **potassium** are far better absorbed and regulated from plants than from animals; calcium from leafy greens, potassium from bananas, beans and nuts.

Zinc can be a problem for vegans: animal zinc is more absorbable than plant zinc (not necessarily a good thing). Plus, as we'd expect with metal accumulation increasing up the "food" chain, animals have lots of zinc in them, with oysters at #1. (The loss of zinc in ejaculate is part of what gives oysters their reputation as aphrodisiacs.) Getting at the zinc from oysters without also getting the PCBs, dioxins and heavy metals is problematic. "Food is a package deal." Planters should just eat plenty of grains, beans, nuts and seeds: food. Plant zinc and iron become more bioaccessible when eaten with "mineral absorption enhancers" such as garlic and onions.

Of the vitamins, **B_9** (folate), **C** and **E** are found only in plants; **D** is made by the action of sunlight on human and other animal skin.

Vitamin K comes overwhelmingly from leafy green vegetables. The top 100 sources in the National Nutrient Database list for vit. K doesn't contain a single animal item that's not a Chinese restaurant dish that also contains confounding veggies.

The top sources of **vitamin A** are animals, but there's plenty in dark green leafies, and in yellow, orange and red veggies. Deficiency in the 1st World is almost unheard of, so there's no reason to poison ourselves with animals to get it. As with several other animal issues such as protein, the problem with vitamin A is getting too much, rather than too little.

There's also plenty of **vitamin B_{12}** in animals, but unfortunately we'd have to eat the animals to get the B_{12}, which is the health equivalent of eating monkey droppings to get at an undigested peanut: the peanut's tasty, but not worth eating shit for.

Which leaves four B vitamins, 1, 2, 3 and 6; thiamine, riboflavin, niacin and pyridoxine. (The other two B vitamins, vitamin B_5 (pantothenic acid) and vitamin B_7 (biotin) are the only two of the 13 acknowledged vitamins not to make it into this exclusive list of "17 nutrients of public health importance," probably because they don't play hard to get.)

This 2011 study, in which 13,292 people took part, compared the diets of vegetarians to non-vegetarians:

(B. Farmer, B. T. Larson, V. L. Fulgoni III, A. J. Rainville, G. U. Liepa. A vegetarian dietary pattern as a nutrient-dense approach to weight management: An analysis of the national health and nutrition examination survey 1999-2004. *J Am Diet Assoc.* 2011 111(6):819 – 827, abstract available at http://www.ncbi.nlm.nih.gov/pubmed/21616194.)

Farmer et al start by saying: "Population-based studies have shown that vegetarians have lower body mass index than non-vegetarians, suggesting that vegetarian diet plans may be an approach for weight management. However, a perception exists that vegetarian diets are deficient in certain nutrients."

In other words, we Meaters think you semi-Planter vegetarians are deficient in a bunch of stuff. Let's see if that's true.

Instead, they found that "**Mean intakes of fiber, vitamins A, C, and E, thiamin, riboflavin, folate, calcium, magnesium, and iron were higher for all vegetarians than for all non-vegetarians.**"

Better in every single nutrient tested, including calcium and iron. Also more magnesium: fewer sudden cardiac deaths.

That takes care of **vitamins B_1** and **B_2**. The people who ate the fewest animals had the best thiamin and riboflavin levels. Not optimal, but better – after all these were vegetarians, not vegans.

The researchers concluded: "These findings suggest that vegetarian diets are nutrient dense, consistent with dietary guidelines, and could be recommended for weight management without compromising diet quality."

I think they could have been slightly less underwhelming, considering how much more favorable the results were for mere vegetarians than Meaters.

They could have said, quite truthfully: "A whole-food vegan diet is the most nutrient-dense, and the only logical diet for humans."

Next up: niacin.

I'm pleased, as one of part-English descent, to say that the top source of **niacin (B_3)** per 100g in the USDA database is "yeast extract spread." That sounds suspiciously like Marmite or Vegemite to me, two yeast extract spreads well known in Britain and the colonies, with the look and acquired taste of coal tar waste, long-fermented in a Scottish peat bog. I eat lots of it, so I'm niacinically sorted. The top database entry per household, a turkey breast weighing 1.1171 kg contains 1.1171 mg of niacin, while 0.984 kg vegetarian stew contains 118.56 mg. The stuff's everywhere in food; we shouldn't have a problem getting enough of it, even if absorption may vary.

Pretty much everyone gets enough **vitamin B_6 (pyridoxine),** so I'm not sure why our researchers were more concerned about it than magnesium, of which almost 98% of Americans are deficient. (Hey, wait a minute; almost 2% of the population is now vegan. Is there a connection? Of course, there is. I'm not saying all vegans get enough magnesium, but we're far more likely to when we're vegan.) As with potassium, there's plenty of B_6 in bananas, beans and nuts. (Having enough B_6 helps keep homocysteine levels in check, to suppress inflammation, particularly in the brain.)

Summary of the 17 nutrients of concern

If we're rooting for the Meater nutrient team, it's fourth down with 99 yards to go, with seconds on the clock, our 3rd string quarterback just got crocked, so the water boy had to take his place, and our team is trailing by 30 points. It's not a strong position. (Yet people bet on it all the time.)

Just as we saw with the 50 animal deficiencies I noted earlier, getting one's nutrients from animals is either impossible (because they don't contain them) or fraught with danger, if they do: vitamin B_{12} is a good thing; vitamin B_{12} from animals is anything but. Calcium is a necessary thing; calcium from dairy is not.

Of the 17 nutrients studied, only zinc, B_{12} and D may take some thought for Planters to achieve optimal levels. We do this by eating a wide range of whole plants, by taking a daily or weekly B_{12} supplement, and getting enough sun exposure; failing which, a supplement.

For Meaters, problems abound, starting with growth hormone-promoting, carcinogenic animal protein; continuing with free radical-causing, carcinogenic heme iron; going further with fiber-, folate-, C-, E-and K-poor or –absent animals.

In their paper above, published in the staunchly pro-Meater *Journal of the American Dietetic Association*, of all places, Farmer et al showed that the Plantier we are, the better our intake of "fiber, vitamins A, C, and E, thiamin, riboflavin, folate, calcium, magnesium, and iron."

We achieve optimal nutrition when we Plant… with the single exception of the limp noodle with which Meaters try to stove in Planters' heads: vitamin B_{12}.

And yet, eating the whole-food way Planters do, we can remedy all of our nutrition problems simply by taking a harmless tablet once a week while the plants do the rest.

Eating the way Meaters do, we can certainly avoid taking those dreadful B_{12} supplements, sure, but then we'd have to take statins and aspirin and warfarin for our heart conditions, and zoloft or prozac for our depression, and viagra for our erectile dysfunction, and diuretics (water pills) or ACE inhibitors or angiotensin II receptor blockers or beta blockers or calcium channel blockers or renin inhibitors for our hypertension, and metformin for our diabetes (hi, Prof. Noakes), and tamoxifen or aromatase inhibitors for our breast cancer, and fosamax for our osteoporosis, and cetuximab for our metastatic colorectal cancer, and this for our triglycerides, and that for our gout, and the other thing for our kidney stones, and… and… and… all to combat the symptoms of Meating, world without end.

B_{12} is an embarrassing argument to use *in favor of* Meating and *against* Planting.

As we've seen, Meating truly is a nutrient-poor disaster of a diet.

To quote Prof. T. Colin Campbell one more time: "There is no nutrient in animals that's not better supplied by plants…" and there are tens of thousands of plant nutrients of which animals are totally bereft.

If we're humans, we're Planters. Planting is our God- and/or evolution-given nature.

Anyone who needs a little extra convincing should check out Dr. Milton Mills' excellent *The Comparative Anatomy of Eating*. It's available at http://www.adaptt.org/Mills%20The%20Comparative%20Anatomy%20of%20Eating1.pdf

After examining our facial muscles, jaw type, jaw joint location, jaw motion, major jaw muscles, mouth opening vs. head size, teeth (incisors), teeth (canines), teeth (molars), chewing, saliva, stomach type, stomach acidity, stomach capacity, length of small intestine, colon, liver, kidneys and nails (vs. claws), he says:

> "In conclusion, we see that human beings have the gastrointestinal tract structure of a "committed" herbivore. Humankind does not show the mixed structural features one expects and finds in anatomical omnivores such as bears and raccoons. Thus, from comparing the gastrointestinal tract of humans to that of carnivores, herbivores and omnivores we must conclude that humankind's GI tract is designed for a purely plant-food diet."

Planters… that's what we are.

When it comes to the rapid encephalization of *H. & F. sapiens* in our primeval past, my money's on Rachel Carmody and Richard Wrangham, with their theory that the control of fire, which allowed greater energy from cooked plants, particularly the USOs or underground storage organs (such as tubers) which Nathaniel Dominy is so keen on.

Paleonutrition is a stimulating subject. However, it's entirely irrelevant to the study of modern nutrition, for the simple reason that only whole plants are food, to whom and where and when it matters - to us modern human beings, living right here, right now.

Even in the extremely unlikely event that eating animals made us human by causing our sugar-powered brains to put on a growth spurt millennia ago, our digestive tracts and arteries, hearts and brains still can't tolerate animals today. So we should just say thank you to our hominin ancestors whose subsistence on animal emergency rations may have given us our modern brains, and now that we're not constrained in our eating choices, let normal plant-food service resume.

~

Part 5 (Summary): Why Animals Aren't Food

When the Cows Come Home to Roost: The Consequences of Meating

Robert Louis Stevenson: "Everybody, soon or late, sits down to a banquet of consequences."

In Part 1 of this book, ANIMALS, THEMSELVES, I described

- the CONSTITUENTS of animals
- the MECHANISMS whereby Meating sickens us
- the EATIOLOGY of degenerative "diseases", now known to be symptoms of Meating

I showed that Meating and Junking are responsible for 90% of all the "Diseases" of Western Civilization, and that what we think of as diseases are usually reversible symptoms of Meating and Junking.

In Part 2 (~~FOOD~~BORNE PATHOGENS), I described the life forms that come packaged with animals. These include:

- Viruses
- Bacteria and their toxins
- Parasites
- Fungi, including yeasts
- Prions

I showed that Meating is responsible for at least 90% of the illnesses, hospitalizations and deaths due to microbes, because of the extraordinary load of pathogens Meating introduces.

In Part 3 (~~FOOD~~BORNE CONTAMINANTS), I described the inert pollution with which animals become contaminated, including:

- Industrial pollutants, inserted accidentally and
- "Food" and feed additives, contaminants inserted on purpose.

I showed how the biological processes of bio-accumulation and bio-magnification are why Meating introduces more than 90% of environmental pollutants into our bodies.

In Part 4 (ANIMAL DEFICIENCIES), or Missing in Action, I described some of the nutrients that animals and junk lack, including fiber, carbohydrates, vitamins, phytates and other phytonutrients.

I showed that hyper-processed plants and animals have an Eatiology ("disease"-causing effect) that's very similar in many ways. Processed junk behaves more like processed animals than it does like whole plants.

In Part 5 (SUMMARY), it's my intention to put all the pieces together. After one last section of reductionist science - almost seventy pages of references to and discussions of landmark studies in biomedicine - I'm going to switch gears and practice nutrition science as it ought to be practiced - in a holistic or wholistic way.

A Turd's Eye View of an Animal Meal describes what happens when we eat a meal of animals, from when we ingest them to when we excrete them, pointing out the harmful effects they have on our digestion, metabolism and overall health.

After that we'll be well-armed with both reductionist and wholistic nutrition science with which to view the world and to see - because we'll know to the depths of our being that animals aren't food - that as individuals we need to make changes if we'd like to thrive, and that, as a species, we're going to need to make changes if we're to survive.

Here now is the last of the reductionist science…

References: Landmarks in medical and nutrition research

Blaise Pascal is supposed to have apologized to a friend that he hadn't had the time to write a shorter letter. I apologize that five years hasn't been enough time for me to condense everything I wanted to say about Meater and Junker mal-nutrition into fewer than the 800-odd pages it's taken me.

As a result, and because my sources are liberally sprinkled throughout the text, I'm not going to do what Michael Greger did in his *How Not to Die* and supply you with more than a hundred pages of references. In 70-odd pages, I'm going to hit the high notes, and I'm going to provide some commentary too. This section contains references to papers about the biggies like diabetes, hypertension, auto-immune conditions, cancer, stroke, heart "disease" and Alzheimer's but not to studies about more obscure maladies such as ankylosing spondylitis or abdominal aortic aneurysm.

But don't worry: everything's connected… ankylosing spondylitis is an auto-immune condition and, with a few exceptions such as celiac disease and rheumatic heart disease, they're usually ailments with the same Meater Eatiology. And AAA is inseparable from atherosclerosis and hypertension, which are also the same thing – it's not possible to give ourselves one without the other – and we give them to ourselves by Meating and Junking.

What's the most important illness in the world? It's the one we have.

If you'd like to read good primary sources about a condition of interest and I haven't cited it in this reference section or in the body of the book, you could do worse than start where I did five years ago, at nutritionfacts.org. Type in, say, polyps, then follow the links to the videos or articles about your topic; then click on the 'sources' link and read the original papers in *The New England Journal of Medicine* or *The Lancet* or wherever they may lurk.

Now let's take a look at the extraordinary source materials behind the lifestyle medicine and plants-only nutrition renaissance. If you watch carefully, you'll notice that all the best new evidence shows the same thing in two different ways: Meating and Junking make us ill, while Planting prevents, stops or heals what Meating and Junking and other things cause. And please note that we're going to measure real health outcomes here, like reversal of illness and extension of life. We're not merely going to manipulate biomarkers as low-carbers are wont to do.

References to papers on animal and junk components (with a few pathogens thrown in for good measure)

First, a quick word about scientific language. Scientists, like judges, hate to have their opinions overturned on appeal, so they speak circumspectly. We shouldn't be fooled by their heavy use of words like 'may' and 'can.' In our minds we should substitute 'will' and 'do.'

For example, when G. Brewer says: "This copper is potentially toxic because it may penetrate the blood/brain barrier," we can be darn certain that copper *is* toxic because it *does* enter the brain. And when Abrahamsson et al say: "Diet modifications may be one breast cancer prevention strategy," we know that diet modification (Planting) *is* the best strategy.

I won't pussyfoot around: if the best science tells us it's so, I'll say so. If later, better evidence shows that I'm wrong a time or two, I'll let you know. The overall ill-effects of Meating and Junking will endure the picayune.

Acrylamide

M Stott-Miller, ML Neuhouser, JL Stanford. Consumption of deep-fried foods and risk of prostate cancer. *Prostate.* 2013 73(9):960 – 969.

Stott-Miller et al say that "Regular consumption of select deep-fried foods is associated with increased PCa (prostate cancer) risk."

As a prostate owner, I say acrylamide's a good reason to avoid crispy carbs.

Alpha-gal

SP Commins, TAE Platts-Mills. Delayed anaphylaxis to red meat in patients with IgE specific for galactose alpha-1,3-galactose (alpha-gal). *Curr Allergy Asthma Rep.* 2013 13(1):72 – 77.

"Anaphylaxis is a severe allergic reaction that can be rapidly progressing and fatal… delayed onset anaphylaxis 3-6 hours after ingestion of mammalian food products (e.g., beef and pork)."

For 99% of us, food doesn't do this. The exceptions are a tiny fraction of the population that has an issue with gluten and those with allergies to whole plants such as some nuts or seeds or members of the nightshade family).

Ammonia

A Birkett, J Muir, J Phillips, G Jones, K O'Dea. Resistant starch lowers fecal concentrations of ammonia and phenols in humans. *Am J Clin Nutr.* 1996 May;63(5):766-72.

"…RS [resistant starch] significantly attenuates the accumulation of potentially harmful byproducts of protein fermentation in the human colon."

Resistant starch is found in whole plants and it combats the bacterial formation of ammonia from animal proteins in our intestines.

Amyloid, cholesterol and Alzheimer's

Ortiz D, Shea TB. Apple juice prevents oxidative stress induced by amyloid-beta in culture. *J Alzheimers Dis.* 2004 Feb;6(1):27-30.

"Increased oxidative stress contributes to the decline in cognitive performance during normal aging and in neurodegenerative conditions such as Alzheimer's disease… the antioxidant potential of apple products can prevent Amyloid-beta-induced oxidative damage."

An apple a day… plus berries plus citrus plus… no animals or junk.

B Reed et al. Associations between serum cholesterol levels and cerebral amyloidosis. *JAMA Neurol.* 2014 Feb;71(2):195-200.

"Elevated cerebral Aβ [amyloid-beta] level was associated with cholesterol fractions in a pattern analogous to that found in coronary artery disease."

The same cholesterol that causes heart "disease" helps cause Alzheimer's "disease".

"Animal calories" ~ Brown fat or brown adipose tissue

M Saito, T Yoneshiro. Capsinoids and related food ingredients activating brown fat thermogenesis and reducing body fat in humans. *Curr Opin Lipidol.* 2013 Feb;24(1):71-7.

"As human BAT [brown adipose tissue] may be inducible, a prolonged ingestion of capsinoids would recruit active BAT and thereby increase energy expenditure and decrease body fat. In addition to capsinoids, there are numerous food ingredients that are expected to activate BAT and so be useful for the prevention of obesity in daily life." And they're all in plants. Capsaicin is the hot stuff in chilies.

Animal carbohydrates (lactose and galactose)

A. Stang et al. Adolescent milk fat and galactose consumption and testicular germ cell cancer. *Cancer Epidemiol. Biomarkers Prev.*, 15(11):2189-2195, 2006.

"Recent case-control studies suggested that dairy product consumption is an important risk factor for testicular cancer… Our results suggest that milk fat and/or galactose may explain the association between milk and dairy product consumption and seminomatous testicular cancer."

Got milk? Got ball cancer.

Animal fats (Saturated fats and trans fats)

D Estadella et al. Lipotoxicity: effects of dietary saturated and transfatty acids. *Mediators Inflamm.* 2013;2013:137579.

"The ingestion of excessive amounts of saturated fatty acids (SFAs) and transfatty acids (TFAs) is considered to be a risk factor for cardiovascular diseases, insulin resistance, dyslipidemia, and obesity... The saturated and transfatty acids favor a proinflammatory state leading to insulin resistance. These fatty acids can be involved in several inflammatory pathways, contributing to disease progression in chronic inflammation, autoimmunity, allergy, cancer, atherosclerosis, hypertension, and heart hypertrophy as well as other metabolic and degenerative diseases."

Animals and junk aren't food.

Animal proteins

MF McCarty. Vegan proteins may reduce risk of cancer, obesity, and cardiovascular disease by promoting increased glucagon activity. *Med Hypotheses.* 1999 Dec;53(6):459-85.

"An unnecessarily high intake of essential amino acids – either in the absolute sense or relative to total dietary protein – may prove to be as grave a risk factor for 'Western' degenerative diseases as is excessive fat intake."

The right question to ask about protein isn't "Where do we get it?"

It's "How do we not get too much of it?" or "How do we avoid animal proteins?" Plant proteins are superior.

Arachidonic acid

G Esposito et al. Imaging neuroinflammation in Alzheimer's disease with radiolabeled arachidonic acid and PET. *J Nucl Med.* 2008 Sep;49(9):1414-21.

"Incorporation coefficients (K*) of arachidonic acid (AA) in the brain are increased in a rat model of neuroinflammation, as are other markers of AA metabolism. Data also indicate that neuroinflammation contributes to Alzheimer's disease (AD)…. K* for AA is widely elevated in the AD brain…"

AA could stand for "animals alone" instead of arachidonic acid.

Biogenic amines

A. J. Vargas et al. Dietary polyamine intake and risk of colorectal adenomatous polyps. *Am. J. Clin. Nutr.* 2012 96(1):133–141.

"Putrescine, spermidine, and spermine are the polyamines required for human cell growth... This study showed a role for dietary polyamines in colorectal adenoma risk."

Carcinogenic polyamines, or biogenic amines form in the dead flesh we eat.

Bones

Peonim V, Udnoon J. Left subclavian arterioesophageal fistula induced by chicken bone with upper gastrointestinal hemorrhage and unexpected death: report of a case. *J Med Assoc Thai.* 2010 Nov;93(11):1332-5.

"Postmortem examination revealed a chicken bone embedded in middle part of esophagus with fistula between the esophagus and the left subclavian artery."

The fibrous skeleton of plants doesn't kill us.

Calcium

Heaney RP, Weaver CM. Calcium absorption from kale. *Am J Clin Nutr.* 1990 Apr;51(4):656-7.

"Absorption of calcium from intrinsically labeled kale was measured in 11 normal women and compared in these same subjects with absorption of calcium from labeled milk. The average test load was 300 mg. Fractional calcium absorption from kale averaged 0.409... and from milk, 0.321... In contrast with the poor absorption previously reported for spinach calcium, kale, a low-oxalate vegetable, exhibits excellent absorbability for its calcium."

Calcium is better absorbed from low-oxalate plants, plus there's no pus, shit, estrogens, cholesterol, lactose, galactose, saturated butterfat, casein, casomorphins, bacteria, antibiotics or pesticides in organic kale.

Carnitine

RA Koeth et al. Intestinal microbiota metabolism of l-carnitine, a nutrient in red meat, promotes atherosclerosis. *Nat Med.* 2013 Apr 7.

"Intestinal microbiota metabolism of choline/phosphatidylcholine produces trimethylamine (TMA), which is further metabolized to a proatherogenic species, trimethylamine-N-oxide (TMAO). Herein we demonstrate that intestinal microbiota metabolism of dietary L-carnitine, a trimethylamine abundant in red meat, also produces TMAO and accelerates atherosclerosis… Intestinal microbiota may thus participate in the well-established link between increased red meat consumption and CVD risk."

Note: There isn't just a postulated link between Meating and cardiovascular "disease" – there's a "well-established link." Everyone in nutrition seems to understand this except the Low-Carb Bullshit Artists, who'd like us to carry on eating the choline in eggs, poultry, dairy and fishes, and the carnitine in red flesh.

Casein

Karina Arnberg et al. Skim Milk, Whey, and Casein Increase Body Weight and Whey and Casein Increase the Plasma C-Peptide Concentration in Overweight Adolescents.

"Outcomes were BMI-for-age Z-scores (BAZs), waist circumference, plasma insulin, homeostatic model assessment, and plasma C-peptide… high intakes of skim milk, whey, and casein increase BAZs in overweight adolescents and that whey and casein increase insulin secretion."

Milk is food for baby cows, not baby humans. Not adult humans either.

Casomorphin

Z Sun et al. Relation of beta-casomorphin to apnea in sudden infant death syndrome. *Peptides*. 2003 Jun;24(6):937-43.

"Beta-CM is an exogenous bioactive peptide derived from casein, a major protein in milk and milk products, which has opioid activity. Mechanistically, circulation of this peptide into the infant's immature central nervous system might inhibit the respiratory center in the brainstem leading to apnea and death."

Cows' milk causes crib death, a.k.a. SIDS (sudden infant death syndrome). Cows' milk kills human babies.

Ceramide

AB Awad, SL Barta, CS Fink, PG Bradford. Beta-Sitosterol enhances tamoxifen effectiveness on breast cancer cells by affecting ceramide metabolism. *Mol Nutr Food Res*. 2008 52(4):419–426.

"The objective of this study was to investigate the effects of the dietary phytosterol beta-sitosterol (SIT) and the antiestrogen drug tamoxifen (TAM) on cell growth and ceramide (CER) metabolism in… human breast cancer cells."

Drugs and phytonutrients both combat ceramide, a metabolite of saturated fats found in animals and junk.

Cholesterol

Low-Carb Bullshit Artists love to bang on about how cholesterol doesn't cause heart "disease". Okay then, let's take a look instead at cholesterol's role in causing cancer, followed by some examples of phytonutrients that help prevent cancer.

C Danilo, PG Frank. Cholesterol and breast cancer development. *Current Opinion in Pharmacology*. 2012 12(6):677–682.

"Breast cancer is the most commonly occurring type of cancer in the world… laboratory studies… indicate that cholesterol is capable of regulating proliferation, migration, and signaling pathways in breast cancer… The recognition of cholesterol as a factor contributing to breast cancer development identifies cholesterol and its metabolism as novel targets for cancer therapy." Or novel targets for Planting.

BJ Grattan Jr. Plant sterols as anticancer nutrients: Evidence for their role in breast cancer. *Nutrients*. 2013 5(2):359 – 387.

"… specific food components have been identified which are uniquely beneficial in mitigating the risk of specific cancer subtypes. Plant sterols are well known for their effects on blood cholesterol levels… the cholesterol modulating actions of plant sterols may overlap with their anti-cancer actions."

What Meating breaks, Planting fixes.

AS Vadodkar, S Suman, R Lakshmanaswamy, C Damodaran. Chemoprevention of breast cancer by dietary compounds. *Anticancer Agents Med Chem*. 2012 12(10):1185 – 1202.

"… daily consumption of dietary phytochemicals reduces the risk of several cancers."

There are zero studies showing that eating animals helps prevent cancer. Natural Products – "novel potent molecules as anticancer agents" – are found only in plants (24 of which we met on page 620). Are the Low-Carb Bullshit Artists the ultimate misogynists, that they simply refuse to present this information that could save millions of women's lives each year?

Copper

G. J. Brewer. The risks of copper toxicity contributing to cognitive decline in the aging population and to Alzheimer's disease. *Journal of the American College of Nutrition*, 28(3):238, 2009.

"In this brief review I advance the hypothesis that copper toxicity is the major cause of the epidemic of mild cognitive impairment and Alzheimer's disease engulfing our aging population... The epidemic is associated with the use of copper plumbing, and the taking of copper in multi-mineral supplements. Food copper (organic copper) is processed by the liver and is transported and sequestered in a safe manner. Inorganic copper, such as that in drinking water and copper supplements, largely bypasses the liver and enters the free copper pool of the blood directly. This copper is potentially toxic because it may penetrate the blood/brain barrier."

The animals we eat are also often contaminated with inorganic copper from pesticides, particularly in the USA, which is lax about testing for pesticide residues. (Why? Because the USDA and FDA et al cater to corporate interests, not the well-being of the public they're supposed to serve.)

Creatine

Benton D, Donohoe R. The influence of creatine supplementation on the cognitive functioning of vegetarians and omnivores. *Br J Nutr.* 2011 Apr;105(7):1100-5.

"...in vegetarians rather than in those who consume meat, creatine supplementation resulted in better memory."

Planters and Meaters started out with the same memory abilities. Planters' memories improved when they took a creatine supplement; Meaters' didn't. So should Planters take supplements? Probably not, because of contamination with other unhealthy stuff.

Creatinine

Holland RD, Gehring T, Taylor J, Lake BG, Gooderham NJ, Turesky RJ. Formation of a mutagenic heterocyclic aromatic amine from creatinine in urine of meat eaters and vegetarians. *Chem. Res. Toxicol.* 2005 18(3):579–590.

"Creatinine and 2-aminobenzaldehyde are likely precursors of IQ[4,5-b]. The detection of IQ[4,5-b] in the urine of both meat eaters and vegetarians suggests that this HAA may be present in nonmeat staples or that IQ[4,5-b] formation may occur endogenously within the urinary bladder or other biological fluids."

Or it may be because vegetarians eat things that vegans don't, such as eggs, dairy and fishes, all of which can contain heterocyclic amines. (Why do researchers waste their time and energy on studying vegetarians?)

Diabetogens

PT Fujiyoshi, JE Michalek, F Matsumura. Molecular epidemiologic evidence for diabetogenic effects of dioxin exposure in U.S. Air force veterans of the Vietnam war. *Environ Health Perspect.* 2006 114(11):1677–1683.

Fujiyoshi et al found "a diabetogenic shift occurred in the biochemistry of adipose tissues from Vietnam veterans who were exposed to dioxin-containing Agent Orange herbicide preparations."

Thank you, Monsanto, for making diabolical chemicals and giving diabetes to Vietnam veterans and multitudes of others.

(Also in Monsanto's arsenal along with Agent Orange, Roundup and GM organisms are these devilish products - saccharin (beginning in1901), PCBs and bovine growth hormone. Maria Rodale writes in her excellent-for-a-doesn't-quite-get-it-Meater *Organic Manifesto*: "Every single one of the company's lines of business have wrought disaster, and yet it still survives and thrives."

And how bad must Monsanto's GM shit be if, as Rodale tells us, their CEO Hugh Grant told an interviewer in 2008 that he ate only organic food?)

Diacyl-glycerol

E W Kraegen, G J Cooney. Free fatty acids and skeletal muscle insulin resistance. *Curr Opin Lipidol.* 2008 Jun;19(3):235-41.

"Muscle lipid metabolites such as long chain fatty acid coenzyme As, diacylglycerol and ceramides may impair insulin signaling directly."

Saturated fats from animals and junk help cause diabetes.

Empty calories

Empty calories come from junk (and animals too.) The opposite concept is 'nutrient density.' Plants are high in nutrients, low in energy.

Sarter B, Campbell TC, Fuhrman J. Effect of a high nutrient density diet on long-term weight loss: a retrospective chart review. *Altern Ther Health Med.* 2008 May-Jun;14(3):48-53.

"An HND [high nutrient density, i.e. high-plant] diet... may be the most health-favorable and effective way to lose weight... Of the 19 patients who returned after 2 years, the mean weight loss was 53 lbs... , mean cholesterol fell by 13 points, LDL by 15 points, triglycerides by 17 points, and cardiac risk ratio dropped from 4.5 to 3.8. Changes in systolic and diastolic blood pressure were highly significant..."

We can choose how we lose weight: healthily with plants or unhealthily with lots of animals.

Endotoxins

Erridge C, Attina T, Spickett CM, Webb DJ. A high-fat meal induces low-grade endotoxemia: evidence of a novel mechanism of postprandial inflammation. *Am J Clin Nutr.* 2007 Nov; 86(5):1286-92.

"Bacterial endotoxin [lipopolysaccharide (LPS)], [is] a potently inflammatory bacterial antigen that is present in large quantities in the human gut... [There is]... increased circulating plasma endotoxin after a high-fat meal in healthy subjects. Increased postprandial LPS may contribute to the development of the postprandial inflammatory state, endothelial cell activation, and early events of atherosclerosis."

Dead bacteria or bacterial metabolites in the animals we eat cause after-meal inflammation and arterial "disease".

Endocrine disruptors (EDs)

Environmental hormone-disrupting chemicals enter our bodies mainly when we put the environment inside us: when we eat animals.

A. Bergman et al. The impact of endocrine disruption: A consensus statement on the state of the science. *Environ. Health Perspect.* 2013 121(4):A104-6.

"Many endocrine-related diseases and disorders are on the rise." The authors list

- low semen quality
- The incidence of genital malformations, such as non-descending testes (cryptorchidisms) and penile malformations (hypospadias), in baby boys
- The incidence of adverse pregnancy outcomes, such as preterm birth and low birth weight
- Neurobehavioral disorders associated with thyroid disruption

- [Increasing rates of] endocrine-related cancers (breast, endometrial, ovarian, prostate, testicular and thyroid)
- Earlier onset of breast development in young girls… a risk factor for breast cancer.
- [Dramatically increased] prevalence of obesity and type 2 diabetes… over the last 40 years.

Endocrine disruption's contribution to these disorders is a direct result of Meating.

Animal Estrogens

A Abrahamsson, V Morad, N M Saarinen, C Dabrosin. Estradiol, tamoxifen, and flaxseed alter IL-1β and IL-1Ra levels in normal human breast tissue in vivo. *J Clin Endocrinol Metab.* 2012 Nov;97(11):E2044-54.

"Sex steroid exposure increases the risk of breast cancer by unclear mechanisms. Diet modifications may be one breast cancer prevention strategy… The objective of this study was to elucidate whether estrogen, tamoxifen, and/or diet modification altered IL-1 levels in normal human breast tissue."

What did they find? Estrogens from animals cause breast cancer. Flax seeds (containing phyto-, or xenoestrogens) help combat breast cancer. As usual, Planting fixes what Meating causes.

Feces/Manure/Shit

J. L. W. Rademaker, M. M. M. Vissers, and M. C. T. Giffel. Effective heat inactivation of mycobacterium avium subsp. paratuberculosis in raw milk contaminated with naturally infected feces. *Appl. Environ. Microbiol.*, 73(13):4185-4190, 2007.

"High concentrations of feces from cows with clinical symptoms of Johne's disease were used to contaminate raw milk in order to realistically mimic possible incidents most closely."

You can't make this stuff up. Just so you're not missing the point here: to represent reality, these researchers took shit from sick cows and added it to milk.

Fish oil

There's evidence pro and con fish oil's role in the prevention of heart "disease" and cancer, largely on the basis of the long chain fatty acids DHA and EPA, with the most recent studies showing negative results. But what else is in fishes besides their fatty acids? Not anything good. Meaters say we should eat fishes for omega 3s is a bit like me saying Stalin was alright because he had a terrific moustache.

J M Ritchie et al. Organochlorines and risk of prostate cancer. J *Occup Environ Med.* 2003 Jul;45(7):692-702.

"...organochlorines... oxychlordane and PCB 180 were associated with an increased risk of prostate cancer."

That's the kind of stuff that's in fishes and the oils pressed from their dead bodies.

Free fatty acids

M Roden et al. Mechanism of free fatty acid-induced insulin resistance in humans. *J Clin Invest.* Jun 15, 1996; 97(12): 2859–2865.

Roden et al found that "that free fatty acids induce insulin resistance in humans by initial inhibition of glucose transport/phosphorylation which is then followed by an ~50% reduction in both the rate of muscle glycogen synthesis and glucose oxidation." Free fatty acids are a Meater issue.

Galactose

L A Batey et al. Skeletal health in adult patients with classic galactosemia. *Osteoporos Int.* 2013 Feb;24(2):501-9.

"Bone density in adults with galactosemia is low, indicating the potential for increased fracture risk."

If people with a genetic predisposition to high blood levels of this milk sugar have more osteoporosis, why would people who add dietary galactose also not be more osteoporotic? In fact, as we'll see under Osteoporosis later, milk drinkers are more prone to having brittle bones.

Gluten ~ Gliadin ~ Wheat protein

G De Palma et al. Effects of a gluten-free diet on gut microbiota and immune function in healthy adult human subjects. *Br J Nutr.* 2009 Oct;102(8):1154-60.

"... the GFD [gluten-free diet] led to reductions in beneficial gut bacteria populations and the ability of faecal samples to stimulate the host's immunity."

The tiny minority of people with celiac disease should avoid gluten because their lives depend on it. However, people without celiac disease are damaging their health by not eating gluten. As go our gut flora, so go we.

Harmane

E D Louis et al. Blood harmane, blood lead, and severity of hand tremor: Evidence of additive effects. *Neurotoxicology* 2011 32(2):227 – 232.

"Blood harmane and lead concentrations separately correlated with total tremor scores. Participants with high blood concentrations of both toxicants had the highest tremor scores, suggesting an additive effect of these toxicants on tremor severity."

That's why Essential Tremor is essentially a Meater condition: "Harmane (1-methyl-9H-pyrido[3,4-β]indole) is a potent β-carboline alkaloid [found] esp. in animal protein," and lead bioaccumulates in the fat of animals.

Heme iron

J C Fernandez-Cao et al. Heme iron intake and risk of new-onset diabetes in a Mediterranean population at high risk of cardiovascular disease: an observational cohort analysis. *BMC Public Health.* 2013 Nov 4;13:1042.

"The evidence examining the association between heme iron intake and CVD risk is limited to a few studies which suggest overall that high intakes of heme iron are associated with increased CVD risk. However it is possible that this could be due to other components of meat (the main source of heme iron) associated with CVD risk, such as saturated fats or other dietary and lifestyle factors associated with meat intake."

Well, okay then. It *may not* be the heme iron in animals that causes cardiovascular "disease"; it may be something else in the animals. Or something else as well as heme iron. Does it matter? Next time you order a steak, try asking your waitron to "hold the iron and the saturated fats and the animal proteins," see where that gets you.

Geoffrey C. Kabat, Thomas E. Rohan. Does excess iron play a role in breast carcinogenesis? an unresolved hypothesis. *Cancer Causes & Control* December 2007, Volume 18, Issue 10, pp. 1047-1053.

"In addition to its independent role as a pro-oxidant, high levels of free iron may potentiate the effects of estradiol, ethanol, and ionizing radiation—three established risk factors for breast cancer… Iron overload favors the production of reactive oxygen species, lipid peroxidation, and DNA damage, and may contribute to breast carcinogenesis…"

Heterocyclic amines (PhIP, MeIQx, IQ and IQ4,5b)

AE Norrish et al. Heterocyclic amine content of cooked meat and risk of prostate cancer. *J Natl Cancer Inst.* 1999 Dec 1; 91(23):2038-44.

"Meat doneness was weakly and inconsistently associated with prostate cancer risk for individual types of meat, but increased risk was observed for well-done beefsteak (relative risk = 1.68…)"

High Fructose Corn Syrup (HFCS)

George A Bray, Samara Joy Nielsen, and Barry M Popkin. Consumption of high-fructose corn syrup in beverages may play a role in the epidemic of obesity. *Am J Clin Nutr* 2004;79:537–43.

"It is becoming increasingly clear that soft drink consumption may be an important contributor to the epidemic of obesity, in part through the larger portion sizes of these beverages and through the increased intake of fructose from HFCS and sucrose."

The combination of meat + sweet is what fattens, sickens and kills us.

Homocysteine

S Seshadri et al. Plasma homocysteine as a risk factor for dementia and Alzheimer's disease. *N Engl J Med.* 2002 Feb 14;346(7):476-83.

M Hoffman. Hypothesis: hyperhomocysteinemia is an indicator of oxidant stress. *Med Hypotheses.* 2011 Dec;77(6):1088-93.

A H Ford, O P Almeida. Effect of homocysteine lowering treatment on cognitive function: a systematic review and meta-analysis of randomized controlled trials. *J Alzheimers Dis.* 2012;29(1):133-49.

Three papers that show the harms of Meating and the benefits of Planting.

Hydrogen sulfide

E Magee. A nutritional component to inflammatory bowel disease: the contribution of meat to fecal sulfide excretion. *Nutrition.* 1999 Mar;15(3):244-6.

"Dietary protein from meat is an important substrate for sulfide generation by bacteria in the human large intestine."

Animal protein is the very stuff meat is made from… and it's poisonous, because our gut flora turn it into a carcinogen. After millions of years of coexisting with us, our intestinal bacteria still don't like eating animals.

IGF-1 (Insulin-like growth factor-1)

M F McCarty. A low-fat, whole-food vegan diet, as well as other strategies that down-regulate IGF-1 activity, may slow the human aging process. *Med Hypotheses*. 2003 Jun;60(6):784-92.

"If down-regulation of IGF-I activity could indeed slow aging in humans, a range of practical measures for achieving this may be at hand. These include a low-fat, whole-food, vegan diet, exercise training, soluble fiber, insulin sensitizers, appetite suppressants, and agents such as flax lignans, oral estrogen, or tamoxifen that decrease hepatic synthesis of IGF-I. Many of these measures would also be expected to decrease risk for common age-related diseases."

Say no to the drugs and yes to the food. Animal proteins stimulate IGF-1 production and rapid cell division, leading to more cancer and faster aging.

Junk

R Moodie, D Stuckler, C Monteiro, N Sheron, B Neal, T Thamarangsi, P Lincoln, S Casswell, Lancet NCD Action Group. Profits and pandemics: prevention of harmful effects of tobacco, alcohol, and ultra-processed food and drink industries. *Lancet*. 2013 Feb 23;381(9867):670-9.

This is an extraordinary paper. Junk like salt and industrial sugar (sucrose) and corn syrup are three of the foremost (non-animal) killers in the industrial "food" supply.

"The 2011 UN high-level meeting on non-communicable diseases (NCDs) called for multisectoral action including with the private sector and industry. However, through the sale and promotion of tobacco, alcohol, and ultra-processed food and drink (unhealthy commodities), **transnational corporations are major drivers of global epidemics of NCDs**. What role then should these industries have in NCD prevention and control? We emphasise the rise in sales of these unhealthy commodities in low-income and middle-income countries, and consider the **common strategies that the transnational corporations use to undermine NCD prevention and control**. We assess the effectiveness of self-regulation, public–private partnerships, and public regulation models of interaction with these industries and conclude that **unhealthy commodity industries should**

have no role in the formation of national or international NCD policy. Despite the common reliance on industry self-regulation and public–private partnerships, there is no evidence of their effectiveness or safety. Public regulation and market intervention are the only evidence-based mechanisms to prevent harm caused by the unhealthy commodity industries." [Emphases added]

And get this – we don't often hear such courageous speaking of truth to power:

"**In industrial epidemics, the vectors of spread are not biological agents, but transnational corporations**. Unlike infectious disease epidemics, however, these **corporate disease vectors implement sophisticated campaigns to undermine public health interventions**. To minimise the harmful effects of unhealthy commodity industries on NCD prevention, we call for a substantially scaled up response from governments, public health organisations, and civil society to regulate the harmful activities of these industries."

Big "Food" and Big Chemical are lying us to death today just the way Big Smoke did for decades, and they're being abetted by their cronies in governmental, pharmaceutical and medical circles.

Lactose

PCRM. Understanding Lactose Intolerance.
www.pcrm.org/sites/default/files/pdfs/health/faq_lactintol.pdf

"Approximately 70 percent of African Americans, 90 percent of Asian Americans, 53 percent of Hispanic Americans, and 74 percent of Native Americans were lactose intolerant."

75% of the world's population cannot tolerate lactose. Consuming it leads to flatulence, constipation or diarrhea, at least.

LDL cholesterol

Spence JD. Fasting lipids: the carrot in the snowman. *Can J Cardiol.* 2003 Jul;19(8):890-2.

"Dietary cholesterol (one egg yolk), though it increases fasting low density lipoproteins by only about 10%, increases oxidized low-density lipoproteins by 34%... The current paradigm for the management of lipids is focused almost entirely on fasting lipid levels. However, most of the day is spent not in a fasting state, but in a postprandial [post-eating] state. Meals high in animal fat impair endothelial function for 4 hours… It is time to stop focusing only on fasting lipid levels and to begin paying more attention to outcomes."

How true. Measuring our cholesterol levels after a night's sleep, when most of the stuff has cleared our systems, gives artificially low readings. It's as if our water meter doesn't measure the amount we use after dark. Someone who thinks they're in the safe zone because their fasting LDL levels are "only" 100 may have real LDL levels much higher than that.

Methionine

B. C. Halpern, B. R. Clark, D. N. Hardy, R. M. Halpern, R. A. Smith. The effect of replacement of methionine by homocystine on survival of malignant and normal adult mammalian cells in culture. *Proc. Natl. Acad. Sci. USA* 1974 71(4):1133 - 1136.

In several cancers there is an "apparent absolute dependence of the malignant cells on preformed methionine," an amino acid found mainly in animals. "Absolute methionine dependence" is yet another good reason to be a pure Planter. We've known this for more than forty years.

Neu5Gc

Padler-Karavani V, Yu H, Cao H, Chokhawala H, Karp F, Varki N, Chen X, Varki A. Diversity in specificity, abundance, and composition of anti-Neu5Gc antibodies in normal humans: potential implications for disease. *Glycobiology*. 2008 Oct;18(10):818-30.

"As dietary Neu5Gc is primarily found in red meat and milk products, we suggest that this ongoing antigen-antibody reaction may generate chronic inflammation, possibly contributing to the high frequency of diet-related carcinomas and other diseases in humans."

This single animal component, which always causes a reaction from our immune system, is enough to disqualify animals as food.

Nitrites

Huncharek M, Kupelnick B. A meta-analysis of maternal cured meat consumption during pregnancy and the risk of childhood brain tumors. *Neuroepidemiology*. 2004 Jan-Apr;23(1-2):78-84.

"The data provide support for the suspected causal association between ingestion of NOCs [N-Nitroso compounds] from cured meats during pregnancy and subsequent CBT [childhood brain tumors] in offspring."

That's a long-winded, sciency way of saying that Meater mothers can give their babies cancer of the brain because of the nitrites in animals.

Nitrosamines and Nitrosamides/N-nitroso-compounds (NOCs)
N Ramirez, M Z Ozel, A C Lewis, R M Marce, F Borrull, J F Hamilton. Exposure to nitrosamines in third-hand tobacco smoke increases cancer risk in non-smokers. *Environ Int.* 2014 Oct;71:139-47.

"In addition to passive inhalation, non-smokers, and especially children, are exposed to residual tobacco smoke gases and particles that are deposited to surfaces and dust, known as third-hand smoke (THS)… The maximum risk from exposure to all nitrosamines measured in a smoker occupied home was one excess cancer case per one thousand population exposed. The results presented here highlight the potentially severe long-term consequences of THS exposure, particularly to children…"

If this is what nitrosamines do, why would we feed our kids hot dogs?

According to press release no. 240 of the WHO's International Agency for Research into Cancer on 26 October 2015, "Processed meat was classified as carcinogenic to humans (Group 1), based on sufficient evidence in humans that the consumption of processed meat causes colorectal cancer."

Cigarettes and animals are carcinogens. I'll say it again: Meating = Smoking.

PhIP
C. Wilson, A. Aboyade-Cole, O. Newell, E. Darling-Reed, E. Oriaku, R. Thomas. Diallyl sulfide inhibits PhIP-induced DNA strand breaks in normal human breast epithelial cells. *Oncology Reports* 2007 17(NA):807-811.

"Heterocyclic amines (HCAs) are formed when meat products such as beef, chicken, pork and fish are cooked at high temperatures. The most abundant HCA found in the human diet is 2-amino-1-methyl-6-phenylimidazo[4,5-b] pyridine (PhIP). PhIP… is associated with an increased risk of developing colon, breast, and prostate cancer … DAS inhibits PhIP-induced DNA strand breaks by inhibiting the production of reactive oxygen species. Therefore, we propose that DAS can prevent PhIP-induced breast cancer."

The PhIP in cooked flesh damages our DNA. Garlic prevents it. If we'd prefer not to have breast cancer, we should eat no animals and plenty of veggies, particularly alliums such as garlic, leeks and onions.

Phthalates

Meeker JD, Calafat AM, Hauser R. Urinary metabolites of di(2-ethylhexyl) phthalate are associated with decreased steroid hormone levels in adult men. *J Androl.* 2009 May-Jun;30(3):287-97.

"…urinary metabolites of DEHP [di(2-ethylhexyl) phthalate] are inversely associated with circulating steroid hormone levels in adult men."

Phthalates bioaccumulate in animals, and they're part of the reason why Meater men have lower testosterone levels than Planters. Phthalates can also lead to the feminization of male genitalia, or the 'undervirilization' of Meater males.

Phosphorus

R. A. Sherman, O. Mehta. Dietary phosphorus restriction in dialysis patients: Potential impact of processed meat, poultry, and fish products as protein sources. *Am. J. Kidney Dis.* 2009 54(1):18 - 23.

"Dietary intake of phosphorus is derived largely from protein [i.e. animal] sources and is a critical determinant of phosphorus balance in patients with chronic kidney disease."

R. A. Sherman, O. Mehta. Phosphorus and potassium content of enhanced meat and poultry products: Implications for patients who receive dialysis. *Clin J Am Soc Nephrol* 2009 4(8):1370 - 1373.

"The impact of addition of phosphorus to EMPP [enhanced meat and poultry products] is likely to be clinically significant, especially so in view of the probability that phosphorus in food additives is much better absorbed than phosphorus that is contained in unprocessed foods."

For healthy kidneys, we shouldn't eat animals. And then, if our kidneys are shot because we ate animals, we definitely shouldn't eat any more animals.

Polycyclic aromatic hydrocarbons (PAHs)

Chen JW, Wang SL, Hsieh DP, Yang HH, Lee HL. Carcinogenic potencies of polycyclic aromatic hydrocarbons for back-door neighbors of restaurants with cooking emissions. Sci Total Environ. 2012 Feb 15;417-418:68-75.

"In the present study, 21 polycyclic aromatic hydrocarbon (PAH) congeners were measured in the exhaust stack of 3 types of restaurants: 9 Chinese, 7 Western, and 4 barbeque (BBQ)…The total benzo[a]pyrene… concentrations… were highest in Chinese restaurants…, followed by Western... and BBQ-type restaurants... We further developed a probabilistic risk model to assess the incremental lifetime cancer risk (ILCR) for people exposed to carcinogenic PAHs."

Just living down-wind from Meaters can kill us.

Purines

Y Zhang, C Chen, H Choi, C Chaisson, D Hunter, J Niu, T Neogi. Purine-rich foods intake and recurrent gout attacks. *Ann Rheum Dis* 2012 71(9):1448 – 1453.

"The study findings suggest that acute purine intake increases the risk of recurrent gout attacks by almost fivefold among gout patients. Avoiding or reducing amount of purine-rich foods intake, especially of animal origin, may help reduce the risk of gout attacks."

High-fructose corn syrup also causes gout. Cherries fix it.

Pus

P. C. B. Vianna, G. Mazal, M. V. Santos, H. M. A. Bolini, and M. L. Gigante. Microbial and sensory changes throughout the ripening of prato cheese made from milk with different levels of somatic cells. *J. Dairy Sci.*, 91(5):1743-1750, 2008.

"The lower overall acceptance of the cheeses from high-SCC [somatic cell count; pus] milk may be associated with texture and flavor defect…"

Strange, that: people found that low-pus cheese tastes better.

Salt/sodium

He FJ, MacGregor GA. Effect of modest salt reduction on blood pressure: a meta-analysis of randomized trials. Implications for public health. *J Hum Hypertens*. 2002; 16:761–770.

"This meta-analysis strongly supports other evidence for a modest and long-term reduction in population salt intake, and would be predicted to reduce stroke deaths immediately by approximately 14% and coronary deaths by approximately 9% in hypertensives, and reduce stroke and coronary deaths by approximately 6 and approximately 4%, in normotensives, respectively."

The manufacturers of a drug this effective would own the world.

Steroids ~ sex hormones

L Aksglaede et al. The sensitivity of the child to sex steroids: possible impact of exogenous estrogens. *Hum Reprod Update.* 2006 Jul-Aug;12(4):341-9.

"Disrupted sex hormone action is… believed to be involved in the increased occurrence of genital abnormalities among newborn boys and precocious puberty in girls… Because no lower threshold for estrogenic action has been established, caution should be taken to avoid unnecessary exposure of fetuses and children to exogenous sex steroids and endocrine disruptors, even at very low levels."

In other words, pregnant mothers and their children shouldn't eat any animals at all.

TMA and TMAO

WHW Tang et al. Intestinal Microbial Metabolism of Phosphatidylcholine and Cardiovascular Risk. *N Engl J Med* 2013; 368:1575-1584.

"The production of TMAO from dietary phosphatidylcholine is dependent on metabolism by the intestinal microbiota. Increased TMAO levels are associated with an increased risk of incident major adverse cardiovascular events."

If we like eating eggs, we better enjoy them a whole lot because the choline in them increases our risk of heart attack, stroke and death.

The un-credible, indelible chemical egg.

Sidebar: Bacon and eggs - Eggs Bernays?

Edward Bernays, nephew of Sigmund Freud, the "Father of public relations" and author of *Propaganda* and *Crystallizing Public Opinion*, invented the dish we know as "bacon and eggs" in the 1920s to boost sales of bacon for the Beech-Nut Packing Company. Bernays co-opted "White Coat" "third party authorities" to say that "a heavy breakfast was sounder from the standpoint of health." (He tells the story, with no small self-satisfaction, at https://www.youtube.com/watch?v=KLudEZpMjKU.)

Ad slogans such as "4500 physicians urge bigger breakfast" [including bacon and eggs] sound eerily like the "More doctors smoke Camels than any other cigarette" jingle that would later help maim and kill millions more through lung cancer.

Apparently the devil takes care of his own. This highly influential, repugnant human being died in 1995, aged 103.

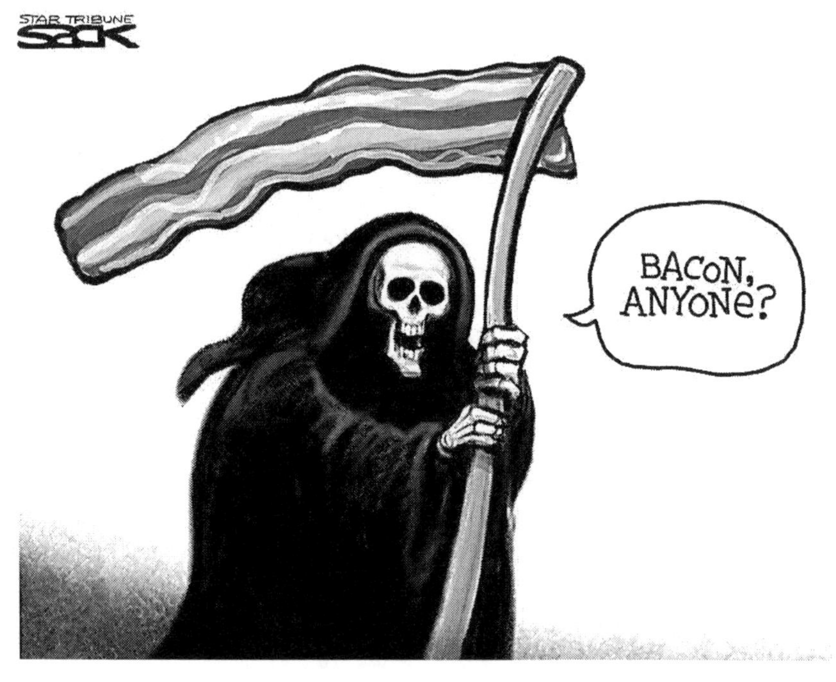

Cartoon, "Processed meat," thanks to Steve Sack, Star Tribune, 27 October 2015, following the WHO's announcement on the previous day that bacon and other processed meats are Group 1 carcinogens.

References to papers on "diseases" Meating causes

Acne

Loren Cordain, PhD; Staffan Lindeberg, MD, PhD, Magdalena Hurtado, PhD, Kim Hill, PhD, S. Boyd Eaton, MD and Jennie Brand-Miller, PhD. Acne Vulgaris: A Disease of Western Civilization. *Arch Dermatol* 2002,138:1584-1590.

"It is possible that low-glycemic diets may have therapeutic potential in reducing the symptoms of acne, a disease virtually unknown to the Aché and Kitavans."

Acne barely exists amongst people who don't eat lots of animals and junk… trust paleofantasist Cordain to emphasize the latter.

B Melnik. Milk consumption: Aggravating factor of acne and promoter of chronic diseases of western societies. *J Dtsch Dermatol Ges*, 7(4):364-370, 2009.

If the reader remembers just one fact from this book, there are few better than this: Acne = heart "disease" = cancer = hypertension = diabetes. They're all manifestations of the same thing: Meating and Junking.

In this brilliant paper, Bodo Melnik writes: "Milk is a complex fluid that developed over the course of mammalian evolution. Its primary function is to support growth and cell proliferation… Consumption of cow's milk and cow's milk protein result in changes of the hormonal axis of insulin, growth hormone and insulin-like growth factor-1(IGF-1) in humans."

These are not good things, and food shouldn't do them unless we're infants drinking our mother's breast milk.

"The epidemic incidence of adolescent acne in Western milk-consuming societies can be explained by the increased insulin- and IGF-1-stimulation of sebaceous glands mediated by milk consumption. Acne can be regarded as a model for chronic Western diseases with pathologically increased IGF-1-stimulation," which is also one of the pathways of cancer formation. We do *not* need alien hormones sloshing around in us and bossing us around.

Aggression

B. A. Golomb, M. A. Evans, H. L. White, J. E. Dimsdale. Trans fat consumption and aggression. *PLoS ONE* 2012 7(3):e32175

"Dietary trans fatty acids (dTFA) are primarily synthetic compounds that have been introduced only recently… Greater dTFA were strongly significantly associated with greater aggression, with dTFA more consistently predictive than other assessed aggression [and irritability] predictors… If the association is causal, the findings provide one further potential explanation for the recognized association between hostile/aggressive behaviors and heart disease. Trans fats could serve as common cause for both outcomes."

Trans fats are found in animals and junk, not in whole plants. Meating and junking make us irritable and aggressive.

Aging

D Ornish, J Lin, J Daubenmier, G Weidner, E Epel, C Kemp, M J M Magbanua, R Marlin, L Yglecias, P R Carroll, E H Blackburn. Increased telomerase activity and comprehensive lifestyle changes: a pilot study. *Lancet Oncol.* 2008 Nov;9(11):1048-57.

Dean Ornish does it yet again: first Planting conquered heart "disease" (1990), then prostate cancer (2005) and now it slows down cellular aging (2008), by increasing the length of our telomeres, the caps of our chromosomes. And that's great because:

"Telomere shortness in humans is emerging as a prognostic marker of disease risk, progression, and premature mortality. The aspect of cellular ageing that is conferred by diminished telomere maintenance seems to be an important precursor to the development of many types of cancer. Shortened telomeres predict poor clinical outcomes, including increased risk of metastasis in patients with breast cancer, increased risk of bladder, head and neck, lung, and renal-cell cancers, worse progression and prognosis of patients with colorectal cancer, prostate-cancer recurrence in patients undergoing radical prostatectomy, and decreased survival in patients with coronary heart disease and infectious disease."

Alzheimer's "disease"

Neal D. Barnard et al. Dietary and lifestyle guidelines for the prevention of Alzheimer's disease. *Neurobiology of Aging* 35 (2014) S74-S78.

Seven guidelines for the prevention of Alzheimer's emerged from The International Conference on Nutrition and the Brain, Washington, DC, July 19-20, 2013. The first two are:

"1. Minimize your intake of saturated fats and trans fats. Saturated fat is found primarily in dairy products, meats, and certain oils (coconut and palm oils). Trans fats are found in many snack pastries and fried foods and are listed on labels as "partially hydrogenated oils.""

In other words, no Meating or Junking.

"2. Vegetables, legumes (beans, peas, and lentils), fruits, and whole grains should replace meats and dairy products as primary staples of the diet."

In other words, whole Planting.

I guess none of the blithering idiots at the 'Nutrition and the Brain' conference bought Dr. David Perlnutter's idiotic, best-selling *Grain Brain.*

Amputations and Gangrene

MG Crane & C Sample. Regression of Diabetic Neuropathy with Total Vegetarian (Vegan) Diet. *Journal of Nutritional Medicine* Volume 4, Issue 4, 1994, pages 431-439.

Let's talk about diabetic neuropathy, the destruction of our peripheral or distal nerves in our limbs, which is the main cause of amputations. The authors speak of "systemic distal polyneuropathy (SDPN)."

On a Total Vegetarian Diet (TVD) – a vegan diet high in fiber and low in fat - plus exercise:

"Complete relief of the SDPN pain occurred in 17 of the 21 patients in 4 to 16 days… Follow-up studies of 17 of the 21 patients for 1-4 years indicated that 71% had remained on the diet and exercise programme as advised in nearly every item. In all except one of the 17 patients, the relief from the SDPN had continued, or there was further improvement."

These patients' blood glucose was "under good control [from] about the 10th day." When the diabetes goes away, the nerve damage goes away, and so does the risk of amputations. Planting does it routinely.

Angina

Göran K. Hansson and Peter Libby. The immune response in atherosclerosis: a double-edged sword. *Nature Reviews Immunology* volume 6 July 2006; 508-519.

"Although thrombi [blood clots] cause most of the acute complications of atherosclerosis, the gradual formation of stenoses [narrowings] that impede blood flow causes many of the chronic symptoms of atherosclerotic disease, such as angina pectoris (chest discomfort precipitated typically by physical or emotional stress)."

The authors call angina a "reversible attack of chest discomfort." It's permanently reversible on a Planter diet.

Asthma

L G Wood et al. Manipulating antioxidant intake in asthma: A randomized controlled trial. *Am J Clin Nutr.* 2012 96(3):534-543.

"Modifying the dietary intake of carotenoids alters clinical asthma outcomes. Improvements were evident only after increased fruit and vegetable intake, which suggests that whole-food interventions are most effective."

Whole plants help asthma sufferers; not animals, not junk, not supplements.

Atherosclerosis

W. C. Roberts. The cause of atherosclerosis. *Nutr Clin Pract,* 23(5):464-467, 2008.

"In summary, the connection between cholesterol elevation and atherosclerotic plaques is clear and well established. Atherosclerosis is a cholesterol problem! If one has elevated cholesterol, has an elevated blood pressure, smokes cigarettes, or has an elevated blood sugar, these additional factors serve to amplify the cholesterol damage but they by themselves do not produce atherosclerotic plaques! Societies with a high frequency of systemic hypertension or a high frequency of cigarette smoking but low cholesterol levels rarely get atherosclerosis."

As Roberts writes elsewhere, "It's the cholesterol, stupid." [http://www.ncbi.nlm.nih.gov/pmc/articles/PMC3012294/]

"No one has produced atherosclerosis experimentally by increasing the arterial blood pressure or glucose levels or by blowing smoke in the faces of rabbits their entire lifetime or by stressing these animals. The only way to produce atherosclerosis experimentally is by feeding high-cholesterol and/or high-saturated-fat diets to herbivores."

Roberts has been Editor–in–Chief of *The American Journal of Cardiology* since 1982.

Birth defects

S. J. Genuis. Nowhere to hide: Chemical toxicants and the unborn child. *Reprod. Toxicol.*, 28(1):115-116, 2009.

"…maternal exposure to toxic chemical compounds may be associated with various congenital defects, pediatric problems, skewed gender ratios, lethal cancers in children and teens, psychosexual challenges, as well as reproductive and endocrine dysfunction in later life. Just as endogenous hormones such as insulin, testosterone or estrogen have physiological or developmental effects at parts per billion, toxicants can also exert bioactive influence at exceedingly low levels."

In particular, "Gestational consumption of contaminated seafood remains a potential source of toxicant exposure, including mercury, for the developing child."

Dioxins, PCBs, DDT, heavy metals… I've devoted an entire section of this book to showing that the chemicals that cause birth defects and developmental disorders enter our bodies almost entirely through the animals we eat, mostly the fishes.

And if anyone's going to continue with the nonsense that we need to eat fishes to 'get' omega-3 fatty acids, please consider this study:

AW Turunen et al. Dioxins, polychlorinated biphenyls, methyl mercury and omega-3 polyunsaturated fatty acids as biomarkers of fish consumption. *Eur J Clin Nutr*, 64(3):313-323, 2010.

A biomarker is something we can measure that gives us a good idea about something else, which we usually can't measure as easily. In this study, Turunen et al present us with different ways of telling how many fishes someone eats. Now, if we measure our blood levels of omega-3s, that should be a good biomarker of fish consumption, right? Fishes are touted as a good source of omega-3s. The only problem with this is that there are better biomarkers for fish consumption: the toxic chemicals fishes have bio-accumulated in their flesh which we then bio-accumulate when we predate upon them.

"According to multiple regression modeling and LMG metrics, the most important fish consumption biomarkers were **dioxins** and **PCBs** among the men and **MeHg** [methyl mercury] among the women… Environmental contaminants seemed to be slightly better fish consumption biomarkers than omega-3 PUFAs in the Baltic Sea area."

It's no use eating fishes – even wild fishes – for the supposed benefits of their fats when their fats are so contaminated with chemical pollutants which more than undo the purported benefits of eating omega-3s.

Fishes aren't food, not even if one of their ingredients is supposedly beneficial. "Food is a package deal" and lethal pollutants are now an unavoidable part of the fish package.

Perhaps when the people at the Mayo Clinic get around to reading the Turunen paper, they'll remove salmon from their list of Top 10 Healthy Foods - Why They Are Good For You (Mayo Clinic News 1 August 2006).

Of salmon they say: "This fish is an excellent source of omega-3 fatty acids, which are believed to provide heart benefits. Salmon is also low in saturated fat and cholesterol and is a good source of protein. If possible, choose wild salmon, which is less likely to contain unwanted chemicals such as mercury."

Pretty much utter bollocks – 20th Century nutrition thinking. There is no safe lower intake of saturated fats or cholesterol (or mercury – not for our kids' brains.)

We'd all be better off eating the remaining 9 real foods on the Mayo list, though why they say wheat bran and vegetable juice instead of whole grains and whole vegetables is beyond me: Apples, Almonds, Broccoli, Blueberries, Red beans, Spinach, Sweet potatoes, Vegetable juice, Wheat germ.

Body odor

J. Havlicek and P. Lenochova. The effect of meat consumption on body odor attractiveness. *Chem. Senses* 31(8):747-752, 2006.

"Results of repeated measures analysis of variance showed that the odor of donors when on the nonmeat diet was judged as significantly more attractive, more pleasant, and less intense. This suggests that red meat consumption has a negative impact on perceived body odor hedonicity."

Without knowing it, Meaters smell bad. (There's a metaphor in there.)

Breast cancer

BJ Grube et al. White button mushroom phytochemicals inhibit aromatase activity and breast cancer cell proliferation. *J Nutr.* 2001 Dec;131(12):3288-93.

"Estrogen is a major factor in the development of breast cancer… diets high in mushrooms may modulate the aromatase activity and function in chemoprevention in postmenopausal women by reducing the in situ production of estrogen."

S. Choudhary, S. Sood, R. L. Donnell, H.-C. R. Wang. Intervention of human breast cell carcinogenesis chronically induced by 2-amino-1-methyl-6-phenylimidazo[4,5-b]pyridine. *Carcinogenesis* 2012 33(4):876 - 885

"More than 85% of breast cancers are sporadic and attributable to long-term exposure to environmental carcinogens, such as those in the diet, through a multistep disease process progressing from non-cancerous to premalignant and malignant stages. The chemical carcinogen 2-amino-1-methyl-6-phenylimidazo[4,5-b]pyridine (PhIP) is one of the most abundant heterocyclic amines found in high-temperature cooked meats and is recognized as a mammary carcinogen."

PhIP provides just one of the many Meater mechanisms of breast cancer.

Breast cancer healed or prevented

BR Goldin et al. Estrogen excretion patterns and plasma levels in vegetarian and omnivorous women. *N Engl J Med.* 1982 Dec 16;307(25):1542-7.

"We conclude that vegetarian women have an increased fecal output, which leads to increased fecal excretion of estrogen and a decreased plasma concentration of estrogen."

Planter women get less breast cancer because we out-poop our Meater sisters.

Adams LS, Chen S. Phytochemicals for breast cancer prevention by targeting aromatase. *Front Biosci.* 2009 Jan 1;14:3846-63.

Adams et al "discuss whole food extracts and the common classes of phytochemicals which have been investigated for potential aromatase inhibitory activity."

The isoflavones in soy exert a phytoestrogenic effect that counters animal estrogens. This is one probable reason why Asian women were free of breast cancer until their recent nutrition transition to Meating and Junking.

Cancer

D. Boivin et al. Antiproliferative and antioxidant activities of common vegetables: A comparative study. *Food Chem.*, 112(2):374-380, 2009.

"These results thus indicate that vegetables have very different inhibitory activities towards cancer cells and that **the inclusion of cruciferous and Allium vegetables in the diet is essential for effective dietary-based chemopreventive strategies**."

In other words, the broccoli and onion-&-garlic families prevent cancer.

Also: "…individuals who eat five servings or more of fruits and vegetables daily have approximately half the risk of developing a wide variety of cancer types, particularly those of the gastrointestinal tract."

EK Silbergeld, K Nachman. The environmental and public health risks associated with arsenical use in animal feeds. *Ann. N.Y. Acad. Sci.*, 1140:346-357, 2008.

"Arsenic exposures are among the most important environmental health risks in many regions of the world. Arsenic is a human carcinogen, and is also associated with increased risks of several noncancer endpoints, including cardiovascular disease, diabetes, neuropathy, and neurocognitive deficits in children."

Chickens and eggs are most contaminated, and it's added on purpose. But that's not all that's in chickens…

ES Johnson et al. Mortality from malignant diseases-update of the Baltimore union poultry cohort. *Cancer Causes Control.* 2010 Feb;21(2):215-21.

We've met the sad Baltimore union poultry cohort before. Johnson et al told us that oncogenic viruses in chickens are mainly responsible for their extraordinarily high cancer rates. "Other potentially carcinogenic occupational exposures include exposure to fumes emitted from the wrapping machine, nitrosamines during the curing of poultry, and to smoke or aerosol emitted during smoking or cooking of poultry products that contain polycyclic aromatic hydrocarbons and heterocyclic amines."

Animals themselves are poisonous; they contain other poisons; and cooking them creates still others.

"Compared to the US general population, an excess of cancers of the buccal and nasal cavities and pharynx (base of the tongue, palate and other unspecified mouth, tonsil and oropharynx, nasal cavity/middle ear/accessory sinus), esophagus, recto-sigmoid/rectum/anus, liver and intrabiliary system, myelofibrosis, lymphoid leukemia and multiple myeloma was observed in particular subgroups or in the entire poultry cohort. We hypothesize that oncogenic viruses present in poultry, and exposure to fumes, are candidates for an etiologic role to explain the excess occurrence of at least some of these cancers in the poultry workers."

If we eat poultry, we can add penis cancer to the list.

Collins AR, Harrington V, Drew J, Melvin R. Nutritional modulation of DNA repair in a human intervention study. *Carcinogenesis*. 2003 Mar; 24(3):511-5.

"Kiwifruit provides a dual protection against oxidative DNA damage, enhancing antioxidant levels and stimulating DNA repair. It is probable that together these effects would decrease the risk of mutagenic changes leading to cancer."

Kiwifruits are not alone among plants that provide this dual protection against cancer.

S Rohrmann et al. Consumption of meat and dairy and lymphoma risk in the European Prospective Investigation into Cancer and Nutrition. *Int J Cancer*. 2011 Feb 1;128(3):623-34.

In the EPIC study, Rohrmann et al found "that men and women with a high consumption of processed meat are at increased risk of early death, in particular due to cardiovascular diseases but also to cancer. In this population, reduction of processed meat consumption to less than 20 g/day would prevent more than 3% of all deaths."

In the USA, that would translate into about 75,000 fewer deaths each year… just from cutting out deli meats.

Loh YH, Jakszyn P, Luben RN, Mulligan AA, Mitrou PN, Khaw KT. N-Nitroso compounds and cancer incidence: the European Prospective Investigation into Cancer and Nutrition (EPIC)-Norfolk Study. *Am J Clin Nutr*. 2011 May;93(5):1053-61. Epub 2011 Mar 23.

N-nitroso compounds, or nitrosamines, are carcinogens found in animals, particularly highly processed animals, and cigarette smoke.

"Dietary [nitrosamines (NDMA) [N-nitrosodimethylamine] was associated with a higher gastrointestinal cancer incidence, specifically of rectal cancer."

Got meat? Got smoking? Got cancer of the butt.

This is the third time I'm saying this: Meating = Smoking.

Cardiovascular "disease"

SK Park et al. Fruit, vegetable, and fish consumption and heart rate variability: The veterans administration normative aging study. *Am. J. Clin. Nutr.*, 89(3):778-786, 2009.

"Conclusion: These findings suggest that higher intake of green leafy vegetables may reduce the risk of cardiovascular disease through favorable changes in cardiac autonomic function."

In other words, green leafy vegetables help keep our hearts beating.

JD Spence, DJ Jenkins, J Davignon. Dietary cholesterol and egg yolks: not for patients at risk of vascular disease. *J. Can J Cardiol.* 2010 Nov;26(9):e336-9.

"Dietary cholesterol, including egg yolks, is harmful to the arteries. Patients at risk of cardiovascular disease should limit their intake of cholesterol. Stopping the consumption of egg yolks after a stroke or myocardial infarction would be like quitting smoking after a diagnosis of lung cancer: a necessary action, but late. The evidence presented in the current review suggests that the widespread perception among the public and health care professionals that dietary cholesterol is benign is misplaced, and that improved education is needed to correct this misconception."

So, who's at risk of vascular "disease", according to Spence et al? Everyone who's eating the Standard American Diet of animals and junk.

Cataracts

PN Appleby, NE Allen, TJ Key. Diet, vegetarianism, and cataract risk. *Am J Clin Nutr.* 2011 May;93(5):1128-35.

"Vegetarians were at lower risk of cataract than were meat eaters in this cohort of health-conscious British residents."

Now imagine if they'd studied Planters.

Colon cancer ~ Colorectal cancer

O'Keefe SJ, Kidd M, Espitalier-Noel G, Owira P. Rarity of colon cancer in Africans is associated with low animal product consumption, not fiber. *Am J Gastroenterol.* 1999 May;94(5):1373-80.

"The low prevalence of colon cancer in black Africans cannot be explained by dietary "protective" factors, such as fiber, calcium, vitamins A, C and folic acid, but may be influenced by the absence of "aggressive" factors, such as excess animal protein and fat, and by differences in colonic bacterial fermentation."

When it comes to healthy outcomes of eating, it's either the good effects of Planting or the absence of the bad effects of Meating and Junking. The "differences in colonic bacterial fermentation" between cancer-provoking animal-fed gut flora and cancer-preventing, fiber-fed gut flora are immense.

Constipation

G Iacono et al. Intolerance of cow's milk and chronic constipation in children. *N Engl J Med.* 1998 Oct 15;339(16):1100-4.

Iacono et al tell us that "the concomitant presence of other manifestations of intolerance of cow's milk (**bronchospasm**, **dermatitis**, and **rhinitis**) increases the probability that constipation will be found to be a symptom of intolerance of cow's milk… clinical examination of the children in our study showed a very high frequency of severe **anal fissures**. Because these lesions reappeared after the reintroduction of cow's milk and before the onset of constipation, we hypothesize that they are one of the mechanisms causing constipation. **Pain on defecation** can cause retention of feces in the rectum, with consequent dehydration and hardening of the stools, thus aggravating constipation."

Does this muck sound like food? "Forty-four of the 65 children (68 percent) had a response while receiving soy milk." In other words, they got better when they stopped drinking cows' milk and started drinking plant milk – no more problems with breathing, skin conditions, hay fever, constipation or anal fissures.

Sanjoaquin MA, Appleby PN, Spencer EA, Key TJ. Nutrition and lifestyle in relation to bowel movement frequency: a cross-sectional study of 20630 men and women in EPIC-Oxford. *Public Health Nutr.* 2004 Feb;7(1):77-83.

"In conclusion, we have identified several nutritional and lifestyle factors that were associated with the frequency of bowel movements. The strongest associations were seen with having a vegetarian or vegan diet, dietary fibre intake, fluid intake and vigorous exercise."

Planters poop more often (and more) and, as a result, get sick less often and live longer. It's as basic as that. We shouldn't need any more information when deciding on a dietstyle.

COPD (chronic obstructive pulmonary "disease")

E Keranis et al. Impact of dietary shift to higher-antioxidant foods in COPD: a randomised trial. *Eur Respir J.* 2010 Oct;36(4):774-80.

"…a dietary shift to higher-antioxidant food intake may be associated with improvement in lung function, and, in this respect, dietary interventions might be considered in COPD management."

Plants are antioxidants; animals are oxidants – animals make it hard for people with emphysema to breathe.

Crohn's "disease"

C L Roberts et al. Translocation of Crohn's disease *Escherichia coli* across M-cells: contrasting effects of soluble plant fibres and emulsifiers. *Gut.* 2010 Oct;59(10):1331-9.

"Crohn's disease is common in developed nations where the typical diet is low in fibre and high in processed food… Translocation of *E coli* across M-cells is reduced by soluble plant fibres, particularly plantain and broccoli, but increased by the emulsifier Polysorbate-80."

Whole plant fibers ameliorate Crohn's "disease". Emulsifiers (such as dishwashing liquids and P-80 in junk) make matters worse.

Depression

M Berk et al. So depression is an inflammatory disease, but where does the inflammation come from? *BMC Med.* 2013 Sep 12;11:200.

"A range of factors appear to increase the risk for the development of depression, and seem to be associated with systemic inflammation; these include psychosocial stressors, poor diet, physical inactivity, obesity, smoking, altered gut permeability, atopy [allergies], dental cares, sleep and vitamin D deficiency. Most [of these] sources of inflammation may play a role in other psychiatric disorders, such as bipolar disorder, schizophrenia, autism and post-traumatic stress disorder."

Besides 'psychosocial stressors' ("Stuff happens"), Meating makes most depression factors worse, while Planting improves them. For example:

M E Payne et al. Fruit, vegetable, and antioxidant intakes are lower in older adults with depression. *J Acad Nutr Diet.* 2012 Dec;112(12):2022-7.

"These associations may partially explain the elevated risk of cardiovascular disease among older individuals with depression. In addition, these findings point to the importance of antioxidant food sources [i.e. whole plants] rather than dietary supplements."

Type 1 Diabetes

G. Dahlquist. The aetiology of type 1 diabetes: An epidemiological perspective. *Acta Paediatr Suppl.* 1998 425:5-10.

"Risk factors that may initiate the autoimmune process include early exposure to cow's milk proteins, nitrosamines or early foetal events such as blood group incompatibility or foetal viral infections."

There are no casein, nitrosamines or viruses in plants.

Type 2 Diabetes

M. A. Hyman, D. Ornish, M. Roizen. Lifestyle medicine: Treating the causes of disease. *Altern Ther Health Med* 2009 15(6):12 - 14.

"…the recent "EPIC" study published in the Archives of Internal Medicine studied 23 000 people's adherence to 4 simple behaviors (not smoking, exercising 3.5 hours a week, eating a healthy diet [fruits, vegetables, beans, whole grains, nuts, seeds, and limited amounts of meat], and maintaining a healthy weight [BMI <30]). In those adhering to these behaviors, 93% of diabetes, 81% of heart attacks, 50% of strokes, and 36% of all cancers were prevented."

Lifestyle medicine works better than any other medical intervention… and it's free. The authors conclude: "If lifestyle medicine becomes central to the practice of medicine, our sick care system will be transformed into a healthcare system."

A. Vang, P. N. Singh, J. W. Lee, E. H. Haddad, and C. H. Brinegar. Meats, processed meats, obesity, weight gain and occurrence of diabetes among adults: Findings from adventist health studies. *Ann. Nutr. Metab.*, 52(2):96-104, 2008.

"Our findings raise the possibility that meat intake, particularly processed meats, is a dietary risk factor for diabetes."

So why does Dr. Mark Hyman promote animals as food? I have no idea.

Neal D Barnard, Heather I Katcher, David JA Jenkins, Joshua Cohen, and Gabrielle Turner-McGrievy. Vegetarian and vegan diets in type 2 diabetes management. *Nutrition Reviews*® Vol. 67(5):255–263.

According to Dr. Neal Barnard et al, "Several possible mechanisms may explain the effect of low-fat, plant-based diets on glycemic [sugar] control:

- Weight loss...
- Changes in intramyocellular lipid [fat inside muscle cells]...
- Reductions in saturated fat intake...
- Reduced glycemic index...
- Increased intake of dietary fiber...
- Reductions in iron stores."

Of the six mechanisms, low-carbers can provide weight loss and reduced glycemic load. Only Planting produces all six mechanisms for preventing diabetes. This is why many low-carbers remain or become diabetic even when they're skeletally thin on the outside: they're fiber-deficient and fat where it counts in nutrition – inside.

Planters have the best glycemic control, the least insulin resistance, the least diabetes and the fewest degenerative "diseases" overall.

WJ Crinnion. The role of persistent organic pollutants in the worldwide epidemic of type 2 diabetes mellitus and the possible connection to Farmed Atlantic Salmon (*Salmo salar*). *Altern Med Rev.* 2011 16(4):301 – 313.

"Recent studies reveal that the presence of several persistent organic pollutants (POPs) can confer greater risk for developing the disease than some of the established lifestyle risk factors [poor nutrition, obesity, lack of exercise]. In fact, evidence suggests the hypothesis that obesity might only be a significant risk factor when adipose tissue contains high amounts of POPs... Obesity is one of the most well-known risk factors associated with developing T2DM. The evidence on POPS and T2DM suggests that increased body fatness with low in vivo POPs levels does not place a person at increased risk, while increased adiposity with high levels of POPs does."

If this is true, it helps explain why Meaters have far worse insulin resistance and far more diabetes than Planters. It's partly because the animals they eat biomagnify POPs to obscene levels. As usual, carnivorous fishes such as salmons are the most contaminated.

And lastly, please note the title of the following paper – "Higher insulin sensitivity in vegans..."

J Gojda et al. Higher insulin sensitivity in vegans is not associated with higher mitochondrial density. *Eur J Clin Nutr*. 2013 Dec;67(12):1310-5.

I won't go into the details of this paper. What's important to grasp is that the baseline from which competent biomedical researchers work is this: Vegans have the highest insulin sensitivity, the least insulin resistance, and therefore the least diabetes. As usual, people on extremely high whole-carb diets have the best health outcomes.

Why more needs saying?

Gestational diabetes

C Qiu et al. Risk of gestational diabetes mellitus in relation to maternal egg and cholesterol intake. *Am. J. Epidemiol.* 2011 173(6):649 - 658.

"...high egg and cholesterol intakes before and during pregnancy are associated with increased risk of GDM [gestational diabetes mellitus]... relative risk... 2.52 for consumption of ≥10 eggs/week."

Diabetic retinopathy

N Cheung, P Mitchell, T Y Wong. Diabetic retinopathy. *Lancet.* 2010 Jul 10;376(9735):124-36.

"Optimum control of blood glucose, blood pressure, and possibly blood lipids remains the foundation for reduction of risk of retinopathy development and progression."

Who have the lowest blood glucose and cholesterol levels, and the lowest blood pressure? Planters. Who have the least diabetes and therefore the least diabetic retinopathy? Planters.

Diarrhea

X Xia et al. Presence and characterization of shiga toxin-producing *Escherichia coli* and other potentially diarrheagenic *E. coli* strains in retail meats. *Appl Environ Microbiol*, 76(6):1709-1717, 2010.

"...retail meats, mainly ground beef, were contaminated with diverse STEC strains."

Diarrheagenic bacteria such as *E. coli*, *C. diff* and *Y. enterocolitica* are animal-borne pathogens. No wonder Meaters get diarrhea so often.

Disc degeneration & herniation

U G Longo et al. Symptomatic disc herniation and serum lipid levels. *Eur Spine J*. 2011 Oct;20(10):1658-62.

"When comparing the two groups, patients with symptomatic herniated lumbar disc showed statistically significant higher triglyceride concentration… and total cholesterol concentration… Serum lipid levels may be a risk factor for IVD [intervertebral disc] pathology."

Meating damages the discs between the vertebrae of our spines.

Diverticulosis and Diverticulitis

NS Painter, DP Burkitt. Diverticular disease of the colon: a deficiency disease of Western civilization. *Br Med J.* 1971 May 22;2(5759):450-4.

Neil Painter and Denis Burkitt say: "We present a hypothesis as to the cause of diverticulosis coli which is consistent with its geographical distribution, its recent emergence as a medical problem, and its changing incidence.

Diverticulosis appears to be a deficiency disease caused by the refining of carbohydrates which entails the removal of vegetable fibre from the diet. Consequently we consider it to be preventable.

Diverticulitis first became a clinical problem at the turn of the century, and the term "diverticulosis" first appeared in 1914. As recently as 1916 the disease was not important enough to merit a mention in textbooks."

Both animals and junk are deficient or entirely lacking in fiber. Other consequences of fiber deficiency include constipation and all the resulting 'pressure diseases,' plus a host of other Western conditions.

Lisa L. Strate et al. Nut, Corn, and Popcorn Consumption and the Incidence of Diverticular Disease. *JAMA.* 2008;300(8):907-914.

"Patients with diverticular disease are frequently advised to avoid eating nuts, corn, popcorn, and seeds to reduce the risk of complications. However, there is little evidence to support this recommendation… In this large, prospective study of men without known diverticular disease, nut, corn, and popcorn consumption did not increase the risk of diverticulosis or diverticular complications. The recommendation to avoid these foods to prevent diverticular complications should be reconsidered."

Drug resistance

AE Waters et al. Multidrug-Resistant *Staphylococcus aureus* in US Meat and Poultry. *Clin Infect Dis.* 2011 May;52(10):1227-30.

"Conventional concentrated animal feeding operations (CAFOs) provide all the necessary components for the emergence and proliferation of multidrug-resistant zoonotic pathogens. In the United States, billions of food animals are raised in densely stocked CAFOs, where antibiotics are routinely administered in feed and water for extended periods to healthy animals. NARMS [the National Antimicrobial Resistance Monitoring System] has shown that multidrug-resistant *E. coli* and *Enterococcus* species are prevalent among US meat and poultry products. Our findings indicate that multidrug-resistant *S. aureus* should be added to the list of antimicrobial-resistant pathogens that routinely contaminate our food supply."

Eating animals is bringing us more infectious diseases, while simultaneously removing our ability to treat them.

Erectile dysfunction ~ Impotence

DR Meldrum et al. The link between erectile and cardiovascular health: The canary in the coal mine. *Am. J. Cardiol.* 2011 108(4):599-606.

I've said this a few times in different ways, but it bears saying again: Heart "disease" = acne = erectile dysfunction = lower back pain. They're all symptoms of Meating. If we have one, it's almost certain we have others, even if they're not yet clinically detectable.

"In men aged <60 years and in men with diabetes or hypertension, erectile dysfunction can be a critical warning sign for existing or impending cardiovascular disease and risk for death… by better understanding the complex factors influencing erectile and overall vascular health, physicians can help their patients prevent vascular disease and improve erectile function, which provides more immediate motivation for men to improve their lifestyle habits and cardiovascular health."

For men, passion is hydraulic, and Meating messes with our fluid pipes.

Fatty liver "disease"

There are two variants of fatter liver "disease" - alcoholic and nonalcoholic. What causes the latter, which now provides the majority of cases? Would you be surprised to hear 'Animals and Junk?'

A K Leamy, R A Egnatchik, J D Young. Molecular mechanisms and the role of saturated fatty acids in the progression of non-alcoholic fatty liver disease. *Prog Lipid Res.* 2013 Jan;52(1):165-74.

"…saturated fatty acids are more toxic than their unsaturated counterparts, resulting in a progressive lipotoxic cascade… fatty acid saturation plays a critical role in determining cell fate under lipotoxic conditions."

M K Hellerstein. Mitigating factors and metabolic mechanisms in fructose-induced nonalcoholic fatty liver disease: the next challenge. *Am J Clin Nutr.* 2012 Nov;96(5):951-2.

"Fructose homes in like a laser beam on the liver and its glycolytic pathways, with ~90% of fructose uptake by the liver. Fructose intake results in hepatic release of lactate, storage of glycogen, and stimulation of de novo fatty acid synthesis. Fructose shares this liver tropism with galactose [milk sugar], but perhaps a better analogy is ethanol. Like ethanol, fructose increases de novo lipogenesis (DNL), inhibits fatty acid oxidation, and has been implicated in NAFLD."

The 3 dietary villains in nonalcoholic fatty liver "disease"? Animal fats, animal sugar and junk sugar. Whole grains and oatmeal are protective.

Gallstones

Portincasa P, Moschetta A, Palasciano G. Cholesterol gallstone disease. *Lancet.* 2006 Jul 15;368(9531):230-9.

The title of this paper sums up gallstones: Cholesterol gallstone disease.

"Gallstones are abnormal masses of a solid mixture of cholesterol crystals, mucin, calcium bilirubinate, and proteins… In Western societies, cholesterol gallstones account for 80–90% of the gallstones found at cholecystectomy [surgical removal]. Precipitation of excess cholesterol in bile as solid crystals is a prerequisite for cholesterol gallstone formation."

And high levels of blood cholesterol (the result of eating saturated and trans fats and cholesterol) are a prerequisite for causing the "precipitation of excess cholesterol in bile as solid crystals" or stones in our gall bladders. Ouch. It's too bad that the agony of Meating is usually atopic and atemporal, occurring elsewhere and else-when, becoming evident only after years of eating non-meals.

Glaucoma

AL Coleman et al; Study of Osteoporotic Fractures Research Group. Glaucoma risk and the consumption of fruits and vegetables among older women in the study of osteoporotic fractures. *Am J Ophthalmol.* 2008 Jun;145(6):1081-9.

"A higher intake of certain fruits and vegetables may be associated with a decreased risk of glaucoma."

Gout

Under Purines earlier, Zhang et al told us we should avoid eating animals because of the purines they contain if we want to avoid gout.

Choi HK, Willett W, Curhan G. Fructose-rich beverages and risk of gout in women. *JAMA*. 2010 Nov 24;304(20):2270-8.

"Although sugar-sweetened beverages contain low levels of purine (i.e. the precursor of uric acid), they contain large amounts of fructose, which is the only carbohydrate known to increase uric acid levels."

Gout comes from animal purines and junk fructose, because they raise uric acid levels. As Falstaff says in 2 Henry IV: "A pox of this gout! or, a gout of this pox! For the one or the other plays the rogue with my great toe."

Think on Shakespeare's wordplay: Falstaff - fall staff - means erectile dysfunction, and ED = obesity = gout = stroke = heart "disease" etc.

Guillain-Barré syndrome

TA Hardy et al. Guillain-barré syndrome: modern theories of etiology. *Curr Allergy Asthma Rep*. 2011 Jun;11(3):197-204.

"Guillain-Barré syndrome (GBS) is a classic failure of the immune system with a life-threatening attack upon a critical self-component… Triggers for GBS include infection… particularly [with] *Campylobacter jejuni*."

How do we become infected with *Campylobacter*?

Mainly by eating chickens.

Nachamkin I, Allos BM, Ho T. *Campylobacter* species and Guillain-Barré syndrome. *Clin Microbiol Rev*. 1998 Jul;11(3):555-67.

"*C. jejuni* is the most common cause of bacterial gastroenteritis in the United States, surpassing *Salmonella* in most studies. It is estimated that over 2.5 million cases occur each year in the United States."

'Playing chicken' takes on a new meaning when it comes to total paralysis.

Heart "disease" (Coronary artery "disease", Cardiac "disease")

W. F. Enos, R. H. Holmes, J. Beyer. Coronary disease among United States soldiers killed in action in Korea preliminary report. Journal of the American Medical Association 1953 152(12):1090 - 1093.

Back in the early 1950s, way, way, way before today's Low-Carb Bullshit Artists say we became fat and sick because of all the sugar we're eating, autopsied American soldiers in the Korean police action, with an average age of 22.1 years old, were found to be riddled with heart "disease". And it wasn't because of all the smoking they were doing. As the Japanese population used to prove, before their lethal transition to the SAD diet, high smoking rates allied with low animal-eating rates lead to low cancer and heart "disease" rates.

According to Enos et al: "In 77.3% of the hearts, some gross evidence of coronary arteriosclerosis was found. The disease process varied from "fibrous" thickening to large atheromatous plaques causing complete occlusion of one or more of the major vessels." At 22 years old.

Here's another oldie but goody: A. G. Shaper, K. W. Jones. Serum-cholesterol, diet, and coronary heart-disease in Africans and Asians in Uganda: 1959. *Int J Epidemiol.* 2012 41(5):1221-1225.

"In the African population of Uganda coronary heart disease is almost non-existent… In the Asian community, on the other hand, coronary heart disease is a major problem."

Interesting. What's going on here? Is it genetic? Or is it the food?

It's the food, with the healthy indigenous African population eating the following and staying heart attack-free:

"The staple foods, green plantain and sweet potatoes, are steamed in banana leaves; cassava, yams, maize, and millet are also staple commodities in particular of the non-Baganda groups, while pumpkins, tomatoes, and green leafy vegetables are taken by all. The adequacy of protein in the diet depends almost entirely on the extent to which pulses, groundnuts, and cereals are used. Most meals are served with a sauce made of groundnuts, beans, and a mixture of vegetables, and occasionally meat or fish, and these are fried in very small amounts of fat…" Sounds almost ideal.

Ornish D, Brown SE, Scherwitz LW, Billings JH, Armstrong WT, Ports TA, McLanahan SM, Kirkeeide RL, Brand RJ, Gould KL. Can lifestyle changes reverse coronary heart disease? The Lifestyle Heart Trial. *Lancet.* 1990 Jul 21;336(8708):129-33.

"Overall, 82% of experimental-group patients had an average change towards regression. Comprehensive lifestyle changes may be able to bring about regression of even severe coronary atherosclerosis after only 1 year, without use of lipid-lowering drugs."

Those two dry sentences changed the world, or should have... In just one year of Planting (+ relaxation and exercise and other desirable but non-essential lifestyle changes), four out of five patients' heart conditions improved. No drugs, no surgery… and Lifestyle Medicine was born.

That the entire medical community hasn't sat up and taken notice of this landmark of medical landmarks is a scandal that will resound down the ages.

Esselstyn CB Jr. Resolving the Coronary Artery Disease Epidemic Through Plant-Based Nutrition. *Prev Cardiol.* 2001 Autumn;4(4):171-177.

Another genius, confirming Ornish's work… Here's his opening paragraph:

"The world's advanced countries have easy access to plentiful high-fat food; ironically, it is this rich diet that produces atherosclerosis. In the world's poorer nations, many people subsist on a primarily plant-based diet, which is far healthier, especially in terms of heart disease. To treat coronary heart disease, a century of scientific investigation has produced a device-driven, risk factor-oriented strategy. Nevertheless, many patients treated with this approach experience progressive disability and death. This strategy is a rear-guard defensive one. In contrast, compelling data from nutritional studies, population surveys, and interventional studies support the effectiveness of a plant-based diet and aggressive lipid lowering to arrest, prevent, and selectively reverse heart disease. In essence, this is an offensive strategy. The single biggest step toward adopting this strategy would be to have United States dietary guidelines support a plant-based diet. An expert committee purged of industrial and political influence is required to assure that science is the basis for dietary recommendations."

Esselstyn concludes: "We are fortunate to possess the knowledge of how to prevent, arrest, and selectively reverse this disease. [Planting.] However, we are not fortunate in the capacity of our institutions to share this information with the public. The collective conscience and will of our profession is being tested as never before. Ties to industry and politics result in conflict within our private and governmental health institutions, compromising the accuracy of their public message. This is in total violation of the moral imperative of our profession. Now is the time for us to have the courage for legendary work. Science — not the messenger — must dictate the recommendations."

And, finally, a word from the man beloved of Low-Carb Bullshit Artists for his development of the Glycemic Index…

DJ Jenkins et al. The Garden of Eden – plant based diets, the genetic drive to conserve cholesterol and its implications for heart disease in the 21st century. *Comp Biochem Physiol A Mol Integr Physiol.* 2003 Sep;136(1):141-51.

"We conclude that reintroduction of plant food components, which would have been present in large quantities in the plant based diets eaten throughout most of human evolution into modern diets can correct the lipid abnormalities associated with contemporary eating patterns and reduce the need for pharmacological interventions."

In a short video called "Dr. David Jenkins discusses the glycemic index of foods," he says: The glycemic index "is a difficult horse to ride. You can be thrown off quite easily." Like me, Jenkins thinks low-carb and paleo diets are a load of horse feathers, and that low-carb cowboys are 'all hat, no cattle' greenhorns who can't stay astride the frisky GI pony.

Hemorrhoids

Denis P. Burkitt. Some Diseases Characteristic of Modern Western Civilization. *British Medical Journal*, 1973, 1, 274-278.

"A number of diseases of major importance are characteristic of modern Western civilization. These diseases are rare or unknown in communities who have deviated little from their traditional way of life, and a rise in their frequency follows adoption of Western customs… Haemorrhoids are believed to be present to some degree in nearly half of all people over the age of 50."

It's not just the fiber in the diet that prevents piles. It's many different phytonutrients working together in concert within a high-fiber diet.

Neither Meating nor Junking is a high-fiber diet.

Hiatus hernia

Continuing with Burkitt (1973, above):

"Hiatus Hernia and Faecal Arrest

The close epidemiological relationship between hiatus hernia and a low-residue diet could well be accounted for by the raised intra-abdominal pressures consequent on such a diet. Constrictive clothing and adiposity have been considered to be causes of increased intra-abdominal pressures contributing to hiatus hernia, but these must cause insignificant pressure change compared with straining at stool."

Meating and Junking are constipating and cause the 'pressure diseases.'

Hyperactivity ~ ADHD (Attention Deficit Hyperactivity Disorder)
D McCann et al. Food additives and hyperactive behaviour in 3-year-old and 8/9-year-old children in the community: a randomised, double-blinded, placebo-controlled trial. *Lancet*, Vol 370, #9598, 1560 - 1567, 3 Nov 2007.

"Artificial colours or a sodium benzoate preservative (or both) in the diet result in increased hyperactivity in 3-year-old and 8/9-year-old children in the general population."

Junk isn't food, so why do we feed it to our precious children?

Hypertension
F M Sacks, E H Kass. Low blood pressure in vegetarians: effects of specific foods and nutrients. *Am J Clin Nutr*. 1988 Sep;48(3 Suppl):795-800.

"Strict vegetarians, who eat little if any animal products and lactovegetarians, who regularly eat dairy products, have lower blood pressures than the general population… modest intake of animal products may be a marker for a large intake of other potentially beneficial nutrients from vegetable products."

Hey, this paper was written in 1988, so let's cut the authors some slack. A quarter century later, we can say that cutting out all animal products leads to normotension, i.e. normal blood pressure.

J Stamler et al; INTERMAP Research Group. Glutamic acid, the main dietary amino acid, and blood pressure: the INTERMAP Study. *Circulation*. 2009 Jul 21;120(3):221-8.

"Dietary glutamic acid may have independent BP lowering effects, possibly contributing to the inverse relation of vegetable protein to BP."

The more plants we eat, the lower our blood pressure. Flaxseeds are terrific at countering hypertension.

Hypertensive retinopathy
Walter Kempner, MD. Treatment of Hypertensive Vascular Disease with Rice Diet. *American Journal of Medicine* 1948 pp. 545-577.

"Vascular retinopathy has been found to disappear with the rice diet. The retinal improvement does not necessarily coincide with decrease in blood pressure. Very severe retinopathy has disappeared in patients when the blood pressure remained at a constant high level or showed only an insignificant reduction."

Tiny arteries in the eye may benefit from Planting way before systemic blood pressure comes down.

"Those patients in whom the retinopathy remained unchanged had been on the diet from one to three and one-half months except for one patient with exudative stippling who was on the rice diet for nineteen months. The patients in whom the retinopathy cleared up only partially had been on the rice diet from one to seventeen months, an average of five months. The period of time in which the retinal changes disappeared completely ranged from two to thirty months, an average of fourteen months."

Plants are powerful healers.

Iatrogenic deaths

J Lazarou et al. Incidence of adverse drug reactions in hospitalized patients: a meta-analysis of prospective studies. *JAMA*. 1998 Apr 15; 279(15):1200-5.

The objective was to "estimate the incidence of serious and fatal adverse drug reactions (ADRs) in hospital patients… We estimated that in 1994 overall 2 216 000 hospitalized patients had serious ADRs and 106 000 had fatal ADRs, making these reactions between the fourth and sixth leading cause of death."

And that's just deaths of people taking the correct on-prescription meds, prescribed by physicians… no medical errors or in-hospital infections.

Infectious "diseases"

D W Eyre et al. Diverse sources of *C. difficile* infection identified on whole-genome sequencing. *N Engl J Med.* 2013 Sep 26;369(13):1195-205.

"It has been thought that *Clostridium difficile* infection is transmitted predominantly within health care settings. However, endemic spread" is on the rise. "Over a 3-year period, 45% of *C. difficile* cases in Oxfordshire were genetically distinct from all previous cases."

In other words, 45% of *C. diff* infections are now spreading within the community at large.

Where are the bacteria coming from? They're in the "food" supply, particularly in the pigs we eat.

Why? Because of fecal contamination among densely packed pigs in farrowing crates and other situations in which animals are hyper-confined.

The same applies to a multitude of other animal-borne pathogens.

Infectobesity

Pasarica M, Dhurandhar NV. Infectobesity: obesity of infectious origin. *Adv Food Nutr Res.* 2007;52:61-102.

"Of the several etiological factors [of obesity], infection, an unusual causative factor, has recently started receiving greater attention. In the last two decades, 10 adipogenic pathogens were reported, including human and nonhuman viruses, scrapie agents, bacteria, and gut microflora."

Chickens are the main host of obesity-causing viruses, principally avian adenovirus SMAM-1.

Kidney failure

Lin J, Hu FB, Curhan GC. Associations of diet with albuminuria and kidney function decline. *Clin J Am Soc Nephrol.* 2010 May; 5(5):836-43.

"Higher dietary intake of animal fat and two or more servings per week of red meat may increase risk for microalbuminuria [protein in the urine, a sign of kidney failure]. Lower sodium and higher B-carotene intake may reduce risk for eGFR [Estimated Glomerular Filtration Rate] decline."

More animals + more junk = more decline in kidney function.

Kidney stones

C R Tracy, S Best, A Bagrodia, J R Poindexter, B Adams-Huet, K Sakhaee, N Maalouf, C Y Pak, M S Pearle. Animal protein and the risk of kidney stones: a comparative metabolic study of animal protein sources. J Urol. 2014 Jul;192(1):137-41.

"Consuming animal protein is associated with increased serum and urine uric acid in healthy individuals. The higher purine content of fish compared to beef or chicken is reflected in higher 24-hour urinary uric acid. However, as reflected in the saturation index, the stone forming propensity is marginally higher for beef compared to fish or chicken. Stone formers should be advised to limit the intake of all animal proteins, including fish."

Who forms kidney stones? People who eat animals. Meaters. So they should be advised not to eat animals.

MD Sorensen et al, Women's Health Initiative Writing Group. Dietary intake of fiber, fruit and vegetables decreases the risk of incident kidney stones in women: a Women's Health Initiative report. *J Urol.* 2014 Dec;192(6):1694-9.

What do you know? Planting can prevent kidney stones. Why? More of the good PLUS less of the bad:

"Greater intake of fruits, vegetables, and fiber likely contributes to decreased intake of foods that are high in calories, sodium, fat, and animal protein."

Lou Gehrig's "disease" ~ ALS ~ Amyotrophic Lateral Sclerosis
W Holtcamp. The Emerging Science of BMAA: Do Cyanobacteria Contribute to Neurodegenerative Disease? *Environ Health Perspect.* 2012 Mar; 120(3): a110–a116.

"In addition to protein misincorporation, high levels of unbound BMAA can continually overstimulate glutamate receptors on cells, leading to neuronal injury… **BMAA and methylmercury** – a common pollutant in seafood – both **deplete glutathione**, the main endogenous antioxidant in the body, and they act synergistically to harm nerve cells."

β-Methylamino-L-alanine, or BMAA, is an amino acid that's made by blue-green algae and which then becomes concentrated in the fatty flesh of sea animals – fishes, oysters, mussels, crabs. And when we eat them, BMAA becomes concentrated in our fatty brains, and especially in the brains of people suffering from neurodegeneration, such as Alzheimer's and Parkinson's victims.

Macular degeneration
S. Beatty et al. Macular pigment and risk for age-related macular degeneration in subjects from a Northern European population. *Invest. Ophthalmol. Vis. Sci.* 2001 42(2):439 - 446.

"Human macular pigment (MP) consists of the two hydroxycarotenoids, lutein (L) and zeaxanthin (Z), with concentrations that peak at the center of the fovea. MP is an effective filter of damaging blue light, which causes photo-oxidative retinal injury… Further, L and Z are powerful antioxidants… Consequently, it has been hypothesized that MP protects against AMD [age-related macular degeneration]… The macular pigment is entirely of dietary origin…"

The macular pigment of our eyes is made entirely out of the plants we eat.

JM Stringham et al. The influence of dietary lutein and zeaxanthin on visual performance. *J Food Sci.* 2010 Jan-Feb;75(1):R24-9.

"…the [plant] pigments protect the retina and lens, and perhaps even help to prevent age-related eye diseases such as macular degeneration… and cataract."

L Ma et al. Lutein and zeaxanthin intake and the risk of age-related macular degeneration: A systematic review and meta-analysis. *Br. J. Nutr.* 2012 107(3):350 - 359.

"…an increase in the intake of these carotenoids may be protective against late AMD."

We need to eat lots of plants if we want to see well when we're old.

Metabolic syndrome

Rizzo NS, Sabaté J, Jaceldo-Siegl K, Fraser GE. Vegetarian dietary patterns are associated with a lower risk of metabolic syndrome: the adventist health study 2. *Diabetes Care.* 2011 May;34(5):1225-7.

"A vegetarian dietary pattern is associated with a more favorable profile of MRFs [metabolic risk factors]… (HDL, triglycerides, glucose, blood pressure, and waist circumference)… and a lower risk of MetS [metabolic syndrome].

Mood

Beezhold BL, Johnston CS, Daigle DR. Preliminary evidence that vegetarian diet improves mood. American Public Health Association annual conference, November 7-11, 2009. Philadelphia, PA.

"An omnivorous diet is typically higher in fat and protein, and contains less healthy fatty acid proportions than vegetarian diets. Research has shown that these dietary factors can promote subtle but adverse changes in the brain that impair mood state…

FISH participants significantly increased their EPA/DHA intakes and decreased their saturated fat intake but mood scores were not significantly reduced.

Conclusion: The complete restriction of flesh foods significantly reduced mood variability in omnivores."

Arachidonic acid is a polyunsaturated omega-6 fatty acid found in animals that causes brain inflammation.

Beezhold BL, Johnston CS, Daigle DR. Vegetarian diets are associated with healthy mood states: a cross-sectional study in seventh day adventist adults. *Nutr J.* 2010 Jun 1;9:26.

"Vegetarians reported significantly less negative emotion than omnivores… participants with low intakes of EPA, DHA, and AA and high intakes of ALA and LA had better mood.

Conclusions: The vegetarian diet profile does not appear to adversely affect mood despite low intake of long-chain omega-3 fatty acids."

Mortality ~ Death

If there's one thing that Meaters and Junkers are better at than Planters, it's dying. It's not fair: Meaters and Junkers get so much more practice.

R. Sinha et al. Meat intake and mortality: a prospective study of over half a million people. *Arch Intern Med.* 2009 March 23; 169(6): 562–571.

"Red and processed meat intakes were associated with modest increases in total mortality, cancer mortality and CVD mortality."

Meating kills, so my modest proposal for increased longevity is that we shouldn't eat animals.

P. N. Singh, J. Sabaté, and G. E. Fraser. Does low meat consumption increase life expectancy in humans? *American Journal of Clinical Nutrition*, 78(3):526, 2003.

"Current prospective cohort data from adults in North America and Europe raise the possibility that a lifestyle pattern that includes a very low meat intake is associated with greater longevity… a longer duration ($\geq$ 2 decades) of adherence to this diet contributed to a significant decrease in mortality risk and a significant 3.6-year increase in life expectancy."

How much is 3.6 years of life worth to you? I guarantee you, when you're sucking your last gasp you'll be willing to give everything you own for 3.6 more minutes.

Baer HJ, Glynn RJ, Hu FB, Hankinson SE, Willett WC, Colditz GA, Stampfer M, Rosner B. Risk factors for mortality in the nurses' health study: a competing risks analysis. *Am J Epidemiol.* 2011 Feb 1; 173(3):319-29.

"Age, body mass index at age 18 years, weight change, height, current smoking and pack-years of smoking, glycemic load, cholesterol intake, systolic blood pressure and use of blood pressure medications, diabetes, parental myocardial infarction before age 60 years, and time since menopause were directly related to all-cause mortality, whereas there were inverse associations for physical activity and intakes of nuts, polyunsaturated fat, and cereal fiber."

Inverse associations means that being active and eating plants are associated with living longer lives. Meating, Junking, smoking, being older, taking medications and having bad genes are associated with dying sooner.

H. Noto, A. Goto, T. Tsujimoto, M. Noda. Low-carbohydrate diets and all-cause mortality: A systematic review and meta-analysis of observational studies. *PLoS ONE* 2013 8(1):e55030.

I cited this study earlier to show why hyper-Meaters die more often. Here's another quote from Noto et al:

"...low-carbohydrate diets tend to result in reduced intake of fiber and fruits, and increased intake of protein from animal sources, cholesterol and saturated fat, all of which are risk factors for mortality and CVD [cardiovascular disease]... Our meta-analysis supported long-term harm and no cardiovascular protection with low-carbohydrate diets."

Why would one bother with questionable low-carb diets when there is no question about the long-term benefits of whole-food veganism?

How important is it to eat fruits and vegetables?

A Bellavia et al. Fruit and vegetable consumption and all-cause mortality: A dose-response analysis. *Am J Clin Nutr.* 2013 98(2):454 – 459.

"In comparison with 5 servings FV/d [fruits and vegetables per day], a lower consumption was progressively associated with shorter survival and higher mortality rates. Those who never consumed FV lived 3 y shorter... and had a 53% higher mortality rate... than did those who consumed 5 servings FV/d. Consideration of fruit and vegetables separately showed that those who never consumed fruit lived 19 mo shorter... than did those who ate 1 fruit/d. Participants who consumed 3 vegetables/d lived 32 mo longer than did those who never consumed vegetables…

Conclusion: FV consumption <5 servings/d is associated with progressively shorter survival and higher mortality rates."

There's a dose-response between added fruits and vegetables and extra years of life. This finding was confirmed by the massive Global Burden of Disease study, funded by the Bill and Melinda Gates Foundation, but in the negative: the biggest killer on planet Earth may be **not eating enough fruits and vegetables**, responsible for 4.9 million deaths around the world each year. Who doesn't eat enough whole plants? Junkers, poor people, and wealthy low-carb/paleo twits.

R Lozano et al. Global and regional mortality from 235 causes of death for 20 age groups in 1990 and 2010: a systematic analysis for the Global Burden of Disease Study 2010. *The Lancet.* Volume 380, No. 9859, p2095–2128, 15 December 2012.

"…dietary risk factors and physical inactivity were responsible for the largest disease burden… in 2010. Of the individual dietary risk factors, the largest attributable burden in 2010 was associated with diets **low in fruits** (4·9 million… deaths… followed by diets **high in sodium** (4·0 million…), **low in nuts and seeds** (2·5 million…), **low in whole grains** (1·7 million…), **low in vegetables** (1·8 million…), and **low in seafood omega-3 fatty acids** (1·4 million…)"

I think they're out to lunch about seafood omega-3s, because if we were all Planters almost no one would die of an omega deficiency, but let's not quibble. Most deaths are caused by plant deficiencies – 10.9 million people – followed by high-Junk diets.

More than 14.9 million of us humans die each year because we're not whole-food vegans.

Mucus production

Bartley J, McGlashan SR. Does milk increase mucus production? *Medical Hypotheses.* 2010 Apr;74(4):732-4.

Yes, for many: "a subgroup of the population, who have increased respiratory tract mucus production, find that many of their symptoms, including asthma, improve on a dairy elimination diet."

Multiple sclerosis

R. L. Swank, B. B. Dugan. Effect of low saturated fat diet in early and late cases of multiple sclerosis. *Lancet* 1990 336(8706):37-39.

"144 multiple sclerosis patients took a low-fat diet for 34 years. For each of three categories of neurological disability (minimum, moderate, severe) patients who adhered to the prescribed diet (≤20 g fat/day) showed significantly less deterioration and much lower death rates than did those who consumed more fat than prescribed (>20 g fat/day). The greatest benefit was seen in those with minimum disability at the start of the trial; in this group, when those who died from non-MS diseases were excluded from the analysis, 95% survived and remained physically active."

Since Dr. Roy Laver Swank started publishing his findings about the healing power of whole plants for sufferers of MS, such as "Multiple sclerosis: a correlation of its incidence with dietary fat," in *The American journal of the medical sciences* (1950), there has been no better treatment found. Dr. John McDougall continues his pioneering work today. My best guess is that his cutting out the fishes and fish oils Swank allowed will lead to improved results. It's too soon to tell.

Obesity

Rosell M, Appleby P, Spencer E, Key T. Weight gain over 5 years in 21,966 meat-eating, fish-eating, vegetarian, and vegan men and women in EPIC-Oxford. *Int J Obes* (Lond). 2006 Sep;30(9):1389-96.

"Men and women who changed their diet in one or several steps in the direction meat-eater → fish-eater → vegetarian → vegan showed the smallest mean annual weight gain of 242… and 301 g, respectively… During 5 years follow-up, the mean annual weight gain in a health-conscious cohort in the UK was approximately 400 g. Small differences in weight gain were observed between meat-eaters, fish-eaters, vegetarians and vegans. Lowest weight gain was seen among those who, during follow-up, had changed to a diet containing fewer animal foods."

We saw this earlier with the studies of 7th Day Adventists: vegans weigh substantially less and get less diabetes, hypertension – you name it – and live years longer:

S. Tonstad, T. Butler, R. Yan, and G. E. Fraser. Type of vegetarian diet, body weight, and prevalence of type 2 diabetes. *Diabetes Care*, 32(5). 791-796, 2009.

"Mean BMI was lowest in vegans (23.6 kg/m^2) and incrementally higher in lacto-ovo-vegetarians (25.7 kg/m^2), pesco-vegetarians (26.3 kg/m^2), semi-vegetarians (27.3 kg/m^2), and nonvegetarians (28.8 kg/m^2)… The 5-unit BMI difference between vegans and nonvegetarians indicates a substantial potential of vegetarianism to protect against obesity." [I think scientists compete for the driest tone while announcing startling findings.]

Any diet book that doesn't mention how whole-food veganism is the best weight maintenance tool is ripping us off. Fat vegans become and stay fat by eating junk instead of food… and by not exercising enough, if at all.

A Vergnaud et al. Meat consumption and prospective weight change in participants of the EPIC-PANACEA study. *Am J Clin Nutr.* 2010 Aug;92(2):398-407.

"Total meat consumption was positively associated with weight gain in men and women, in normal-weight and overweight subjects, and in smokers and nonsmokers. With adjustment for estimated energy intake, an increase in meat intake of 250 g/d (eg, one steak at '450 kcal) would lead to a 2-kg higher weight gain after 5 y (95% CI: 1.5, 2.7 kg). Positive associations were observed for red meat, poultry, and processed meat… Our results suggest that a decrease in meat consumption may improve weight management."

Osteoporosis

P. Appleby, A. Roddam, N. Allen, T. Key. Comparative fracture risk in vegetarians and nonvegetarians in epic-oxford. *Eur J Clin Nutr*, 61(12):1400-1406, 2007.

Here's some contradictory evidence… there are vegans in the UK who're not eating enough leafy greens and other calcium-containing plants, and the result is increased risk of bone fracture:

"The higher fracture rate among vegans in this study appears to reflect their markedly lower mean calcium intake… The percentage of subjects consuming less than 700 mg/day calcium was 15.0 for meat eaters, 15.9 for fish eaters, 18.6 for vegetarians and **76.1 for vegans**." That's an astonishing difference – what are you vegans eating in the UK, for crying out loud? There can't be many Planters among you; and plenty of Junkers. Get a grip, dear Limey vegans – you're making the rest of us look bad.

Also of interest from this paper: "Meat eaters had the highest mean BMI [weighed the most] and tended to be the least active group, with vegans having the lowest mean BMI whilst reporting the highest levels of walking, cycling and vigorous exercise."

K Michaelsson et al. Milk intake and risk of mortality and fractures in women and men: cohort studies. *BMJ*. 2014 Oct 28;349:g6015.

"What this study adds: A high milk intake in both sexes is associated with higher mortality and fracture rates and with higher levels of oxidative stress and inflammatory biomarkers. Such a pattern was not observed with high intake of fermented milk products."

This study confirms the epidemiology of osteoporosis, which shows that the populations who consume the most dairy products have some of the brittlest bones. Keeping in mind that lactose tolerance is a genetic quirk found mainly among people of northern European descent, it's instructive then that the women of the following European nations all suffer high rates of bone disease (>300 per 100,000): The UK, Ireland, Iceland, Norway, Sweden, Denmark, Switzerland, Germany, Czech Republic, Italy, Slovenia, Slovakia, Hungary, Greece and Turkey. The women of Portugal, Spain, France and the Netherlands all have medium rates (>200 per 100,000).

Milk defenders and promoters will say that it's all the sugar these people eat. I agree: it's the milk sugar (and the milk proteins and… and… and…)

There's an interesting map showing this information at http://www.iofbonehealth.org/facts-and-statistics/hip-fracture-incidence-map.

Indians consume mainly fermented milk products, which aren't as bone-destructive as whole milk. Africans have strong bones and consume very little milk. Ditto for China. Sadly, the Chinese living in Taiwan have really taken to dairy products recently – "One local dairy farm imported 1,200 heifers in 2011, which is expected to boost production over the medium term" and "On the import side, the United States overtook New Zealand as the largest supplier of cheese to Taiwan during the first seven months of 2012," according to the USDA'S Foreign Agricultural Service GAIN Report Number TW12032 – and the lactose-intolerant, cheese-eating Taiwanese too have high rates of osteoporosis.

While the lactase mutation may have been beneficial to some of us in prehistory, it's definitely not worth taking advantage of now.

(And I didn't even mention the aging and inflammatory effects of milk's D-galactose.)

Parkinson's "disease"

H. Chen, E. O'Reilly, M. L. McCullough, C. Rodriguez, M. A. Schwarzschild, E. E. Calle, M. J. Thun, and A. Ascherio. Consumption of dairy products and risk of parkinson's disease. *Am. J. Epidemiol.*, 165(9):998-1006, 2007.

"Diet may play an important role in the etiology of Parkinson's disease, either by altering the oxidative balance in the brain or by serving as a vehicle for environmental neurotoxins… dairy consumption may increase the risk of Parkinson's disease, particularly in men."

Dairy, because of what's in it naturally and because of environmental toxins. Coffee is protective against Parkinson's.

Pre-diabetes

J Tuomilehto et al. Prevention of type 2 diabetes mellitus by changes in lifestyle among subjects with impaired glucose tolerance. *New England Journal of Medicine* 2001 344(18):1343–1350.

"Type 2 diabetes can be prevented by changes in the lifestyles of high-risk subjects… Each subject in the intervention group received individualized counseling aimed at reducing weight, total intake of fat, and intake of saturated fat and increasing intake of fiber and physical activity."

Planting plus exercise stops pre-diabetes progressing to diabetes. Actually, they reverse pre-diabetes, a "disease" in its own right. Here's one of the ways Planting rids us of pre-diabetes:

S Chuengsamarn et al. Curcumin extract for prevention of type 2 diabetes. *Diabetes Care.* 2012 Nov;35(11):2121-7.

"…curcumin extract was able to substantially and significantly prevent T2DM development in the prediabetic population (**0% of curcumin-treated subjects developed DM**, whereas 16.4% of placebo-treated subjects developed DM). In addition, we found that curcumin intervention improved β-cell functions… curcumin treatment may result in better β-cell function in the prediabetic population."

Turmeric and other spices are highly concentrated stores of phytochemicals and have remarkable preventive and healing properties.

Premature puberty

K. Maruyama, T. Oshima, and K. Ohyama. Exposure to exogenous estrogen through intake of commercial milk produced from pregnant cows. *Pediatr Int*, 52(1):33-38, 2010.

"The present data on men and children indicate that estrogens in milk were absorbed, and gonadotropin secretion was suppressed, followed by a decrease in testosterone secretion. Sexual maturation of prepubertal children could be affected by the ordinary intake of cow milk."

Cow's milk is not food for humans; not if it makes 8-year-old girls start growing adult breasts. Ten-year-old minds in 20-year-old bodies is what drives STDs, teenage pregnancies and much of the abortion demand.

It's the milk, stupid, with its huge load of hormones… and the phthalates… and the other endocrine disruptors…

Prostate cancer

Ornish D, Weidner G, Fair WR, Marlin R, Pettengill EB, Raisin CJ, Dunn-Emke S, Crutchfield L, Jacobs FN, Barnard RJ, Aronson WJ, McCormac P, McKnight DJ, Fein JD, Dnistrian AM, Weinstein J, Ngo TH, Mendell NR, Carroll PR. Intensive lifestyle changes may affect the progression of prostate cancer. *J Urol.*, 174(3):1065-9; discussion 1069-70, 2005.

"…intensive changes in diet and lifestyle may beneficially affect the progression of early prostate cancer… Patients with low grade prostate cancer were able to make and maintain comprehensive lifestyle changes for at least 1 year, resulting in significant decreases in serum PSA and a lower likelihood of standard treatment."

Planting has the power to reverse prostate cancer.

Ornish D, Magbanua MJ, Weidner G, Weinberg V, Kemp C, Green C, Mattie MD, Marlin R, Simko J, Shinohara K, Haqq CM, Carroll PR. Changes in prostate gene expression in men undergoing an intensive nutrition and lifestyle intervention. *Proc Natl Acad Sci U S A.* 17;105(24):8369-74, 2008.

"In conclusion, the GEMINAL study suggests that intensive nutrition and lifestyle changes may modulate gene expression in the prostate."

Planting is epigenetically beneficial; Meating never is.

Rheumatoid arthritis

P Tangvoranuntakul et al. Human uptake and incorporation of an immunogenic nonhuman dietary sialic acid. *Proc Natl Acad Sci U S A.* 2003 Oct 14;100(21):12045-50.

"The small amounts of Neu5Gc in normal tissues also raise the possibility that anti-Neu5Gc antibodies are involved in autoimmunity. In this regard, it is interesting that vegetarian diet has been suggested to improve rheumatoid arthritis."

Neu5Gc is an "inflammatory meat molecule" made by the mammals we eat but not by us. Not for two or three million years or so.

J. McDougall et al. Effects of a very low-fat, vegan diet in subjects with rheumatoid arthritis. *J Altern Complement Med*, 8(1):71-75, 2002.

"...patients with moderate-to-severe RA, who switch to a very low-fat, vegan diet can experience significant reductions in RA symptoms."

Planting improves inflammatory conditions such as arthritis; Meating makes them worse.

Sciatica

P Leino-Arjas et al. Serum lipids in relation to sciatica among Finns. *Atherosclerosis.* 2008 Mar;197(1):43-9.

"Atherosclerosis of arteries supplying the lumbar region has been suggested as a mechanism leading to intervertebral disc degeneration and sciatica... Independent of BMI and other possible confounders, clinically assessed sciatica in men was associated with levels of atherogenic serum lipids."

The cholesterol Low-Carb Bullshit Artists tell us not to worry about is what causes sciatica and spinal degeneration... and erectile dysfunction... and...

Sexual dysfunction

K Esposito et al. Hyperlipidemia and sexual function in premenopausal women. *J Sex Med.* 2009 Jun;6(6):1696-703.

"Women with hyperlipidemia [high cholesterol] have significantly lower FSFI-domain scores [Female Sexual Function Index] as compared with age-matched women without hyperlipidemia... women with hyperlipidemia reported **significantly lower arousal, orgasm, lubrication, and satisfaction** scores than control women. Based on the total FSFI score, 51% of women with hyperlipidemia had scores of 26 or less, indicating sexual dysfunction, as compared with 21% of women without hyperlipidemia."

Esposito et al set very high LDL-cholesterol levels, so the chances are the 21% mentioned above also weren't Planters (who are the only people to have optimum animal fat and cholesterol intakes of zero.)

SIDS (Sudden Infant Death Syndrome) ~ Crib Death

J Wasilewska et al. Cow's-milk-induced infant apnoea with increased serum content of bovine β-casomorphin-5. *J Pediatr Gastroenterol Nutr.* 2011 Jun;52(6):772-5.

"We report a case of a breast-fed infant with recurrent apnoea episodes, which have always been preceded by his mother's consumption of fresh cows' milk. A biochemical examination has revealed a high level of β-casomorphin-5 (BCM-5) in the child's serum. We speculate that it is an opioid activity that may have a depressive effect on the respiratory centre of the central nervous system and induce a phenomenon called milk apnoea."

This is how the casomorphin in cows' milk depresses the breathing center in the brains of infants, causing them to die suddenly in their sleep.

Stroke (Cerebrovascular "disease")

JD Spence, DJA Jenkins, J Davignon. Egg yolk consumption and carotid plaque. *Atherosclerosis* 2012 224(2):469–473.

"TPA [total plaque area, a measure of ill-health in the carotid arteries supplying blood to the brain] increases exponentially with smoking pack-years [a measure of cigarette smoking]. TPA increases exponentially with egg-yolk years. The effect size of egg yolks appears to be approximately 2/3 that of smoking. Probably egg yolks should be avoided by persons at risk of vascular disease."

Who's at risk of vascular "disease", putting themselves at risk of stroke? Meaters and Junkers. And Smokers. So, to prevent strokes, who shouldn't eat eggs? People who eat eggs!

Sudden Cardiac Death

Kong MH, Fonarow GC, Peterson ED, Curtis AB, Hernandez AF, Sanders GD, Thomas KL, Hayes DL, Al-Khatib SM. Systematic review of the incidence of sudden cardiac death in the United States. *J Am Coll Cardiol.* 2011 Feb 15;57(7):794-801.

"In the United States, cardiovascular disease was the underlying cause of one of every 2.9 deaths occurring in 2006. The proportion of these deaths that is sudden has been estimated to be as high as 50%, making sudden cardiac death (SCD) the most common cause of death in this country."

One of several reasons why Meaters and Junkers are more prone to SCD is because of a deficiency in magnesium, the metal at the heart of the chlorophyll molecule. Understandably, as chlorophyll is the green pigment in plants, Planters aren't deficient in magnesium.

M Guasch-Ferre et al, PREDIMED Study Group. Dietary Magnesium Intake Is Inversely Associated with Mortality in Adults at High Cardiovascular Disease Risk 1. *J Nutr.* 2014 Jan;144(1):55-60.

"Dietary magnesium intake was inversely associated with mortality risk in Mediterranean individuals at high risk of CVD [cardiovascular disease].

Ulcerative colitis

A Birkett, J Muir, J Phillips, G Jones, K O'Dea. Resistant starch lowers fecal concentrations of ammonia and phenols in humans. *Am J Clin Nutr.* 1996 May;63(5):766-72.

"During the high-RS [resistant starch] diet daily excretion of fecal nitrogen increased… and excretion of fecal phenols fell … Fecal concentrations of ammonia decreased… and phenols decreased… pH decreased from 6.4… to 6.2… during the high-RS period. These results suggest that RS significantly attenuates the accumulation of potentially harmful byproducts of protein fermentation in the human colon."

For colon health, Meating bad, Planting good.

SU Christi et al. Antagonistic effects of sulfide and butyrate on proliferation of colonic mucosa: a potential role for these agents in the pathogenesis of ulcerative colitis. *Dig Dis Sci.* 1996 Dec;41(12):2477-81.

"…feces of patients with ulcerative colitis uniformly contain sulfate reducing bacteria. Sulfide produced by these bacteria… may be involved in the pathogenesis of ulcerative colitis… Our data support a possible role of sulfide in the pathogenesis of UC and confirm the role of butyrate in the regulation of colonic proliferation and in the treatment of UC."

Again, Planting feeds our gut bacteria and they produce beneficial butyrate, while Meating produces pathogenic hydrogen sulfide.

Urinary tract infections (UTIs)

L. Jakobsen et al. Is Escherichia coli urinary tract infection a zoonosis? Proof of direct link with production animals and meat. *Eur. J. Clin. Microbiol. Infect. Dis.* 2012 31(6):1121 – 1129.

"This study showed a clonal link between E. coli from meat and humans, providing solid evidence that UTI is zoonosis [animal-borne disease]."

Bacteria from animals, particularly chickens, cause urinary tract infections in ten million American Meater women each year.

Bacterial vaginosis

N. Ahluwalia, H. Grandjean. Nutrition, an under-recognized factor in bacterial vaginosis. *J. Nutr.* 2007 137(9):1997 - 1998

"…lower serum concentrations of vitamins A, C, and E, and b-carotene were associated with BV, and lower iron status… was associated with increased prevalence of Candida colonization."

The more nutrient-dense our diet is, and the higher the pH of our vaginas remains, the less we'll suffer from bacterial infections of the vagina. In other words… the more Planter our diet is, the healthier our vaginas.

Being high in saturated fats, both Junking (cakes and cookies) and Meating (dairy and chickens) tend to raise vaginal pH and encourage unhealthy bacteria to blossom.

Yeast infections ~ *Candida*

LA David et al. Diet rapidly and reproducibly alters the human gut microbiome. *Nature* 505, 559–563 (23 January 2014).

"Significant increases in *Penicillium*-related fungi were observed, along with significant decreases in the concentration of *Debaryomyces* and a *Candida* sp."

Part of the reason why Planters get fewer yeast infections is that our gut bacteria are unfriendly to pathogenic species of yeasts and friendly to beneficial species. *Candida albicans* et al can only flourish and 'bloom' in conditions made propitious for them by Meating or Junking.

~

References to papers on animal deficiencies

MH Carlsen et al. The total antioxidant content of more than 3100 foods, beverages, spices, herbs and supplements used worldwide. *Nutr J*. 2010 Jan 22;9:3.

"…there are several thousand-fold differences in antioxidant content of foods. Spices, herbs and supplements include the most antioxidant rich products in our study, some exceptionally high. Berries, fruits, nuts, chocolate, vegetables and products thereof constitute common foods and beverages with high antioxidant values.

This database is to our best knowledge the most comprehensive Antioxidant Food Database published and it shows that **plant-based foods introduce significantly more antioxidants into human diet than non-plant foods** [animals]."

Also, it's important to "understand the role of dietary phytochemical antioxidants in the prevention of cancer, cardiovascular diseases, diabetes and other **chronic diseases related to oxidative stress**."

The animals we eat **cause oxidative stress** and are pathetically deficient in antioxidants. Some plants contain more than one hundred thousand times as many antioxidants as animals do; but to be fair, on average, the common food plants we eat most often contain about 64 times more antioxidants than their animal counterparts.

Animals are poor food substitutes and should be treated as emergency rations only.

Nishi K, Kondo A, Okamoto T, Nakano H, Daifuku M, Nishimoto S, Ochi K, Takaoka T, Sugahara T. Immunostimulatory in vitro and in vivo effects of a water-soluble extract from kale. *Biosci Biotechnol Biochem*. 2011;75(1):40-6.

"Since IgA [immunoglobulin A, an antibody produced by plasma, or white blood cells] is the predominant Ig in normal intestinal mucosa, accounting for 70-90% of all Igs in GALT [gut-associated lymphoid tissue, the gastrointestinal tract's immune system] and thus plays a pivotal role in host defense, the intake of kale might provide a beneficial effect on humans to enhance the defense against such pathogens as viruses, bacteria and toxins [all of which come overwhelmingly from animals]. The immune-stimulating effect will provide an additional advantage of kale, as well as its antioxidative capacity and other effects."

Animals provide the antigens, or foreign attackers; plants provide the antibodies, or local defense force. So which is food?

Chen T, Yan F, Qian J, Guo M, Zhang H, Tang X, Chen F, Stoner GD, Wang X. Randomized phase II trial of lyophilized strawberries in patients with dysplastic precancerous lesions of the esophagus. *Cancer Prev Res* (Phila). 2012 Jan;5(1):41-50.

Strawberries are protective against esophageal cancer. Not this or that or the other extracted, refined chemical from strawberries: whole strawberries.

Animals cause cancers; plants heal them.

SS Percival et al. Bioavailability of Herbs and Spices in Humans as Determined by ex vivo Inflammatory Suppression and DNA Strand Breaks. *J Am Coll Nutr.* 2012 31(4):288-294.

Don't get put off by the technical language; just take in the fact that the named herbs and spices protect us against DNA damage and cancer:

"Herbs and spices that protected PBMCs against DNA strand breaks were **paprika**, **rosemary**, **ginger**, heat-treated **turmeric**, **sage**, and **cumin**. **Paprika** also appeared to protect cells from normal apoptotic processes... **Clove**, **ginger**, **rosemary**, and **turmeric** were able to significantly reduce oxidized LDL-induced expression of TNF-α.

Serum from those consuming **ginger** reduced all three inflammatory biomarkers. **Ginger**, **rosemary**, and **turmeric** showed protective capacity by both oxidative protection and inflammation measures."

Plants are anti-oxidant, anti-inflammatory and DNA-protective; animals are oxidizing, inflammatory and DNA-disruptive.

Bailey SJ, Winyard P, Vanhatalo A, Blackwell JR, Dimenna FJ, Wilkerson DP, Tarr J, Benjamin N, Jones AM. Dietary nitrate supplementation reduces the O_2 cost of low-intensity exercise and enhances tolerance to high-intensity exercise in humans. *J Appl Physiol.* 2009 Oct;107(4):1144-55.

Now this would seem to be a very important nutrition and sports physiology paper, but I've never seen or heard it mentioned by a single Low-Carb Bullshit Artist, even the world-famous sports physiologists among them.

It appears that beets, beet greens, arugula and other high-nitrate plants can boost our arterial production of NO (nitric oxide) and cause our arteries to dilate to such an extent and supply our muscle cells with so much oxygen that we can do remarkable athletic feats, previously thought to be impossible. For one, we can perform the same amount of work while using less oxygen. For another, we can significantly extend our time to exhaustion while doped up with leafy greens.

Endurance athletes should be greening up as well as carbo-loading. As Michael Greger puts it: "Beets [have been] found to significantly improve athletic performance while reducing oxygen needs, upsetting a fundamental tenet of sports physiology." It's a wee bit technical, but I urge anyone interested in peak performance to read this paper.

Bailey et al say: "It should be stressed that the remarkable reduction in the O_2 cost of submaximal cycle exercise following dietary supplementation with inorganic nitrate in the form of a natural food product cannot be achieved by any other known means, including long-term endurance exercise training."

I'll translate into English from Bailey's low-key science-speak: "This is freaking amazing! We thought this was impossible… rewrite all the sports physiology books."

Animals don't do this, because they're not food. Only whole plants truly nourish human beings.

And that's me done with providing references to great 'microscopic' science. It's time now to break out our endoscopes… our gastroscopes and enteroscopes, depending on which end we're going to scope, front or rear, top or bottom.

~

All together now…

Now that we've gotten all the reductionist science out of the way, let's look at the big picture of nutrition.

We don't eat single 'nutrients'; we eat foods or non-foods; plants or animals and junk, and they contain different groups of nutrients and non-nutrients.

Studying each dietary 'ingredient' individually, in a reductionist manner, is obviously helpful, but we need to see how they all work together if we're to understand how the human organism works as a gestalt.

We don't eat saturated or trans fats or cholesterol on their own. The animals that contain these non-nutrients also harbor cadaverine, putrescine, alpha-gal, amyloid, arachidonic acid, estrogens, harmane, purines, sulfur-containing amino acids and dozens of the other malefic Meater components which we met in Part 1; plus some of the dozens of pathogenic germs and worms we met in Part 2, plus a whole slew of the environmental poisons we met in Part 3. And they all collaborate to harm us, their total carnage being way worse than the sum of their toxic parts.

Imagine for a moment that we're in an auto workshop. A mechanic is working there on a PVT, a 'post-vintage thoroughbred,' a beaut of a car not old enough to be called vintage. [Like me.] She's taken all the pieces apart, and laid them lovingly out on a giant tarp, ready to check and refurbish and oil them, before she puts the whole thing back together again. It looks like a real-life exploded diagram, only without the labels.

Okay, that's what I've done so far with animals and, to a lesser extent, junk. I've laid out all the parts, like the TMAO, the heme iron, the heterocyclic amines – they're all lying there, waiting for me to reassemble them.

All that's passed has been prolog to this moment, in which I try to emulate Prof. T. Colin Campbell's *Whole* approach to nutrition. Keeping in mind that the processes I'm about to describe take place together or shortly after each other, and that some of the processes can build up over decades of Meater mal-nutrition, let's see what happens when we put pieces of animal in our mouths and swallow them.

Here goes…

Down the hatch…

A Turd's Eye View of an Animal Meal

Meating's effects on ingestion, digestion, metabolism and excretion

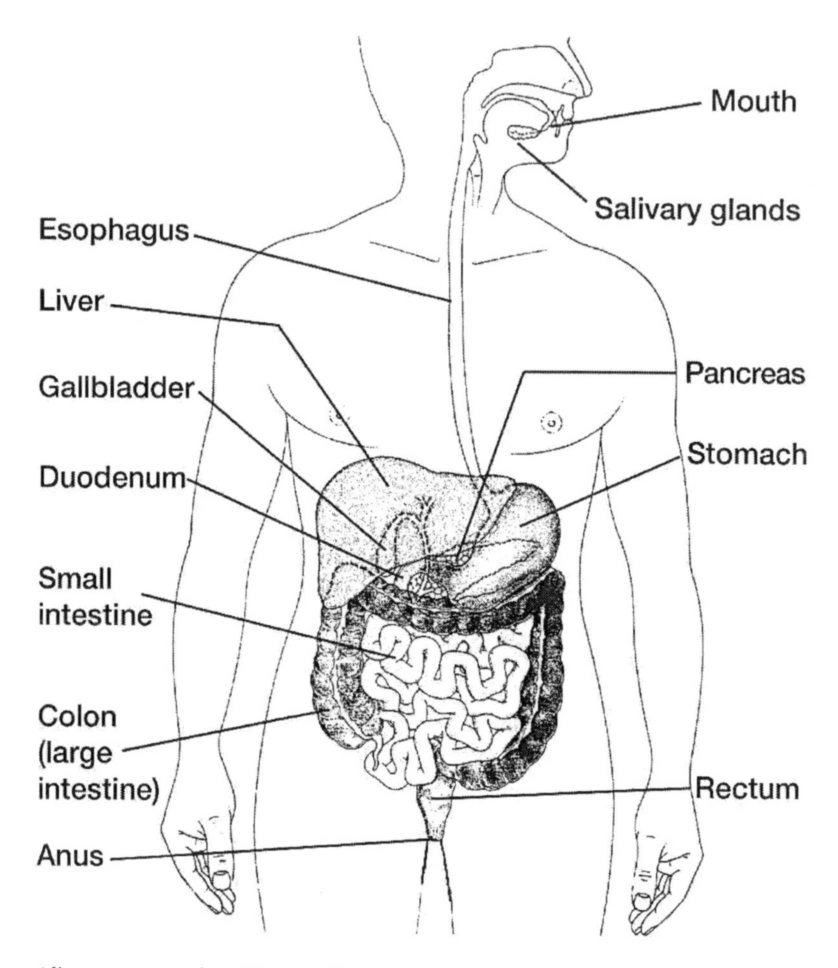

Alimentary, my dear Watson (Source unknown – my apologies – please let me know if it's yours and I'll remedy the situation.)

The Mouth

If we recall from the opening paragraph of Michael Moss's *Salt Sugar Fat*, "Our bodies are hard-wired for sweets." Our mouths are all about sugar. Carbohydrate digestion begins immediately. There are barely any sugars in animals besides some glycogen in their muscles and lactose, so only milk-fed human babies begin digesting energy-rich animal sugars straight away. In adults, sugars come from whole plants, or should.

There are three types of salivary glands in the mouth: the sublingual (below the tongue), the submandibular (below the lower jaw bone, or mandible) and the parotid, the largest ones in our cheeks. Their watery secretions contain the carb-cracking enzyme salivary amylase, a.k.a. ptyalin.

Our teeth – of which we have two matching plates of 16, top and bottom – are outstanding slicers and grinders of fibrous plants, with their tough cellulose cell walls. They're not very well adapted to tearing and chewing animals, the cells of which have outer membranes rather than walls.

The shape and size and spacing of our teeth, and our jaw musculature and hinging, allowing for side-to-side motion, also reflect our essential Planter nature.

On page 5 of his "The Comparative Anatomy of Eating," Dr. Milton Mills says:

> "Human teeth are also similar to those found in other herbivores with the exception of the canines (the canines of some of the apes are elongated and are thought to be used for display and/or defense). Our teeth are rather large and usually abut against one another. The incisors are flat and spade-like, useful for peeling, snipping and biting relatively soft materials. The canines are neither serrated nor conical, but are flattened, blunt and small and function like incisors. The premolars and molars are squarish, flattened and nodular, and used for crushing, grinding and pulping non-coarse foods."
>
> Human saliva contains the carbohydrate-digesting enzyme, salivary amylase. This enzyme is responsible for the majority of starch digestion."

On page 2, Dr. Mills says:

> "The saliva of carnivorous animals does not contain digestive enzymes. When eating, a mammalian carnivore gorges itself rapidly and does not chew its food. Since proteolytic (protein-digesting) enzymes cannot be liberated in the mouth due to the danger of autodigestion (damaging the oral cavity), carnivores do not need to mix their food with saliva; they simply bite off huge chunks of meat and swallow them whole."

We don't have to travel very far through the digestive tract to realize that – based on our physiology and anatomy – we're not Meaters. Just because we practice omnivorism doesn't make us functional omnivores.

(That some Meaters claim we're supposed to eat animals because we have teeth called canines is hilarious. Our canines are sometimes called 'eye teeth.' Does that mean I'll be able to see in the dark if I walk around with my mouth open?)

Nevertheless (after we've stabbed the beast with our steely knives instead of using our teeth for the initial slicing), our jaws and teeth are versatile enough to allow us to break down animals mechanically into swallowable pieces. And then our saliva coats them and makes them easier to swallow.

Before that happens, the introduction of unfriendly bacteria can disturb the beneficial bacteria that live around our tongues, which are responsible for nitrate metabolism and NO production, so important for arterial dilation.

A mouthful of animal alerts our immune system to the presence of antigens (foreign invaders) and may start producing antibodies. Aphthous ulcers, or canker sores are, most often, an immune response to dairy products.

When it's time to swallow, our tongues and cheeks and palates all get in on the action, and the mouthful moves past the epiglottis, through the pharynx (preferably not into the larynx, or wind pipe in front of it) and into…

The Esophagus

The esophagus is a muscular, pink 18-inch-long tube that connects our throats to our stomachs. Proving that we come from outer space, our esophagi can propel food upward against gravity, when we're upside down, by muscular contractions similar to peristalsis in our intestines. (Kidding.) Its narrow diameter is best adapted to passing well-chewed fibrous plants, not large chunks of flesh. 99.9999% of the time, or so, Meaters survive the swallowing process. Occasionally we choke to death on a gobbet of flesh, if un-Heimliched, or we get punctured by a bone.

The esophagus passes through our chest cavities, in between the lungs, then behind our hearts and through the sheet of muscle that controls our breathing – the diaphragm – and so into our stomachs, in our abdomens. The hole in the diaphragm through with the esophagus passes is called the esophageal hiatus. At the bottom of the esophagus is a ring of muscles that closes up to prevent acid from the stomach refluxing into the esophagus.

We'll come back to hiatus hernia and gastro-esophageal reflux disease later.

The Stomach

When a bolus, or ball of anything we eat hits our stomach after transiting the esophagus, protein digestion begins. Our stomach linings are amazing. They're made out of proteins and yet they're able to secrete hydrochloric acid and a stew of protein-cracking enzymes – pepsin, trypsin and chymotrypsin – without auto-digesting themselves.

They do this in a most cunning way. There are mucus-secreting cells that provide a barrier against the food/acid/enzyme mix and, also, the acid is secreted in such a way that it only becomes activated in the lumen, or chamber, of the stomach. Amazing.

Protein breakdown happens in three ways – via acid and enzymes, and also by the churning action of the stomach. It's a muscular pouch and its internal surface has folds, or rugae, which act in the same way as the turbulence-creating vertical fins in blenders to mix things up well.

While quite acidic, our gastric juices are nowhere as low in pH (more acidic) as those of omnivores or carnivores. Even so, the higher protein load of animals is problematic, in that it requires a more acidic environment and a longer time to break down the peptide chains of amino acids. Meaters are more prone to ulceration. (Aspirin-taking Meaters are much more prone to ulcers than Planters, who get their salicylic acid from plants.)

Animals stay in our stomachs for longer than plants, because Meaters are getting up to triple the amount of proteins than Planters do, and both groups in the US are eating more than is necessary. "Getting our protein" is a persistent myth. It would take great skill to plan a diet that didn't provide enough proteins if we're eating enough calories.

Going back to the esophagus. Over time, a constant assault of animals and junk such as hot beverages, alcohol, phosphoric acid-containing sodas and overly hot (as in spicy) foods can damage the relatively weak muscles of the lower esophageal sphincter (LES), allowing stomach acid to reflux into the esophagus, especially when we lie down.

Unlike the stomach, the esophagus has no mucous barrier to acid, and the acid can burn the inner lining of cells and cause bleeding, a condition called esophagitis, and, if it continues, cause a long-term inflammatory condition known as GERD, or gastro-esophageal reflux disease, which in turn can become chronic Barrett's esophagus or even lethal esophageal cancer.

Fortunately, we can minimize the dangers of these conditions. The main reason we create stomach acid is to deal with proteins. Firstly, animals contain more than plants. Secondly, we eat way more animals than we need. So, if we're Planting we get about half the proteins that Meaters consume (and that's probably still more than we need). That's helpful when we're faced with GERD or cancer.

In his terrific video, *Digestion Made Easy – A Journey Through Your Amazing Digestive System*, Michael Klaper, MD, suggests we do the following to combat GERD:

- raise the head of our beds 4 to 6 inches to prevent reflux at night;
- eat high-protein meals early in the day; high-carb in the evenings;
- try "herbal considerations" such as slippery elm, deglycyrrhizinated licorice (DGL) and cabbage juice;
- get a test done for *Helicobacter pylori*, an ulcer-causing bacterium;
- as a last resort, use acid-blocking drugs for the six weeks or so it takes our esophagi to rejuvenate.

The other problem I alluded to before – hiatus or hiatal hernia – is one of the pressure "diseases" we encountered earlier when we discussed constipation. Constipation (which is common among Meaters and Junkers) or being obese (not a Planter condition) can create sufficient pressure to force a part of our stomach or esophagus (which are supposed to stay below our diaphragms in our abdomens) up through the esophageal hiatus – the gap in the diaphragm through which the esophagus passes – and into our chest cavities or thoraxes. The LES, or lower esophageal sphincter then loses all function and reflux occurs as a matter of course, and most every time we lie down.

Meating + Junking → constipation + obesity → hiatus hernia → esophagitis → GERD → esophageal cancer.

We need to snap this chain, as early as possible. To me that doesn't mean taking fiber supplements or going on a weight-loss diet; it means stopping Meating and Junking.

Our meal is now ready to leave the stomach. The animal parts we're following have had their proteins cracked into smaller peptide units, made up of shorter strings of amino acids. Nothing much has happened to fats other than being churned into smaller droplets: no chemical breakdown yet.

(Carbohydrate digestion, which starts in the vaguely alkaline mouth, lies dormant in the highly acidic stomach, as the amylase enzyme is diluted and deactivated.)

The next stop on the digestion train is the small intestine, specifically the C-shaped first 12 inches called the duodenum (the Greek for 12 inches being 'duodeni.') The last station in the stomach is the very strong muscular sphincter at the bottom end of the stomach, the pyloric sphincter. But there's a problem.

The Duodenum

Form follows function… and the function of the duodenum is to continue cracking carbs and proteins, while starting to crack fats. It works best at an alkaline pH. Because of its function, the duodenum's form lacks mucus-secreting cells, so how are we going to keep it safe from the acid we're about to inject?

Ladies and gentlemen, I give you…

The Pancreas

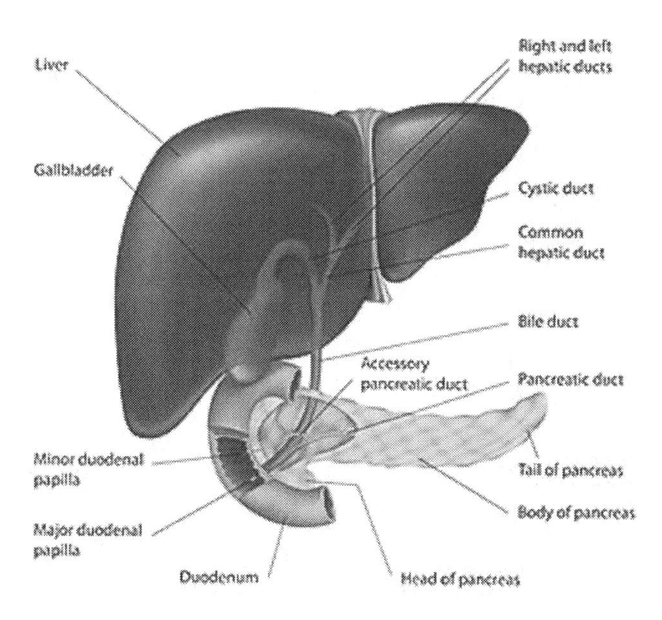

Liver, gallbladder et al. http://images.medicinenet.com/images/appictures/liver-disease-s2-what-is-liver-disease.jpg

The pancreas is a glandular organ that nestles within the curve of the duodenum, behind the stomach

When the stomach's work is done, the pyloric sphincter opens briefly and it jets through a tablespoon or two of chyme, a gruel of semi-digested, acidified nutrients, into the duodenum.

At the same time, our new friend, the pancreas, secretes a dose of digestive enzymes into the duodenum, along with a spritz of bicarbonate, which has a pH of 8.8. When chyme meets pancreatic juices, pancreatic juices win and neutralize the acid, and the pH of the duodenum settles down to about 8.0, which is the perfect alkalinity for carbohydrate digestion to continue. (7 is neutral.)

The glands that make up the pancreas come in two varieties: endocrine (which secrete their hormones directly into the bloodstream) and exocrine (which secrete their enzymes into ducts). The digestive enzymes come from the pancreas's alpha- or exocrine glands; two hormones – insulin and glucagon – come from the beta- or endocrine cells in the islets of Langerhans within the pancreas.) We'll have a lot more to say later about insulin and it's less famous reciprocal, glucagon.

The pancreas secretes about 8 cups of juice a day. The digestive enzymes in it are

- Amylase, which continues the breakdown of carbohydrates (starch) into simple sugars, begun by salivary amylase;
- Proteases, which break proteins and peptides into amino acids. They also help combat parasites such as yeast, bacteria and protozoa (which are made out of proteins); and
- Lipase, which helps break down fats.

That's the order in which digestion proceeds – carbs first, then proteins, then fats – and that should give us some idea about their relative physiological importance: carbs to power us; proteins for making enzymes and (a little) for meat-making; and fats for future energy storage, and other jobs like maintaining cell membranes and nerve sheaths.

So, in the duodenum, starch and protein digestion continue, and fat digestion begins. Again, fats are more complicated than starch and protein.

Our intestines and bloodstreams are watery, or aqueous environments, and oil and water don't mix. So we need a detergent to emulsify the fats to make them water-soluble. Enter…

The Liver and Gallbladder

The liver is our "master chemist": it takes in all the nutrients we eat and digest and take up in our blood, and from them it creates thousands of different useful compounds. (There is a porous membrane which allows just-about-everything to enter the liver – this makes it susceptible to damage by toxins such as industrial pollutants and alcohol.)

One hepatic compound we're interested in for digestion is a yellowish fluid called bile, or gall. The liver takes cholesterol and makes bile out of it.

When some chyme enters the duodenum, our pancreases release alkaline pancreatic juices full of enzymes. The lipase starts fat breakdown, releasing smaller fat droplets.

At the same time, the liver releases bile into its duct system, it flows down (past a turnoff to the gallbladder, the between-meal storage depot for bile) and enters the duodenum at the sphincter of Oddi. Bile is electrically charged, with positive and negative ends. The negative ends attach to fat droplets, leaving the positive ends to interact with water (consisting of H^+ and O^- ions.) The fats are now soluble in the water and can be absorbed into the bloodstream and transported to the liver.

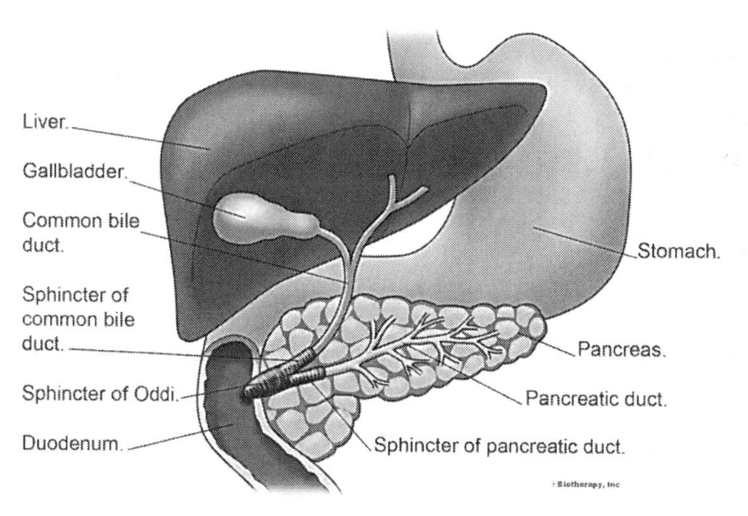

The Sphincter of Oddi, at the end of the common bile duct and the pancreatic duct - irishdysautonomia.wordpress.com

When we've finished processing the entire meal, bile continues to collect in the bile duct system above the sphincter of Oddi. When it meets the turnoff to the gallbladder, instead of backing up into the liver, it heads up the side duct and gets stored in the gallbladder. At the onset of digestion of the next meal, the gallbladder squeezes a spritz of bile back down the duct and into the duodenum.

Gallstones

Meating and Junking cause problems in the biliary system by providing excess cholesterol. When we eat animal and junk fats (saturated and trans fats, and hydrogenated oils) we stimulate the liver to produce excess cholesterol. There's only so much cholesterol that bile salts can hold in solution and, when the bile is saturated, cholesterol crystallizes out and forms gallstones. Besides being excruciating – imagine the feeling when the gallbladder contracts and tries to shove large crystalline stones down a narrow pipe – the stones get covered with intestinal bacteria, causing inflammation and infection. Over time, the gallbladder lining is destroyed and loses all function. Every year >700,000 American Meaters and Junkers have their gallbladders surgically removed.

Gallstones aren't the only problem though…

Animals and junk contain no fiber. Fiber is the indigestible-by-humans-but-digestible-by-healthy-gut-bacteria starch found in whole plants. Not only does it have valuable, unique nutrients bound to it; not only does it bulk out our stools and make them easy to pass; fiber acts as a brush that sweeps through our intestines, binding up excess cholesterol and heavy metals and other nasties, and otherwise keeping our guts (and us) healthy.

Fiber performs a host of important functions:

- Because whole plants are low in energy and high in bulk, our stomachs fill up sooner, giving us a sense of fullness or satiety
- It bulks out our stools, making them activate the pressure receptors in our bowels, telling peristaltic waves to move our garbage along
- It holds more moisture, making our stools softer and easier to evacuate
- It binds up heavy metals, excess cholesterol and carcinogenic bile acids
- It removes excess carcinogenic estrogens from our system

- It creates a health gut flora, which keeps pathogenic strains of microbes in check, preventing intestinal and extra-intestinal infections; the ones which kill tens of thousands of Meaters annually, and
- It feeds our gut flora, which in turn produce cancer-fighting substance such as butyrate and lignans.

High fiber diets and healthy intestines are synonymous. Meating and Junking are potentially lethal fiber-deficiency diseases.

What we eat affects our

Transit time

When we're Planters, a meal takes 24 hours to enter our mouths, be digested and absorbed, and for our fecal waste to exit our poop chutes. Meaters and Junkers can take a week or more to expel a meal. That's asking for trouble: days of extra, unnecessary exposure to carcinogens, parasites and toxins. Constipation helps cause cancer.

We're not just what we eat. And we're not just what we absorb. We are what we don't excrete. When we're constipated, we don't excrete a whole lot… which you can read either way you like.

Meating creates constipation. Anyone who isn't having at least one excellent bowel movement a day is ill. To have only a single bowel movement a week, as happens to many Meaters, isn't only to be full of shit; it's to court dis-ass-ster [dis-arse-ster in the UK]. Sorry, it's not a laughing matter.

If we're constipated, we know we're malnourished, and mal-nutrition is what causes heart "disease", stroke, cancer, hypertension, and the endless roll call of "diseases" of Western civilization. We're eating ourselves to death, and constipation is a fire alarm that should cause us to exit the building; instead, to our peril, we switch off the smoke detector with drugs or supplements and ignore it.

Our health is in our own hands. We can either eat whole plants, especially water- and fiber-rich fruit, and not cause constipation or cancer, or we can buy supplements from the Atkins or paleo punters to try and reverse the constipating and cancer-causing conditions their dietstyles cause.

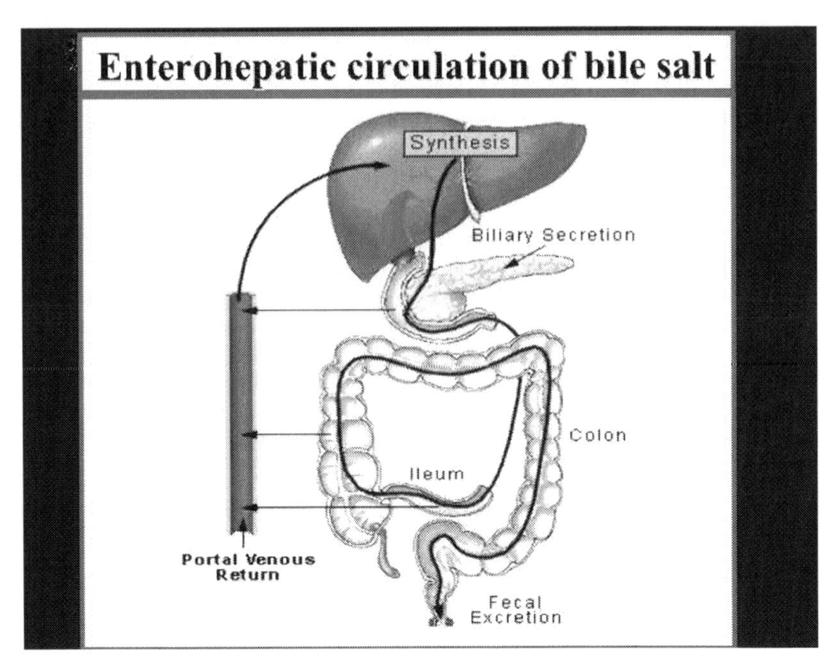

Enterohepatic circulation of bile salt. Image: slideshare.net

Our bodies are conservative, in more ways than one. They don't do radical. And they conserve the nutrients and metabolites they need. Why excrete stuff if you can use it again?

The enterohepatic circulation of bile

Enterohepatic means 'gut – liver.' Most of our bile gets recycled. Before the end of the small intestine, which we're about to get up close to, the bile passes through the gut wall along with absorbed nutrients and gets collected in larger and larger veins until the portal vein enters the liver, where it then fans out and floods our liver cells with nutrients. Our hepatocytes (liver cells) extract the bile and send it back into the duct system for reuse. Excess bile gets discharged into the fecal stream in the large intestine and gets pooped out. Which is good because excess causes cancer. Meaters and Junkers have far more in their feces, and it spends more time there. Hence, their increased risk of colorectal and other cancers.

Breast and prostate cancer

As we saw earlier, women who have few bowel movements are at much greater risk of developing breast cancer. Excess carcinogenic bile acids and carcinogenic cholesterol and carcinogenic estrogens don't get swept out of us when we're fiber-deficient Meaters and Junkers; they re-enter our blood and become hyper-concentrated in breast and prostate tissue at 100x the external level. When we're Planters we have lots of fiber in our guts, which flush out these noxious chemicals. Breast cancer is largely an eating disorder.

Not only does everything happen at once; all parts of us are connected to all the other parts of us – our blood flows everywhere – and what happens in our bowels affects all our body systems. Moving on…

The Small Intestine

The small intestine is the miraculous place where macro-nutrient absorption takes place. By now we've broken down our proteins, starch and fats into their basic units. The small intestine is where these units pass through the gut wall and enter the blood, and make their way to the liver for metabolism.

The small intestine, of which the duodenum is the first foot, is 22 to 30 feet long (or 7 to 9 meters) and its inner lining consists of bajillions of sea anemone-like projections called villi that increase its absorptive area by orders of magnitude. According to Michael Klaper, we each have 'half an NFL football field' of absorptive area in our small intestines.

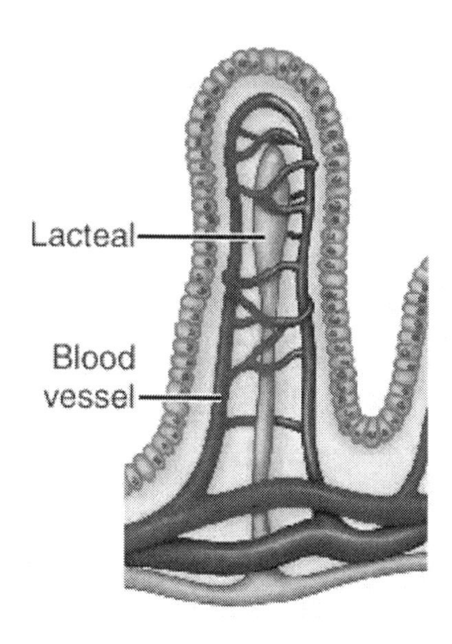

A villus. http://medical-dictionary.thefreedictionary.com/villus

Sugars and amino acids pass through the villi walls and get taken up in the venous return system and make their way to the liver. Fats definitely suffer from the fear of being ordinary: their absorption is different to starch and protein. Instead of entering the veins in the villi, they enter lacteals.

A lacteal is a lymphatic vessel that conveys chyle. And chyle, according to Dorland's Medical Dictionary is "the milky fluid taken up by the lacteals from food in the intestine, consisting of an emulsion of lymph and triglyceride fat (chylomicrons); it passes into the veins by the thoracic duct and mixes with blood," and then makes its way to the liver. There's always one…

The mesenteric system, or the hepatic portal system

As nutrients get absorbed into the villi's veins and lacteals, the blood flows into ever-larger mesenteric veins, which eventually join in our guts' Amazon river, the hepatic portal vein – the doorway to the liver.

By the time we reach the end of the narrow, long small intestine, all of the macronutrients have been absorbed, and most of the bile acids have been reabsorbed.

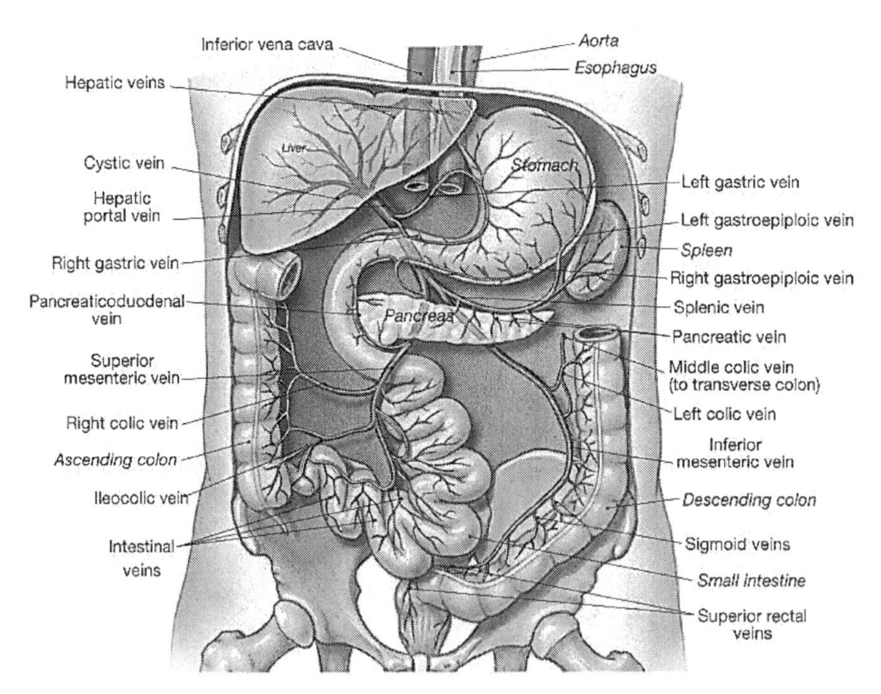

The mesenteric venous system: http://droualb.faculty.mjc.edu/

The terminal end of the small intestine – the ileum – meets the much wider, shorter larger large intestine, or colon, at the ileocecal junction. The first part of the large intestine is called the cecum.

In Planters, about 6 hours have gone by. Meaters and Junkers, with more fats and proteins to process, take hours longer.

PCRM describes the consequences of a high-fat meal very well. High-fat meals are usually Meater- and Junker-catered… Planters should be wary of vegetable oils – they're 100% fat.

The Good Stuff? Think Again…

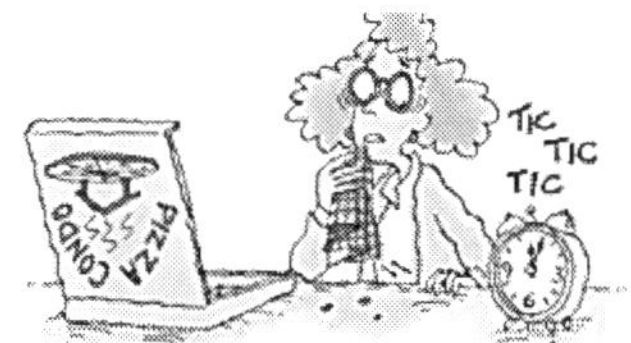

What Happens after Only One High-Fat Meal?

So you've just finished your high fat dinner of a hamburger, cheese pizza or chicken…
What's next?

Immediately…
- Your triglyceride levels, a measurement of fat in your bloodstream, are rising.
- Your cholesterol levels are increasing, contributing to plaque formation.
- Clotting factors in your blood have been activated.

Two hours later…
- Your triglycerides have increased by 60 percent.
- Your blood flow has decreased by half.

Three hours later…
- The lining of your arteries has lost elasticity impeding blood flow.
- Blood vessel function has become abnormal.

Four hours later…
- Your blood has gotten thicker, flowing even slower than it was 2 hours ago.

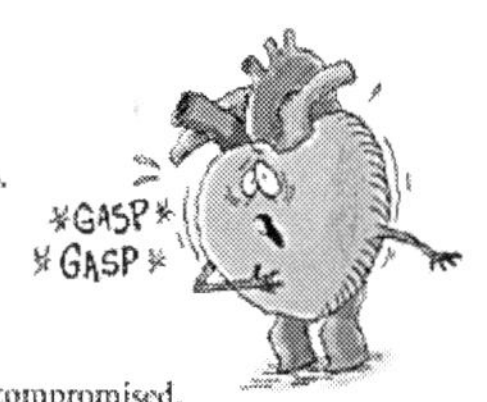

Five hours later…
- Your triglyceride levels have now increased by 150 percent.

Six hours later…
- The anti-inflammatory effect of "good" cholesterol has been significantly compromised.

Consumption of high-fat foods over days, weeks, months, years…
- Saturated fat in your diet has promoted the continuous buildup of plaque in your arteries, reducing blood flow even further.
- Decreased blood flow leads to decreased oxygen supply, which can lead to a heart attack.
- You are in danger of developing fatty liver disease.

Larsen LF, Bladbjer EM, Jespersen J, Marckmann P. Effects of dietary fat quality and quantity on postprandial activation of blood coagulation factor VII. *Arterioscler Thromb Vasc Biol.* 1997;17:2904-2909.

Vogel RA, Corretti MC, Plotnick GD. Effect of a single high-fat meal on endothelial function in healthy subjects. *Am J Cardiol.* 1997; 79:350-354.

Nicholls SJ, Lundman P, Harmer J, et al. Consumption of saturated fat impairs the anti-inflammatory properties of high-density lipoproteins and endothelial function. *J Am Coll Cardiol.* 2006; 48: 715-720.

Hozumi T, Eisenberg M, Sugioka K, et al. Change in coronary flow reserve on transthoracic Doppler echocardiography after a single high-fat meal in young healthy men. *Ann Intern Med.* 2002:136:523-528.

Post-prandial lipemia.
Source: PCRM (Physicians Committee for Responsible Medicine)

Now's a good time to talk about

Insulin resistance – pre-diabetes - diabetes

Besides producing digestive juices in its exocrine glands, the pancreas produces two hormones in its endocrine glands, which it secretes directly into our blood.

When glucose appears in our blood, it's the role of hormone #1, insulin, to deliver glucose to individual cells. Insulin uses a key to open a door in our cell membranes, it takes glucose through the door, and then, inside the city, it takes glucose to the cell's power plants, organelles called mitochondria. In the presence of oxygen, glucose gets burned up and produces energy molecules called ATP.

It's insulin's job to deal with glucose when it arrives. It lowers our blood sugar level.

Hormone #2 – glucagon – is the anti-matter to insulin's matter. It raises our blood sugar level when it falls too low. It does this by mobilizing sugar from glycogen, the small short-term sugar store in our muscles.

Insulin and glucagon work together to keep our blood sugar levels within a narrow healthy band.

Normally, glucose comes packaged with fiber and other phytonutrients, and it takes time to break down the starches. Normally, there's a slow, extended release of glucose over many hours. Junking – eating fiber-depleted plants – presents our bodies with an immediate blast of pre-digested glucose. Our blood sugar level spikes up – bang – causing our insulin level to spike up to remove the sugar from our blood – bang – then our blood sugars plummet again – bang – often dropping back below where we started, leaving us exhausted.

It's like teenage sex… wham, bam, thank you, ma'am, over in a flash, then you lie around, depleted, not knowing where to look or what to say.

Over the course of years, we may need to produce more insulin to get the same result. Sugar's just like any drug, that way. By constantly assaulting our pancreases with sugar, we may become resistant to insulin, and set ourselves up for diabetes.

But… that's only the Junker part of the story. Here's the Meater part.

It's not just sugar that causes us to release insulin. Because of the animal fats they contain, which insulin is responsible for ferrying into fat cells, and because of the amino acids they contain, which insulin moves into other body cells for growth and repair, the animals we eat cause an insulin spike similar to that caused by high-glycemic, processed carbs like white sugar. Even though they don't contain any carbs. Insulin isn't only about glucose. Try to find that tidbit in a Low-Carb Bullshit Artist's nutrition comic book.

Then, animal and junk fats cause insulin resistance. Fats block insulin's ability to ferry glucose into our muscle cells, and block insulin from ferrying glucose to our mitochondria inside our cells, causing our pancreases to increase insulin secretion and leading, long-term, to reduced sensitivity and type II diabetes. Nasty sequelae of diabetes – a Meater and Junker affliction – include arterial damage, heart "disease", blindness (diabetic retinopathy), kidney failure, amputations because of gangrene, and dementia.

And while the animal proteins may be damaging and lowering the effectiveness of our pancreatic insulin-making cells (even in cases where type 1 diabetes doesn't arise), the animal fats are sludging up our blood, coating our blood cells and making peripheral circulation difficult, gradually allowing the build-up of crut where it doesn't belong, damaging our eyes with drusen, and other delicate organs with lactic acid and other metabolites.

Insulin resistance is about 'meat + sweet.' It's about the two non-foods: animals *and* junk. Even if we avoid eating animals, we've still got to avoid Junking. Eating high-glycemic, highly processed, industrialized starches and sugars is a sure-fire recipe for IR, diabesity and diabetes.

For Meaters to blame diabetes entirely on 'carbs' is outright wrong. (Planters, the people who eat the highest whole-carb diets have the least obesity, diabetes, heart "disease", stroke, cancer and… you name it.) Still, it's possible for high-animal eaters to be healthy-looking in the short term, when they cut out Junking. Paleo dieters are essentially Planter/Meater hybrids, and they're healthy to the extent that they've cut out Junking, and to the extent that their Planting temporarily masks the ill-effects of Meating.

The process of diabetes can takes place over years and decades, so we're fooled into thinking we're healthy and strong until middle age arrives and, all of a sudden, things start going wrong. Not always decades though: kids now get 'adult onset' diabetes – it's the animals AND it's the junk, and it's the lack of vitamin X - exercise.

We shouldn't let the Low-Carb Bullshit Artists bullshit us that whole carbs cause diabetes. They don't.

Whole carbs are the only food.

Next stop…

The Large Intestine

The large intestine is described as having 5 parts:

- Ascending colon
- Transverse colon
- Descending colon
- Sigmoid colon [S-shaped]
- Rectum [Straight]

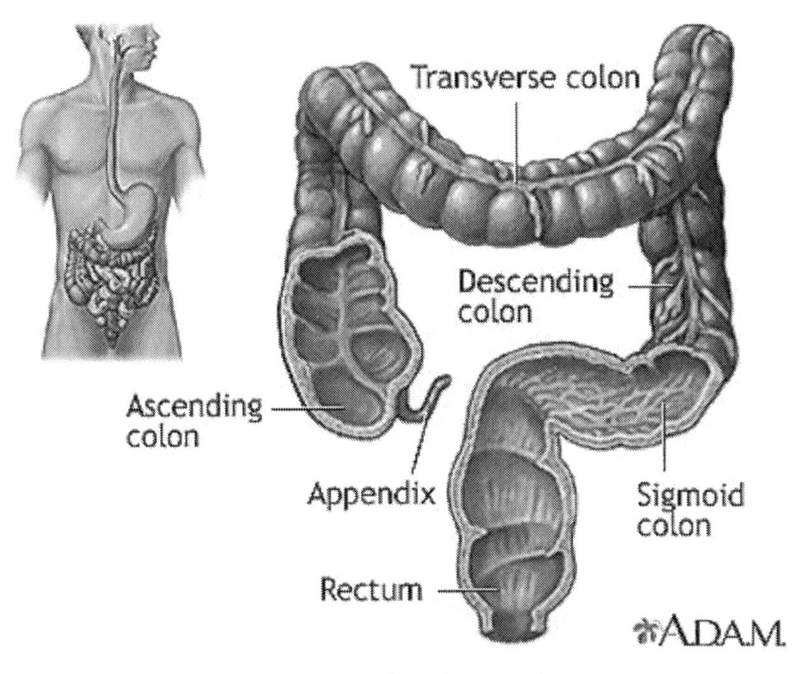

Large intestine:
MedlinePlus Medical Encyclopedia Image www.nlm.nih.gov

Again, form follows function. The colon's main job is to reabsorb water and to absorb electrolytes, so it doesn't need villi to maximize absorption. Most nutrient absorption happens in the small intestine. Compared to the rifled barrel of the small intestine, the colon is a smooth-bore shotgun. It does have concertina-like folds called haustra, which act like baffles to slow down the fecal stream, to maximize water absorption.

If it's taken 6 hours for a Planter mouthful to make it this far, the military principle now kicks in – hurry up and wait – and it'll take another 18 hours to travel the last 6 feet (or 2 meters). The 6 or so quarts (or liters) of water we reabsorb are crucial for us to stay alive: if we lose this precious water through diarrhea, we die, as do thousands of 3rd World children each day because of contaminated drinking water.

Several bad things go wrong for Meaters and Junkers in their colons because of inadequate fiber and inadequate water. Instead of having large, soft fiber-packed stools in their colons, Meaters have small, dense, impacted, fiber-depleted, hard stools. Our muscular guts move our shit along by contracting in waves. This is called peristalsis, which means 'to wrap around.' Our gut walls contract in segments and this segmentation squeezes our poop to the next station, which in turn segments.

Constipation makes it harder for our guts to move our shit towards the exit.

Water is the true macro-nutrient… water and air. Without water we die, quickly. So our bodies will instruct our colons to extract every last drop it can, when it's running low. This sets up a vicious cycle. The more water we extract from our feces, the harder they become and the more difficult it becomes to move them, and the longer they stay in our colons. So we become more dehydrated and our bodies reabsorb more water, and so on.

The Appendix

There's a hollow, worm-like, six-inch long appendage hanging off the bottom of the ascending colon. It's called the appendix, and it's not an unnecessary relic – it's an integral part of our immune system and a source of healthy gut bacteria, from which we can recolonize our colons after a bout of antibiotics wipes them out.

When our colons become filled with hard and hard-to-budge feces, the opening to the appendix can become blocked with shit – especially as the pressure we exert when we're constipated is far higher than is healthy. Inflammation and infection can result, causing us to double over in pain, sometimes vomit, and then end up on a surgeon's table undergoing an appendectomy. This happens frequently to Meaters and Junkers; rarely to Planters.

Fruit is the natural antidote to constipation (and therefore to appendicitis). Besides being full of phytonutrients, fruits are full of water and fiber.

Our fecal stream now moves up the ascending colon, across the transverse, and down the descending colon. (Masseurs learn to rub up on the right-hand side of our abdomens, across, and then down on the left, so that they're not going against the flow.) Most of the pressure problems we experience show up in the last foot or so of our colons, 80% of them from the sigmoid on.

Diverticulosis ~ diverticulitis

When we're 'straining at stool,' we're pushing hard wide masses into a narrow rectal chamber, with an even narrower anus door at the far end. Something's gotta give… and sometimes the something is our intestinal wall. Little pockets get blown out at weak points, forming one diverticulum, several diverticula.

(**Polyps** are something else. They're bumps in the colon which develop out of epithelial cells and may be precursors to cancer. Berries are great at regressing what Meating causes.)

As we'd expect, these balloons can fill up with shit, become enflamed and infected. Diverticulosis has morphed into diverticulitis. If a diverticulum ruptures, it can spill shit out into our abdominal cavities, cause a condition of sepsis known as peritonitis and kill us.

Because of its location, diverticulitis is sometimes called 'left-sided appendicitis.' Diverticulitis and appendicitis happen in different parts of the colon, but they have the same Meater/Junker Eatiology.

Diverticula also set us up for colorectal cancer, which erases tens of thousands of Meaters and Junkers each year.

Meating and Junking → fiber and water deficiency → constipation → pressure "diseases" including diverticulitis → colorectal cancer.

Diverticular "disease" goes away on a Planter diet. The diverticula close up and wither away. Why would that surprise us? They're caused by Meating and Junking.

Hemorrhoids (Piles)

Not all things hemorrhoidal are bad: we have hemorrhoidal arteries and veins at the end of our poop chutes, around our anuses. When we apply pressure to hard turds in our rectums, we can cut off the blood flow in our hemorrhoidal veins. The back pressure causes them to bulge and become permanently varicose, or distended. We can get hemorrhoids internally or externally, or both, and sometimes the internal ones can 'prolapse' or fall out of our asses, requiring someone to stuff them back in again.

If we undergo any of the many procedures to remove piles, while continuing to Meat and Junk, we haven't done anything to remove the underlying cause... we haven't removed from our butts the things that wrecked 'em to begin with.

Hemorrhoids go away on a Planter diet.

Other pressure "diseases"

The Meater and Junker pressure "diseases" we've met so far are:

- Constipation
- hiatal hernia
- (appendicitis)
- diverticulosis and –itis; peritonitis
- ulcerative colitis
- hemorrhoids

The same high pressure mechanism causes varicose veins in our legs. Sometimes people exert so much pressure when they're straining to poop, they burst blood vessels... and aneurysms can be deadly. Colorectal cancer may follow from colitis.

Constipation can be lethal. Meaters and Junkers are full of it. Planters go with the flow...

Fiber and our gut flora

Planting activates our immune system in our intestines – alerting us to an encounter with the outside environment. And Planting beneficially interacts with our DNA to epigenetically up- and down-grade the expression of a multitude of genes. Planting does one other amazing thing: it creates and maintains the **organ** known as the **microbiome**. Synonyms are gut flora; beneficial bacteria; good bacteria, etc.

Our microbiome is what separates the amateur eaters from the pros. Here, for the umpteenth and last time in this book, is my role model, Dr. Michael Greger, on the subject of the microbiome:

"Health-promoting effects of our good bacteria include boosting our immune system, improving digestion and absorption, making vitamins, inhibiting the growth of potential pathogens, and keeping us from feeling bloated, but should bad bacteria take roost, they can produce carcinogens, putrefy protein in our gut, produce toxins, mess up our bowel function, and cause infections."

[See: http://nutritionfacts.org/video/microbiome-the-inside-story/]

Planting gives us a healthy microbiome organ that makes anti-cancer and anti-inflammatory substances like lignans, butyrate, acetate and propionate. A low level of butyrate in our colons, which is indicative of low fiber intake (i.e. a low level of Planting) and a depleted gut flora, is what starts the inflammatory cascade that leads to inflammatory bowel "diseases" such as ulcerative colitis and Crohn's "disease", and colorectal cancer. Planting, in effect, controls our enteric immune system, keeping it off and keeping us healthy when fiber is abundant; switching it on and attacking our guts when we're fiber-deficient. Meating and Junking are fiber-free disaster zones.

Fiber- and phytate-deficient Junking and Meating also provoke our microbiome to emit H_2S (because of the animal proteins) and to create TMAO (from the carnitine and choline), causing cancer and damaging our entire arterial tree.

Planting acknowledges that we – humans, that is – are outnumbered in our own bodies by bacteria, which live mainly in our colons. Not to feed them the fiber they thrive on is to be at war with ourselves. They're Planters; we're Planters. The only way to eat sanely and be well is to co-operate with the fellow components of our bodies.

Planting acknowledges that there's ~150 to 300 times more bacterial DNA in us than there is human DNA. Not to feed our bacteria the plants that benefit both 'us' and 'them' epigenetically is to be schizophrenic and sick. They are us; we are them; and we all thrive on the same whole plants.

I think that everyone would agree that taking antibiotics constantly would be terribly bad for our health, particularly for the health of our intestinal bacteria. But wait a moment… eating animals *is* like taking antibiotics all the time. Meating kills our beneficial bacteria in exactly the same way as taking antimicrobial drugs! The animals we eat *are* antibiotics.

The microbiome at the terminus of our digestive tracts is fed and nourished by Planting. It responds by feeding and nourishing us. To be a Meater or a

Junker is to live in a house divided and, as Jesus says: "If a house is divided against itself, that house cannot stand."

Jesus' code of ethics includes "Thou shalt not kill" and "Do unto others as you would have them do unto you," golden rules that ethical Planters abide by naturally on all levels.

The Buddha says that to be a Planter "is to step into the stream which leads to nirvana."

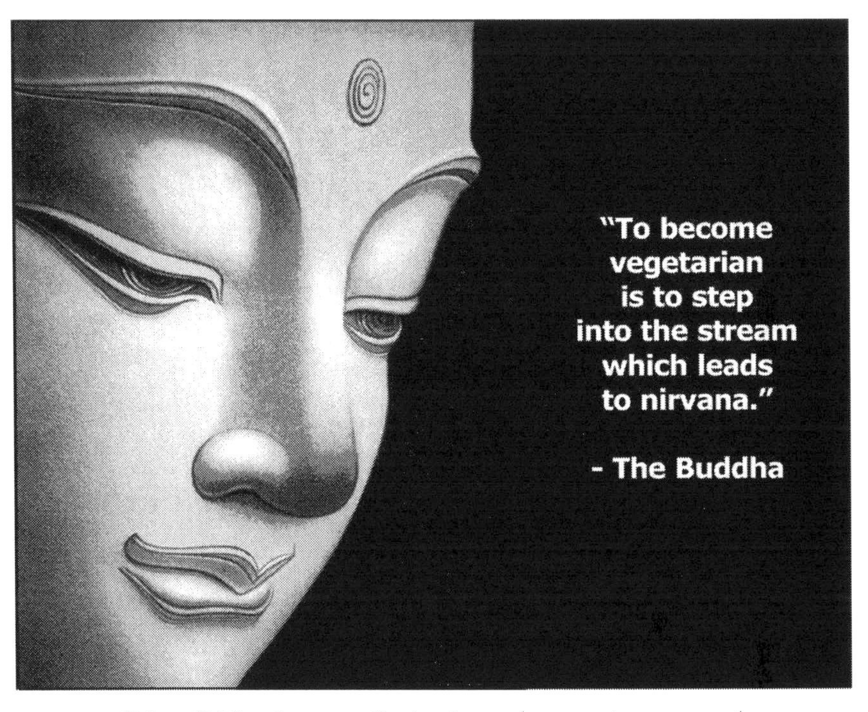

Prince Siddhartha. www.facebook.com/compassionateeaters/

In the Bhagavad Gita, Krishna says: "One who is not envious but who is a kind friend to all living entities… he is very dear to Me."

According to Isaiah, prophet to Muslims, Jews and Christians, Yahweh asks: "Of what use are all your sacrifices to Me? I have had enough of the roasted carcasses of Rams and of the fat of fattened Beasts. I take no pleasure in the blood of Calves, Lambs and Goats. When you spread out your hands, I close My eyes to you; despite however much you pray, I will not listen. Your hands are full of blood! Wash yourselves clean! Put away your misdeeds from before My eyes and stop doing evil."

Mahavira says: "Non–violence and kindness to living beings is kindness to oneself. For thereby one's own self is saved from various kinds of sins and resultant sufferings and is able to secure his own welfare."

And in the Quran we read: "There is not an animal on the earth, nor a flying creature on two wings, but they are people like unto you."

In our great religious teachings, the gut bone connects to the soul bone - animals aren't food; nor are they ours to think of as food.

~

Looking back

Okay, we've come to the end of Mr. Turd's wild ride through our colons. We need to go back now and study a few more of the trains Meating and Junking shunted into sidings or derailed along the tracks.

Fatty liver "disease"

As we saw earlier, alcohol, high-fructose, cholesterol and animal fats all contribute to fatty liver "disease". Healthy liver cells 'drop out' and gradually get replaced with fat cells. In time, scar tissue forms throughout the liver, and when the scar tissue contracts, the outer margins of the liver take on the scalloped appearance characteristic of cirrhosis. Now we have an irreversibly dysfunctional liver. Before that, Planting can reverse liver "disease". The liver is a marvel of regeneration, an absolute champion, when we feed it nothing but whole plant nutrients. Alcohol isn't a nutrient.

Kidney failure

'Meat + sweet' is what kills our kidneys. Industrial sugars, animal fats and animal proteins cause hyper-filtration and protein leakage. Planting keeps our kidneys healthy.

Gout and non-oxalate kidney stones are a product of eating industrial sugars and purines– Meating and Junking. Oxalate kidney stones form in the acid conditions Meating supplies – high-oxalate plants don't cause kidney stones.

Auto-immune conditions

For rheumatoid arthritis and other animal-borne auto-immune responses, let's go back a few steps to where the animals are first getting absorbed in our small intestine. The fatty acids have been released from the fats, and the amino acids have been semi-released from their proteins. Products of incomplete digestion, peptide chains are strings of amino acids that are still linked together. One such peptide in casein, the main protein in cow's milk, consisting of 17 amino acids, is identical to a peptide in the beta-cells of our pancreases, which are responsible for manufacturing insulin. In a friendly fire auto-immune attack, our immune system can wipe out the beta cells and cause irreparable type I diabetes.

Meating causes auto-immune responses. Therefore, animals cannot be food.

The Eatiology of most auto-immune "diseases" is similar: it's a reaction to the introduction of animal proteins which our bodies rightly consider to be inimical to our health. Lupus, MS and rheumatoid arthritis are Meater conditions, symptoms not diseases, and they improve on a pure Planter diet.

Atherosclerosis & cardiovascular "disease"

Animal fats (and processed plant fats) provoke our livers to produce more cholesterol, to go along with the cholesterol we eat. Now, cholesterol, as we know by now, is a substance vital for good health, used in cell membranes and nerve cell sheaths, etc., but it's not a nutrient. We have zero need to eat cholesterol. Our bodies make it; always have, always will. In fact, cholesterol is another animal ingredient that provokes an immune response.

The beginning stage of atherosclerosis is when immune system cells called macrophages are galvanized into gobbling up cholesterol. The macrophages become full of cholesterol, they get sequestered in our arterial walls, becoming foam cells; the foam cells become fatty streaks; over time, our arteries become narrowed, enflamed and stiffened.

Anything we eat that causes an immune response in us has never been food. Both animal proteins and animal cholesterol disqualify animals on the ground that they cause our immune systems to try to destroy them

Animal proteins can do their damage relatively quickly, in weeks or months. Sadly, for us herbivores and the herbivores we eat, our auto-immune response to cholesterol (exacerbated by animal and junk fats) takes decades to manifest clinically. Sub-clinically, if we've been eating animals for years, we've all got heart and arterial "disease". Pure Planters are immune.

Atherosclerosis of the brain's arteries is what sets the stage for dementia, such as Alzheimer's, with animal-borne amyloidosis and metal deposits joining in the destruction.

Leaky gut

Saturated fats play another malefic role in the Meater Eatiology. They compromise the tight junctions of the enterocyte cell lining of our gut walls, allowing endotoxins – dead bacteria in animals – to penetrate where they don't belong and to enter our bloodstreams, causing endotoxemia – blood poisoning. With every bite we take, in microscopic amounts.

A crippling wave of 'stiffness' flows through our entire arterial tree after we eat a single high-fat meal, whether of animal or junk origin. BARTs (brachial artery reflex tests) show that it takes 6 or more hours for our arteries to return to baseline after a high-fat meal, by which time we're ready to repeat the procedure with more animals and junk.

Loosening our tight junctions, by allowing pathogens and large protein fragments free passage out of our guts, makes immune responses worse, and also makes Meaters more susceptible to allergic reactions such as hay fever and eczema (which they are). Meating causes a 'leaky gut,' a condition far more serious than its jokey-sounding name.

Over decades, atherosclerosis – an entirely Meater and Junker condition – causes insidious, unnoticed, under-diagnosed damage. Most people who die from heart attacks and strokes, do so suddenly, mysteriously, seemingly out of the blue. "But she looked so well…" "I can't believe it, he was so fit…" That's because even skinny, healthy-looking people can be fat on the inside, where it counts, in our heart and blood vessels. Like jogging guru Jim Fixx.

Cholesterol levels, as set by our foremost health authorities – read: Meaters – are criminally high. That's because healthy, low cholesterol levels are only possible with a pure Planter dietstyle. To be safe from heart attack and stroke, our total cholesterol levels need to be below 150 (3.9 in the UK) and LDL needs to be below 70-75 (1.9). That's it. Planters with cholesterol below those levels are "heart attack-proof," says Dr. Caldwell Esselstyn.

It doesn't matter whether we believe in cholesterol or not; cholesterol believes in us. It causes our immune systems to attack it when we eat or make it in excess. It's not food.

Saturated fats aren't the only culprit – fiber deficiency leads to a decrease in the number of good bacteria like *F. prausnitzii* in our colons, which leads in turn to a thinning of the protective mucous intestinal lining and damaged tight junctions, allowing pathogens to penetrate the gut wall, resulting in increased immune response and inflammation, and more inflammatory bowel "disease". Meating seems always to have redundant systems to cause harm.

Hypertension

Back to atherosclerosis… As Meating makes our arteries stiffer and narrower and less elastic, our blood pressure gradually rises. With narrower hose pipes, our hearts have to beat harder. Acute high blood pressure becomes permanent, chronic, even malignant hypertension, perhaps the best indicator we have for ill-health and imminent death; better even than high cholesterol levels. (High cholesterol shows that bad stuff could happen; hypertension shows it has already happened.)

Hypertension in turn sets us up for hemorrhagic stroke, while atherosclerosis is setting us up for ischemic stroke, two of our biggest killers… but these so-called diseases are all merely symptoms of the underlying Meating.

So, Meating causes inflammation, constriction of our arteries, elevated blood pressure… The narrowing of our arteries causes hypoperfusion in the tissues and organs our blood bathes: a reduction in blood flow, meaning a reduction in oxygen and nutrients.

Dementia

Our brains make up less than 2% of our body weight, but they receive about 20% of our blood flow. Hypoperfusion of our brains over time sets the stage for dementia. Atherosclerosis of the brain, caused by Meating, is what lays the table for Alzheimer's and other forms of dementia. At the same time that cholesterol is assaulting the blood-brain barrier and causing a 'leaky brain,' atherosclerosis is reducing brain blood supply, and increasing the possibility of infarctions and minor strokes. The other damage comes later, with misfolded animal proteins called amyloids, forming plaques and tangles, and metals like copper and iron complicating the mess that Meating started with coronary artery and carotid artery "disease".

Stiffened, diseased arteries – system-wide, not just in our hearts – can't dilate properly. Animals, deficient in nitrates, are unable to produce nitric oxide, the signaling molecule emitted by our endothelial cells to cause our vessels to dilate. Nitrates come from veggies, leafy greens in particular. Meaters are kept healthy to the extent we also include Planting.

Cancer

Meaters swallow excess hormones. Cow's milk in particular interferes with our own signaling systems. If we think of hormones as the chemical versions of our nervous system, carrying information and instructions from glands to muscles or other organs, would we eat a foreign species' nerves if they started ordering us around?

That's what we do when we drink animals' milk – we swallow their liquid nerves, and these alien hormones start ordering our bodies around. Milk is something we're only adapted to utilizing when we're infants: it's our growth-signaling stimulus. We have zero need of growth stimulus in adulthood. The hormones in milk – particularly the estrogens, some 15 of them – are what incite the "sexual cancers" in humans – cancers of breast, ovary, vagina, uterus and prostate.

Animal proteins are carcinogenic: when a load of animal proteins arrives in us, our livers – programmed to receive breast milk protein only in infancy – see protein bricks arrive and think, hell, it must be building time. So our livers start pumping out IGF-1, insulin-like growth factor, our human growth hormone.

Allied to the animal growth hormones we're Meating – plus the huge load of external chemical endocrine disruptors bio-magnified in animals – our own hormones + animal hormones + chemical hormone-like substances all promote cancer growth. Inappropriate stimulus of cell growth in us promotes cancer… And more rapid aging. The more hormones we eat (i.e., the more animals we eat), the more cancers we'll get. Cancer and rapid aging are symptoms of Meating.

Animal protein is carcinogenic. So too are the poultry and other oncogenic viruses that are in the animals. So too are the environmental chemicals that come packaged with the animals: the arsenic and lead and mercury and PCBS and phthalates and… and… and…

Cancer thrives on inflammation. Well, atherosclerosis does a good job of that, producing inflamed, ulcerated, pustular lesions in our arteries. Animal proteins cause inflammation. Animal fats promote inflammation through leaky guts. So does fiber deficiency. Animal blood iron (heme iron) causes inflammation. Arachidonic acid in animals causes inflammation. Neu5Gc causes so much inflammation it's known as the "inflammatory meat molecule." Meating initiates some tumors. The tumors that Meating causes use the inflammation Meating supplies to grow, and Meating promotes cancer, then makes tumors more invasive, causes angiogenesis in tumors (providing them with a blood supply), and finally promotes metastasis and spread to other parts of the body.

Obesity

Meating is also obesogenic: it makes us fat. So too is Junking. Planters are the only sector of society that's not overweight. Meating and Junking are both nutrient-poor and energy-dense. It's vice versa for Planting. Already too rich in calories, Meating also provides chemical and biological obesogens that make us fatter – endocrine-disrupting pollutants and obesogenic viruses, found most often in chickens. Meating even provides us with infectobesity – obesity as an animal virus-borne "disease". (I find this concept astonishing.)

Obese people's fat cells create estrogens of their own, thereby completing the circle of why obesity and cancer are so strongly linked. The spillover effect causes obese people to constantly have high levels of circulating blood fats, even when not eating much food, completing the circle of why obesity and insulin resistance go together; their partnership sometimes called diabesity. These are Meater and Junker conditions, not Planter.

Lung health

When we eat lots of animal proteins, our stomachs secrete obscene amounts of acid. Acid reflux can cause problems to the esophagus, as we saw earlier. In our mouths, the acid can eat away the enamel on our teeth and can cause a persistent cough and damage to our throats - giving us a hoarse, Lauren Bacall-like voice - and chronic exposure of our lungs to acid can lead to asthma and even emphysema.

The high sulfur content of animal proteins is what gives Meaters their characteristic bad breath, redolent of rotten eggs, and also their repellent, meaty body odor. Occidental Meaters smell rank to the Orientals who're still eating their traditional low-animal diets (and to Planters eating their traditional no-animal diets). Uber-meaters on ketogenic diets also exhale ketones, giving them 'rotten apple breath' to go along with the stench of putrescent eggs.

Aging

Methionine and leucine, two of the sulfur-containing amino acids found predominantly in animals, a surfeit of calories (found in both Meating and Junking) and a generally acidified, oxidized and inflammatory state are the main reasons we age prematurely. (There's a very lengthy description of aging in Part 1B (Mechanisms).)

All of these Eatiological mechanisms are in play at the same time, affecting every single part of our bodies, sapping our immune systems and making us more susceptible to illness.

The Meater abyss

The Meater pit is bottomless. Just when we think we've scraped the bottom with animals as food, new research comes in to add another layer of evidence of their anti-food nature. Every month I read papers showing things like… Animal proteins overload our kidneys and cause them to decline in function. Animal fats cause fatty liver "disease" and set us up for hepatitis and liver failure or cancer. Animal arachidonic acid causes inflammation in our brains. Animal casomorphins, made from the beta-casein in cows' milk, kill infants via crib death (sudden infant death syndrome or SIDS). The hormones in milk cause acne, another biomarker for heart "disease" and early death. The HAs and PAHs that form when we incinerate animals cause cancer. And on, and on, with never any peer-reviewed science to show a benefit of Meating. Plenty out there in the blogosphere and from non-researchers with books to sell to the credulous; none done by reputable scientists untainted by industry money. None. Ever. How can I be so sure? Because it's not possible - animals aren't food.

Death

With Meaters and Junkers, it's a race… It's only a matter of chance which symptom of Meating and Junking gets to the finishing line first: will we die of a heart attack, or will the piece of atheroma that breaks off lodge in our brains and kill us with a stroke? Or will the hypoxia brought about by atherosclerosis cause a tumor, which meatastasizes into our bone marrow and does us in, before our liver shrivels and quits? It doesn't matter what the coroner writes in the book – Sudden Cardiac Death, stroke, malignant neoplasm, hepatitis – the real ur-causes of death are Meating and Junking.

Animals themselves, via their three main inbuilt mechanisms of atherosclerosis, oncogenesis and auto-immunity, degrade our systems, slowly sickening and killing us.

Animals introduce most of the chemical pollutants, which we then need to detoxify and expel; sometimes they sicken and kill us.

Animals introduce most of the pathogens, which we then need to combat and kill; sometimes they win, and they sicken and kill us.

Animals are almost entirely deficient in beneficial nutrients, while being saturated with lethal ingredients and overly-endowed with energy and sulfurous proteins.

It's a sad fact that our constitutions are too resilient for our own good. If the animals we eat were to incite more violent and acute symptoms in us instead of the insidious chronic, almost invisible symptoms that they do, we'd all be better off. Non-human animals would be too. Our bodies' resistance to the daily onslaught of Meating is nothing short of miraculous.

> "What a piece of work is a [hu]man!
> How noble in reason, how infinite in faculty!
> In form and moving how express and admirable!
> In action how like an angel, in apprehension how like a god!
> The beauty of the world. The paragon of animals.
> And yet, to me, what is this quintessence of dust?
> Man delights not me. No, nor woman neither, …"

Not when we betray our angelic natures by ignorantly stuffing ourselves full of the bodies of dead animals. We are not paragons then; we are not then like a god. When we eat animals, we become fallen angels. Then we're beneath bestial, for every beast knows what is and what isn't food.

Except humans.

As smart as we are, we're exceptionally stupid when it comes to eating, a most basic of animal functions.

We Americans in particular *are* exceptional. Not because outdated or silly ideas like Manifest Destiny or "the end of history" made us so; because of our Meater and Junker mal-nutrition. We're exceptionally ignorant about food and, as a result, we're exceptionally fat and diseased. We spend more on healthcare than the next gazillion countries put together [numbers can be numb-ers – they numb us] and still we have worse health than 30-odd countries, coming in roughly the same as Cuba, a country we've embargoed for a half-century, peevishly driving their economy into the rubble because they chose to be free of us. And yet, despite their economic disadvantages, they have good health… partly because they eat so many plants and so few animals, and partly because there's a shortage of pharmaceutical drugs. Both are unforeseen benefits of our suffocating their industrialization.

Meating is what harms us; Planting is what makes us whole.

We can only become "noble in reason" again, and "infinite in faculty" when we re-learn how to eat. The scientific evidence is in: animals aren't food.

I hope this brief synopsis of a Meater meal serves to show how dangerous Meating and Junking are. Obviously, I've just pointed out the molehill – there's far more going on underground than I've had the skills or the space to describe. But you get the drift...

Meating kills, dear hearts. Animals aren't food. Should I say it again? Ah, what the heck… Animals aren't food.

ONCE YOU COME TO TERMS WITH WHY YOU DON'T EAT CATS, DOGS, MONKEYS AND DOLPHINS, YOU WILL BEGIN TO UNDERSTAND WHY I DON'T EAT COWS, PIGS, CHICKENS AND LAMBS.
~EDWARD SANCHEZ
EVOLVE!

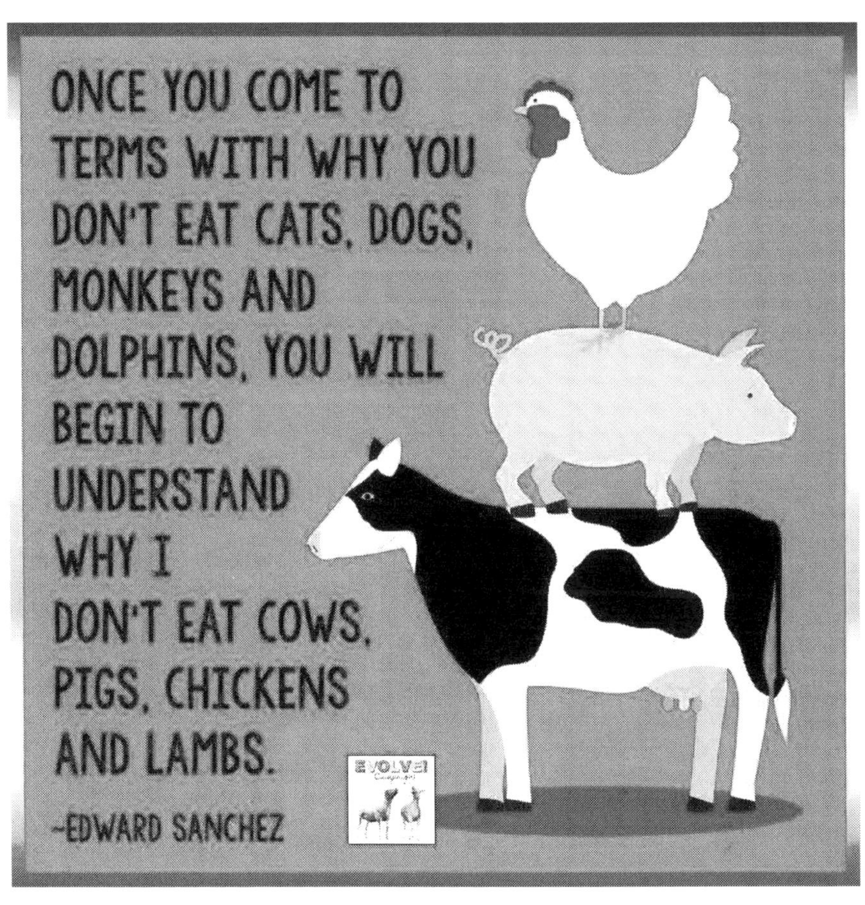

Edward Sanchez quote. Image, with thanks: Evolve! Campaigns

On Silver Bullets & Coffin Nails

Here's a list of ten silver bullets that shoot down the ghoul of Meating; or ten coffin nails that seal the lid of the gruesome, abusive, pointless practice. These are ten truths that, each on their own, should be enough to show that animals aren't food. When taken in their totality they make it certain that they're not. Certain, that is, to eaters who're willing to follow the Eatiology and nothing but the Eatiology to its logical conclusion.

#1 is **animal protein**. Animal protein causes a whole slew of auto-immune responses in those who eat it, such as type I diabetes, rheumatoid arthritis and multiple sclerosis. *They're* animals; *we're* animals; our bodies can't tell the difference. Foods don't cause auto-immune responses.

#2 is **animal protein**. Eating animal proteins after infancy, when we should have been weaned off animals, signals our bodies to release IGF-1, thus initiating cancer and speeding up aging.

#3 is **heme iron**. Our bodies lack a regulatory mechanism for inflammatory heme iron. Animal blood is thus "evolutionarily novel" to us, still unprocessable after millions of years.

#4 is **cholesterol**. Atherosclerosis is a condition found naturally only in herbivores. We get atherosclerosis when we eat animals. Therefore, we are herbivores. Atherosclerosis is our bodies' immune response to cholesterol, potentiated by animal and junk fats. Anything that causes an immune response isn't food.

#5 is **Neu5Gc**, another animal component that causes an immune response in us, leads to a cascade of inflammation, and conditions that thrive in inflammatory conditions, such as cancer. Arachidonic acid and alpha-gal, also found only in animals, are other similar examples of Meater silver bullets, but I throw them in here for free.

#6 is our **small intestines' immune function**. Even though Meating provides more than 90% of the toxic load of hundreds of CONSTITUENTS, PATHOGENS and CONTAMINANTS, the small gut's immune system is activated especially by cruciferous plants, proving that plants formed the overwhelming majority of the diets of proto-humans, and, probably, that our remote ancestors ate nothing but plants.

#7 is our **colonic gut flora**. Though made up of trillions of separate micro-organisms, our gut flora is tantamount to a separate human organ. Meaters have high-sulfur gut flora that produce H_2S and TMAO, with a resulting torrent of "disease", while Planters' gut bacteria produce health-promoting butyrate, acetate and propionate. Eating high-fiber whole plants keeps our immune systems well-calibrated, and us free from inflammatory "diseases".

#8 is **zeaxanthin+lutein**. These plant pigments are our eye pigments. When we eat leafy green vegetables, these two phytonutrients make a beeline for the retinas and lenses of our eyes, and take up residence there. They become us; we are them. (Miraculous chlorophyll, a blood tonic and carcinogen interceptor, is another Planter silver bullet freebie.)

#9 is **dietary intervention studies**, the gold standard of practical nutrition science. Instead of looking at a single variable such as cholesterol, as reductionists are wont to do, when we change people's entire diet to Pure Planting, conditions such as type II diabetes, heart "disease", prostate cancer, auto-immune conditions… aging!... slow down, stop, and sometimes even reverse. Lifestyle practitioners such as Nathan Pritikin, Roy Swank, Walter Kempner, Dean Ornish, Caldwell Esselstyn Jr., Neal Barnard, Brenda Davis and John McDougall have proved this over and over again, for fifty years and more.

#10 is the **Adventist Studies**. These are like dietary intervention studies at the population level, and they show that the longest-lived people ever studied are the vegans among the 7th Day Adventist community in and around Loma Linda, CA. Outliving the general populace by 10 to 14 years, exercising, non-smoking, non-drinking, non-Junking Loma Linda vegans are the longest-lived people ever recorded. They never eat animals.

With the gradual addition of animals to their diet, Adventists, just like the rest of us, become, by quantum leaps, fatter, more diabetic, more osteoporotic and hypertensive, more heart-diseased and shorter-lived. The Proof is in the Planter Pudding.

Taken as a group of ten inescapable facts about Meating, these final ten truths are the nails in the Meater coffin:

Animals aren't food.

~

The Pointlessness of Meating

If I've done my job, we now agree that animals and other junk aren't food.

If animals aren't food, isn't much of what we do pointless?

We smash down rain forests – the lungs of our planet – so we can eat cheap non-foods.

We strip-mine our oceans so we can eat the non-foods we quarry there.

In order to feed the animals we eat, we pour gigatons of chemicals on our land, which end up killing our waterways and oceans.

We give massive subsidies to non-food farmers to grow "food" that kills us, and a mere pittance to food farmers who heal us.

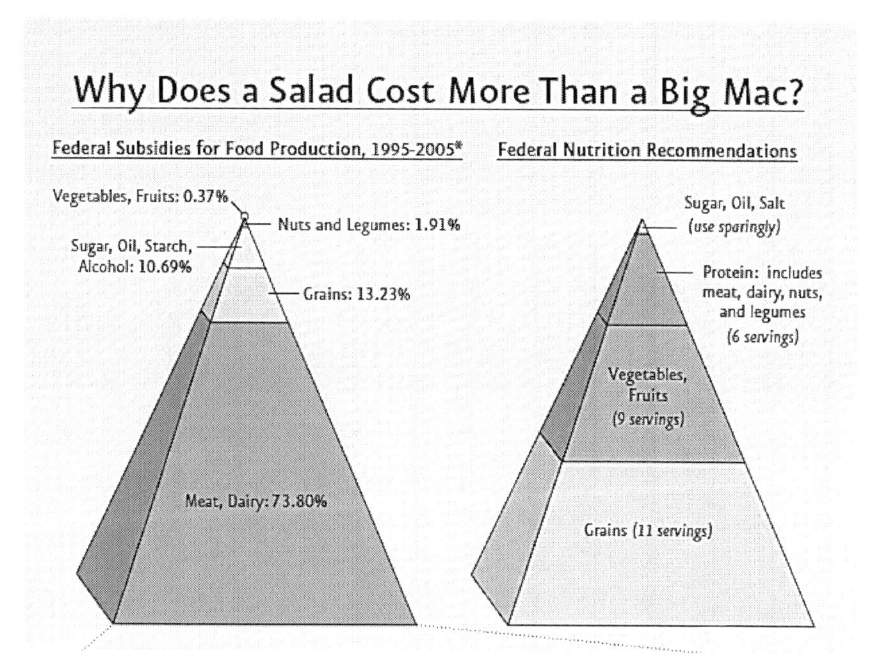

Why does a salad cost more than a Big Mac? Source: PCRM

With the US government, money speaks louder than words: 85% of subsidies go to Meating and Junking, 15% to food.

We give 85% of agricultural subsidies to the non-food sector that causes 90% of our health care costs, which are bankrupting us, as families and as a nation. Our Meater government gives our money to their Meater cronies who're killing us, and when we inevitably become sick it gives our money to their pals in the insurance and medical industries that refuse to heal us with plants.

We feed most of the healing plants we grow to non-human animals that sicken us. Especially corn, even though cattle can't digest it.

We feed tons of antimicrobial drugs to animals so that they can grow faster; so our children may die quicker when the drugs become impotent.

We spend billions on drugs to counter our own impotence, instead of stopping eating animals, which is what makes us impotent.

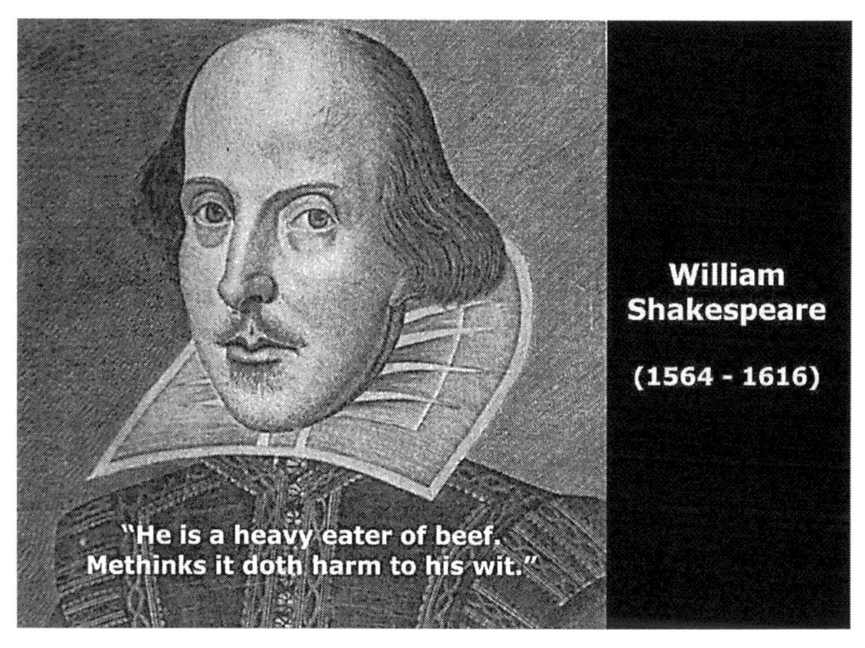

Billy Waggledagger, as my mother Fay used to call him....
www.facebook.com/compassionateeaters/

We rent out vast tracts of public land to non-food farmers at pennies on the dollar. We have a government department that kills all the wildlife that competes with non-food farmers on their cheap public land. Orwell would have approved of its doublespeak name – The Department of Wildlife Services.

We have states in which it's illegal to "disparage" "foods" even though they're not plants and, therefore, not foods.

Our federal government has passed an Animal Enterprise Terrorism Act to protect animal wrongs activists, or animal abusers perpetrating "generally accepted practices," from the sane indignation of animal rights activists.

We have states which will jail us for taking photos of the wretched places where they disassemble animals to produce non-foods.

We have a Department of Agriculture that subsidizes, publicizes and promotes non-foods, even though 'truth in advertising' laws don't allow them to call these products 'healthy' or 'nutritious' or even 'safe.'

We have 5-yearly Nutrition Guidelines Committees, staffed by industry-owned Junkers and Meaters, that kill us by recommending we eat non-foods; those at the pinnacle of their "Food" Pyramids or on MyPlates. (To show a glass of milk next to MyPlate is asinine.)

We have a CDC that purports to control and prevent diseases, while remaining ignorant of Planting's ability to control and prevent "disease", and ignorant of the prime and choice roles Meating plays in the Eatiology of infections.

We have an NIH that tells us such bizarre rubbish as "Most adults do not get enough dairy products." Unbelievably crass, this nightmarish nutrition advice comes from the NIH's National Institute on Aging.

We have a Food and Drug Administration that's all about drugs (to combat the effects of Meating) and nothing about foods (which naturally avoid the effects of Meating).

As Wendell Berry says: "People are fed by the food industry, which pays no attention to health, and are treated by the health industry, which pays no attention to food."

We have a government that's besieged by armies of lobbyists of special interest groups, whose interests aren't special to the overwhelming majority of Americans, who just aren't special enough. The siege analogy is wrong, for the armies are ensconced within the citadel. We're on the outside.

We have a supreme court that's enshrined the rights of corporations, without defining any of their responsibilities beyond profit-making. While corporations remain "legal persons" and aren't constrained in the amounts of money they can contribute to election campaigns, we're all in trouble. The money will continue to flow into the pockets of elected officials who care nothing for public opinion or the truth about food.

We spend far many more billions of dollars on advertising and phony scientific studies for non-foods than it costs to produce them. Just as the tobacco companies used to do. In fact, they're the same people: the companies themselves and their gun-for-hire scientific and PR assassins. "Doubt is their product."

The parent company of Registered Dieticians – The Academy of Dietetics and Nutrition (AND) – is a morally bankrupt, quasi-owned subsidiary of Big Animal, Big Chemical and Big Junk, forced by their sell-out to their corporate sponsors such as Monsanto, Pepsi, Coke, Lay's and MacDonald's to tell us such preposterous whoppers as "There are no good or bad foods."

We eat more animals than any human population that's ever existed. And more junk.

Because we're suffering from Meater and Junker mal-nutrition, other dominoes fall…

We're the fattest, sickest people who've ever lived.

70% of us are taking at least one medication and 10%, five or more.

With 2.5 million Americans in jail, we have the largest prison population that's ever existed; many incarcerated for victimless crimes… drug crimes which I (as an ex-addict) think stem from our greatest addiction of all: eating animals.

We're a violent people, made so by our Meating.

We have as many guns in the US as we have people, which doesn't bother me as much as the fact that we're Meaters and nothing loath to use our guns on other animals and other people. Planters don't kill animals, either non-human or human.

We have the largest land, sea, air and special forces the world has ever seen. We have five thousand military bases in the continental USA and another thousand overseas in more than 150 countries. Not including its sand castle atolls in the South China Sea, China has one overseas base. Russia has three.

We kidnap our perceived enemies [rendition], smuggle them into prisons [black sites] and then torture them [extraordinary interrogation techniques], even though we know that the intel gained from torture is useless. Guantanamo remains open for business.

We have thousands of drones that patrol the skies ceaselessly, piloted by Meaters half a world away, murdering some perceived enemies, while murdering many more unlucky bystanders, who we shrug off as "collateral damage." We have a president who personally selects targets for drone strikes, including US citizens, as if he's playing video games, and to hell with the 9 unlucky passersby who don't vote.

We kill 100 billion land animals and maybe a trillion sea creatures each year… collateral damage to our societal ignorance about what is and what isn't food.

We have ten or eleven aircraft carrier groups that patrol the oceans continuously; each with enough firepower to destroy entire nations. We do this to maintain a constant flow of energy, which is the lifeblood of Empire, and then we squander the energy on inefficient cars and an inefficient, insane way of eating.

We put more energy into rearing non-foods than we get back from eating them. We transport some of the things we eat thousands of miles before eating them.

We may generate up to half of greenhouse gases in putting dead animals on our plates. For our eating pleasure, almost 100 million cattle share America with 320 million humans, and each of those animals contributes (fill in a numb-er (say) thirty) times more environmental waste than a human animal.

We use [fill in a numb-er, say 2 or 10 or 20] times as much water to grow one non-food meal than a food meal with the same energy content.

And our drinkable water is ~~running out~~ being pumped out; the high mountain snowpacks are dwindling; the glaciers are melting; the prehistoric aquifers are being siphoned dry, and the water tables are plummeting. We're flinging the water out carelessly on the land to grow crops to feed to animals, and then it disappears into the salt seas, lost for human use.

We use (say) 10 times as much fuel; 10 times as much land; 10 times as many inputs such as poisonous energy-dense fertilizers and pesticides for growing genetically modified crops to feed the animals we eat, compared to Planting.

In effect, it takes the food of 10 to 20 Planters to feed 1 Meater. In effect, a population of 320 million Meater Americans is eating the food of between 3.2 and 6.4 billion Planter humans. Or only 1.6 billion. What does it matter?

We're still eating way more than our fair share. (Perhaps that's the freedom we're hated for, little Georgie Jr?)

We're eating our planet to death, so that we can eat ourselves to death with non-foods.

We 1st Worlders are malnourished with too much, while the remaining 80% of humanity survive on our leftovers, and at least a billion people are malnourished because they have too little. When we eat ourselves to death on animals, we're also eating to death those to whom we've denied grains by feeding them to animals who can't digest them.

In the words of my beloved Thay… Thich Nhat Hanh:

> "Every day forty thousand children die in the world for lack of food. We who overeat in the West, who are feeding grains to animals to make meat, are eating the flesh of these children."

All pointless… Because animals aren't food, dear gorgeous people.

It's not too late to wake up.

To be a Planter is to be awake and on the side of the angels.

~

Meating and Earth's Climate

Near the end of the 20th Century, well-known Cornell ecologist David Pimentel told us: "If all the grain currently fed to livestock in the United States were consumed directly by people, the number of people who could be fed would be nearly 800 million." It's probably a billion people by now.

Cornell Chronicle Aug. 7, 1997.
http://www.news.cornell.edu/stories/1997/08/us-could-feed-800-million-people-grain-livestock-eat

Meanwhile, Meater climate change activist Bill McKibben (founder of 350.org) wants us to lower atmospheric carbon dioxide to 350 parts per million, while he continues to scarf down liverwurst sandwiches, as he does in *The End of Nature* (the book that first alerted us to climate change).

Al Gore, another well-known climate change activist, found Meating too inconvenient a truth to mention in his documentary, *An Inconvenient Truth.*

As film director James Cameron says, it's not possible to be an effective environmentalist *and* a Meater, Bill and Al. It's one or the other. And if you're a Planter now, Al, you need to bite the bullet and include Planting in your message – it's far more effective than keeping our car tires pumped up or installing special light bulbs or driving hybrid cars.

Actually, our inability to reach anything near peak performance while we carry on Meating is true of all occupations. It goes for conservationists and ecologists and ethologists and anthropologists and game park rangers and oceanographers and marine biologists (as confirmed by the wonderful Sylvia Earle - "There's still time, but not a lot, to turn things around"), and it goes for veterinarians and nutritionists and dieticians and chefs and physicians and public health officials and farmers and scientists and hospital administrators and caterers and athletes and bodybuilders and doulas and spiritual guides of all denominations… and… and… and… especially economists (still seeking infinite growth on our finite planet).

We only become truly human when we stop eating an inhuman diet of animals and junk. It's the difference between being easily, unconsciously humane and trying to make conscious humane choices; the difference between unconscious mastery and conscious incompetence.

To try to be healthy while continuing to Junk and Meat is to pee into a hurricane – there's bound to be lots of blowback.

Hospitals selling McDonald's "food," schools using milk or egg board indoctrination materials, alphabet-soup governmental organizations such as the CDC, the USDA, the NIH, the EPA and FDA, sundry organizations devoted to individual maladies like heart "disease," diabetes and cancer … all of these groups are complicit in keeping Meating unobjectionable. All of them should get their acts together, for the sake of our individual and societal health.

When it comes to planetary health, Meating is just as culpable. Here's some info about greenhouse gases from the Center for Climate and Energy Solutions, which shows that, while eliminating industrial coolants and refrigerants etc. is necessary, the best way to stop and reverse climate change is by eradicating animal agriculture.

Greenhouse Gas	Chemical Formula	Anthropogenic Sources	Atmospheric Lifetime[1] (years)	GWP[2] (100 Year Time Horizon)
Carbon Dioxide	CO_2	Fossil-fuel combustion, Land-use conversion, Cement Production	~100[1]	1
Methane	CH_4	Fossil fuels, Rice paddies, Waste dumps	12[1]	25
Nitrous Oxide	N_2O	Fertilizer, Industrial processes, Combustion	114[1]	298
Tropospheric Ozone	O_3	Fossil fuel combustion, Industrial emissions, Chemical solvents	hours-days	N.A.
CFC-12	CCL_2F_2	Liquid coolants, Foams	100	10,900
HCFC-22	CCl_2F_2	Refrigerants	12	1,810
Sulfur Hexaflouride	SF_6	Dielectric fluid	3,200	22,800

Main greenhouse gases.
Source: http://www.c2es.org/facts-figures/main-ghgs

We see that the GWPs (global warming potentials) of the Meater greenhouse gases – methane and nitrous oxide (CH_4 and N_2O) – are 25 and 298 respectively. That is, they are 25 and 298 times more damaging than CO_2, the benchmark gas. [Or 78 or 12 or whatever… a *lot*…]

Removing the nitrous oxide is equivalent to removing more than three hundred times as much CO_2, because it persists 1.14 times as long.

Removing methane has a double benefit. While it's 'only' 25 times more potent than CO_2, its 'atmospheric lifetime' is a mere 12 years, in comparison to CO_2's 100. So, over the course of a century, removing one molecule of methane is equivalent to removing 25 x 100 ÷ 12 = 208 molecules of CO_2.

Plus, when we look at the next table we see that methane is the gas that has built up the most in the troposphere since the industrial revolution began:

	Pre-1750 Tropospheric Concentration[3] (parts per billion)	Current Tropospheric Concentration[4] (parts per billion)
Carbon Dioxide	280,000[5]	388,500[6]
Methane	700[7]	1,870 / 1,748[8]
Nitrous Oxide	270[5]	323 / 322[8]
Tropospheric Ozone	25	34
CFC-12	0	.534 / .532[8]
HCFC-22	0	.218 / .194[10]
Sulfur Hexaflouride	0	.00712 / .00673[8, 10]

Changes in tropospheric concentrations of greenhouse gases.
Source: http://www.c2es.org/facts-figures/main-ghgs

While CO_2 levels have gone up 38.75% since 1750, N_20 levels have gone up 19.63%. But methane levels have catapulted up by 167.14%... Atmospheric methane is 2 and 2/3 times as bad now as it was back then, plus methane is 25 times as harmful as carbon dioxide.

Methane is the main climate changer; not CO_2, and not the CFCs, the HCFCs or the sulfur hexafluoride, which have all gone up infinitely, because they didn't exist in 1750, but which we produce in much smaller quantities.

Thank heavens for that. What good news.

Why? Because:

1. Methane is the most harmful greenhouse gas;
2. Confined animals are the biggest source of methane, and the one most easily stopped;

3. Animals aren't food, so (2) is unnecessary (even suicidal);
4. Methane survives in the atmosphere for only 12 years; so
5. If we stop creating MEAThane, we can limit climate change in just over a decade, and perhaps even stop it.

The best way to prevent climate change – now, before the frozen northern tundra releases its giga-load of methane – is to stop eating animals.

There's no other strategy that comes close to the effectiveness of this one (which also happens to be the healthiest choice for us): we'll preserve the Earth as we know it, when we stop killing other animals and ourselves.

Not to mention the metaphysical liberation and the spiritual joy that become possible when we stop the screams of the tens of billions of land animals we kill each year, which I imagine resounding through space instead of the Music of the Spheres or Johann Strauss's 'Beautiful Blue Danube,' which played during the unforgettable scene in *2001: A Space* Odyssey in which Discovery One glides out past Jupiter.

This is why angels don't like to come here any more – they have sensitive hearing and they can't bear the cacophony of animal bellowing emanating from Earth. Have you seen any angels lately? I haven't. (Do angels have delicate, hollow bones like birds? Why are their wings and arms separate structures?)

Just as Planters aren't serial killers, neither are we the main cereal killers – Meaters top those lists. The Cornell Chronicle article about David Pimentel, quoted earlier, says: "From one ecologist's perspective, the American system of farming grain-fed livestock consumes resources far out of proportion to the yield, accelerates soil erosion, affects world food supply and will be changing in the future."

The very near future.

Either we change the climate now, by stopping Meating, or Meating will continue to change our climate and stop us. The planet will be just fine; we may not be so lucky.

Our recognition that animals aren't food is crucial to our species' future wellbeing. The World Health Organization acknowledged this on 26 October 2015, when they confirmed that processed animals are Group 1 carcinogens – on a par with arsenic, asbestos, alcohol and cigarette smoke – and that less-processed animals cause a lower level of carcinogenicity.

"Overall, the Working Group classified consumption of processed meat as "carcinogenic to humans" (Group 1) on the basis of sufficient evidence for colorectal cancer… The Working Group classified consumption of red meat as "probably carcinogenic to humans" (Group 2A)."

See: Véronique Bouvard, Dana Loomis, Kathryn Z Guyton, Yann Grosse, Fatiha El Ghissassi, Lamia Benbrahim-Tallaa, Neela Guha, Heidi Mattock, Kurt Straif, on behalf of the International Agency for Research on Cancer Monograph Working Group. Carcinogenicity of consumption of red and processed meat. *Lancet Oncol* 2015 Published Online October 26, 2015 http://dx.doi.org/10.1016/ S1470-2045(15)00444-1

(Look, we've known this for decades – while vested interests have fought us tooth and nail, just as they did with asbestos and smoking, using the same mercenary White Coats to confuse matters – but it's great that our most authoritative public health organizations are now stating the facts. The WHO publishing in *The Lancet*… it doesn't get much better than that.)

This gives us a wonderful opportunity to continue to eat fewer animals (the way the industrialized world has been doing for the last decade) and to stop the acceleration of Meating that's happening among the nouveau riche, promoted by external Western corporations who also pushed smoking and banned pesticides there when sales fell off back at home.

For our own personal health and for the health of our planetary home, there is no more important realization:

Animals aren't food.

~

The Good News

It's not all doom and gloom. There is good news. Great news, in fact.

Planting fixes just about everything that ails us.

It restores us to health.

It's the best weight management program around, without an Oprah, yoyo effect. It's permanent.

It removes our most fundamental addiction, making it easier for other addictions to melt away.

It restores our sanity. It makes us less violent, more serene.

It restores us to our true selves, removing the cognitive dissonance which blinds us when we say we love animals, while we eat them. We can only truly love animals when we're Planters.

When our circle of compassion lassos all species, and encircles even Meater humans, then we become more embracing, less chauvinist, less bellicose.

If we need to love ourselves before we can love others, we love ourselves best by being Planters.

Planting restores Nature, and allows us to relax into the food web, instead of clawing our way to the top of an imaginary, self-imposed food chain.

It makes wild animals numinous again; if they're not food, then they're holy. Precious; not trophies, not game, not meat.

Planting solves the problems of peak oil and how to feed a growing world population. It's an antidote to consumerism.

It helps stop climate change, whether we believe in it or not.

It stops deforestation and soil erosion and desertification.

It stops the acidification and eutrophication of our seas and lakes and streams.

It preserves the ancient water in our aquifers.

It preserves the ancient sunlight, our dwindling hydrocarbon reserves.

It preserves the quality of our air.

It would stop the current great extinction event, the only one in billions of years perpetrated by one species upon millions of others.

It stops the extinction of the antibiotics which have been such a boon to us, and whose loss may condemn millions to death in a bleak future.

It stops the development and spread of zoönotic plagues, from hyper-confined non-humans to hyper-confined humans.

When we stop our pointless eating of animals, we heal our most basic wounds: our estrangement from the other sentient beings with whom we share this beautiful blue world, and our estrangement from our best selves.

Meating was our opportunistic past…

Junking is our ignorant present…

Planting is our beautiful future.

I hope to see you there.

~

Acknowledgments

I wouldn't have been able to write this book were it not for the work of the extraordinary Dr. Michael Greger, who's done more than any other person to bring the intricacies of nutrition science to a lay audience. His website – www.nutritionfacts.org – is a resource without peer. I urge you to seek it out, if you don't already know it. I'll go so far as to call it a service to humanity. It's totally free, a 501c3 nonprofit charity supported by donations, and I encourage anyone who benefits from its brilliance to contribute.

I also recommend Dr. Greger's groundbreaking new book: *How Not to Die: Discover the Foods Scientifically Proven to Prevent and Reverse Disease*. Definitive.

Every year Dr. Greger "reads through every issue of every English-language nutrition journal in the world so [we] don't have to." His annual, hour-long presentation previewing his work of the year to come is an eagerly awaited event, and the back editions can be found on nutritionfacts.org or YouTube. Besides being densely informative, they're entertaining (and wickedly funny!)

(His jest that "if there's one thing we know about hot dog eaters, it's that they're picky about what goes in their food" always cracks me up.)

On Mondays, Wednesdays and Fridays of each week, Dr. Greger posts a short new video on an aspect of nutrition and health that he and his team have gleaned from their reading. All back numbers are archived and efficiently searchable by keyword, of which there are more than a thousand.

On Tuesdays and Thursdays, Dr. Greger posts an article. He lists all the sources he cites in his videos and articles, and clicking the hyperlinks takes us straight to the relevant papers, in such prestigious journals as the *New England Journal of Medicine*, *The Lancet*, the *American Journal of Clinical Nutrition* and hundreds of others, some quite obscure, so we can read and verify the primary materials for ourselves, if we so wish.

I did so wish, and it was Dr. Greger who inspired my nutrition education and the writing of this book. If I've quoted Dr. Greger or nutritionfacts.org a hundred times in this book, I wouldn't be surprised. I can't claim to have read all the papers he's referenced, but I do have a burgeoning collection of "landmark" masterpieces such as Dr. Dean Ornish et al's 1990 *Lancet* paper which first proved that a pure plant diet can reverse heart "disease". I date the beginning of modern lifestyle medicine from the day – 21 July 1990 – on which Dr. Ornish and his co-workers posed the question: "Can lifestyle changes reverse coronary heart disease?"

The answer was a resounding "yawp" of a yes. At that time, modern medicine had degenerated into mere symptom management, via chemistry, radiation and surgery (where it still languishes, for the most part). Then Ornish showed us that healing *is* possible, not by suppressing symptoms, but by removing root causes. And the way we heal is through Right Nutrition… through Planting. And Planting removes multiple, multiple maladies, as I've shown, as much through the life-affirming benefits of Planting as through ending the habitual, repetitive injuries of Meating and Junking.

I have any number of Planter heroes. Those with whom I've studied, and through whom I've gained some modest accreditation in nutrition science and dietstyle counseling, include Prof. T. Colin Campbell of Cornell, eCornell and the T. Colin Campbell Foundation; Dr. Neal Barnard of PCRM, Food for Life, The Plantrician Project and The George Washington University; Dr. John McDougall of *The Starch Solution*, Dr. McDougall's Health and Medical Center and the McDougall Research & Education Foundation; Mary-Ann and Mark Shearer of The Natural Way, and Will Tuttle, PhD, author of *The World Peace Diet – Eating for Spiritual Health and Social Harmony* [required reading for all eaters everywhere, everywhen], and leading light of Prayer Circle for Animals and the World Peace and Yoga Jubilee … astonishingly wonderful humans, all.

I owe you all a debt of gratitude for the decades of work you've put into making our world a healthier, happier, holier place. Kudos to you all, and to all my fellow Planters, those of us who're already here and those of us who're yet to be.

~

Bibliography - Recommended reading for Planters

Some of the great thinkers who've formed my mind

Anything by Jonathan Balcombe. *Pleasurable Kingdom: Animals and the Nature of Feeling Good* is my favorite, so far. [Animal emotions made visible.]

Anything by Dr. Neal Barnard. *Breaking the Food Seduction*, *Turn Off the Fat Genes*, etc. [All excellent books on the science of nutrition.]

Gene Baur. *Farm Sanctuary: Changing Hearts and Minds About Animals and Food* [Opening our hearts and homes to other species.]

Marc Beckoff and Jessica Pierce. *Wild Justice: The Moral Lives of Animals* [Overturning the Cartesian view of animals as insensate machines.]

T. Colin Campbell and Howard Jacobson. *Whole : Rethinking the Science of Nutrition* [How we should practice nutrition science - absolutely demolishes the reductionist approach favored by Low-Carb Bullshit Artists. Essential.]

T. Colin Campbell & Thomas Campbell II. *The China Study* [Foundational.]

Dr. Gabriel Cousens *There Is a Cure for Diabetes* [I call it Planting.]

Brenda Davis and Vesanto Melina. *Becoming Vegan: The Complete Guide to Adopting a Healthy Plant-based Diet* [Excellent how-to manual for newbies.]

Gail Eisnitz. *Slaughterhouse: The Shocking Story of Greed, Neglect and Inhumane Treatment Inside the U.S. Meat Industry* [Heartbreaking; almost unendurable.]

Dr. Caldwell Esselstyn, Jr. *Prevent and Reverse Heart Disease.* [Magnificent.]

Jonathan Safran Foer. *Eating Animals* [Slaughterhouses and fisheries; the violence and the devastation.]

Dr. Joel Fuhrman. *Eat to Live: The Revolutionary Formula for Fast and Sustained Weight Loss* [The Nutritarian way to health via eating for nutrient density.]

Dr. Michael Greger. *How Not to Die: Discover the Foods Scientifically Proven to Prevent and Reverse Disease.* [The best guide to optimal eating. Extraordinary.]

Jenny Hall and Iain Tollhurst. *Growing Green: Animal-Free Organic Techniques* [Veganic farming made clear.]

Anything by Chris Hedges. [An ethical vegan, he out-Chomskys Chomsky.]

Julia Butterfly Hill. *The Legacy of Luna: The Story of a Tree, a Woman and the Struggle to Save the Redwoods* [Activism = patriotism. Inspirational.]

Ellen Jaffe Jones. *Eat Vegan on $4 a Day: A Game Plan for the Budget-Conscious Cook* [Terrific resource for all of us, not just budget-conscious vegans.]

Melanie Joy, PhD. *Why We Love Dogs, Eat Pigs and Wear Cows* [Carnism, the psychology of Meaterialism - Joy defines & describes it better than anyone.]

Dr. Michael Klaper. *Vegan Nutrition: Pure and Simple*
[Does, most entertainingly, what it says on the label.]

Douglas Lisle, PhD and Alan Goldhamer, DC. *The Pleasure Trap - Mastering the Hidden Force That Undermines Health and Happiness* [Addiction explained.]

Jim Mason. *An Unnatural Order: Why We Are Destroying the Planet and Each Other* [The consequences of Meating laid bare.]

Dr. John McDougall. *The Starch Solution* [Brilliant population studies.]

Isa Chandra Moskowitz & Terry Hope Romero. *Veganomicon: The Ultimate Vegan Cookbook.* [Yum yum yum.]

Marion Nestle. *Food Politics: How the Food Industry Influences Nutrition, and Health* [A landmark in consumer watchdoggery.]

Ingrid Newkirk. *One Can Make a Difference* [A primer in activism.]

Dr. Dean Ornish. *Dr Dean Ornish's Program for Reversing Heart Disease* [Outstanding, as befits the dean of lifestyle medicine practitioners.]

Any Colleen Patrick-Goudreau [Compassionate cooking; film; literature.]

Charles Patterson. *Eternal Treblinka: Our Treatment of Animals and the Holocaust* [Insightful comparison of humans' treatment of animals and each other.]

Anything by John Robbins. *Healthy at 100: The Scientifically Proven Secrets of the World's Healthiest and Longest-Lived Peoples*, my favorite. Inspirational.

Maria Rodale. *Organic Manifesto* [Excellent coverage of chemical company and government corruption. A drawback: she thinks veganism a 'fad.']

Matthew Scully. *Dominion: The Power of Man, the Suffering of Animals, and the Call to Mercy* [Outs our scabrous justifications of animal exploitation.]

Anything by Paul Shepard, Dr. Terry Shintani, Vandana Shiva, Isaac Bashevis Singer and so many others… just under S.

Will Tuttle, PhD. *The World Peace Diet – Eating for Spiritual Health and Social Harmony* [The consequences of Meating. Brilliant and indispensible.]

Paul Watson. *Ocean Warrior: My Battle to End the Illegal Slaughter on the High Seas* [The activist's activist.]

Zoe Weil. *So, You Love Animals: An Action-Packed, Fun-Filled Book to Help Kids Help Animals* [Humane education: guiding the young to a sane future.]

Glossary ~ Terminal Terminology

These are some terms I've found useful as nutrition aides-de-cogitation:

- **UFOs** – Un-digestible Food-like Objects: Animals or junk.
- **In-digestion** – illness brought about by eating indigestible or poorly digested components or contents of animals and junk.
- **Mal de merde** – illness brought about by eating shit (and shit-eating bacteria), which we do with almost every mouthful of animal.
- **Affluenza** – A constellation of maladies caused by eating a rich diet, rich in animals and junk, rich in calories, but poor in nutrients, poor in exercise. A.k.a. **"Diseases" of affluence** or **Western "diseases"** or **"Diseases" of civilization**.
  Symptoms, not diseases.
- **Effluenza** is a combo of mal-de-merde and affluenza… us rich folk dying from animal-shit-borne diseases thanks to the powerful industrial forces that cater to our addiction to eating animals. OK, at the very least a habit.
- **Wreck-creational eating** – the practice of eating ourselves to death for fun when we eat animals and junk. Barbecuing is a perfect example; so too are Junkers' french fries and potato chips.
- **Unrest-aurants** – very lucrative eating establishments that rarely serve food. To meet my definition of restaurant, they should serve nothing but food. Otherwise they're providing "wreck creation" for us and cannon fodder for our medical establishment. They cause unrest.
- **Chili-con-carnage** – the devastation we cause to ourselves, to animals and to the biosphere, by mistakenly mixing animals in with our beans.
- **Brotein** – Something only Meater bro-scientists worry about.
- **Meatabolic syndrome** – an expansion of metabolic syndrome to include all the maladies induced by Meating: type II diabetes, hypertension, atherosclerosis, heart "disease", stroke, dementia, plus the kitchen sink. Not diseases; symptoms.

- **Freudian slap** – the accidental or unexpected buffet we often need to receive to shock us to our senses; akin to a "Zen blow." My dietstyle Freudian slap was a benign meningioma. And a lovely velovegan ex. (Hi, Andi.)
- **Dietstyle** – a perfectly integrated way of eating and living, akin to Right Eating, a candidate for inclusion in the Buddha's Noble Eightfold Path. How are we to Catch Bull at Four if we don't eat right? Dietstyle can also refer to what Meaters and Junkers do, with a negative connotation.
- **Wurst class proteins** – In archaeo-nutrition dating back to the 19th Century, long before the discovery of the vitamins and other phytonutrients, animal proteins were called "first class proteins" because they're most like human animal proteins and thus more easily assimilated. It turns out that their near resemblance to us is a serious drawback, causing autoimmune conditions; their high sulfur content is acid-forming and gut flora-disruptive; and their IGF-1 stimulation is aging and cancer-stimulating. It turns out that first class proteins are worst class proteins.
- **Zoöphages** and **Zoöphagy** – animal eaters; animal eating. I was pretty chuffed with myself when I thought I'd coined these words, but apparently they've been around since at least 1877.
- **Phytophages** and **Phytophagy** – plant eaters; plant eating; 1913.
- **Meaterialism** – our prevailing, hyper-violent Western worldview that's built on our mistaken belief that animals are food. The origin of Materialism and consumerism; akin to the great Melanie Joy's concept of Carnism, the "invisible belief system, or ideology, that conditions people to eat certain animals." (Required reading: Joy's brilliant *Why We Love Dogs, Eat Pigs and Wear Cows.*)
- **Omnivoraciousness** – Omnivorism connotes treating and eating all kinds of things as food, even though we're not anatomical or physiological omnivores. Omnivoraciousness is the quality that Meating creates in us: we become like hungry ghosts, mythical creatures from the Buddhist canon, with tiny gullets and enormous bellies, forever insatiable. We devour and despoil the world – as we see animal agriculture doing to our lakes and forests – and all for

no good reason, once we understand animals aren't food. ("Ethical omnivorism" is not. "Ethical omnivorism" is an oxymoron, as practiced by oxy morons trying to put a positive spin on a vicious practice they want to feel virtuous about continuing.)

- **Oxy morons** – When we're Meaters we're so imbedded in the matrix of Meating that we can unconsciously juxtapose totally irreconcilable words cheek-by-jowl, without feeling the vaguest frisson of psychic distress or discordance. Oxy morons seem to feel nary a twinge of cognitive dissonance when using oxymorons such as "fast food," "ethical omnivorism," "happy cows" and "humane slaughter." (It pains me that the word slaughter contains laughter.)
- **Club Medical** – The intersection of Big Pharma, modern (non-nutritional) medical practice and the sickness insurance industry, each driven by the new Hippocratic oath, which the cynic in me describes as "First, do no harm to the bottom line." Chronic "disease" is Big Business. There's little money in healing or curing; symptom management is where corporations make the big bucks. Repeat business, with each brainwashed customer hooked on multiple, lifelong medications (which – bad for business! – kill more than 105,000 Americans each year, even when taken correctly. I wonder: do drug company execs get pissed off with each other for killing their cash cows? I can picture threats like this one: "I'm warning you, man. You'd better pull that statin of yours – it's killing too many of my diabetes customers.") Planting heals… for free… and for good, so we never need to go back. The bean counters don't know beans about healing. The bean counters also don't like beans: they're too healthy and they're not profitable.
- **"First do no ham"** – My vegan ethical code. All else follows.
- **Aggro-culture** – Our hyper-violent methods of ripping up the Earth and sousing it with lethal chemicals, then perpetrating zoö-genocide on hundreds of billions of self-aware animals each year, to provide ourselves with toxic animal calories.
- **The Mootrix** – Not my word. The Meater culture in which we're imbedded which makes us oblivious to the carnage Meating causes. But, when we take the red pill… A.k.a. The Meatrix. (Check out the Mootrix videos on YouTube. They're fun.)

- **Phood** or **pHood** – The word 'food,' which now includes animals and junk, no longer means what it should: vital, healthy, and long-life-producing fuel and medicine, all in one package. Since food became contaminated with animals and junk, it's no longer food. Instead of the initial eff, pHood uses the phi φ of φυτόν, phyton, the old Greek word for plant, indicating that it's the whole plant and nothing but the plant. (The pH has the added value of telling us that real food brings about the right pH, and isn't acid-forming like animals.)
- **The En-lightenment Dietstyle**: Awakening compassion for all beings includes the ultimate keep-it-off-for-good weight loss program, leaving us spiritually and bodily en-lightened. It doesn't cost a dime – we've got to eat – so we may as well eat phood.
- **Mung beans** – Human beings. Silly, I know, but one of the benefits of aging is that, like *Mad*'s Alfred E. Neuman, sometimes I just shrug and say: What, me worry? I use it sometimes to remind myself that eating plants is what makes us human and humane.
- **Phyting fit** – a non-violent way of being healthy, by eating nothing but whole plants, and getting plenty of exercise.

~

"What's next?" and "Staying in touch"

One of the worst disease vectors infecting our planet today is a group of individuals who, for reasons best known to themselves, are spreading deadly low-carb and paleo diets. I've made it my life's mission to out these propagandists, confusionists and denialists for the scientific frauds they are.

Because animals aren't food, as I've just demonstrated via hundreds of animal components, harmful mechanisms, pathogens, contaminants and deficiencies, the Low-Carb Bullshit Artists are forced to use any means, usually foul, to whitewash Meating. I hope you'll join me in my next book, ***The Low-Carb Bullshit Artists Are Lying Us to Death***, which details the many ways these un-empathic, even psychopathic killers go about their slimy business.

Why Animals Aren't Food consumed five years of my life. I looked everywhere for a compilation of the science showing the harmfulness of eating animals, but there wasn't one, so I realized I'd have to write it myself.

Now, when I'm not busy revising this book and writing the next, I'm going to ramp up my first love, which is public speaking. I really enjoy thinking and talking about nutrition. Interacting with people about how to eat is what really blows my hair back - what there is of it - and it's rewarding to coax an audience into appreciating the glories of Planting and the miseries of Meating.

I also enjoy coaching a select few motivated over-achievers, helping them to gain even more edginess, the Planter way.

Nutrition science is only now entering its Planter Renaissance after the Meater Middle Ages, and there's a ferment of Planter nutrition science constantly brewing, so if you enjoyed **Why Animals Aren't Food** please go to *WAAF*'s Facebook page at https://www.facebook.com/whyanimalsarentfood/, and if you Like the page, you'll receive the updates I plan to make in the future.

The address for the *WAAF* website is **www.whyanimalsarentfood.com**.

I manage two other Facebook pages besides *WAAF*'s. One is a community page called **Compassionate Eaters** and it contains images of and sayings by inspirational vegan and near-vegan role models down the ages, to help keep vegans inspired and proud of our awesome lineage, stretching back to

Pythagoras and beyond. You can find us "accentuating the positive" at https://www.facebook.com/compassionateeaters/.

My "eliminating the negative" page is called **The Pinoakesio Diet** and it's an evidence-based critique of one particular Low-Carb Bullshit Artist and, more broadly, it's a science-based refutation of all promoters of high-animal diets, from Atkins, Banting, Cordain, Dukan, Eades, Fallon… to Yudkin and Zone. We're at https://www.facebook.com/The-Pinoakesio-Diet-1661390480774740/.

My LinkedIn profile is at **https://za.linkedin.com/in/rohan-millson-46872126**. On Twitter, I'm **@rohanmillson**.

Other projects with which I'm involved are Greyton Transition Town (GTT), in South Africa, of which I'm currently the secretary, and Greyton Farm Animal Sanctuary, where 16 rescued sheep, 19 pigs, 2 geese, 3 fluffy white chickens and 1 brindled cow (at the time of writing) have me very well-versed in their dietary foibles and sleeping arrangements. Both of these organizations were founded by my extraordinary ex-wife, eternal friend, and Tabularasa Farm partner, Nicola Vernon.

(Our 100-acre farm is off-the-grid, solar-powered, and we built the houses ourselves with the help of eight unconventional builders we trained after spending our honeymoon learning how, from Bill and Athena Steen at the Canelo Project in Arizona; mostly out of straw bales, clay, recycled wood, rock, sand and water. And not in a Fred Flintstone manner either - because their Gaia-friendly materials are within the two-foot-thick clay-plastered walls they're not obvious.)

Greyton Transition Town is the first such sustainable community in Africa. It's our goal to make our surrounding region more resilient in the face of peak oil, climate change and economic instability, and to ameliorate years of racial inequality. Decent housing for all is our #1 priority, followed by humane education in our schools and a host of other projects. If you're interested in seeing more of what we do, or how you can be involved, please visit https://www.greytontransition.co.za.

The **Friends of Greyton Transition Town** congregate at https://www.facebook.com/groups/GTTfriends/. Visitors can stay, inexpensively and comfortably, at GTT's **Greyton EcoLodge** (https://www.facebook.com/ecolodgeatgreyton/), and **Pure Café**

Greyton has a vegan menu and a farmers' market of locally grown produce (https://www.facebook.com/PureCafeGreyton/).

As Nicky and I are both card-carrying vegans, fully aware of the sad pointlessness of eating animals, we've done our best to provide a permanent home for rescued farm animals, who often arrive traumatized or at death's door, or a temporary home for injured or orphaned wild animals, many of whom we've successfully eased out into the wilderness again once they're ready, willing and able to go.

You can find **The Greyton Farm Animal Sanctuary** at https://www.facebook.com/greytonanimals/. City dwellers, in particular, might enjoy sponsoring one of our beautiful babies as a way of contributing towards the animal liberation movement. Our finances are constrained (shall we say?) and many of our sweeties need parents, so please help out, perhaps even consider adopting one of our babbas from afar [tele-adoption?], if you'd like a simple way to make a big difference in someone else's life. We welcome visitors, and we find that visiting children are often the key that unlocks their parents' hearts (and stomachs).

Devoted animal lovers may like to stay over on the farm, to take part in the pre-dawn feeding of the pigs and geese and other critters. You can find our inexpensive shepherd's hut and barn accommodation on **www.airbnb.com**, under **Shepherd's Hut,** in Greyton, Western Cape, South Africa.

Nicky and I are both firm believers in community building, so please reach out and make contact with us, especially if your motto is also "For the animals…" Also, despite my best efforts, in a book of this size and ambition there are bound to be errors of commission and omission, of grammar and fact: please let me know my mistakes, and I'll gratefully fix 'em. Naturally, I welcome all *constructive* criticisms and corrections. Thanks. You can send emails to **whyanimalsarentfood@gmail.com**.

So, that's what my present looks like, and what I have mapped out for the near future… Of course, the Great Unknowable has a whimsical sense of humor and may have entirely different plans for me.

Till later… Be happy, be healthy, be Planter, bye bye.

The End

Parting Snapshot… here's some of my family members at the Greyton Farm Animal Sanctuary on Tabularasa Farm outside Greyton in the Western Cape region of South Africa. It was so cold a Chukchi in Siberia might have spoken of a "three dog night" (as in William Burroughs' *Climate Change in Prehistory*). In this case, it was a six piggy night, with Bella, Michelle, Gracie, Dulcie, Margot and Rudi generating the body heat wave.

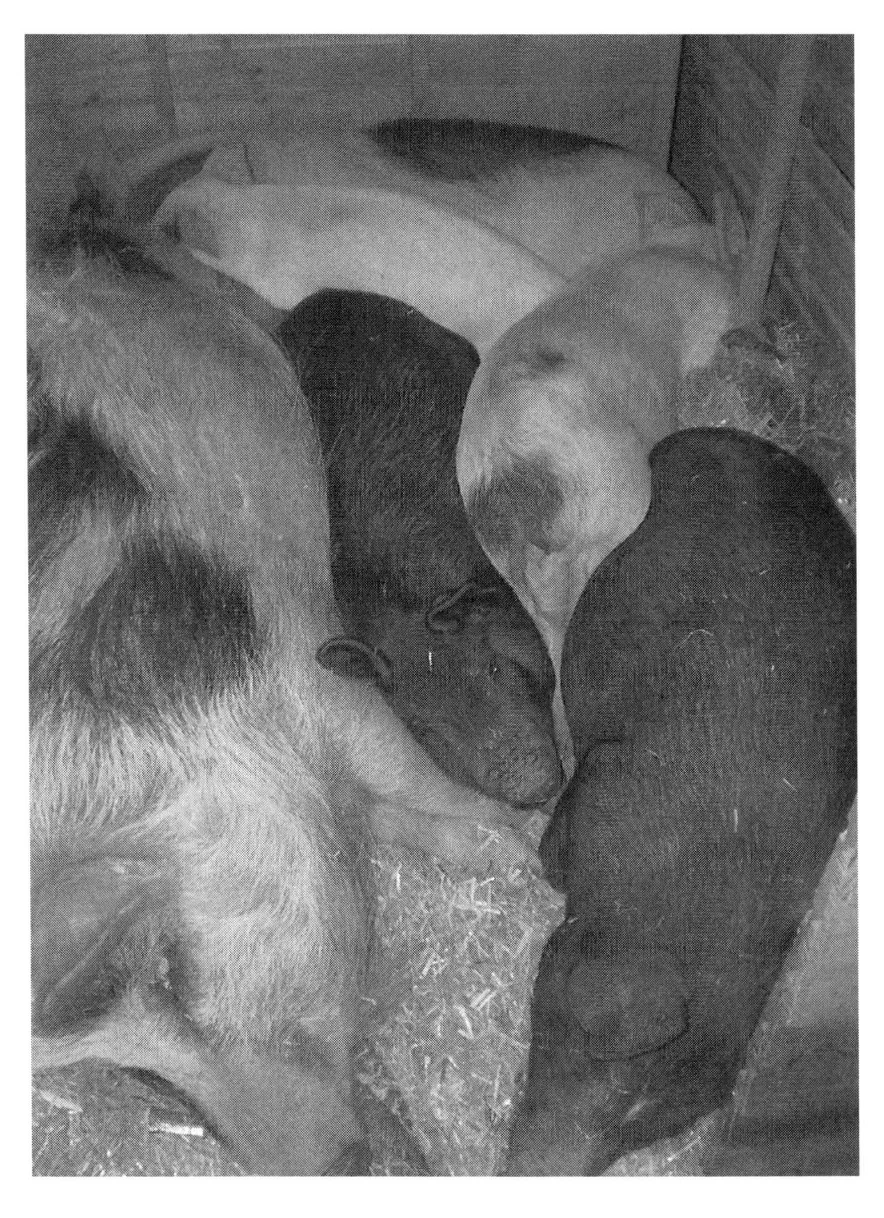

Extended Table of Contents

~

Index

A listing of the major topics and personalities in *Why Animals Aren't Food*

~

NOTES

Made in the USA
Charleston, SC
17 April 2016